1,000,000 Books

are available to read at

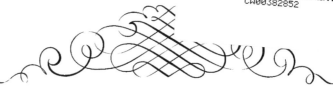

---◆---

www.ForgottenBooks.com

---◆---

Read online
Download PDF
Purchase in print

ISBN 978-1-5283-3787-8
PIBN 10911842

This book is a reproduction of an important historical work. Forgotten Books uses
state-of-the-art technology to digitally reconstruct the work, preserving the original format
whilst repairing imperfections present in the aged copy. In rare cases, an imperfection in
the original, such as a blemish or missing page, may be replicated in our edition. We do,
however, repair the vast majority of imperfections successfully; any imperfections that
remain are intentionally left to preserve the state of such historical works.

Forgotten Books is a registered trademark of FB &c Ltd.
Copyright © 2018 FB &c Ltd.
FB &c Ltd, Dalton House, 60 Windsor Avenue, London, SW19 2RR.
Company number 08720141. Registered in England and Wales.

For support please visit www.forgottenbooks.com

1 MONTH OF
FREE
READING

at

www.ForgottenBooks.com

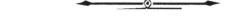

By purchasing this book you are
eligible for one month membership to
ForgottenBooks.com, giving you
unlimited access to our entire
collection of over 1,000,000 titles via
our web site and mobile apps.

To claim your free month visit:

www.forgottenbooks.com/free911842

* Offer is valid for 45 days from date of purchase. Terms and conditions apply.

English
Français
Deutsche
Italiano
Español
Português

www.forgottenbooks.com

Mythology Photography **Fiction**
Fishing Christianity **Art** Cooking
Essays Buddhism Freemasonry
Medicine **Biology** Music **Ancient**
Egypt Evolution Carpentry Physics
Dance Geology **Mathematics** Fitness
Shakespeare **Folklore** Yoga Marketing
Confidence Immortality Biographies
Poetry **Psychology** Witchcraft
Electronics Chemistry History **Law**
Accounting **Philosophy** Anthropology
Alchemy Drama Quantum Mechanics
Atheism Sexual Health **Ancient History**
Entrepreneurship Languages Sport
Paleontology Needlework Islam
Metaphysics Investment Archaeology
Parenting Statistics Criminology
Motivational

READINGS ON
AMERICAN FEDERAL
GOVERNMENT

EDITED BY

PAUL S. REINSCH

PROFESSOR OF POLITICAL SCIENCE IN THE UNIVERSITY OF WISCONSIN
AUTHOR OF "WORLD POLITICS," "COLONIAL GOVERN-
MENT," "AMERICAN LEGISLATURES"

GINN AND COMPANY
BOSTON · NEW YORK · CHICAGO · LONDON

READINGS ON
AMERICAN FEDERAL
GOVERNMENT

EDITED BY

PAUL S. REINSCH

PROFESSOR OF POLITICAL SCIENCE IN THE UNIVERSITY OF WISCONSIN
AUTHOR OF "WORLD POLITICS," "COLONIAL GOVERN-
MENT," "AMERICAN LEGISLATURES," ETC.

GINN AND COMPANY
BOSTON · NEW YORK · CHICAGO · LONDON

Copyright, 1909

By PAUL S. REINSCH

———

ALL RIGHTS RESERVED

894

The Athenæum Press

GINN AND COMPANY · PRO-
PRIETORS · BOSTON · U.S.A.

INTRODUCTION

THE present collection of materials for the study of American government was suggested to the Editor by his own experience in studying the processes of American government with a large university class. It was apparent that students could derive great benefit from reading extensively in documentary sources, but the difficulty of obtaining access to the latter even in a well stocked library proved so great that only a very limited use could be made of this method. So it occurred to the Editor that if a number of characteristic selections were to be made from articles and statements written by representative men, a body of information could be brought together which would be exceedingly helpful not only to the student in course, but to the general reader who might desire to inform himself somewhat in detail about the manner in which public affairs are actually managed.

The materials contained in this book are selected almost without exception from the spoken or written work of men actually engaged in the business of government, — presidents, legislators, administrative officials, and judges. On account of their special value, there are included a few articles by writers who do not have this particular qualification. With this exception, the material is taken from the *Congressional Record*, from official reports, messages, and public addresses. It is fashionable to sneer at the *Congressional Record* as a congeries of undigested and uninteresting material pouring itself out in liberal volume for the benefit of an occasional country editor. But while there may be few constant and faithful readers of this formidable document, it nevertheless constitutes a valuable record of able thought upon the public problems of the day. The debates of Congress, it is true, suffer from various drawbacks. In the Senate the legal and juristic side of public action is given perhaps too great a predominance. The question most frequently asked is "what can we do under the constitution," rather than "what is the wisest policy for a great nation to pursue." It is, of course, not to be expected that Senators should be experienced in all the detailed pursuits and interests that at present call for federal legislation. They are, however, nearly all capable of dealing with the legal aspects of the matter. This constitutes the common meeting ground of discussion, and so it is not surprising that questions of policy are in the Senate usually treated in the terms of legal thought and of constitutional limitation. But with this qualification in mind, the reader may judge for himself of the value of Senatorial discussions and of the grade of ability displayed by the participants.

The House of Representatives is in an unfavorable position as a forum of argument. In the Senate there is constant debating, a constant meeting of minds, a persistent hammering out of policies and legal theories. In the House real debates are rare. When great measures are up for discussion, the time allotted is usually so short that the individual speakers can do no more than merely indicate their line of thought; moreover, the bulk of time is usually taken up by fencing for parliamentary position under the rules, rather than by a discussion of the merits of the legislation. Very thoughtful and valuable speeches are indeed written by members of the House, who often welcome any opportunity to get them into the *Record*. Thus a member may take advantage of five minutes falling to him in the discussion of the Diplomatic and Consular Appropriation Bill, to deliver himself of a speech upon the iniquities of the tariff or upon the desirability of further restrictions to emigration. During the last session of Congress the distribution of the President's message was made a question of debate almost until the end of the session. Whatever the member lacks time to say in the three or five minutes allotted to him he may, nevertheless, print in the *Record*, or he may even obtain leave to print a speech no part of which has ever been delivered on the floor of the House. That such arrangements defeat the spontaneity of discussion will be evident. Yet there are many able and experienced men in the House, who occasionally do get an opportunity for an actual discussion of public policies; and even the speeches which are written for partial delivery are frequently worth reading. The discussions which take place under the five-minute rule in Committee of the Whole, when appropriation bills are under consideration, are unfortunately often characterized by a somewhat petty sedulity in matters of detail. It is somewhat discouraging to have great measures, upon which the national welfare depends, disposed of in a two hours' debate, while nearly the same time may be given to the question as to whether the salary of a clerk in some department shall be $1,100 or $1,300. However, notwithstanding all these disadvantages and drawbacks, the debates in the House are often very valuable and informing.

In this collection special attention has been given to the procedure in the House of Representatives and in the Senate. Congressional procedure is, indeed, highly technical, but it is most desirable that the nation should thoroughly inform itself upon this matter. The procedure in the National Legislature ought to be such as would facilitate the discussion of really important national problems and would encourage and bring forward those men who are truly representative of the people and of their common interests. It is very questionable whether the methods of procedure now prevailing sufficiently subserve these purposes.

INTRODUCTION

The collection before the reader has been confined to material illustrating the actual working of the American government in our day. It may, indeed, be said that for a thorough study of American government a knowledge of the historical development of political institutions is indispensable. Yet it is equally essential that there should be a clear conception of what is actually being done at the present time. On account of the limitations of space and in order to preserve the unity of the collection, purely historical accounts have not been admitted. For similar reasons there have been excluded purely legal arguments and controversial discussions of suggested reforms. But some discussions of a legal nature have been admitted because they served directly to illustrate the actual workings of the government. To reveal actualities rather than historical developments or future tendencies is the purpose of this collection. From this point of view, much critical matter has been included, for the reason that opposition serves to make us conscious of many facts which otherwise we might have overlooked. Thus the details of the centralized organization in the House of Representatives would not have become matters of public knowledge but for the opposition which this system has evoked. Of course, in the use of such material the reader will exercise caution, making allowance for the heat of party controversy, and forming his own conclusions as to how far the views of the individual writer or speaker may have been colored by a specific political purpose.

Though the Editor has aimed to steer clear of purely partisan discussions, it appeared impossible to exclude everything tinged with a party bias without reducing the collection to a neutral and inane level. It is exactly the personal equation in discussion and argument that lends value when backed by character and experience. In order to feel at home in the actual world of political thought and action, the student should be familiar with the controversial methods that he will encounter at every turn, — he should be trained in distinguishing political fact from political opinion. However, in most of the important matters dealt with in this collection the principle of party allegiance may be regarded as non-essential. The details of House procedure have been attacked by men of all political faiths. Men of all parties have been united upon the necessity of public control of corporations. As a matter of fact, of recent years, controversies in our legislative bodies have rarely taken on the form of pure party action.

The Case Method which has been used with great success in the study of private and public law may be applied to the study of institutions in general. The student should read a certain group of selections and then reason out for himself the implications therein contained, analyze the discussions and debates, separate the essential from the non-essential, and avoid false analogies, making allowance for personal and political bias. Thus he will arrive at his own conclusions, relying upon his own judgment, as he must whenever confronted by the facts of the actual world. This method has some great advantages over that of getting ready-made conclusions from text-books, although it does not in the study of political science supersede the latter. The process while irksome at the beginning will soon have the same exhilarating effect upon the mind that brisk physical exercise has on the body. The Editor, in the notes accompanying the selections, has avoided making summaries or drawing conclusions. He has merely given the general setting of the selection, and indicated its relation to other matters. In cases where parts of articles are printed, the material omitted is usually historic or of an incidental nature, while the part reproduced deals directly with present day methods of government.

The Editor desires to make special acknowledgments to various publishers and authors who have permitted him to make selections from articles or works, published or written by them. He desires in the first place to mention the " Autobiography of Senator Hoar," published by Scribner's Sons and Company, an admirable treasure-house of political reminiscence, to be compared among recent books only to the Memoirs of Carl Schurz. The same publishers have permitted the use of portions of articles published in *Scribner's Magazine*, by Mr. Frank A. Vanderlip on the Treasury, General W. H. Carter on the War Department, Mr. S. P. Langley on the Scientific Work of the Government, and Governor Magoon on the War Department. Secretary Root permitted the use of his address on Local Self-Government of the States; and Judge Charles F. Amidon, that on the Nation and the Constitution. Acknowledgments are further due the following publications and writers: The *Atlantic Monthly*, for articles by Mr. S. W. McCall, on the Power of the Senate and on the Fifty-Ninth Congress; Judge F. C. Lowell, on American Diplomacy; as well as Mr. A. P. Dennis, on Our Changing Constitution. The *North American Review* permitted the use of articles by Mr. A. Maurice Lowe, on the Oligarchy of the Senate, and Mr. Albert D. Currier, on Government by Executive Rulings. The *Political Science Quarterly* is entitled to acknowledgment for those by Mr. Harold M. Bowman, on American Administrative Tribunals, and Mr. A. P. Dennis, on the Democratic Convention of 1904; the *Independent* for that by Mr. Albert Halstead on The President at Work; the *Outlook* for the article by Mr. Huntingdon Wilson, on the Foreign Service of the United States. The *Review of Reviews* permitted the use of the article by Mr. W. B. Shaw, on The Civil Service under Roosevelt, and of Mr. Bowker, on the Post Office; *McClure's Magazine* of that by President Cleveland, on The Government in the Chicago Strike of 1894; The *Forum*, that by Mr. H. L. West, on the Senate; and the *Michigan Law Review*, that on The Department of Justice by Professor J. A. Fairlie. The Editor is further greatly obliged to the publishers of the *New York Evening Post* for the permission to reproduce a number of valuable articles and editorials from that journal. Two articles have been taken from foreign Reviews, that by Professor S. J. McLean, on President Roosevelt and the Trusts and by Mr. Frederic Harrison, on the Inauguration of President McKinley. The Presidents, Senators, Representatives, Judges and Government Officials whose careful and authoritative statements in Congressional debates and public documents form the great bulk of this collection are also entitled to the personal thanks of students of American Government for their lucid contributions towards its description.

The Editor also desires to express his obligation to Mr. William L. Bailey and to Professor R. B. Scott, for looking over the proofs.

CONTENTS

Page

READINGS ON
AMERICAN FEDERAL GOVERNMENT

I

THE PRESIDENT

[The inauguration of the President has perhaps never been described in a more attractive manner than by Mr. Frederic Harrison. The date of the inauguration is so early that the inclemency of the weather at that time often makes the occasion a trying one to the health of the participants. It has therefore been suggested that the date should be changed so as to fall on the memorial day of Washington's first inauguration, April 30th. — The essay by Mr. Halstead, now Consul at Birmingham, gives an account of the methods of despatching business in the Executive Office.]

THE INAUGURATION OF PRESIDENT McKINLEY, 1900

By Frederic Harrison [1]

THE Ceremony of the Inauguration of the President and Vice-President at Washington on the 4th of March is, indeed, a characteristic and suggestive function. I had the good fortune to witness it this year under the most favorable conditions, and was deeply impressed with all it represented. It summoned up the vast extent and power of the United States, its absolute democracy, the simplicity, ease, and homeliness of its government, its contempt of forms, its entire confidence in itself and perfect satisfaction with its own ways. In the grand Capitol of the noble city of Washington, than which no finer edifice or city exists in the Old World, were gathered the men chosen by the adult citizens of a nation of some seventy millions, scattered over a vast continent. The President, Vice-President, senators, and representatives elected on this enormous ballot, entrusted with this stupendous power and wealth, sate indistinguishable from the ordinary citizens around them — clerks,

---

[1] From "Impressions of America" in *The Nineteenth Century*, 49: 922.

secretaries, journalists, and casual friends, who were crowded pell-mell on the floor of the Senate House itself.

To this miscellaneous body, which might be any average county council or borough board, there entered a long file of ambassadors and ministers in all the finery of European and Oriental courts; uniforms blazing with gold lace, plumes, velvet or fur, swords, sabres, and helmets; the Austro-Hungarian magnate, the stately ambassadors of Great Britain, Germany, France, and Russia, in their court uniforms; Minister of China, in his buttoned headdress uniform; the envoys of the smaller Powers of Europe, and then the diplomatists of the South American and Central American and West Indian States; black men, brown men, whitey-brown men, in various gaudy uniforms; the Minister of the Sultan in his fez, those of Siam and Korea in their national dress — more than thirty in all, in every color, adornment, and style, representing men of every race from every part of the planet.

This brilliant and motley group may be seen at St. Stephen's, or at the functions of Berlin and St. Petersburg, where it is only a natural part of similar bravery and feudal splendor. But here, in a hall crowded with sober citizens in broadcloth, without a star, a ribbon, or a sword between them, the effect was almost comic. Siam, Korea, Hungary, and Portugal as gay as butterflies. McKinley and Roosevelt matter-of-fact civilians, as if they were Chairman and Vice-Chairman of the London County Council! And around them were the chosen delegates of the great Republic, jostled in their own hall by pressmen, secretaries, and curious strangers like myself. The shirt-sleeve theory of government could hardly go farther, and, perhaps, need not go quite so far. My own republican soul was stirred when I set myself to think which of the two forms would prevail in the centuries to come. I thought first of the Roman Senate (according to the old myth), sitting immovable as statues in their white togas, when the Gauls of Brennus, in their torques and war-paint, dashed into the Senate House; and then I began to think, Were these quiet citizens seated there to see a comic opera at the Savoy Theatre?

Not that the representatives of the Republic are wanting in personal bearing. The President sate through the ceremonies with placid dignity, his fine features, in their stern repose, looking like a bronze figure of the Elder Brutus or Cato the Censor. But at a personal reception in the White House Mr. McKinley will show as much grace and courtesy of demeanour as any Sovereign by divine right, and his smile and his voice are pronounced (not only by women) to be perfectly winning. The diplomatists of Europe agree in assuring us that nothing can exceed the tact and "correctness" which distinguish Mr. Hay, the accomplished Secretary of State. It is true that Congressmen (in their shirt sleeves) have not that repose of manner which marks the caste of Vere de Vere. But the men who are charged to speak in the name of the State will usually be found to rise to the occasion with that facility which enables every genuine American to adapt himself to play a new part, and to fulfil an unaccustomed duty.

It is no easy task to combine the conduct of vast interests, the representation of enormous power, with the ultra-democratic traditions of the absolute equality of all citizens. No sooner had the President summoned before him the splendiferous envoys of the whole world, than he passed out to the historic steps of the Capitol, to pronounce his Inaugural Address. As I stood near him, and listened to the clear and keenly-balanced sentences, which the cables and telegraphs of the civilized world were carrying to expectant nations, I noticed how the crowd, a few feet only below him, was a miscellaneous gathering from the streets like a knot in the Park listening to a Salvation preacher or a Socialist orator on a Sunday, negroes and lads not the least vociferous in their applause, whilst on a platform fifty yards off there were mounted a dozen batteries of photographers, from kodaks to life-size lenses. The American public man — even the private man and private woman — has always to reckon with the man in the street, journalists, and kodaks.

It is needless to point the moral of the difference between the Inaugural Address of a President, delivered in the open air to a miscellaneous crowd, and the speech of an European Sovereign opening Parliament. The one is an elaborate State paper, spoken by a citizen in frock coat to a mob of his fellow-citizens in the street; the other is usually conventional platitudes, pronounced in a gorgeous palace with a scene of medieval pageantry. It is the contrast between the monarchical survival and Republican realism. Kodaks, mobs, and vociferous negroes are not a necessary part of the government of a State. But the Presidential address from the steps of the Capitol is certainly more like that of Pericles on the Pnyx, or of Scipio and Marius on the Rostra, than our House of Lords; and it is conceivable that it may prove more agreeable to the practice of future republics in the ages to come. The President of the United States expounds his policy in a reasoned argument to all citizens who choose to hear him. The European monarch performs a traditional ceremonial to a crowd of state courtiers who possess office without power and honor without responsibility.

The White House, as the executive mansion is called, is interesting for its historic associations, which exactly cover the nineteenth century, with its portraits and reminiscences of Presidents and statesmen, and its characteristic simplicity and modest appointments. It is not a convenient residence for a President with such great responsibilities. But, as the term of residence is usually so short, and the associations of the house are so rich, it would be a pity to change it for a pretentious modern palace. In the meantime the quiet old mansion, merely a fine Georgian country house in a pleasant park, serves to remind the American citizen of the democratic origin of his Chief Magistrate, who is certainly not yet an emperor. The White House was a residence suitable for men like Jefferson, Lincoln, and Grant; and it seems a not unfitting office for their successors.

The Capitol at Washington struck me as being the most effective mass of public buildings in the world, especially when viewed at some distance, and from the park in which it stands. I am well aware of certain constructive defects which have been insisted on by Ferguson and other critics; and no one pretends that it is a perfect design of the highest order either in originality or style. But as an effective public edifice of a grandiose kind, I doubt if any capital city can show its equal. This is largely due to the admirable proportions of its central dome group, which I hold to be, from the pictorial point of view, more successful than those of St. Peter's, the Cathedral of Florence, Agia and Sophia, St. Isaac's, the Pantheon, St. Paul's, or the new Cathedral of Berlin. But the unique effect is still more due to the magnificent site which the Capitol at Washington enjoys. I have no hesitation in saying that the site of the Capitol is the noblest in the world, if we exclude that of the Parthenon in its pristine glory. Neither Rome nor Constantinople, nor Florence, nor Paris, nor Berlin, nor London possesses any central eminence with broad open spaces on all sides, crowned by a vast pile covering nearly four acres and rising to a height of nearly three hundred feet, which seems to dominate the whole city. Washington is the only capital city which has this colossal center or crown. And Londoners can imagine the effect if their St. Paul's stood in an open park reaching from the Temple to Finsbury Circus, and the great creation of Wren were dazzling white marble, and soared into an atmosphere of sunny light.

Washington, the youngest capital city of the world, bids fair to become, before the twentieth century is ended, the most beautiful and certainly the most commodious. It is the only capital which has been laid out from the first entirely on modern lines, with organic unity of plan, unencumbered with any antique limitations and confusions. The spacious avenues, intersected by very broad streets, all lined with maple and elm, and radiating from a multitude of "circles," its numerous parks and squares, with fountains, monuments, and equestrian statues at each available junction, its semitropical climate, for it is in the latitude of Lisbon and Palermo, its freedom from the disfigurements of smoke, trade, and manufactures, its singular form of government under a State autocracy without any municipal representation, give it unique opportunities to develop. As yet it is but half completed, owing to local difficulties as to rights of property; and it still has the air of an artificial experiment in city architecture. But within two or three generations, when its vacant sites are filled up, and public buildings, monuments, and statues continue to be raised with all the wealth, resources, and energy of the Republic, if the artists of the future can be restrained within the limits of good sense and fine taste, Washington may look more like the Rome of the Antonies than any city of the Old World.

Of all that I saw in America, I look back with the most emotion to my visit to Mount Vernon, the home and burial place of George Washington. I saw it on a lovely spring day, amidst thousands of pilgrims, in the Inauguration week. On a finely wooded bluff, rising above the grand Potomac River, stands the plain but spacious wooden house of the Founder of the Republic. It has been preserved and partly restored with perfect taste, the original furniture, pictures, and ornaments supplemented by fit contemporary pieces. It enables one perfectly to conjure up an Image of the homely, large, and generous life of the President before the war called him to the field, and after he had retired from all cares of state. We fancy him sitting under the spacious eastern portico with its eight tall columns, looking out over the broad landscape of forest and river, or lying in his last sleep in the simple bed, with its dimity coverlet, and then laid to rest in the rural tomb below the house, which he ordered himself, and in which his descendants have insisted on keeping his remains. General Grant lies beside the Hudson at New York in a magnificent mausoleum palpably imitated from the tomb of Napoleon in the Invalides. How infinitely more fitting and more touching is the Spartan simplicity of Washington's burial place — an austere cell within his own ancestral ground; yet not a morning's drive from the splendid capital which the nation has named after its heroic founder — how much more fitting and more touching is this than is the imperial mausoleum to which they have carried the bones of the tyrant who ruined France! It has been frequently attempted to remove the sarcophagus in which Washington lies from Mount Vernon, his home, to place it under the dome of the Capitol. But as yet it has been wisely decided to do nothing that can impair the unique legend which has gathered round the memory of the Western Cincinnatus.

THE PRESIDENT AT WORK [1]

By Albert Halstead

While the Presidency is, of necessity, a laborious office, its cares may be much lessened if the Secretary to the President is capable and diplomatic, able to relieve his chief of many burdens, a good counselor who is broad and big enough mentally to make an efficient Cabinet officer. President McKinley has such a man in George B. Cortelyou, who is not only his secretary, but his trusted friend. Though a staunch Republican, Mr. Cortelyou was not selected through political influence, but because

[1] From the *Independent*, Sept., 1901. Reprinted in part, by permission.

he had proved himself efficient and trustworthy. In this difficult position
he makes friends rather than enemies for the President. He is the most
popular secretary who has served a President in a quarter of a century.
When it is remembered how many people he must disappoint each day;
that he must tell the newspaper correspondents what they should know
without seeming to suppress information; that he must remember every
public man he has ever met; that he must be quick to grasp what each
caller wants and be fully informed on every subject, and that he must
be the buffer between the President and the public, it becomes apparent
that unusual talents are required of him. Mr. Cortelyou has earned
the President's confidence, and he does more executive work than any
previous secretary. He has been so successful in systematizing the work
of his office that it is better and more promptly done than ever before.

The extent of President McKinley's correspondence can be appreciated from the fact that four hundred thousand communications were
received and disposed of at the executive offices in his first term. Mr.
Cortelyou, with a force composed almost exclusively of stenographers,
who read each others' notes with facility, has dispensed with an immense
amount of unnecessary work. When a letter or document is received
a memorandum, to show what is to be done with it, is written in shorthand in its upper left hand corner. This is to be kept on the paper until
it comes back to the secretary for approval. A letter is then written by
a clerk in conformity with the memorandum. Thus in most of the correspondence there is no dictation. A "precedent index," prepared by
Secretary Cortelyou, covering practically every case that is likely to
arise, serves as a guide to the clerks in answering correspondence and
lessens the work materially. When a letter is of sufficient importance to
be filed in the executive offices the shorthand notes are preserved with
it, so the exact action taken can be learned at a glance. Every important
paper is briefed in typewriting, and when necessary this brief is filed
with the papers, giving an accurate record. Appreciating the importance of expediting business, Mr. Cortelyou prepared and had printed
a number of indorsement papers, which are attached to papers referred
to other departments. Consequently when a communication comes to
the White House that should go to the Department of State, a paster
referring it there is attached and, thus indorsed, it is forwarded. A rule
of the executive offices requires that the work of each desk be finished
on the day of its receipt. This prevents an accumulation of work and
keeps it up to date.

When the President makes a journey his secretary and several members of the White House clerical force accompany him. All speeches
made on the trip are reported stenographically. Copies are furnished
the newspaper men with the party, and a special copy is preserved for
the office records. Telegraphers from the office force are also with the
President, and he is kept in constant touch with Washington. The

"war room," where several telegraphers are always on duty, puts the President in communication with every part of the world. Here cipher despatches are received and he is kept advised of every important event. With such a system, so much work and such a force there is no idling in the executive offices.

President McKinley is rather an early riser. He breakfasts at eight and reads the papers until shortly before ten, when he goes to the Cabinet room, which he makes his private office. There on his desk he finds a neat, typewritten paper, headed: "The President's Engagements," and dated. Upon this is the name of each caller who has a specific engagement, and a line stating the purpose of the visit. Mr. McKinley receives his caller at the head of the Cabinet table, often, however, stepping forward to meet him. A cordial handgrasp is given and he waits for the visitor to state his business. He usually remains standing during the interview, but if he sits down it is time to retire when he arises. On his desk the President finds papers relating to the questions that are apt to come up, as well as others that require immediate attention. His engagements are subject to interruption by the arrival of a Cabinet officer, a Senator or Representative. Each visitor is made to feel that he is welcome. More than any recent President he has caused his political opponents to find it a pleasure to call. At times he persuades them of the desirability of something he wishes done, so it is often difficult to muster an aggressive opposition to his policies among the minority. Bitterly as he may be criticized by the minority, there is no one who is not on friendly terms with him.

Of the many thousand letters addressed to him the President probably has less than one per cent brought to his personal attention. They are opened in the executive offices and those of importance selected. Mr. Cortelyou signs, or has stamped with a fac-simile of his signature, every official letter, except a few which the President may prefer to sign. Of even the small percentage of letters laid before him he reads few. His secretary states briefly the contents of each and he gives the necessary directions or dictates an answer.

Since the beginning of his first administration President McKinley has made very few personal appointments. Practically every selection is now made upon the recommendation of a Senator; sometimes a Representative's wish is influential, while a Cabinet officer's approval is final. Generally the President is not personally acquainted with his appointees, though it is not unusual for an applicant for office to be presented to the Executive. This furnishes an opportunity to take his measure. The President has become very adept in judging character. The papers in a case are briefed at the department to which the office is attached, showing the names of those indorsing a candidate and the Secretary's view. These are then forwarded to the President and, if the office is a local one, the appointment is made without delay. It is

remarkable that in so many instances the President has some knowledge of the candidate, due to his own long public service and wide acquaintance. Where the office to be filled is sought by men of different
States, each with strong political backing, the selection is more difficult.
The better man is then usually chosen. Small things will decide for or
against an applicant. Too many indorsements, showing an undue
anxiety for office, have proved fatal; too much importuning, until the
President is tired of the candidate's name, has killed many a man's
chances. Where there are no complications a vacancy is filled as soon as
it occurs. When claims conflict more time is required, but the President seldom delays long in making an appointment, desiring to be relieved of the pressure and to get his difficulties behind him.

Seldom does a State paper go without the President's personality impressed upon it. If he does not prepare it himself he generally inspires
it. When a Cabinet officer prepares a paper for him it is invariably
altered by the President in some phrase or expression, better to express
or qualify a meaning. When he makes a change it is usually an improvement, no matter who happened to prepare the document. Cabinet
officers say in private that they cannot write anything that will pass
muster with the President unless he makes some effective correction.
He is particularly careful with proclamations. Now, a Thanksgiving
proclamation may seem to be easily drafted, but it is a difficult task.
It ought to be original, but so many have been issued that originality
is almost impossible. Mr. McKinley begins early on such a task, and
he may lay the first or second draft aside for a week, but when it comes
forth it is a gem, emphasizing that for which the nation should be most
thankful.

In writing his messages President McKinley takes the greatest pains.
His methods of preparation vary somewhat each year. He may dictate
almost an entire message, or write most of it himself with pen or pencil.
The first draft simply begins the work. Long before it is written notes
have been made, thoughts jotted down and a list of subjects is prepared.
That is often changed. It is a guide to the message. Every note is so
marked as to be easily identified. The President may be in his room,
when an idea strikes him; it is noted; he may be walking or driving
and a phrase or epigram, exactly expressing some thought or expression
that can be advantageously used is not lost but is stored away for future
use. This is one of his methods in writing speeches.

About the third week in October the real work of getting a message
ready begins. Each subject is placed under a separate head. It is
copied on tinted slips, about four by eight inches, with broad spacing,
so as to leave ample room for alterations. Each slip is numbered, dated,
and its subject noted thus: "Tariff-Draft I, Page I, October 17th, 1900."
The notes from which this is copied are also marked so as to be identified; then if the paper is lost it can be duplicated or identified. Where

figures are used blanks are left in the slips for them; afterward they are secured at the Treasury Department, which is held responsible for their accuracy. Every figure or statement is verified. If it concerns the Treasury, it is proved by Secretary Gage through his Secretary. If a mistake is made the Treasury Department is held to account. The Department of State prepares for the Message an accurate account of the conduct of foreign affairs for the year. It is not generally used in the exact form in which it comes. It may be too long, or some subject may require a more cautious or a more vigorous handling. Other departments furnish live matter and the President takes what he wants, but it is all rewritten and condensed. The President has been known to use just three short paragraphs out of a statement ten thousand words long, giving in detail the work of a department for a year, and even then Congress did not suffer from a lack of information. A President's message, at least a McKinley message, is not, then, a patchwork, but is a product of much labor and painstaking care.

The President dictates very rapidly. He has a splendid vocabulary, and is never at a loss for a word. This dictation, after being typewritten, is most carefully revised. The material is then rearranged, if necessary, and copied again. Then it goes to the printer, who, after it is set up, takes a proof on unusually wide paper, so that at the sides, at the top, and at the bottom, there is ample room for corrections. This revised proof is then corrected by the printer and another proof made — with every revision there is a new proof. Sometimes portions of the message are revised ten times. It is hard, patience-trying work, but the President takes pains, weighs every word and studies every phrase with scrupulous care, correcting or rewriting his copy until he is perfectly satisfied with it. The greater part of the message stands, however, as at first prepared. Ordinarily the first and last paragraphs are not written until a day or two before the message goes to Congress, but when it is finished it is a complete document in which every word has a specific purpose. President McKinley's messages have varied from thirteen to twenty-two thousand words, depending upon what must be said; but the tendency is for messages to grow in length as more subjects must receive treatment.

Considering the amount of work involved, ever-present and onerous responsibilities that cannot be shifted, importunities for place, unceasing demands upon his time and patience, difficult problems pressing for solution, unending routine, criticisms, misunderstandings, and frequent evidences of ingratitude, the President's salary is inadequate. This is more evident when it is recalled that out of it the expenses for entertaining, that custom requires, must be paid. And yet these drawbacks do not interfere with cultivation of the Presidential bee by every man in the country, who would, by any stretch of the imagination, be regarded as eligible.

II

POWERS OF THE EXECUTIVE

[There has recently been much discussion of the proper extent of the executive powers, especially in the national government, where there has taken place a great expansion of executive functions. By many men this tendency has been attacked as dangerous, while others see in it only that growth of governmental power which would naturally accompany the increase in national wealth and population. The speeches of Senator Rayner and Representative Towne, directing themselves against the expansion of the executive power, will serve to bring out clearly the matter in controversy. Allowance being made in all Congressional speeches for partisan bias, the attacks of the opposition will often bring out most clearly new political developments. Senator Rayner's speech was made in the debate upon the President's action with respect to San Domingo. Mr. Towne was speaking on party politics during the discussion of the Consular and Diplomatic Appropriation Bill. For a good general treatment of this subject see Ford, " Rise and Growth of Am. Politics," 275.]

FROM A SPEECH OF SENATOR RAYNER [1]

Now let us look for a moment at the result of the President's construction of his prerogative. A new sect of political scribes have commenced to edit a revised edition of the Constitution. They call it the unwritten Constitution. They are framing an apocryphal collection of epistles and are promulgating their heresy from academic chairs and lecture platforms. The President is the prophet of this new creed and the Messiah of this strange hallucination. They do not propose to add any additional chapters to the original manuscript, but they insist that under the general-welfare clause, which is simply a repetition of the phrase that was used in the Articles of Confederation, this Government has implied powers not enunciated in the charter. They seem to forget that Hamilton's proposition in the Constitutional Convention which provided that Congress was to have power to pass all laws whatsoever, subject to the Executive veto, and the outline that he communicated to Mr. Madison that the Legislature of the United States shall have power to pass all laws which they shall judge necessary to the common defense

[1] *Congr. Record,* Jan. 31, 1907.

and welfare of the Union, were not even referred to the committee, and that it was in the plan presented by Patterson and by Randolph and by Pinckney that there was finally evolved that immortal scheme that can never be recast under the plastic touch of political necromancers and enchanters.

When they approach the executive department the implication becomes unlimited, and under the distribution of Executive power the President can perform all functions not allotted to other branches of the Government.

I know that Congress has enacted a great many laws enabling the President to perform the duties confided to him by the Constitution. It has done this under Article I, section 8, subsection 18, of the Constitution, which provides that —

Congress shall have power . . . to make all laws which shall be necessary and proper for carrying into execution the foregoing powers and all other powers vested by this Constitution in the Government of the United States, or in any department or officer thereof.

Hamilton, in discussing this clause of the Constitution, said that —

The declaration itself, though it may be chargeable with tautology or redundancy, is at least perfectly harmless.

There has been a considerable diversity of opinion upon this point. Chief Justice Marshall illumined the proposition in this manner. He said:

Should Congress in the execution of its powers adopt measures which are prohibited by the Constitution, or should Congress, under the pretext of executing its powers, pass laws for the accomplishment of objects not entrusted to the Government, it would become the painful duty of this tribunal, should a case requiring such a decision come before it, to say that such an act was not the law of the land. But where the law is not prohibited, and is really calculated to effect any of the objects entrusted to the Government, to undertake here to inquire into the degree of its necessity would be to pass the line which circumscribes the judicial department, and to tread on legislative ground. This court disclaims all pretensions to such a power.

And there I stand. No one at this day would demand a literal construction of the Constitution which would deprive the President of performing functions necessary to carry out the powers that are granted to him; on the contrary, he has the broadest field of discretion within which to adopt and exercise whatever methods are proper for this purpose. What I insist upon and contend for is that he must never abuse his constitutional prerogative by invading the domain of other departments, and must never, under color of title, assume authority upon subjects that have no relation to his office, and do not in the remotest degree appertain to the performance of his executive functions.

We know that every word of the Constitution is written. We know that there is not a line or letter that anyone has the right to insert. The Supreme Court may interpret, it may construe according to the spirit, but it can never add to the text. The Supreme Court may hold that a given act of the Executive is not an interference with legislative functions. It may broaden the right of the President to negotiate a treaty, but if it were ever to decide that the President had a right to conclude a treaty without the constitutional ratification its adjudication would lead either to impeachment or revolution. Every judgment, decree, and order that it renders must be under, and not above and beyond, the Constitution. It can set aside an act of Congress, but it can not abridge or extend the limits of the charter. What the Supreme Court can not do by expression the Executive ought not to be allowed to do by implication.

The President has the right to veto any enactment that we may pass. He has the right, if he chooses to do so, to advise with members in reference to legislation, and to make any suggestions that he may deem proper. This is not a constitutional prerogative, and its propriety has been questioned and assailed, but I am willing within proper bounds to regard it as an incident of his executive functions. One thing he has no right to do, and that is to use the vast public patronage at his disposal to compel obedience to his views. Another thing he has no right to do, and that is to make compacts with the Speaker of the House of Representatives or its committees, to accomplish the legislation that he desires, or prevent legislation. And still another thing he has no right to do, and that is beyond his messages, in which he is given the right at any time to suggest any measure he may deem proper or necessary, to interfere with legislation and to force Congress either to adopt his recommendations or if it rejects them to bring about a breach between the legislative and executive departments that is detrimental to the best interests of the country; that constitutes an assumption of dictatorial power which the people of this Republic, in the course of time, will not submit to, I care not how great the achievement or how much it may conduce to their progress and welfare, or what benefit, advantage, or prosperity we may derive from its accomplishment.

In order to show that I have not at all exaggerated the claims and pretensions of this new school of Executive construction, I want now to refer to some extracts from the address of an eminent lawyer,[1] delivered before the New York State Bar Association, in which the doctrines of this creed are announced in such unmistakable and unambiguous terms that we are no longer left in any doubt or uncertainty as to the evolution and development that we are undergoing upon the cardinal

[1] Chas. A. Gardiner, " The Constitutional Power of the President," 1905.

principles of republican government. If the propositions that he maintains reflect the sentiment of the people, then it is safe to say that the
Constitution is a thing of shreds and patches, and the Government that
it created is as much of a monarchical institution as the Government
of Great Britain, or of any other government, with the exception perhaps of those of Russia and Turkey, upon the Continent of Europe.

Listen now for a moment to some of the passages from this delightful
dissertation upon the Executive prerogative.

1. The President is the chief invention of the Constitution, a personal magistrate for a republic. . . . The conversion of an abstract sovereignty into a
concrete sovereign.

2. The executive and magisterial attributes of the Government being invested in the President, it follows inevitably that the President must possess
the executive and magisterial attributes of the people, and that the people retain
no undelegated attributes or passive sovereignties under the tenth amendment
or otherwise.

3. If Southern States abridge the privileges and immunities of Federal negro
citizens, the President, on his own initiative, can and should prohibit such
action, whether Congress legislates on the subject or not. If Southern States
deny the right of suffrage to Federal negro citizens on the ground of race or
color, the President, without waiting for penalizing statutes, can and should
use every means, civil, military, or both, to stop it.

4. To execute all his omnipotent functions the people have given the President absolute control of an irresistible physical force, the Army and Navy of
80,000,000 people.

5. Such are the powers of the President, express and implied. They are
all plenary. The office and power to execute it are in unqualified language.
The power to execute the Constitution is without limitation or restriction.
The power to administer the executive sovereignties is complete, and the implied
powers are coextensive with the express grants. Hence all the powers of the
President are unqualified, plenary, and unlimited.

And now for some of the thrilling climaxes of this remarkable
production.

Thus my ideal of the President coincides with the ideal of the people, a
majestic constitutional figure uncontrolled by Congress, unrestrained by the
courts, vested with plenary constitutional power and absolute constitutional
discretion.

How, then, is it possible for the President to exceed his express constitutional
authority? What Federal act can he perform that he may not claim is in execution of his office and its attributes, of the Constitution and the laws, or of his
executive powers?

Majesty is another attribute. It inheres in every sovereign, be he Czar or
President. Imperium majestasque populi Romani.

The President is invested with an office and the whole of it . . . . Who hath
fixed its bounds? Who hath said, Thus far and no farther? No one has
determined its illimitable extent; no one can determine it so long as the
Republic endures.

And this matchless conglomeration of incoherent absurdities was delivered, Mr. President, before an assemblage, every man of whom was probably conversant with the authorities and decisions that have consistently placed the brand of judicial condemnation upon this frenzied exposition of executive sovereignty.

This demonstrates, Mr. President, that the entire trouble arises from the fact that the Constitution is being perverted upon the grant of executive power. Article II of the Constitution says the executive power shall be vested in a President of the United States of America. This does not vest executive power in any greater degree than Article I vests legislative power when it says that all legislative powers herein granted shall be vested in a Congress of the United States, or than Article III vests judicial power except in the Supreme Court of the United States.

I plant myself upon the proposition that the President derives no authority whatever from this clause. Nearly three-quarters of a century ago the greatest political philosophers who ever illustrated the pages of American history settled before this body this contention so that it has been considered a constitutional axiom until the present day. This provision of the Constitution simply relates to the distribution of governmental functions and can not be considered in the light of a grant.

As luminous a constitutional argument as Webster ever made was upon this precise point. The President must derive his authority from the subsequent provisions of the instrument that contain the grant, and the entire grant of power, and which are not in the slightest degree enlarged by the clause that I have quoted. His school of disciples evidently think that I am wrong upon this point and are bewildering the mind of the rising generation upon this proposition. If we were to pass a law here to-day reposing in the President a governmental function beyond the specifications of the Constitution and not necessary for the exercise of any power contained in the specifications, the enactment would be void. Now, if the law would be void, what power has the President without the sanction of law to trespass beyond the confines of his prerogative? The President is either the executive officer of the Government, vested with unlimited executive functions, or he is the Executive acting under special and delegated powers. Which is he? Is he the general executive agent of the people, or their immediate representative, as was once claimed by one of his predecessors who also had an erroneous conception of his prerogative, or is he a special agent who shall look to his commission and credentials for his authority? There are unlimited executive acts performed by monarchical rulers, the exercise of which the framers of the Constitution never intended to repose in the President, and therefore they circumscribed his functions.

I am aware that persons who are not familiar with the source of organic power are losing sight of fundamental distinctions and are looking to results and not instrumentalities. I am not surprised at this view, but I am surprised that any men occupying the highest positions in the Government and instructors and text writers upon constitutional law should at this hour justify a doctrine that strikes down at its very altar the oracle of our faith and substitutes for it a worship that is only temporary and that can not possibly continue and endure. The day will come, Mr. President, I predict it — it is bound to come — when this illusion will disappear, when the people will retrace their steps, and as they flee from the pagan temple they will bear upon their shoulders the ark of the covenant and the scroll of the ancient law.

FROM A SPEECH OF REPRESENTATIVE TOWNE [1]

It is, I take it, well within the province of a member of this popular representative branch of the National Legislature to examine and, within the limits of the decencies and proprieties of parliamentary discussion, to criticise the official conduct of the President of the United States. The independence of the legislative branch of the Government and the responsibilities of the Executive Office justify and require this liberty of comment.

It is, in my deliberate opinion, a very serious matter, not only as related to pending and immediately prospective public questions, but as concerning the development of our institutions and the preservation of that wise balance of power among the coördinate branches of this Government to which so much importance was originally attached, that the present Chief Executive of the country is disposed to magnify and to personalize his great office and to exercise authority beyond not only the traditional but the legal and constitutional limitations of his place. [Applause from the Democratic side.] This is not the time or the occasion, sir, for anybody, and certainly not for one no more competent to the task than I can claim to be, to attempt anything like an analysis and final judgment upon the character and achievements of Theodore Roosevelt, as to whom future historians, as has been the case with his contemporaries, will undoubtedly differ radically among themselves. There will be panegyrists and detractors hereafter, as there are eulogists and faultfinders now. I shall attempt no ultimate judgment. I shall briefly, however, comment upon certain aspects of his character, and upon certain of his official performances, for the purpose of drawing what seems to me to be necessary and helpful conclusions. There are many things in the character and endowments of that remarkable man that I have admired. There are also, on the other hand, many things that, as a representative of the people in this great body, I feel justified in pronouncing to be of a nature to unfit him for a judicious, careful, just, and deliberate discharge of high executive functions, and under the impul-

[1] *Congr. Record*, June 11, 1906.

sion of which he has time and again gone beyond the legitimate boundaries of his authority. [Applause on the Democratic side.]

This tendency of the Chief Executive is a matter of common knowledge
among members of both Houses of Congress and the representatives of
the newspaper press who are stationed at the capital. It is a serious
misfortune, as I view it, that the unusual vogue enjoyed by the President
imposes upon Senators, Representatives, and correspondents a reticence
in regard to these excesses of Executive authority that would not under
ordinary conditions be observed. In my opinion we ought to be honest
with the people of the United States, and tell them frankly what everybody in this House knows, what every member of the Senate knows,
and what everybody in the press galleries knows, that the President of
the United States endeavors, so far as an almost phenomenal activity
and endurance will permit, to embrace within himself and to exercise
at once almost all of the powers and prerogatives of the three coördinate
branches of this Government. Moreover, he seems to regard the high
and solemn duties of his office not only as in the nature of personal assets
of his own, but as appropriate occasion for the exercise of an indeliberate
and whimsical disposition apparently as little regardful of the momen-
tousness and significance of his action as that of a boy occupied with
his toys.

The reörganization of the Army has emphasized the military aspects
of the Presidency. The President's relation to the Army is not much
different from that sustained by the Emperor William to the German
army. It is notorious that promotions during the present administration have been made in a manner so harmful to the discipline of the
service, and to so great a degree upon grounds of favoritism and personal preference, as to have become the subject of repeated and solicitous
conference among men having knowledge of the situation and concerned
with the preservation of the *morale* of the Army. The diplomatic service has fallen under the same influence. The Secretary of State, although himself a man of great ability and strong personality, has had
many of his functions shorn. The President's relation to the general
body of the service is much more intimate and direct than heretofore,
and we have recently seen how, for the first time in American diplomacy,
the President has referred to a high representative of the United States
at a foreign court as "my ambassador." A similar personal dominance
is asserted in the province of every Cabinet office, and everybody remembers the promulgation of the famous ";order of silence" by which
those high functionaries were forbidden to talk to reporters about their
business, and directed to leave a monopoly of publicity to the head of
the Government.

The civil-service rules have been made conveniently pliant to the
personal and political exigencies of the Chief Executive, and, although
in former days that gentleman filled a great place in the movement for

civil-service reform, the records show that the rules have been set aside during his administration about four times as often as they were during his predecessor's term. The most important considerations of public policy are constantly and customarily made subservient to the personal feelings of the Chief Magistrate. The evidence, for example, to which everybody had access, disclosed that one of his Cabinet officers, some time since resigned, had been engaged, while occupying a high official position with a great railroad system, in repeated violations of the inter-state-commerce law; but the fact of his close official and personal relation to the President not only relieved him from prosecution or censure, but actually won for him an official certificate of innocence in direct contradiction of even his own confession.

*　　*　　*　　*　　*　　*.　　*　　*

In February, 1905, Admiral Walker testified that he and other members of the Panama Canal Commission, on the President's express authorization, charged and received, in addition to their regular compensation, director's fees for attending the meetings of the board of directors of the Panama Railroad. Expenses far beyond those that have scandalized former administrations are incurred by this administration with a gay and easy nonchalance seemingly justified by the entire lack of subsequent public criticism. Whereas wide and unfavorable comment was made upon one of his predecessors for too frequent use of one Government vessel, very little is now said about the employment by the President of the United States of the *Sylph*, the *Dolphin*, and the *Mayflower* together. White House repairs are undertaken and carried out apparently with as little hesitancy as that with which a prosperous farmer would build a wood shed; and $750,000 is spent in alleged increase of the facilities and attractions of the Executive Mansion, where no living architect can possibly see where there was opportunity to disburse more than a seventh of that sum to produce the very unhandsome results. Some of these matters to which I have referred thus cursorily may seem somewhat trivial. The catalogue is not exhaustive even of important considerations. I cite these few only as illustrative of that persistent and irrepressible tendency to personalize his office, to regard it as an appendage to his will, which characterizes the present occupant of that great place.

It is, moreover, inevitable that a man possessing the characteristics of the President should trench upon the traditional and constitutional restrictions of his authority. This natural inclination is unfortunately reënforced by certain considerations growing out of the political conditions of our time. In the first place, there is a necessary reaction upon the methods of our Executive Department by the unavoidable secrecy and arbitrariness with which the affairs of our colonial possessions are conducted. It is yet too soon for us fully to appreciate the irreparable damage done to our peculiar institutions by the rash assumption of the dangers of colonial government. From the commencement of the departure in our experience I have felt the deepest concern for its effect upon that constitutional balance among the different departments of the Government upon which our elder statesmen placed so much stress, and upon whose permanent preservation, as I believe, rests to a very large degree the perpetuity of civil liberty in this country. In the course of a speech on our Philippine policy in the Senate of the United States, on the 28th of January, 1901, I used the following language:

This policy favors the growth of the executive department of the Government at the expense of the other, and is opposed to democratic principles. It involves singleness of authority, celerity of action, secrecy of purpose, irresponsibility; all contrary to the necessary methods of self-government. It begets a superficial admiration for "strong government," and "simple government," which are absolutely inconsistent with liberty. Let me again quote words of wisdom from the speech of Daniel Webster, already cited:

"Nothing is more deceptive or more dangerous than the pretense of a desire to simplify government. The simplest governments are despotisms; the next simplest, limited monarchies; but all republics, all governments of law, must impose numerous limitations and qualifications of authority, and give many positive and many qualified rights. In other words, they must be subject to rule and regulation. This is the very essence of free political institutions.

"The spirit of liberty is, indeed, a bold and fearless spirit; but it is also a sharp-sighted spirit; it is a cautious, sagacious, discriminating, far-seeing intelligence; it is jealous of encroachment, jealous of power, jealous of man. It demands checks; it seeks for guards; it insists on securities; it intrenches itself behind strong defenses, and fortifies itself with all possible care against the assaults of ambition and passion.

"It does not trust the amiable weaknesses of human nature, and, therefore, it will not permit power to overstep its prescribed limits, though benevolence, good intent, and patriotic purpose come along with it. Neither does it satisfy itself with flashy and temporary resistance to illegal authority. Far otherwise. It seeks for duration and permanence. It looks before and after; and, building on the experience of ages which are past, it labors diligently for the benefit of ages to come. This is the nature of constitutional liberty, and this is our liberty, if we will rightly understand and preserve it. Every free government is necessarily complicated, because all such governments establish restraints, as well on the power of government itself as on that of individuals."

A president can not be at one and the same time a constitutional chief magistrate and an autocrat — a President in America, with imperial powers in the Orient.

There is no question in my mind, sir, that the reaction of our absolute government in our distant possessions is partly responsible for the tendency toward Executive excess, at which all close students of our institutions are now gravely concerned. But there is another consideration which reënforces the one just mentioned and the natural characteristics of the President. I refer to the phenomenal popular majority by which the present Chief Magistrate was chosen in the election of 1904. The country had full notice of the personality of the Republican candidate, and was told from every Democratic stump what would be the inevitable tendency of the expression of that personality if it should receive an emphatic electoral indorsement. The recipient of that indorsement can, in one sense, hardly be blamed if he considers the verdict so rendered with such emphasis and after definite notice, as in the nature of a license to exercise his predispositions to the utmost. The result has certainly justified the prognostications. It is only fair to say, however, that these actions since the election of 1904 have merely been of a piece with those that characterized the Presidency of the present incumbent in his first fractional term.

Without attempting a numerous recitation, to say nothing of an exhaustive one, of the matters that may readily be cited in illustration of the proposition I am now considering, I shall mention a few which are of common knowledge.

Everybody remembers the famous "pension order" whereby, while a bill was pending in Congress concerning a classification of claimants before the Pension Office, an Executive order, impatient of the delay by Congress, undertook to perform the function of a legislative act. There has been a practically constant interference from the White House with legislative procedure at the Capitol. It will be recalled how the Irrigation Bill was threatened with a veto unless it should contain certain provisions agreeable to the Executive. The great struggle over the Cuban tariff, the recent controversy about statehood for Indian Territory and Oklahoma and Arizona and New Mexico, and over the provisions of the Railroad Rate Bill are a few among many matters in regard to which the Executive initiative and constant participation in all the complications that attend the progress of a bill from its inception to its passage, might well raise a doubt whether there is any such thing now in our system of government as an independent responsible legislative branch.

The Senate of the United States, in regard to those semi-Executive functions vested in it by the Constitution, has been treated with similar masterfulness. Some fifteen months ago the Arbitration Treaties were withdrawn from the Senate by the President because that body insisted upon the use of the word "treaty" instead of "agreement," thus refusing to countenance the new view that there are certain permanent international compacts into which the President may enter on behalf of this country without the participation of the Senate. In the case of the Santo Domingo treaty an attempt was made by the President of the United States to make a treaty with a foreign government without the action of the Senate, which treaty, moreover, involved a new departure in our diplomacy and the adoption of what the President has called a "development" of the Monroe doctrine potentially fraught with the most momentous consequences to this country.

It seems to me that this is a good connection in which to emphasize the fact that this new doctrine of the responsibility of the United States for the debts and defaults of the South American States, involving on our part the assumption of the duties of constable for the nations of Europe, ought, whatever its merits or demerits, to stand upon its own pretentions and not be permitted to shelter itself behind the designation of "Monroe doctrine."

The Monroe doctrine, properly so called, is a part of the settled policy of this Government, and is very dear to the people of this country. A novel proposition may frequently find acceptance through its success in borrowing the label of one already generally entertained. Whether this new international theory be right or wrong, it ought to stand or fall upon its own claims. It certainly is not "Monroe doctrine." It is just as clearly "Roosevelt doctrine." The original Monroe doctrine of 1823 is very easy to understand. As affirmed by Adams and Monroe, it involved three things. 1. The American continents were not to be subject to colonization by any European power. 2. We could not permit any intervention by any European power in the affairs of the South American Republics "for the purpose of oppressing them or controlling in any other manner their destiny." 3. We could not permit the extension by the allied powers — that is, the members of the "Holy Alliance," formed by the sovereigns of Russia, Austria, and Prussia after the congress of Vienna in 1815 — of their political system to any portion of North or South America.

When, about 1845, President Polk practically took the position that it was the duty of the United States to annex adjacent territory in order to prevent its annexation by European countries; and when, in 1881, Mr. Blaine held, in substance, that the United States was the sole guardian of transit across the Isthmus of Panama and the arbiter of disputes between the Latin-American States; and when, in 1895, Mr. Olney announced that the United States is sovereign in America, that the British colonies in America are temporary, and that these propositions are a part of international law, the prestige of the Monroe doctrine was invoked in favor of these various formulations of our international policy. Yet nothing is clearer than that all these involved distinct variations from the Monroe doctrine. Undoubtedly considerations based on national advantage, duty, and safety could be advanced on the one side and on the other in each of these cases. But that should have been the only method of argument. To introduce the Monroe doctrine was only to confuse both the nature of that doctrine and that of the new problems. The same is true in regard to the Roosevelt doctrine of our general guardianship of the countries to the south of us with responsibilities to their creditors. Whether right or wrong, and I decidedly believe it to be wrong, it is certainly new, and it ought to be examined on its merits without receiving any shelter or warrant whatever from the Monroe doctrine.

This tendency of the Executive, upon which I have been briefly commenting, has involved us in grave national wrong. The conduct of this Government under the lead of the President of the United States in regard to the means by which the independence of Panama was recognized and the arrangements were made for the construction of the Panama Canal is, in my opinion, an idelible stain upon the fair fame and good faith of this Government. In order that the object had in view by the President should be achieved it was necessary to override a statute of the United States, to break a solemn treaty with a foreign government, and to commit an act of war, and without authority of Congress, against a people with whom we were at peace. The law known as the Spooner Act expressly directed the President of the United States to proceed with the construction of the Nicaragua Canal if, within a reasonable time, he could not secure the consent of the Government of the United States of Colombia to the treaty providing for the construction of the canal across the Isthmus of Panama. That consent he did not obtain.

It is beside the question to contend that the United States of Colombia ought to have ratified the treaty. It is an independent government and had a right to reject the treaty if it chose to without giving us any reason whatever. But, upon the rejection of the treaty, instead of proceeding to carry out the plain and specific direction of the act of Congress to construct the Nicaragua Canal, the President of the United States recognized the independence of Panama, a revolted province of the United States of Colombia, used the armed forces of the United States to prevent Colombia from reëstablishing her authority over that territory, despite our solemn engagement in the treaty of 1846 to respect the integrity of her domain; which was unquestionably an act of war upon our part, made a treaty with the new State, and proceeded with what difficulties and scandals the world is aware, to the present stage of the canal construction across the Isthmus. There have not been wanting grave insinuations touching our complicity in the revolution of Panama against Colombia. Certainly the appearance of our gunboats at a time and place when and where Bunau Varilla had promised the revolutionists they should appear, and their effectual action in defeating any attempt by Colombia to recover her province, are circumstances strongly confirmatory of the suspicion; nor does the suspicion involve, if justified, any greater dishonor on our part than that which already attaches to us from the admitted circumstances.

Not long ago, in a remarkable special message to Congress, the President strayed into the judicial reservations of the Constitution by bringing to book a Federal judge (Humphrey) for an opinion rendered by him in the ordinary discharge of his judicial functions, an unprecedented proceeding that would have jarred the credulity of "the fathers."

DEBATE ON THE WAR POWER [1]

[The President's action in dismissing a company of colored soldiers led to a debate in the Senate in which the power of the president as commander in chief of the army was discussed. The main point at issue was the relation of the power of Congress "to make rules for the government and regulation of the land and naval forces," to the functions and powers of the president as commander in chief. The respective arguments are brought out clearly in the following extracts from the debate between Senator Spooner and Senator Bacon.]

MR. SPOONER. Mr. President, my differences with the distinguished Senator from Ohio are upon the legal phases of this matter mainly, and with many of the principles of law which he announces I am entirely in accord with him. That this is a country of law, that no Federal official can be above the Constitution, that the President can lawfully exercise no power which he does not derive from that instrument or the laws of Congress enacted in pursuance of it, of course all must admit. That we may not in some circumstances have what would be in other circumstances autocratic power in this country I can not say, because in its very nature the discipline and conduct of an army requires more or less the summary exercise of power. No one knows that better than the chivalrous and gallant soldier who introduced and advocates this resolution. The very idea of command, which can not be dissociated from a commander in chief, involves more or less autocratic power. Under our system many safeguards have been thrown around its exercise.

I am not opposing the resolution of investigation of the Brownsville affair, properly worded. I do object, however, to the resolution as introduced by the Senator from Ohio and now pending. The inevitable trend of the debate on Saturday and to-day has strengthened me in my objection to it. It has been discussed rather as a case in court than as a legislative function. If the President has, as the Senator from South Carolina, and perhaps others, seem to think, exercised a power which under the Constitution and the laws of the country he does not possess, and in a manner greatly to the prejudice of citizens, it is quite clear to me that the Senate ought not to enter upon an investigation of it. Even if a President abuses the power which he possesses or exercises it with bad motive, I should greatly deplore an attempt by the Senate to investigate it or pass judgment upon it.

In our system the powers of government are distributed among three branches, each coördinate and independent of the other, neither of which is responsible to the other in any manner, except as prescribed by the Constitution. The President is not responsible under the Constitution to the Senate or to the House of Representatives or to both. It is *especially not* the function of the Senate to investigate and determine whether the President has usurped power or abused a power which he possesses,

[1] *Congr. Record*, Jan. 19, 1907.

because under the Constitution the Senate sustains a peculiar relation to the President. Of course it is one of the legislative bodies of the Congress. It is equal in power, in respect of legislation, to the other, with one exception. It is not permitted to originate revenue bills. But, Mr. President, peculiar functions have been conferred upon the House as to some matters, and upon the House alone, and also upon the Senate to the exclusion of the House. None of them are legislative functions. The Senate participates in the making of the laws as a legislative body. It participates, with the President, in appointments, which is not a legislative function. It participates in the exercise of the treaty-making power. But, Mr. President, its most solemn function under the Constitution is a judicial one. Section 3 of the first article provides:

The Senate shall have the sole power to try all impeachments. When sitting for that purpose they shall be on oath or affirmation. When the President of the United States is tried, the Chief Justice shall preside, and no person shall be convicted without the concurrence of two-thirds of the members present.

Section 2 of the same article provides that the House "shall have the sole power of impeachment." The power of *impeachment* is as plainly and exclusively vested in the House of Representatives as is the power to *try impeachments* vested in the Senate. Investigations to determine or which will determine whether an Executive act is violative of the Constitution and beyond the power of a President, or whether, if within his power, it has been abused, if that is the object of the inquiry, surely is properly with the impeaching body, and should not be exercised by the body which alone can constitutionally try and determine. Of course this is an abstraction as to this case and as to this President, but to my mind (I have had occasion to urge it here before) it is a principle which ought not to be disregarded by the Senate, for it would be a horrid thing if when articles of impeachment of an officer reach this Chamber they should be laid before a court which in another capacity, having investigated and considered the same matter, had prejudged it.

Mr. President, so much for that. If a President, whether in his capacity of Chief Executive or as Commander in Chief, has performed an act or made an order which was within his authority to make, I can not see that it is competent for this body or the other, or both, to take testimony as to the wisdom of that executed act, upon which to determine whether it will by *legislative act set it aside*. The Congress, if dissatisfied, may withdraw the power or place additional limitations upon its exercise for the future, but I do not see that it can by legislation render void the act. When a power is possessed by the President or an officer of the Government to do an act in a defined contingency or in his discretion, his decision as to the existence of the contingency or that circumstances are such as to demand the performance of the act is conclusive, and the act can not be impeached or overturned by the Congress because in its opinion the exigency had not arisen or that the power was unwisely exercised. The general rule is well stated by the Supreme Court in the case of *Martin* v. *Mott* (12 Wheat., 19) thus:

Whenever a statute gives a discretionary power to any person, to be exercised by him upon his own opinion of certain facts, it is a sound rule of construction that the statute constitutes him the sole and exclusive judge of the existence of those facts. And in the present case we are all of opinion that such is the true construction of the act of 1795.

Which authorized the President "whenever the United States shall be invaded, or be in imminent danger of invasion from any foreign nation, etc., it shall be lawful for the President of the United States to call forth such number of the militia of the State or States most in danger," etc.

It is no answer that such a power may be abused, for there is no power which is not susceptible of abuse. The remedy for this, as well as for all other official misconduct, if it should occur, is to be found in the Constitution itself. In a free government the danger must be remote, since in addition to the high qualities which the executive must be presumed to possess of public virtue and honest devotion to the public interests, the frequency of elections, and the watchfulness of the representatives of the nation carry with them all the checks which can be useful to guard against usurpation or wanton tyranny.

The principle is peculiarly applicable to a lawful order made by the President as Commander in Chief of the Army and Navy.

I am assuming now that the President possessed the lawful authority to make the order discharging without honor the enlisted men of the battalion of the Twenty-fifth Infantry at Brownsville. The fact that he made such an order does not need investigation. The reports and papers upon which he based it are in the possession of the Senate, and the inquiry into the discharge, and it seems to be limited to that, is as to the wisdom and justness of the order, and the adequacy of the information upon which the President based it; in other words, as it has been put, for the purpose of affording to the enlisted men discharged a day in court.

Aside from the general principle, which is sufficient, I deny that under the Constitution the Congress has any such relation to the Army as permits it to set aside an order lawfully made by the President as Commander in Chief. The provisions of the Constitution which bear upon the subject are few and simple. The Senator from Ohio, who is a very able lawyer, and has said all that can be said by anyone, I think, in support of his contentions, read them.

Congress is given power to declare war, which necessitates the use of an army or navy, or both. Congress is given power to raise and support armies, with the limitation that "no appropriation of money to that use shall be for a longer term than two years." Congress is given power in addition to make *"rules for the government and regulation of the land and naval forces."* The Constitution provides, in section 1 of Article II, that "the executive power shall be vested in a President of the United States," and in section 2 that "the President shall be Commander in Chief of the Army and Navy of the United States, and of the militia of the several States when called into actual service of the United States."

The provisions quoted from the Constitution as to the power of Congress in respect to the Army and Navy are logical and plain. They admirably express the manifest purpose of the framers of the instrument. I will consider them later.

The Constitution has left entirely without definition the scope of the power of the President as Commander in Chief, and the measure of the power was left to be sought elsewhere. I can not agree that the sole Constitutional power of the President is to command the Army in time of war and conduct campaigns. That his power is vastly greater in time of war than in time of peace has been decided, and is not open to dispute. It is largely to be sought in the law of nations and the rules of civilized warfare. But an army and a navy must be commanded in time of peace, as well as in time of war, else neither would be fit for war. What the measure and scope of this power is in time of peace is not necessary at this time to discuss. That it is the power to command, with all that is inherent in the function and necessary to its exercise, can not well be disputed, and that whatever the power is is conferred by the Constitution and can not be interfered with by the Congress will not be denied.

I quite agree with the Senator from Ohio that we need not, even if we may, seek the measure of this power in the power of the King at the time of the adoption of the Constitution. There is something to be said on both sides of the proposition. Some courts have referred to the power of the King as furnishing some guide as to the Constitutional power of the President as Commander in Chief. It is said in the opinion of Judge Knott, speaking for the Court of Claims in the case of *Street* v. *United States* (24 Court of Claims, 230), after referring to the power of the Crown at the time of the adoption of the Constitution exclusively to control the British army, that —

This power of command and control the framers of the Constitution placed in the hands of the President, with only two restrictions set upon it: That Congress should have power "to make rules for the government and regulation of the land and naval forces;" that the appointment of officers should be "by and with the advice and consent of the Senate."

The President can remove any officer of the Army or Navy without cause by appointing, by and with the advice and consent of the Senate, another to supersede him. This was settled in the Mullen case (140 U. S. 240). The practice has wisely made the tenure of military and naval office "practically for life or during good behavior." But I speak of the power.

In Ex parte Milligan (4 Wallace, 2), quoted by the Senator from Ohio, was involved the power of the President to establish martial law in Indiana and the validity of the trial of a citizen by military commission upon the charge practically of giving aid and comfort to the enemy. Milligan and others were sentenced to death by the military commission, and the court held properly that, as Indiana was not in any sense the theatre of war, the civil government there was in full operation, and the courts discharging uninterruptedly their functions, martial law could not lawfully be put in operation in Indiana and that a military commission could not lawfully try and condemn a citizen. In the opinion, upon the general subject which I am discussing, the court say:

Congress has the power not only to raise and support and govern armies, but to declare war. It has, therefore, the power to provide by law for carrying on war. This power necessarily extends to all legislation essential to the prosecution of war with vigor and success, except such as interferes with the command of the forces and the conduct of campaigns. That power and duty belong to the President as Commander in Chief. Both these powers are derived from the Constitution, but neither is defined by that instrument. Their extent must be determined by their nature and by the principles of our institutions.

The power to make the necessary laws is in Congress; the power to execute in the President. *Both powers imply many subordinate and auxiliary powers. Each includes all authorities essential to its due exercise. But neither can the President*, in war more than in *peace*, intrude upon the proper authority of Congress, *nor Congress upon the proper authority of the President*. Both are servants of the people, whose will is expressed in the fundamental law.

It must be certain that where Congress has failed to make rules for the discipline of the Army the power of command lodged in the President carries with it authority in him to issue an order absolutely necessary to the discipline of the Army. An army without discipline, Mr. President, is a mob. Instead of being a shield and a protection to the people it is a menace. It is more dangerous to those who maintain it than it is to the enemies of the country.

* * * * * * * *

Mr. BACON. My opinion, Mr. President, as to the power of the Commander in Chief is this: I do not think every power exercised by the Commander in Chief must be dictated by Congress. I think there are certain natural functions of a commander in chief which, in the absence of restrictions on the part of Congress, any commander in chief can exercise — those which are usually exercised. But at the same time I think there is none which can not be restricted or controlled by Congress.

If the Senator will pardon me for a moment — I fear that I trespass unduly upon his time, but I will take the time with his permission — just to state the proposition that all the clauses of the Constitution in connection with the grant of power to Congress which I have just read indicate the very great solicitude and earnest intention on the part of the framers of the Constitution to take away from any one man the power to wield the Army independently of Congress; and even so jealous were they of the power that they were not willing even that Congress should have an undue exercise of that power, but that, as in the case of the limitation of the length of appropriations, they must go back to the people every two years for the purpose of getting that which alone can sustain an army. Now, let me read those several propositions for the purpose of illustrating the position that the evident purpose of the Constitution was to take away from any one man the dangerous power of unrestrained control and government of the Army. They had too much reason to fear and to dread it.

*   *   *   *   *   *   *   *

I say that all those general grants of power, endeavoring to reach every phase of the important things which relate to the raising of armies and to the government of armies, are laid down in this succession of provisions in a way which, to my mind, clearly points to the purpose of the framers of the Constitution that the great power which would be lodged in one man if he had the power to wield an army without restriction should be denied to the President and should be given the Congress; and that the sole, indefeasible grant of power given to him was that he should be Commander in Chief, to exercise that great office subject to the superior power of Congress to prescribe the rules for the government and regulation of the Army. "Government," I repeat, is a term which can not be qualified. It is complete and entire and does not mean partial government.

The Senator from Wisconsin will pardon me for having trespassed so much upon his time.

Mr. SPOONER. Congress may locate a fort in the State of Georgia. Can Congress pass an act providing that certain troops shall be assigned to that fort?

Mr. BACON. I have not the slightest doubt of it; not a particle.

Mr. SPOONER. What is there to this Commander in Chief?

Mr. BACON. The Commander in Chief is to command the Army, subject to the power of the Congress to prescribe what shall be done in its government. The government of an army refers as much to where it shall be located as to what uniform it shall wear.

Mr. SPOONER. I mean particular troops.

Mr. BACON. I am speaking of particular troops. Congress can prescribe that the uniform of the artillery shall be red ——

Mr. SPOONER. Of course.

Mr. BACON. And the uniform of the cavalry yellow or buff.

Mr. SPOONER. I admit all that.

Mr. BACON. It may prescribe that there shall be so many troops in this place and that many in the other.

With all due respect and the greatest regard for the judgment of the Senator from Wisconsin, I beg to say that I have never heard on the floor of the Senate a doctrine which, to my mind, was more dangerous to the institutions of this country than the doctrine that the President of the United States has any power in the use of the Army which can not be controlled by the law-making power of the land, except the power to command.

Mr. SPOONER. Mr. President, yesterday when I yielded the floor I was in the midst of a colloquy with the Senator from Georgia [Mr. BACON], with whom I agree in part, but with whom I am compelled in part to disagree. I would not minimize, and never have consciously, the power of Congress, nor would I exaggerate in anywise the power of the Executive. My proposition — and I do not intend to spend much time upon it — concedes to Congress the full power which I think it possesses under the Constitution with reference to the Army, and it is very large, of course.

Congress is given power to raise and maintain armies and to provide a navy. The size of the Army is entirely for Congress to determine. The character of the Army as to different branches of the service is entirely for Congress to determine. The grade of officers and the number of officers are for Congress to determine. The oath of enlistment, the contract of enlistment are for Congress to determine. The duration of the term of enlistment is for Congress to determine. The pay and all that is for Congress to determine. The establishment of military tribunals, the definition of military offenses, the method of military trials, and the punishment that is to be administered are for Congress to determine. Congress determines where it will have military posts and where it will not.

Congress may reduce the Army and provide for the muster out of officers, as it has often done, and may provide for the discharge of enlisted men, as it has always done, and which is always a part of the contract of enlistment. Congress can not make a contract for service in the Army with an officer, or, I think, with an enlisted man, which would be a contract protected by the Constitution of the United States against the power of the same or a succeeding Congress to reduce the Army, muster out officers, and discharge enlisted men.

See *Crenshaw* v. *United States*, Mr. Justice Lamar (134 U. S. 99).

The power of Congress to make rules for the government and regulation is a large one, but it is manifestly to be exercised in the manner clearly indicated by the clause itself.

I can not agree with the Senator from Georgia that the Commander in Chief, either in time of peace or war, is under the *supreme* control of Congress. The Constitution need not have made the President the Commander in Chief. Wisely, however, it did so, combining with executive power the power of command. It is conceded by the distinguished Senator from Ohio that in the absence of Congressional rules the President is Commander in Chief. Congress having raised and appropriated money for the support of an army, but having failed to make rules for its government would, *ex necessitate rei,* have the power to make those necessary for the government of the Army and Navy. That would not be simply because of necessity, I think, but because the Constitution has made the President Commander in Chief without defining the functions. This involves the power to do those things which inhere in the office or are necessary to the discharge of the duties of the office.

The Constitution is to be read as a whole, and provisions *pari materia* are to be read together, each in the light of the other. No clause in the Constitution is to be so construed as to destroy another clause or clauses.

Now, I admit the power of Congress over the subject of enlistment. I admit Congress may say properly that no enlisted man shall be discharged before the expiration of his term of enlistment except upon the finding of a board of officers. I admit that the Congress may provide that no man shall be reënlisted unless his service during the preceding term was honest and faithful. This is one of the "rules" made by Congress now in force. I admit that Congress might provide — it would not — that men who shall have been dishonorably discharged by sentence of court-martial may be reënlisted in the Army of the United States upon making satisfactory proof to a board or complying with such other terms as the Congress might provide as showing changed behavior.

But there must be a distinction between the words "Congress may make *rules* for the government and regulation of the land and naval forces" and the words "Congress *shall govern* the land and naval forces." The one would make the power to govern absolute; the other is restrictive as to the manner in which the governmental power of Congress shall be exercised. I repeat on the point a few sentences already read, which certainly declare the law.

It is true that the Constitution has conferred upon Congress the exclusive power "to make rules for the government and regulation of the land and naval forces"; that the two powers are distinct; neither can trench upon the other; the President can not, *under the disguise of military orders,* evade the legislative regulations by which he in common with the Army must be governed, and Congress can not in the disguise of "rules for the government" of the Army impair the authority of the President as Commander in Chief. (28 Court of Claims, 221.)

Mr. FORAKER. Will the Senator give the citation?

Mr. SPOONER. It is 28 Court of Claims, the Swaim case, page 221.

In that case it was held, and affirmed by the Supreme Court, that the President by virtue of his function as Commander in Chief may order a general court-martial.

Now, Mr. President, is there no function that is not subject to the control of Congress involved in the designation Commander in Chief of the Army and Navy of the United States? I have never heard it denied until yesterday that the assignment of officers to particular commands and the disposition of troops throughout the country was not a part of the power of command, and I was amazed that a lawyer of the great ability of my friend from Georgia should suggest — I do not know that he would contend for it — that Congress can provide that a particular officer shall be assigned to a particular troop or that where a regiment or a company has been assigned by the Commander in Chief to a particular State Congress can by resolution, which has the effect of law, countermand that order. If that is correct, it may fix the designation or location to which that command shall be transferred. I never heard it suggested before, Mr. President, that as commander of the Army and Navy the President had not the power to send the war ships hither and yon as in his judgment is best for the country and the people.

The President, as Commander in Chief, acting through the Secretary of War, having lawfully assigned a colored battalion or a colored regiment to Texas for duty, Congress could not constitutionally pass a resolution revoking that order, or, if it had been executed, requiring the President to transfer those troops from Texas to some other State. If the intense construction which the Senator from Georgia puts upon the word "government" in this clause is the law, the Constitution did not constitute the President Commander in Chief of the Army and Navy, but constituted him the *Adjutant-General of the Congress*, and gave him no power to issue a military order in time of peace not revocable and supplantable by a joint resolution of Congress.

Pomeroy says of the powers of the Commander in Chief, *inter alia*, on page 472:

The President's duties in respect to these various subjects may thus be clearly defined and controlled by the legislature —

Indicating matters of Congressional jurisdiction with which I agree —

But in time of peace he has an independent function. He commands the Army and Navy; Congress does not. He may make all dispositions of troops and officers, stationing them now at this post, now at that; he may send out naval vessels to such parts of the world as he pleases; he may distribute the arms, ammunition, and supplies in such quantities and at such arsenals and depositories as he deems best. All this is a work of ordinary routine in time of peace, and is probably left, in fact, to the Secretaries of War and of the Navy and to military officers high in command.

The inevitable effect of the construction contended for by the Senator must lead to its rejection. If the power of Congress over the Army and over the Commander in Chief of the Army is as broad as he suggests, there is no order in time of peace which the President can make himself or through the Secretary of War which can not be countermanded or set aside by an act of Congress dealing solely with that order. If the Commander in Chief makes a lawful order discharging A. B. from the Army for the good of the service, he or some friend appeals to a Senator or Member of Congress to introduce and work for the passage of a joint resolution restoring A. B. to the army, or, in effect, revoking the order of the Commander in Chief. It would be contended that a stigma had been put unjustly upon this man; that he had been discharged from the Army without a hearing; that he had been denied the right, which all men should have, to a "day in court." There would be no limit to the cases in which Congress would be asked to sit as a court of appeals for the review of errors committed by the Commander in Chief in individual cases and to set them aside. All through the Army the Congress, not the Commander in Chief, would be the ultimate power in the minds of enlisted men, and if anything can 'be imagined which would be destructive of discipline in the Army it would be such a system. Does the Senator think that an order lawfully made by the Commander in Chief, discharging without honor A. B. could be revoked by the Congress.

Mr. BACON. I do not want to interrupt the Senator; I did not expect to take any part in this debate; I am agreeing with the Senator upon the conclusion he reaches; but I am simply differing from him as to the particular road over which he travels to reach it. But as the Senator directs himself to me so pointedly in the inquiry he has just propounded, without undertaking to go into any general discussion of the matter — which I am sure he recognizes would be improper and which I would not desire to do at this time — I simply call his attention, in response to the inquiry directly addressed to me by the Senator himself, to the fact that I presume he has in innumerable instances voted to correct the military record of soldiers who have been convicted by courts-martial of desertion.

Mr. SPOONER. Yes.

Mr. BACON. And correcting their record by name, legislating directly upon the point.

Mr. SPOONER. Yes.

Mr. BACON. Of course, the Senator will excuse me from elaborating or answering at large; but I simply suggest the possibility that that may be a reply to the inquiry propounded to me by the Senator.

Mr. SPOONER. Well, Mr. President, there can be no question but that would not be a *rule* for the regulation and government of the Army.

Mr. BACON. No; but, as I understood the Senator, his inquiry was addressed to the point whether or not Congress could legislate as to the particular individual, regarding anything which had been done by the direct order of the President.   An order of a court-martial is under the authority of the President; and when a man is discharged by the judgment of a court-martial, he is practically discharged by order of the President. The inquiry of the Senator was, whether or not Congress could by legislation directly overturn the order of the President dismissing a man. It can overturn the order of a court-martial and restore a man to the rolls with honor, and make him eligible to draw a pension. It seems to me that that probably would be a case such as the Senator suggests.

Mr. SPOONER. No, Mr. President. There are a great many cases, thousands of them, cases that occurred during the war, cases as to officers and cases as to enlisted men, having nothing whatever to do with the *current discipline of the Army,* cases in which, during the excitement and the haste and the tumult of war, injustice has been done to soldiers, dishonorable discharges and dismissals from the Army by the President, and all that, in which Congress has afforded relief. But Congress has never passed an act upon the theory that it restored those men to the Army; that it made void the act of the President or the act of the court-martial.

GROVER CLEVELAND, THE GOVERNMENT IN THE CHICAGO STRIKE OF 1894 [1]

[One of the acts of the federal executive which aroused the greatest amount of discussion was President Cleveland's use of the military forces in the suppression of the Chicago strike of 1894. The action of the President in this matter was carried out under his constitutional power "to take care that the laws be faithfully executed." The interference of the federal government rested upon the necessity of protecting the mail service. The bringing of federal troops into a commonwealth for this purpose aroused strong opposition as it was claimed that the state should have been allowed singly to deal with the disturbance. All phases of this most interesting action and controversy are brought out in the account subsequently written by President Cleveland, the most important parts of which are here reproduced.]

THE President inaugurated on the 4th day of March, 1893, and those associated with him as cabinet officials, encountered, during their term of executive duty, unusual and especially perplexing difficulties. The members of that administration who still survive, in recalling the events of this laborious service, can not fail to fix upon the year 1894 as the most troublous and anxious of their incumbency. During that year unhappy currency complications compelled executive resort to heroic

[1] *McClure's Magazine* (July, 1904), 23 : 227. Reproduced in part, with permission. Copyright 1904, by the S. S. McClure Co.

treatment for the preservation of our nation's financial integrity, and forced upon the administration a constant, unrelenting struggle for sound money; a long and persistent executive effort to accomplish beneficent and satisfactory tariff reform so nearly miscarried as to bring depression and disappointment to the verge of discouragement; and it was at the close of the year 1894 that executive insistence upon the Monroe Doctrine culminated in a situation that gave birth to solemn thoughts of war. Without attempting to complete the list of troubles and embarrassments that beset the administration during this luckless year, I have reserved for separate and more detailed treatment one of its incidents not yet mentioned, which immensely increased executive anxiety and foreboded the most calamitous and far-reaching consequences.

In the last days of June, 1894, a very determined and ugly labor disturbance broke out in the City of Chicago. Almost in a night it grew to full proportions of malevolence and danger. Rioting and violence were its early accompaniments; and it spread so swiftly that within a few days it had reached nearly the entire Western and Southwestern sections of our country. Railroad transportation was especially involved in its attacks. The carriage of United States mails was interrupted, interstate commerce was obstructed, and railroad property was riotously destroyed.

This disturbance is often called "The Chicago Strike." It is true that its beginning was in that city; and the headquarters of those who inaugurated it and directed its operations were located there; but the name thus given to it is an entire misnomer so far as it applies to the scope and reach of the trouble. Railroad operations were more or less affected in twenty-seven states and territories; and in all these the interposition of the General Government was to a greater or less extent invoked.

This widespread trouble had its inception in a strike by the employees of the Pullman Palace Car Company, a corporation located and doing business at the town of Pullman, which is within the limits of the City of Chicago. This company was a manufacturing corporation — or at least it was not a railroad corporation. Its main object was the operation and running of sleeping and parlor cars upon railroads under written contracts; but its charter contemplated the manufacture of cars as well; and soon after its incorporation it began the manufacture of its own cars and, subsequently, the manufacture of cars for the general market.

The strike on the part of the employees of this company began on the 11th day of May, 1894, and was provoked by a reduction of wages.

*　　*　　*　　*　　*　　*　　*　　*

This strike led to a general strike declared by the American Railway Union, and commencing June 26, 1894.

The officers of the Railroad Union from their headquarters in the City of Chicago gave directions for the maintenance and management of the strike, which were quickly transmitted to distant railroad points and were there promptly executed. As early as the 28th of June, two days after the beginning of the strike ordered by the Railway Union at Chicago, information was received at Washington from the Post-Office Department that on the Southern Pacific System, between Portland and San Francisco, Ogden and San Francisco, and Los Angeles and San Francisco, the mails were completely obstructed, and that the strikers refused to permit trains to which Pullman cars were attached to run over the lines mentioned. Thereupon Attorney-General Olney immediately sent the following telegraphic despatch to the United States district attorneys in the State of California:

WASHINGTON, D. C., June 28, 1894.

"See that the passage of regular trains, carrying United States mails in the usual and ordinary way, as contemplated by the Act of Congress and directed by the Postmaster-General, is not obstructed. Procure warrants or any other available process from United States courts against any and all persons engaged in such obstructions and direct the Marshal to execute the same by such number of deputies or such posse as may be necessary."

On the same day, and during a number of days immediately following, complaints of a similar character, sometimes accompanied by charges of forcible seizure of trains and other violent disorders, poured in upon the Attorney-General from all parts of the West and Southwest. These complaints came from post-office officials, from United States marshals and district attorneys, from railroad managers, and from other officials and private citizens. In all cases of substantial representation of interference with the carriage of mails, a despatch identical with that already quoted was sent by the Attorney-General to the United States district attorneys in the disturbed localities; and this was supplemented, whenever necessary, by such other prompt action as the different emergencies required.

I shall not enter upon an enumeration of all the disorders and violence, the defiance of law and authority, and the obstructions of national functions and duties, which occurred in many localities as a consequence of this labor contention, thus tremendously reinforced and completely under way. It is my especial purpose to review the action taken by the Government for the maintenance of its own authority and the protection of the special interests intrusted to its keeping, so far as they were endangered by this disturbance; and I do not intend to especially deal with the incidents of the strike except in so far as a reference to them may be necessary to show conditions which not only justified but actually obliged the Government to resort to stern and unusual measures in the assertion of its prerogatives.

Inasmuch, therefore, as the City of Chicago was the birthplace of the disturbance and the home of its activities; and because it was the field of its most pronounced and malign manifestations, as well as the place of its final extinction, I shall meet the needs of my subject by supplementing what has been already said, by a recital of events occurring at this central point. In doing this, I shall liberally embody documents, orders, instructions, and reports which I hope will not prove tiresome, since they supply the facts I desire to present, at first hand and more impressively than they could be presented by any words of mine.

Owing to the enforced relationship of Chicago to the strike which started within its borders, and because of its importance as a center of railway traffic, Government officials at Washington were not surprised by the early and persistent complaints of mail and interstate commerce obstructions which reached them from that city. It was from the first anticipated that this would be the seat of the most serious complications, and the place where the strong arm of the law would be most needed. In these circumstances it would have been a criminal neglect of duty if those charged with the protection of Governmental agencies and the enforcement of orderly obedience and submission to Federal authority, had been remiss in preparations for any emergency in that quarter.

On the 30th of June the District Attorney of Chicago reported by telegraph that mail trains in the suburbs of Chicago were, on the previous night, stopped by strikers, that an engine had been cut off and disabled, and that conditions were growing more and more likely to culminate in the stoppage of all trains; and he recommended that the Marshal be authorized to employ a force of special deputies who should be placed on trains to protect mails and detect the parties guilty of such interference. In reply to this despatch Attorney-General Olney on the same day authorized the Marshal to employ additional deputies as suggested, and designated Edwin Walker, an able and prominent attorney in Chicago, as special counsel for the Government, to assist the District Attorney in any legal proceedings that might be instituted. He also notified the District Attorney of this action, and enjoined upon him that "action ought to be prompt and vigorous," and directed him to confer with the special counsel who had been employed. In a letter of the same date addressed to this special counsel, the Attorney-General, in making suggestions concerning legal proceedings, wrote: "It has seemed to me that if the rights of the United States were vigorously asserted in Chicago, the origin and center of the demonstration, the result would be to make it a failure everywhere else, and to prevent its spread over the entire country," and in that connection he indicated that it might be advisable, instead of relying entirely upon warrants issued under criminal statutes, against persons actually guilty of the offense of obstructing United States mails, that the courts should be asked to grant injunctions which would restrain and prevent any attempt to commit such offense.

This suggestion contemplated the inauguration of legal proceedings in a regular and usual way to restrain those prominently concerned in the interference with the mails and the obstruction of interstate commerce, basing such proceedings on the proposition that, under the constitution and laws, these subjects were in the exclusive care of the Government of the United States, and that for their protection the Federal courts were competent under general principles of law to intervene by injunction; and on the further ground that under an Act of Congress, passed July 2, 1890, conspiracies in restraint of trade or commerce among the several states were declared to be illegal, and the Circuit Courts of the United States were therein expressly given jurisdiction to prevent and restrain such conspiracies.

On the 1st day of July the District Attorney reported to the Attorney-General that he was preparing a bill of complaint to be presented to the court the next day, on an application for an injunction. He further reported that very little mail and no freight was moving, that the Marshal was using all his force to prevent riots and the obstruction of tracks, and that this force was clearly inadequate. On the same day the Marshal reported that the situation was desperate, that he had sworn in over 400 deputies, that many more would be required to protect mail trains, and that he expected great trouble the next day. He further expressed the opinion that 100 riot guns were needed.

Upon the receipt of these reports, and anticipating an attempt to serve injunctions on the following day, the Attorney-General immediately sent a despatch to the District Attorney directing him to report at once if the process of the court should be resisted by such force as the Marshal could not overcome, and suggesting that the United States judge should join in such report. He at the same time sent a despatch to the special counsel requesting him to report his view of the situation as early as the forenoon of the next day.

In explanation of these two despatches it should here be said that the desperate character of this disturbance was not in the least underestimated by executive officials at Washington; and it must be borne in mind that while menacing conditions were moving swiftly and accumulating at Chicago, like conditions, inspired and supported from that central point, existed in many other places within the area of the strike's contagion.

Of course it was hoped by those charged with the responsibility of dealing with the situation, that a direct assertion of authority by the Marshal and a resort to the restraining power of the courts would prove sufficient for the emergency. Notwithstanding, however, an anxious desire to avoid measures more radical, the fact had not been overlooked that a contingency might occur which would compel a resort to military force. The key to these despatches of the Attorney-General is found in the determination of the Federal authorities to overcome by any lawful and constitutional means all resistance to governmental functions as related to the transportation of mails, the operation of interstate commerce, and the preservation of the property of the United States.

The constitution requires that the United States shall protect each of the states against invasion, "and on application of the legislature, or of the executive (when the legislature cannot be convened) against domestic violence." There was plenty of domestic violence in the City of Chicago and in the State of Illinois during the early days of July, 1894; but no application was made to the Federal Government for assistance. It was probably a very fortunate circumstance that the presence of United States soldiers in Chicago at that time did not depend upon the request or desire of Governor Altgeld.

Section 5,298 of the Revised Statutes of the United States provides that: "Whenever, by reason of unlawful obstructions, combinations or assemblages of persons, or rebellion against the authority of the United States, it shall become impracticable in the judgment of the President to enforce by the ordinary course of judicial proceedings, the laws of the United States within any State or Territory, it shall be lawful for the President to call forth the militia of any or all of the States, and to employ such parts of the land or naval forces of the United States as he may deem necessary to enforce the faithful execution of the laws of the United States, or to suppress such rebellion, in whatever State or Territory thereof the laws of the United States may be forcibly opposed, or the execution thereof be forcibly obstructed;" and Section 5,299 provides that: "Whenever any insurrection, domestic violence, unlawful combinations or conspiracies in any State . . . opposes or obstructs the laws of the United States, or the due execution thereof, or impedes or obstructs the due course of justice under the same, it shall be lawful for the President and it shall be his duty, to take such measures by the employment of the militia, or the land and naval forces of the United States, or of either, or by other means as he may deem necessary, for the suppression of such insurrection, domestic violence or combinations."

It was the intention of the Attorney-General to suggest in these despatches that immediate and authoritative information should be given to the Washington authorities if a time should arrive when, under the sanction of general executive authority, or the constitutional and statutory provisions above quoted, a military force would be necessary at the scene of disturbance.

On the 2d of July, the day after these despatches were sent, information was received from the District Attorney and special counsel that a sweeping injunction had been granted against Eugene V. Debs, president of the American Railway Union, and other officials of the organization, together with parties whose names were unknown, and that the writs would be served that afternoon. The special counsel also expressed the opinion that it would require Government troops to enforce the orders of the court and protect the transportation of mails.

Major-General Schofield was then in command of the army; and, after a consultation with him, in which the Attorney-General and the Secretary of War took part, I directed the issuance of the following order by telegraph to General Nelson A. Miles, in command of the Military Department of Missouri, with headquarters at Chicago:

HEADQUARTERS OF THE ARMY,
WASHINGTON, July 2, 1904.

To the Commanding General,
  Department of Missouri, Chicago, Ill.

You will please make all necessary arrangements confidentially for the transportation of the entire garrison at Fort Sheridan — infantry, cavalry and artillery — to the Lake Front in the City of Chicago. To avoid possible interruption of the movement by rail and by marching through a part of the city, it may be advisable to bring them by steamboat. Please consider this matter and have the arrangements perfected without delay. You may expect orders at any time for the movement. Acknowledge receipt and report in what manner movement is to be made.

J. M. SCHOFIELD, *Major-General Commanding.*

It should by no means be inferred from this despatch that it had been definitely determined that the use of a military force was inevitable. It was still hoped that the effect of the injunction would be such that such an alternative might be avoided. A painful emergency is created when public duty forces the necessity of placing trained soldiers face to face with riotous opposition to the General Government, and in opposition to an acute and determined resistance to law and order. This course, once entered upon, admits of no backward step; and an appreciation of the consequences that may ensue cannot fail to oppress those responsible for its adoption with sadly disturbing reflections. Nevertheless, it was perfectly plain that, whatever the outcome might be, the situation positively demanded such precaution and preparation as would insure readiness and promptness, in case the presence of a military force should finally be found necessary.

On the morning of the next day, July 3d, the Attorney-General received a letter from Mr. Walker, the special counsel, in which, after referring to the issuance of the injunctions and setting forth that the Marshal was engaged in serving them, he wrote: "I do not believe that the Marshal and his deputies can protect the railroad companies in moving their trains, either freight or passenger, including of course the trains carrying United States mails. Possibly, however, the service of the writ of injunction will have a restraining influence upon Debs and other officers of the association. If it does not, from present appearances, I think it is the opinion of all that the orders of the court cannot be enforced except by the aid of the Regular Army."

Thereupon the Attorney-General immediately sent this despatch to the District Attorney:

I trust use of United States troops will not be necessary. If it becomes necessary, they will be used promptly and decisively upon the justifying facts being certified to me. In such case, if practicable, let Walker and the Marshal and United States judge join in statement as to the exigency.

A few hours afterwards the following urgent and decisive despatch from the Marshal, endorsed by a judge of the United States court and the District Attorney, and special counsel, was received by the Attorney-General:

CHICAGO, ILL., July 3, 1894.

HON. RICHARD OLNEY, *Attorney-General*, Washington, D. C.

When the injunction was granted yesterday, a mob of from two to three thousand held possession of a point in the city near the crossing of the Rock Island by other roads, where they had already ditched a mail train, and prevented the passing of any trains, whether mail or otherwise. I read the injunction writ to this mob and commanded them to disperse. The reading of the writ met with no response except jeers and hoots. Shortly after, the mob threw a number of baggage cars across the track, since when no mail train has been able to move. I am unable to disperse the mob, clear the tracks, or arrest the men who were engaged in the acts named, and believe that no force less than the regular troops of the United States can procure the passage of the mail trains, or enforce the orders of the courts. I believe people engaged in trades are quitting employment to-day, and in my opinion will be joining the mob to-night and especially to-morrow; and it is my judgment that the troops should be here at the earliest moment. An emergency has arisen for their presence in this city.

J. W. ARNOLD, *United States Marshal.*

We have read the foregoing and from that information and other information that has come to us, believe that an emergency exists for the immediate presence of United States troops.

P. S. GROSSCUP, *Judge.*

EDWIN WALKER,

THOMAS E. MILCHRIST, *Attys.*

In the afternoon of the same day the following order was telegraphed from Army Headquarters in the City of Washington:

WAR DEPARTMENT,
HEADQUARTERS OF THE ARMY,
WASHINGTON, D. C., July 3, 1894.

To MARTIN, *Adjutant-General,*   4 *o'Clock* P. M.

Headquarters Department of Missouri, Chicago, Ill.

It having become impracticable in the judgment of the President to enforce by the ordinary course of judicial proceedings the laws of the United States, you will direct Colonel Crofton to move his entire command at once to the City of Chicago (leaving the necessary guard at Fort Sheridan), there to execute the orders and processes of the United States court, to prevent the obstruction of the United States mails, and generally to enforce the faithful execution of the laws of the United States. He will confer with the United States Marshal, the United States District Attorney, and ·Edwin Walker, special counsel. Acknowledge receipt and report action promptly. By order of the President.

J. M. SCHOFIELD, *Major-General.*

Immediately after this order was issued, the following despatch was sent to the District Attorney by the Attorney-General:

"Colonel Crofton's command ordered to Chicago by the President. As to disposition and movement of troops, yourself, Walker, and Marshall should confer with Colonel Crofton and with Colonel Martin, Adjutant-General at Chicago. While action should be prompt and decisive, it should of course be kept within the limits provided by the constitution and laws. Rely upon yourself and Walker to see that this is done."

Colonel Martin, Adjutant-General at Chicago, reported the same night at half-past nine o'clock that the order for the movement of troops was, immediately on its receipt by him, transmitted to Fort Sheridan, and that Colonel Crofton's command started for Chicago at nine o'clock.

During the forenoon of the next day, July 4th, Colonel Martin advised the War Department that Colonel Crofton reported his command in the City of Chicago at 10.15 that morning. After referring to the manner in which the troops had been distributed, this officer added: "People seem to feel easier since arrival of troops."

General Miles, commanding the department, arrived in Chicago the same morning, and at once assumed direction of military movements. In the afternoon of that day he sent a report to the War Department at Washington, giving an account of the disposition of troops, recounting an unfavorable condition of affairs, and recommending an increase of the garrison at Fort Sheridan sufficient to meet any emergency.

In response to this despatch General Miles was immediately authorized to order six companies of infantry from Fort Leavenworth, in Kansas, and two companies from Fort Brady, in Michigan, to Fort Sheridan.

On the 5th day of July he reported that a mob of over two thousand had gathered that morning at the stock-yards, crowded among the troops, obstructed the movement of trains, knocked down a railroad official, and overturned about twenty freight cars, which obstructed all freight and passenger traffic in the vicinity of the stock-yards, and that the mob had also derailed a passenger train on the Pittsburg, Fort Wayne and Chicago Railroad and burned switches. To this recital of violent demonstrations he added the following statement: "The injunction of the United States court is openly defied, and unless the mobs are dispersed by the action of the police or they are fired upon by United States troops, more serious trouble may be expected, as the mob is increasing and becoming more defiant."

In view of the situation as reported by General Miles, he was at once directed by General Schofield to concentrate his troops in order that they might act more effectively in the execution of orders theretofore given, and in the protection of United States property. This despatch concluded as follows:

"The mere preservation of peace and good order in the city is, of course, the province of the city and state authorities."

The situation on the 6th day of July was thus described in a despatch sent in the afternoon of that day by General Miles to the Secretary of War:

"In answer to your telegram, I report the following: Mayor Hopkins last night issued a proclamation prohibiting riotous assemblies and directing the police to stop people from molesting railway communication. Governor Altgeld has ordered General Wheeler's brigade on duty in Chicago to support the Mayor's authority. So far, there have been no large mobs like the one of yesterday which moved from 51st Street to 18th Street before it dispersed. The lawlessness has been along the line of the railways, destroying and burning more than one hundred cars and railway buildings, and obstructing transportation in various ways, even to the extent of cutting telegraph lines. United States troops have dispersed mobs at 51st Street, Kensington, and a company of infantry is moving along the Rock Island to support a body of United States marshals in making arrests for violating the injunction of the United States court. Of the twenty-three roads centering in Chicago, only six are unobstructed in freight, passenger, and mail transportation; thirteen are at present entirely obstructed, and ten are running only mail and passenger trains. Large numbers of trains moving in and out of the city have been stoned and fired upon by mobs, and one engineer killed. There was a secret meeting to-day of Debs and the representatives of labor unions considering the advisability of a general strike of all labor unions. About one hundred men were present at that meeting. The result is not yet known. United States troops are at the stock-yards, Kensington, Blue Island, crossing of 51st Street, and have been moving along some of the lines: the balance, eight companies of infantry, battery of artillery, and one troop of cavalry, are camped on Lake Front Park, ready for any emergency and to protect Government buildings and property. It is learned from the Fire Department, City Hall, that a party of strikers has been going through the vicinity from 14th to 41st Streets and Stewart Avenue freight yards, throwing gasoline on freight cars all through that section. Captain Ford, of the Fire Department, was badly stoned this morning. Troops have just dispersed a mob of incendiaries on Fort Wayne tracks, near 51st Street, and fires that were started have been suppressed. Mob just captured mail train at 47th Street and troops sent to disperse them."

On the 8th day of July, in view of the apparently near approach of a crisis which the Government had attempted to avoid, the following Executive Proclamation was issued and at once extensively published in the City of Chicago:

Whereas, by reason of unlawful obstruction, combinations and assemblages of persons, it has become impracticable in the judgment of the President to enforce by the ordinary course of judicial proceedings, the laws of the United States within the State of Illinois, and especially in the City of Chicago within said State; and

Whereas, for the purpose of enforcing the faithful execution of the laws of the United States and protecting its property and removing obstructions to the United States mails in the state and city aforesaid, the President has employed a part of the military forces of the United States: —

Now, therefore, I, Grover Cleveland, President of the United States, do hereby admonish all good citizens, and all persons who may be or may come within the city and state aforesaid, against aiding, countenancing, encouraging, or taking any part in such unlawful obstructions, combinations and assemblages; and I hereby warn all persons engaged in or in any way connected with such unlawful obstructions, combinations and assemblages to disperse and retire peaceably to their respective abodes on or before twelve o'clock, noon, of the 9th day of July instant.

Those who disregard this warning and persist in taking part with a riotous mob in forcibly resisting and obstructing the execution of the laws of the United States or interfering with the functions of the Government, or destroying or attempting to destroy the property belonging to the United States or under its protection, cannot be regarded otherwise than as public enemies.

Troops employed against such a riotous mob will act with all the moderation and forbearance consistent with the accomplishment of the desired end; but the stern necessities that confront them will not with certainty permit discrimination between guilty participants and those who are mingling with them from curiosity and without criminal intent. The only safe course, therefore, for those not actually participating, is to abide at their homes, or at least not to be found in the neighborhood of riotous assemblages.

While there will be no vacillation in the decisive treatment of the guilty, this warning is especially intended to protect and save the innocent.

On the 10th of July, Eugene V. Debs, the president of the American Railway Union, together with its vice-president, general secretary, and one other who was an active director, were arrested upon indictments found against them for complicity in the obstruction of mails and interstate commerce. Three days afterwards our special counsel expressed the opinion that the strike was practically broken. This must not be taken to mean, however, that peace and quiet had been completely restored or that the transportation of mails and the activities of interstate commerce were entirely free from interruption. It meant only the expression of a well sustained and deliberate expectation that the combination of measures already inaugurated, and others contemplated in the near future, would speedily bring about a termination of the difficulty.

On the 17th day of July an information was filed in the United States Circuit Court at Chicago against Debs and the three other officials of the Railway Union who had been arrested on indictment a few days before, but were then at large on bail. This information alleged that these parties had been guilty of open, continued, and defiant disobedience of the injunction which was served on them July 3d, forbidding them to do certain specified acts tending to incite and aid the obstruction of the carriage of mails and the operation of interstate commerce. On the footing of this information these parties were brought before the court to show cause why they should not be punished for contempt in disobeying the injunction. Instead of giving bail for their freedom pending the investigation of this charge against them, as they were invited to do, they preferred to be committed to custody. . . .

That the strike was ended about the time of this second arrest is undoubtedly true; for, during the few days immediately preceding and following the 17th day of July, reports came from nearly all the localities to which the strike had spread, indicating its defeat and the accomplishment of all the purposes of the Government's interference.

I must not fail to mention here as part of the history of this perplexing affair, a contribution made by the Governor of Illinois to its annoyances.

On the 5th day of July, twenty-four hours after our soldiers had been brought to the City of Chicago, pursuant to the order of July 3d, I received a long despatch from Governor Altgeld, beginning as follows:

"I am advised that you have ordered Federal troops to go into service in the State of Illinois. Surely the facts have not been correctly presented to you in this case or you would not have taken the step; for it is entirely unnecessary and, as it seems to me, unjustifiable. Waiving all question of courtesy, I will say that the State of Illinois is not only able to take care of itself, but it stands ready to-day to furnish the Federal Government any assistance it may need elsewhere."

This opening sentence was followed by a lengthy statement which so far missed actual conditions as to appear irrelevant and, in some parts, absolutely frivolous.

This remarkable despatch closed with the following words:

"As Governor of the State of Illinois, I protest against this and ask the immediate withdrawal of Federal troops from active duty in this state. Should the situation at any time get so serious that we cannot control it with the state forces, we will promptly and freely ask for Federal assistance; but until such time I protest with all due deference against this uncalled-for reflection upon our people, and again ask for the immediate withdrawal of these troops."

Immediately upon the receipt of this communication, I sent to Governor Altgeld the following reply:

"Federal troops were sent to Chicago in strict accordance with the constitution and the laws of the United States, upon the demand of the Post-Office Department that obstructions of the mails should be removed, and upon the representation of the judicial officers of the United States that process of the Federal courts could not be executed through the ordinary means, and upon abundant proof that conspiracies existed against commerce between the states. To meet these conditions, which are clearly within the province of Federal authority, the presence of Federal troops in the city of Chicago was deemed not only proper but necessary; and there has been no intention of thereby interfering with the plain duty of the local authorities to preserve the peace of the city."

It became at once evident that the Governor was unwilling to allow the matter at issue between us to rest without a renewal of argument and protest. On the 7th day of July, the day after the date of my despatch, he addressed to me another long telegraphic communication, evidently intended to be more severely accusatory and insistent than its predecessor. Its general tenor may be inferred from the opening words:

"Your answer to my protest involves some startling conclusions, and ignores and evades the question at issue — that is, that the principle of local self-government is just as fundamental in our institutions as is that of Federal supremacy. You calmly assume that the executive has the legal right to order Federal troops into any community of the United States in the first instance, whenever there is the slightest disturbance, and that he can do this without any regard to the question as to whether the community is able to and ready to enforce the law itself."

After a rather dreary discussion of the importance of preserving the rights of the states and a presentation of the dangers to constitutional government that lurked in the course that had been pursued by the Government, this communication closed as follows:

"Inasmuch as the Federal troops can do nothing but what the state troops can do there, and believing that the state is amply able to take care of the situation and to enforce the law, and believing that the ordering out of the Federal troops was unwarranted, I again ask their withdrawal."

I confess that my patience was somewhat strained when I quickly sent the following despatch in reply to this communication:

EXECUTIVE MANSION,
WASHINGTON, D. C., July 6, 1894:

While I am still persuaded that I have neither transcended my authority nor duty in the emergency that confronts us, it seems to me that in this hour of danger and public distress, discussion may well give way to active efforts on the part of all in authority to restore obedience to law and to protect life and property.   GROVER CLEVELAND.

HON. JOHN P. ALTGELD,
   Governor of Illinois.

This closed a discussion which in its net results demonstrated how far one's disposition and inclination will lead him astray in the field of argument.

I shall conclude the treatment of my subject by a brief reference to the legal proceedings which grew out of this disturbance, and finally led to an adjudication by the highest court in our land, establishing in an absolutely authoritative manner and for all time, the power of the National Government to protect itself in the exercise of its functions.

It will be recalled that in the course of our narrative we left Mr. Debs, the president of the Railway Union, and his three associates, in custody of the law, on the 17th day of July, awaiting an investigation of the charge of contempt of court made against them, based upon their disobedience of the writs of injunction forbidding them to do certain things in aid or encouragement of interference with mail transportation or interstate commerce.

This investigation was so long delayed that the decision of the Circuit Court, before which the proceedings were pending, was not rendered until the 14th day of December, 1894. On that date the court delivered an able and carefully considered decision finding Debs and his associates guilty of contempt of court, basing its decision upon the provisions of the law of Congress, passed in 1890, entitled: "An act to protect trade and commerce against unlawful restraint and monopolies;" sometimes called the Sherman Anti-Trust Law. Thereupon the parties were sentenced on said conviction to confinement in the county jail for terms varying from three to six months.

Afterwards and on the 14th day of January, 1895, the prisoners applied to the Supreme Court of the United States for a writ of habeas corpus to relieve them from imprisonment, on the ground that the facts found against them did not constitute disobedience to the writs of injunction and that their commitment in the manner and for the reasons alleged was without justification and not within the constitutional power and jurisdiction of the Circuit Court.

On this application the case was elaborately argued before the Supreme Court in March, 1895; and on the 27th day of May, 1895, the court rendered its decision, upholding on the broadest grounds the proceedings to the Circuit Court and confirming its adjudication and the commitment to jail of the petitioners thereupon.

Justice Brewer, in delivering the unanimous opinion of the Supreme Court, stated the case as follows:

"The United States, finding that the interstate transportation of persons and property, as well as the carriage of mails, is forcibly obstructed and that a combination and conspiracy exists to subject the control of such transportation to the will of the conspirators, applied to one of their courts sitting as a court of equity, for an injunction to restrain such obstructions and prevent carrying into effect such conspiracy. Two questions of importance are presented: First, are the relations of the General Government to interstate commerce and the transportation of the mails, such as authorize a direct interference to prevent a forcible obstruction thereof? Second, if authority exists — as authority in governmental affairs implies both power and duty — has a court of equity jurisdiction to issue an injunction in aid of the performance of such duty?"

Both of these questions were answered by the court in the affirmative; and in the opinion read by the learned justice, the inherent power of the Government to execute by means of physical force through its official agents, on every foot of American soil, the powers and functions belonging to it, was amply vindicated by a process of reasoning, simple, logical, unhampered by fanciful distinctions, and absolutely conclusive; and the Government's resort to the court, the injunction issued in its aid, and all the proceedings thereon, including the imprisonment of Debs and his associates, were fully approved.

Thus the Supreme Court of the United States has written the concluding words of this history, tragical in many of its details, and in every line provoking sober reflection. As we gratefully turn its concluding page those most nearly related by executive responsibility to the troublous days whose story is told may well congratulate themselves especially on their participation in marking out the way and clearing the path, now unchangeably established, which shall hereafter guide our nation safely and surely in the exercise of its functions, which represent the people's trust.

III

THE EXECUTIVE AND CONGRESS

[The relation of the Executive to Congress has been subject to special discussion of late. The strict separation of the three departments in matters of government being impossible, there has in general been a feeling that it is entirely proper for executive officials and the President to interest themselves in legislative measures affecting their particular work. This opinion has, however, not passed without opposition as other men have held that while it is allowable for the executive to suggest legislation, a direct interference in the process of legislative work would lie beyond the proper sphere of executive duty. The following extract from a speech of James A. Garfield discusses the general considerations involved and pronounces in favor of a closer relation between the legislative and the executive. The action of the President in connection with the Railway Rate legislation, which was subjected to much criticism, is defended by Senator Dolliver, and Mr. Adams discusses the part of the Executive in the preparation and passage of the Meat Inspection bill. The views of the opposition are developed by Senator Rayner and Mr. Williams. For earlier discussions of the relations of the President to Congress see President Polk's annual message of December, 1848, and President Buchanan's special messages of March 28, and June 22, 1860.]

JAMES A. GARFIELD ON THE EXECUTIVE AND CONGRESS [1]

NOT the least serious evil resulting from this invasion of the executive functions by members of Congress is the fact that it greatly impairs their own usefulness as legislators. One third of the working hours of Senators and Representatives is hardly sufficient to meet the demands made upon them in reference to appointments to office. The spirit of that clause of the Constitution which shields them from arrest "during their attendance at the session of their respective houses, and in going to or returning from the same," should also shield them from being arrested from their legislative work, morning, noon, and night, by office-seekers. To sum up in a word, the present system invades the independence of the Executive, and makes him less responsible for the character of his

---

[1] From an address on "A Century of Congress" (1877). See Works, II, 483.

appointments; it impairs the efficiency of the legislator by diverting him from his proper sphere of duty, and involving him in the intrigues of aspirants for office; it degrades the civil service itself by destroying the personal independence of those who are appointed; it repels from the service those high and manly qualities which are so necessary to a pure and efficient administration; and finally, it debauches the public mind by holding up public office as the reward of mere party zeal.

To reform this service is one of the highest and most imperative duties of statesmanship. This reform cannot be accomplished without a complete divorce between Congress and the Executive in the matter of appointments. It will be a proud day when an administration Senator or Representative, who is in good standing in his party, can say, as Thomas Hughes said during his recent visit to this country, that, though he was on the most intimate terms with the members of the English administration, yet it was not in his power to secure the removal of the humblest clerk in the civil service of the government.

This is not the occasion to discuss the recent enlargement of the jurisdiction of Congress in reference to the election of a President and Vice-President by the States. But it cannot be denied that the Electoral Bill has opened a wide and dangerous field for Congressional action. Unless the boundaries of its power shall be restricted by a new amendment of the Constitution, we have seen the last of our elections of President on the old plan. The power to decide who has been elected may be so used as to exceed the power of electing.

I have long believed that the official relations between the Executive and Congress should be more open and direct. They are now conducted by correspondence with the presiding officers of the two Houses, by consultation with committees, or by private interviews with individual members. This frequently leads to misunderstandings, and may lead to corrupt combinations. It would be far better for both departments if the members of the Cabinet were permitted to sit in Congress and participate in the debates on measures relating to their several departments, — but, of course, without a vote. This would tend to secure the ablest men for the chief executive offices; it would bring the policy of the administration into the fullest publicity by giving both parties ample opportunity for criticism and defense.

As a result of the great growth of the country and of the new legislation arising from the late war, Congress is greatly overloaded with work. It is safe to say that the business which now annually claims the attention of Congress is tenfold more complex and burdensome than it was forty years ago. For example: the twelve annual appropriation bills, with their numerous details, now consume two thirds of each short session of the House. Forty years ago, when the appropriations were made more in block, one week was sufficient for the work. The vast extent of our country, the increasing number of States and Territories, the legislation necessary to regulate our mineral lands, to manage our complex systems of internal revenue, banking, currency, and expenditure, have so increased the work of Congress that no one man can even read the bills and the official reports relating to current legislation, much less qualify himself for intelligent action upon them. As a necessary consequence, the real work of legislation is done by the committees; and their work must be accepted or rejected without full knowledge of its merits. This fact alone renders leadership in Congress, in the old sense of the word, impossible. For many years we have had the leadership of committees and chairmen of committees; but no man can any more be the leader of all the legislation of the Senate or of the House than one lawyer or one physician can now be foremost in all the departments of law or medicine. The evils of loose legislation resulting from this situation must increase, rather than diminish, until a remedy is provided.

John Stuart Mill held that a numerous popular assembly is radically unfit to make good laws, but is the best possible means of getting good laws made. He suggested, as a permanent part of the constitution of a free country, a legislative commission, composed of a few trained men, to draft such laws as the legislature, by general resolutions, shall direct, which draft shall be adopted by the legislature, without change, or returned to the commission to be amended. Whatever may be thought of Mr. Mill's suggestion, it is clear that some plan must be adopted to relieve Congress from the infinite details of legislation, and to preserve harmony and coherence in our laws.

Another change observable in Congress, as well as in the legislatures of other countries, is the decline of oratory. The press is rendering the orator obsolete. Statistics now furnish the materials upon which the legislator depends; and a column of figures will often demolish a dozen pages of eloquent rhetoric.

Just now, too, the day of sentimental politics is passing away, and the work of Congress is more nearly allied to the business interests of the country and to "the dismal science," as political economy is called by the "practical men" of our time. The legislation of Congress comes much nearer to the daily life of the people than ever before. Twenty years ago, the presence of the national government was not felt by one citizen in a hundred. Except in paying his postage and receiving his mail, the citizen of the interior rarely came in contact with the national authority. Now, he meets it in a thousand ways. Formerly the legislation of Congress referred chiefly to our foreign relations, to indirect taxes, to the government of the army, the navy, and the Territories. Now, a vote in Congress may, any day, seriously derange the business affairs of every citizen.

And this leads me to say that now, more than ever before, the people are responsible for the character of their Congress. It that body be ignorant, reckless, and corrupt, it is because the people tolerate ignorance,

recklessness, and corruptia. If it be intel
because the people deman those high qual
national legislature. Coᵣress lives in th
which beats against the trone.'' The telє
morrow morning announᵤ at a million brє
said and done in Congresto-day. Now, as
the prevailing opinions ad political aspir
wildest delusions of pape money, the crud
passions and prejudices ᵥat find expressio
were first believed and dᵤcussed at the fire
corners of the streets, an in the caucuses a₁
parties.

ᵥe, and pure, iᵗ
ᵗᵨent them in
ᵗhat fierce l'
ᵨe press wil'
ᵥhat has
ᵨress repr
ᵗ people.
ᵗ taxatiᵢ
·e and
ᵢople,
ᵢ of ·

SENATOR DOLIVER ON TH

THE Senate, as in Committee of the Whole,
of the bill (H. R 12987 to amend an act en
commerce," approved ebruary 4, 1887, ɛ
thereof, and to enlarge he powers of the In
mission.

Mr. DOLLIVER. Mr. resident, I have listeɪ
tion and pleasure to thepeech of the honoral
[Mr. Stone], and I do nᵢ rise now for the pu:
the reason that in the min the Senator's rᵢᵢᵢ
the same conclusions tbt have influ⁻
clined to think that whᵢ in the
Missouri of the jurisdicᵢn of the c
the amendment which bs been offerᵤ
Kansas [Mr. Long] is·orrect, a sligᵢ
enters into his statemeɪ.

I have held from the bginning that the
courts have under it exᵢtly the jurisdictiᵢ
them. I have considerl the fixing of a rᵤ
mission as an act of Cᵢgress. I can find n
tion for the exercise ofᵢe power to regulate iᵢ
that power which is ᵢnferred upon the Congᵣᵢ
driven by long meditabn to the conclusion that wᵢ
of the Commission is, ᵢs an act of Congress: for Cᵢ
power conferred by th Constitution to regulate con
States.

 * * * * *

I have risen for a dᵢerent purpose. Much has beᵢ
it with marked solemᵢty and seriousness and some wɪ

<hr>

[1] *Congr. Record*, April 5, 1906.

or
posed to be inv~~~ed in it — about the
nited States in~e work of the Senate.
a certain ra~tion to the legislative
'ed States At any rate, if there
of the U~ted States to publicly
give by the course of this

~ator from Ohio [Mr.
~n, I suppose, of the
~t the President, wrote
~roved it by quoting
~roceedings of the
ly this morning a
's message, and
Senator from
ident's views

which the
's interest
stated
of the
e of
~t-
~

~
out
United States
In the pres~~~
invitation of the legi~~~
in this matter. Among the
Commerce did was to invite him to
mittee explaining to us **our** powers **and** ~~~
thought desirable·in relation to this legislation,
plex, an almost impenetrable subject with whi~
upon **to** deal, and I do not propose to be disparaged or
else to be disparaged by a sneering suggestion th~

recklessness, and corruption. If it be intelligent, brave, and pure, it is because the people demand those high qualities to represent them in the national legislature. Congress lives in the blaze of "that fierce light which beats against the throne." The telegraph and the press will to-morrow morning announce at a million breakfast-tables what has been said and done in Congress to-day. Now, as always, Congress represents the prevailing opinions and political aspirations of the people. The wildest delusions of paper money, the crudest theories of taxation, the passions and prejudices that find expression in the Senate and House, were first believed and discussed at the firesides of the people, on the corners of the streets, and in the caucuses and conventions of political parties.

SENATOR DOLLIVER ON THE PRESIDENT [1]

THE Senate, as in Committee of the Whole, resumed the consideration of the bill (H. R 12987) to amend an act entitled "An act to regulate commerce," approved February 4, 1887, and all acts amendatory thereof, and to enlarge the powers of the Interstate Commerce Commission.

Mr. DOLLIVER. Mr. President, I have listened with very great attention and pleasure to the speech of the honorable Senator from Missouri [Mr. Stone], and I do not rise now for the purpose of replying to it, for the reason that in the main the Senator's researches have brought him to the same conclusions that have influenced my own opinions. I am inclined to think that while in the main the analysis of the Senator from Missouri of the jurisdiction of the courts under the House bill and under the amendment which has been offered to that bill by the Senator from Kansas [Mr. Long] is correct, a slight element of misunderstanding enters into his statement.

I have held from the beginning that the House bill is so framed that the courts have under it exactly the jurisdiction which the Constitution gives them. I have considered the fixing of a railroad rate through the Commission as an act of Congress. I can find no authority in the Constitution for the exercise of the power to regulate interstate commerce except that power which is conferred upon the Congress; and I have been driven by long meditation to the conclusion that whatever else this order of the Commission is, it is an act of Congress; for Congress has the only power conferred by the Constitution to regulate commerce between the States.

    *   *   *   *   *   *   *   *

I have risen for a different purpose. Much has been said — some of it with marked solemnity and seriousness and some with evident appre-

[1] *Congr. Record*, April 5, 1906.

ciation of the humor which is supposed to be involved in it — about the interference of the President of the United States in the work of the Senate. Nobody denies that the President has a certain relation to the legislative business of the Government of the United States. At any rate, if there ever was an excuse given to the President of the United States to publicly explain his views and opinions, it has been given by the course of this debate.

On last Saturday my distinguished friend the Senator from Ohio [Mr. Foraker], responding to a request, or a suggestion, I suppose, of the legislature of that State calling upon him to support the President, wrote a letter that he was supporting the President, and proved it by quoting from the President's message that he desired the proceedings of the Commission to be subject to judicial review. And only this morning a famous newspaper printed an extract from the President's message, and denounced the amendment of my honorable friend the Senator from Kansas on the ground that it was in violation of the President's views and attitude upon this question.

I am not one of those who have been irritated by the interest which the President of the United States has taken in this controversy. His interest has been upon the broadest and highest national ground. He has stated his views and convictions to the American people in every section of the country, and not one line can be attributed to him having in it the trace of a partisan outlook upon this great national question. Therefore whatever interest he has taken in it can certainly not be attributed to a partisan design of any kind or character.

I have been familiar for a good many years with the attitude of the Executive Department of the Government toward the work of Congress. There is a member of the Senate now who, if he were disposed to give his experience, would be able to verify what I say, that it has been for many years the no uncommon practice for the Congress of the United States to take counsel with the Executive Departments in perfecting great acts of national legislation. There are at least five acts of legislation, all of them referring to this and similar questions, that were put through both Houses of Congress in the last five years practically without change, as they came from the office of the Attorney-General of the United States.

In the present controversy the Attorney-General has certainly had the invitation of the legislative branch of the Government to take an interest in this matter. Among the very first things the Committee on Interstate Commerce did was to invite him to give his opinion in writing to the committee explaining to us our powers and making what suggestions he thought desirable in relation to this legislation, It is a difficult, a complex, an almost impenetrable subject with which we have been called upon to deal, and I do not propose to be disparaged or to allow anybody else to be disparaged by a sneering suggestion that we have consulted the

Attorney-General or even the President of the United States. I count it just as respectable and just as perfectly in line with my public duty to take counsel with the President of the United States on these questions as for my colleagues and for others to hold sweet counsel with the presidents of railroad corporations.

Mr. President, I do not propose to submit, without at least a word of protest, to the suggestion that the President of the United States is delivering over this bill to the tender mercies of its enemies. It is a nonpartisan proposition. It has friends on both sides of this Chamber, good friends on both sides of this Chamber. It has possibly enough to perfect the legislation and put it through in an effective and satisfactory form. But whether or not it has that number of members of the Senate in favor of it, its friends do not propose to surrender any principle that is involved in it. They have had a long and arduous fight, and they are ready for a good many years of fighting yet. I undertake to say here that if the Senate of the United States does not conform this measure to the petition of those who have supported it by the million throughout the United States we do not settle this question. Unless the effective legislation which is demanded by the American people is given by the Congress of the United States, instead of settling this issue we merely create the largest national issue with which this generation will have to deal.

Mr. President, there is not a line in the public or private writings of the President of the United States to warrant the suggestion that any man is supporting him or supporting the ideas to which he has given expression during the last two years by so amending this bill as to transfer this power of Congress to the Courts of the United States. The newspaper to which I alluded a moment ago printed an extract from one of the President's speeches, and followed it with a denunciation of the amendment which my friend the Senator from Kansas introduced yesterday, leaving the impression upon the public mind, with a curious mixture of sincerity and satire, that the President of the United States had either changed his position or had never occupied any such position as he would be put in by the amendment of the Senator from Kansas.

Fortunately in connection with the President's messages we have some outside knowledge of what his notions and his ideas have been in respect to these matters, because with a freedom which has been characteristic of his public career, and I think a very admirable part of his idea of public duty, he has taken the American people into his confidence in every section of the United States. It is true that in his message he suggested that the orders of the Commission were to be subject to the review of the courts, and if I have correctly interpreted the purpose of the honorable Senator from Kansas in introducing his amendment, it was for the purpose of defining before the American people exactly what sort of a review the friends of this legislation desire to have.

Not one of them desires to leave this railroad property without redress against a violation of constitutional rights. Not one of them desires an act of oppression or injustice against these carriers, whether committed in malice or through error, to go without a proper redress in the courts of the United States.

The President of the United States in his annual message asked that these orders be made "subject to review in the courts." But for months before that he had been explaining to the American people exactly what jurisdiction he thought the courts should occupy in the matter, and I desire to take the opportunity of putting into the *Record* an extract from a speech made by the President before a Democratic club in the city of Chicago — the Iroquois Club — some time before the last message to Congress was sent, which, in my humble judgment, shows that the President occupies now exactly the position he occupied then, and exactly the position which he explained in his brief recommendation to Congress last December upon this subject. He said:

Personally, I believe that the Federal Government must take an increasing control over corporations. It is better that that control should increase by degrees than that it should be assumed all at once. But there should be, and I trust will be, no halt in the steady progress of assuming such national control. The first step toward it should be the adoption of a law conferring upon some executive body the power of increased supervision and regulation of the great corporations engaged primarily in interstate commerce of the railroads. My views on that subject could not have been better expressed than they were expressed yesterday by Secretary Taft in Washington, and as they were expressed by the Attorney-General in his communication to the Senate committee a couple of weeks ago: "I believe that the representatives of the nation — that is, the representatives of all the people — should lodge in some executive body the power to establish a maximum rate, the power to have that rate go into effect practically immediately, and the power to see that the provisions of the law apply in full to companies owning private cars and private tracks just as much as the railroads themselves. The courts will retain, and should retain, no matter what the Legislature does, the power to interfere and upset any action that is confiscatory in its nature."

Again, in his speech delivered before the Chamber of Commerce of Denver only a few months before the sending of the President's last message to Congress, he used these words:

But with that statement as a preliminary, I wish to urge with all the earnestness I possess, not only upon the public, but upon those interested in the great railway corporations, the absolute need of acquiescence in the enactment of such law. As has been well set forth by the Attorney-General, Mr. Moody, in his recent masterly argument presented to the committee of the Senate which is investigating the matter, the legislators have the right, and, as I believe, the duty, to confer these powers upon some executive body. It can not confer them upon any court, nor can it take away the court's power to interfere if the law is administered in a way that amounts to confiscation of property.

So, from the beginning the President has been clear and straight in his interpretation of his situation, and I doubt very much whether it would have been necessary for him to address these speeches to the country or to take the slightest interest, with those who have been trying, amid a good many difficulties, to perfect legislation, if it were not for the fact that persistently the argument for a review of the orders of the Commission and a trial of the case de novo in the courts, from the beginning of this debate, has taken refuge behind six words in the President's message, to wit, that the order of the Commission should be subject to review in the courts.

I submit in all fairness that it is hardly proper for men who know exactly what the President of the United States has stood for, exactly what he is trying to do, whether they indorse it or nor — it is hardly proper to deal with the American people, with the idea that they are supporting the President, when in point of fact they are urging a proposition that is not only not contained in anything the President has ever said, but reduces the President's recommendation to a practical and legal absurdity before the whole country.

I have spoken in this way, Mr. President, not for the purpose of irritating anybody's feelings. I know that much is said here in the Senate about Executive interference, but I close by suggesting that the institutions and legislation of the American people are much more liable to be damaged here in the Senate of the United States by interference from other quarters than by the friendly and patient suggestions of the President of the United States.

Mr. BAILEY. Mr. President, I belong to that very small class of Senators and Representatives who do not believe that it is proper for them to be influenced in the performance of their legislative duties by the views of the executive department; and it has never been my practice since I had the honor to occupy a seat in Congress to confer with any President, either of my own or of the opposition party, in respect to any legislation.

The only exception I ever made — and that more apparent than real — was in the case of the lamented and martyred McKinley, whose invitation I accepted to confer with him in the hope that we might find a way to avert the war with Spain. Upon a question like that, which was not legislative, I felt that any Member of Congress might properly confer with the Executive of the Republic. But, sir, I have so often seen — and this applies not only to the present President of the United States, but to his predecessors in that great office — I have so often seen the judgment of Congress overruled or controlled by Executive influence that early in my service in the other House I resolved that it should never prevail with me.

I remember when a mere schoolboy reading of a great Virginia Democrat being invited to the White House by a President, of his own party and chosen from his own State, to confer upon an important question pending in the Congress, and I remember how my youthful blood was made to run faster when I read how that great Virginia Democrat said: "Mr. President, the Constitution of the United States has separated the executive and the legislative departments of this Government, and, by the help of God, I intend to keep them separate." I adopted that as my creed and I have lived up to it from that day to this.

But I must say if ever a President was justified in conferring with his friends in Congress, this measure and these circumstances furnish that justification. Earnestly and, as I believe, sincerely striving to put upon the statute book a useful measure, he finds himself confronted with the opposition of his own party. I am safely within the truth when I say that less than one-third of the President's party friends in this Chamber sympathize with this effort to secure the enactment of this legislation.

Mr. ALDRICH. Mr. President ——

Mr. BAILEY. I hope the Senator from Rhode Island is going to include himself in that one-third who help the President.

Mr. ALDRICH. So far as I know, there is no Senator sitting upon this side who does not sympathize fully with the Senator from Texas and the President of the United States in a desire to secure effective and proper legislation with reference to the regulation of railroad rates. That a large part of the Senators on this side do not sympathize either with the President or with the junior Senator from Iowa in an attempt and purpose to so limit and circumscribe the rights of the people of the United States that they can not be effectively secured through the courts of the country I will frankly admit.

Mr. BAILEY. Mr. President, the Senator from Rhode Island always knows exactly what he wants, but he sometimes makes the mistake of supposing that other people do not also know what he wants. I know that a large number of Republican Senators honestly believe that this legislation is unnecessary, and another per cent of gentlemen on that side honestly believe that it will be hurtful. I have no quarrel with them, if that is their honest opinion; and I am one of the men who believe and who dare to say, in spite of all the slanders that fill the air, that a large majority of the men in this body want to do what they think is right. I accord to others the same honesty of purpose and motive that I claim for myself, but it is no impeachment of their patriotism to say that they differ with the President, and their differences with him, I repeat, make it permissible, if it can ever be permissible, for the Executive to seek conferences with the members of the legislative department.

Now, Mr. President, one expression by the Senator from Iowa [Mr. Dolliver] gives me even more concern than the open admission that the President has been striving by conference and suggestion to shape the legislation of Congress on this subject. The Senator from Iowa says that those who have conferred with the President have rendered the country a better service than others who have been conferring with the presidents of railroads. I cordially agree to that statement. But, Mr. President, the Senate is entitled to know who it is here who has been conferring with the presidents of the railroads. If any Senator here has been conferring with the railroads or the presidents of the railroads, with a view to defeating legislation in the public interest, the Senate is entitled to know it, and the country is entitled to know it.

The Senator from Iowa is not given to intemperate or incautious speech, and when he suggests that Senators who are striving to aecomplish the defeat of this bill are consulting with the presidents of railroads with a view to that end, just as he and others who are striving to pass it are consulting with the President of the United States with a view to that end, he utters a serious reflection upon some Senators — not upon the Senate, because no man believes that such conferences as that include the Senate. But if they include any Senator or any Senators, the country and the Senate are entitled to know who these Senators are.

Mr. FORAKER. Mr. President, the Senator from Texas [Mr. Bailey] has only anticipated what I wanted to say. As the Senator from Texas has well said, the charge — for it is not anything short of that — that Senators who are in opposition to the bill he is supporting are in conference here from time to time with presidents of railroads ——

Mr. ALDRICH. With a view of defeating the bill.

Mr. FORAKER. With a view of defeating the bill is a most serious one, and the Senators referred to should be named. I respectfully demand of the Senator from Iowa that he name the Senators, so that if there is a member of this body engaged in such conferences we may know who it is.

Mr. DOLLIVER. I shall take the liberty of not pursuing that controversy.

Mr. FORAKER. Well, Mr. President, it seems to me the Senate has a right to know. I do not imagine the Senator refers to me, but I do know, as every other Senator must know, that the suggestion of the Senator was broad enough to include every member of this body.

Mr. DOLLIVER. I have never dreamed that there was any impropriety in consulting with presidents of railroads. I presume hardly a man here but has sought the counsel and suggestion of those who were practically familiar with railway business. In connection with my honorable friend from Ohio, I spent three months last spring hearing the views of as distinguished a group of railroad managers as ever assembled anywhere in the world, and I have never thought that a man could not talk with railroad presidents without being charged with some form of impropriety. I have no notion that a man can be guilty of the offense of consulting with the Chief Magistrate of the American people without being made the subject of ridicule and misconstruction of his motive.

Mr. FORAKER. I have never complained of anyone who has seen fit to confer with the Chief Magistrate of the nation. I do so whenever I see fit to and he will permit it. I am always glad to do it. I never think of anyone conferring with the President having any improper motive in veiw.

So far as conferences with railroad presidents are concerned, I do not know of any on the part of any member of this body. It is true that when the Senate Committee on Interstate Commerce had hearings, covering five or six weeks last spring, a number of railroad officials appeared before that committee and gave their testimony, just the same as any other witnesses; but I do not know of any member of the committee conferring with those railroad officials at that time. I do not know of any member of that committee or any member of this body conferring at any time or place with any railroad official concerning this proposed legislation.

Now, Mr. President, it will not do for the Senator to say he had no thought or purpose of insinuating that there was anything improper in such conferences, for the Senator said in so many words that Senators had been conferring with railroad presidents in order that they might better know how to defeat this legislation. Only one inference could be drawn from that, and that was that men who do not agree with the Senator from Iowa in his support of this measure were representing in some such way as has been charged railroad interests or railroad officials. I know of no railroad officials having anything whatever to do with this legislation, except only to express their views when they came before the committee. No railroad official, so far as I can recall, has ever talked with me at any time or any place, and I do not believe that any railroad official has ever talked in any improper way with anybody else who is in opposition to this proposed legislation.

Mr. TILLMAN. If the Senator will pardon me, I saw in the newspapers a day or two ago a statement that President Mellen, of one of the New England roads — I have forgotten which — had been to the White House for lunch, conferring with the President about this matter, and rumor had it that he went there to demand that certain features of the Hepburn bill should be stricken out — that part of the bill which relates to requiring the railroads to keep a certain kind of books and no other kind.

While I am on my feet, if the Senator will pardon me, I should like, as one witness, to give some little testimony in this interesting controversy among the brethren on that side as to what took place at the hearings before the Interstate Commerce Committee. I can not recall the date, but I recollect very distinctly that a gentleman came into the committee room and, after shaking hands with a few of his friends, passed on to the inner sanctuary, and I did not see him any more; but I was afterwards informed that he was Mr. A. J. Cassatt, of the Pennsylvania road. Now, what his business was or with whom he conferred I do not pretend to say. I merely state that as a fact.

Mr. FORAKER. Mr. President, I do not know anything about the occasion to which the Senator refers. I never met Mr. Cassatt but once in my life, and I met him at the White House then. He was there calling upon the President.

Mr. President, let me call attention to the fact in this connection, now that Mr. Cassatt has been named in the way he has, that he is one of the railroad presidents of the country who has been favoring this proposed rate making on the part of the Government for the railroads of the country, and Mr. Mellen, who was referred to, is another. They have been advocates of this kind of legislation all the while. There are railroads on both sides of the question. At least, such is the report as to Mr. Cassatt and Mr. Mellen. ·

I have very frequently seen notices of their presence in the city, but never having seen Mr. Cassatt but the one time, of course I do not know what he was here for, except only as the newspapers may have advised. I never met Mr. Mellen; I do not know him at all; but I have noticed that he has been here frequently and that at such times he was usually in conference with the President, and always about railway rate legislation.

I can understand, Mr. President, why Mr. Cassatt, representing the Pennsylvania Railroad, might favor this kind of legislation. He represents a railroad that covers the heart of the country; a railroad so situated and so powerful, having so many advantages, that it could grow inordinately rich on what might destroy other railroad properties. I do not know of anybody else equally fortunately situated. If anybody else is so equally fortunately situated, it is Mr. Mellen and his road; and they are both in favor of this kind of legislation.

REPRESENTATIVE ADAMS ON THE EXECUTIVE [1]

Mr. ADAMS. Mr. Speaker, the gentleman from Mississippi [Mr. Williams] has told the truth, and it is idle to disguise it, that the President of the United States and the Speaker of this House have agreed with reference to the bill which is now before you. The gentleman from Mississippi, with his characteristic intellectual integrity, manifested in this instance, as it has been in many others, accepts the situation, says it is a good bill, and makes no complaint because the President of the United States and the Speaker of this House agree with him.

Now, Mr. Speaker, what has happened? The Secretary of Agriculture sent a committee to Chicago to investigate the conditions under which the packing-house industry of that city was carried on. That committee submitted an elaborate and complete report, covering every

[1] *Congr. Record*, June 19, 1906.

building, covering every room — a report which was simple, direct, concise, evidently prepared without passion and without prejudice, telling the exact truth; and the exact truth was that in the great center of the meat-handling industry of the United States conditions existed which threatened the character and integrity of the meat products of the United States. That report was submitted to the President. In order to confirm it, or not confirm it, he selected two men in whom he had confidence, who did not claim to be experts, who were ordinary, intelligent citizens, having the judgment of ordinary, intelligent citizens, and sent them there to make such an investigation as you and I would make. The report of those two gentlemen confirmed the report that was made to the Secretary of Agriculture. The President of the United States, understanding, as you and I understand, that meat is something which goes into the consumption of every family, knowing, as you and I know, that the great meat industry of the United States exports to foreign lands $200,000,000 worth of meat a year, knowing the importance of this subject, communicated the facts to Congress. Why? In order that public sentiment might be stirred all over the United States, and that the legislative judgment of this body and the other across the Capitol might be stirred to enact into law a provision for governmental inspection, which should insure the healthfulness, the wholesomeness, the cleanliness, the purity, and perfection of American meat products. [Applause.] That is all there is of it.

A bill passed the Senate, passed without consideration, a provision conceived by a gentleman who wished to do good things, who was moved by a good purpose. That bill was imperfect. It came over here and was sent to the Committee on Agriculture. Hearings were had. Representatives of the packers were heard; representatives of the Agricultural Department were heard; the men who went to Chicago to investigate were heard. The committee gave ample consideration to the representatives of all these interests; and I want to say to you, gentlemen, with reference to the truth of the charges which have been made, that when Mr. Wilson, the representative of the packers of Chicago, who came there and very modestly and very clearly stated what he deemed the conditions to be in Chicago, and then, in response to questions, admitted that every solitary conclusion of Mr. Neill and Mr. Reynolds in their report should be carried out, he confessed judgment on the essential points in this controversy. [Applause.] And when the board of health of Chicago sent their representative, under the spur of public feeling that has been applied in this case, into the packing-house district and started to work there, in nearly every establishment the truth of the charges was again sustained. There is no question about it. The committee took up that bill in the utmost good faith, every man actuated with the desire to draw and present to this House a measure which should compel rigid and, in so far as human judgment could make it, perfect inspection of meat, to give us a bill which should not only be just to the producing interests of the United States, but also fair and just to those great manufacturing interests which are handling hundreds of millions of dollars' worth of the meat products of this country. The committee worked in absolute good faith. They have no pride of opinion.   There was but one purpose among the members of that committee and that was to make the bill right.   I disagreed with the majority in the first report which came here, providing for a court review.   I do not believe that every time the Congress of the United States draws a law, under the power which it has over interstate commerce, to regulate some particular kind of business, we must provide in that particular bill for some particular kind of court review.   That provision has gone out of the bill.

It is true that I have consulted with the President.   It is true that the Speaker of this House has taken hold of this thing as a Member of the House and as an American citizen, and has worked with Mr. Roosevelt. Neither has shown any pride of opinion, but a simple desire to yield non-essentials in order that the executive branch of the Government and the legislative branch of the Government and the American people, all of whom want a good law, may have it.   [Applause.]

SENATOR RAYNER ON CONGRESS AND THE EXECUTIVE [1]

WE come now to another and a different scene.   The pivotal point around which the railroad rate bill revolved for months in this Chamber was the character of review that the courts were to assume under its provisions.   One side claimed that the courts should only exercise a constitutional review under the fifth amendment; the other side advocated a full statutory review from the proceedings of the Interstate Commerce Commission.

The President came into the game early.   We realize that no fight is thoroughly equipped upon this floor unless the President is in it.   He longs for a fight as the hart panteth after the water brooks.   It was a match to the finish between the senior Senator from Rhode Island and the President.   They stood respectively in the foremost ranks of their profession.   The Senator from Rhode Island was an expert in the ring and had upon many an occasion in this arena been awarded the victor's prize.   The President, also, was a dean in the art, and had reached a degree of eminence in his calling that made him a dangerous foe to encounter.   It was a most interesting spectacle.   The Senator from Rhode Island time and time again went down beneath the ponderous blows of his opponent, but each time he arose like Aurora, the goddess of the

---

[1] *Congr. Record*, Jan. 31, 1907.   See another part of the speech, *supra*.

dawn, arose from her chariot in the sea. At length science commenced to tell. The Senator from Rhode Island had reserved his strength for the last encounter. The President had changed his tactics so often that he became exhausted and appealed for help. One morning the Senator from Rhode Island appeared in this Chamber with a radiant smile. The President had never penetrated the meaning of that smile. It had lured him like the sirens lure their victims to destruction. The smile indicated that the tournament was over. The Senator from South Carolina looked upon the other side of the Chamber for his promised troops, but they had fled and vanished. An ex-Senator from New Hampshire lay dead upon the field. The President lay entangled in his armor, and his breastplate and his battle-ax were shattered, and above him waved the pennant of Rhode Island, and the Senator from Rhode Island smiled. If the President had only kept out of this fray it would have assumed an entirely different form and ended in an entirely different way. It was impossible, however, for him to do this. He could not remain quiescent in the White House and observe a great struggle like this progressing without taking part in it. So that he got into it, it really did not make much difference to him upon which side he was enlisted. One day he was upon one side and the next day he was upon the other.

Here we were day after day struggling with questions of constitutional law, as if we really had anything to do with their settlement, laboring under the vain delusion that we had the right to legislate; that we were an independent branch of the Government; that we were one department, and the Executive another, each with its separate and well-defined distinctions, imagining these things, and following a vision and a mirage, while the President was at work dominating the legislative will, interposing his offices into the law-making power, assuming legislative rights to a greater extent than he could possibly do if he were sitting here as a member of this body; dismembering the Constitution, and exercising precisely and identically the same power and control as if the Constitution had declared that Congress shall pass no law without the consent of the President; adopting a system that practically blends and unites legislative and executive functions, a system that prevailed in many of the ancient governments that have forever gone to ruin, and which to-day still obtains in other governments, the rebellious protests of whose subjects are echoing over the earth, and whose tottering fabrics I hope are on the rapid road to dissolution.

If I were called upon to select the most wonderful exhibition of the President's power that has occurred within my experience, I would take our action upon the canal bill at the close of the last session of Congress. This was an achievement in which his consummate skill in propelling legislation appeared in its most perfect proportions. We had all heard the argument of the junior Senator from South Dakota in favor of a sea-level canal, and its demonstrative facts and unanswerable logic seemed to carry conviction with its presentation.

All at once a wireless message came from the White House. The President had determined that there was either to be a lock canal or that there should be no legislation upon the subject. I can never forget the day upon which the vote was taken. The biography of the President will perhaps some day be written by the senior Senator from Massachusetts. MacCaulay said that if Boswell had not been the greatest fool who ever lived, he could not have given to the world the greatest biography that was ever written. This will not apply to the Senator from Massachusetts. He wields a master's hand in biographical literature, and when he writes this biography I hope that he will dwell with glowing emphasis upon this surpassing accomplishment. Napoleon at Austerlitz never turned the scales of fortune with greater celerity of movement or audacity of assault than the President threw into this maneuver. How was it done? What subtle force did he employ in the execution of his plan? The day the vote was taken this Chamber presented a most peculiar aspect. The air seemed laden with some narcotic wafting its somniferous essence over this body. When the roll was called the clerk could hardly hear the responses upon the side of the lock canal, and as the answers came they came in whispered accents and with bated breath. The charm had done its work, the deadly vapor had benumbed our faculties and made us pliant slaves to the master will. Even the senior Senator from Ohio who, when his convictions are aroused, has often on this floor displayed the Nemean lion's nerve, fell a victim to the magic power of the love charm that had been concocted at the laboratory of the White House. I would like the Secretary to read a few of the pathetic and funereal passages of the Senator's deliverance upon this occasion.

It shows how the dominating spirit of the President can ride the whirlwind when he has made up his mind to legislate, and how in absolute defiance of the laws of nature he can produce a senatorial vacuum beneath the sweep of his mighty genius.

Mr. FORAKER. Mr. President, I do not care to discuss this question beyond saying something similar to that which has just been said by the Senator from West Virginia.

"I remember, when the proposition was before the Senate some time ago, as to whether we should adopt the Panama or the Nicaragua route, I was greatly influenced in favor of the Panama route, as no doubt many other Senators were by the fact stated at page 11, according to the print I have before me, of Report 783, part 2, Fifty-seventh Congress, first session, where the Interoceanic Canal Committee, or a majority at least of its members — "

Mr. KITTREDGE. A minority.

Mr. FORAKER. Yes; it was a minority report I was looking to see. A minority of the members of that committee set forth the advantages of the

Panama route, as contrasted with the Nicaragua route, and then, after they had enumerated nine specific advantages, they added the following:

"10. It is recognized that a sea-level canal is the ideal. The Panama Canal may be either constructed as a sea-level canal or may be subsequently converted into one. On the other hand, no sea-level canal will ever be possible on the Nicaragua route."

Now, like the Senator from West Virginia, I had remained of the idea ever since until within the last two or three months, when this discussion was commenced, that it was the part of wisdom to build a sea-level canal, and I supposed that would be the result of the investigations that were being made by the committee. I did not have time, because occupied with other work, to follow the hearings before that committee and read the testimony as it was taken and printed from day to day for the benefit of the committee and for the benefit of Senators.

I was, therefore, somewhat unprepared when, a few days ago, it was insisted that we should settle this matter at this time by voting upon it. I then made a request that there might be further time than was proposed to be given us in order that we might investigate this subject and read the testimony to obtain further information.

But we are to vote, and every Senator must speak for himself in a few minutes. There is no time to investigate further, and I propose, although with some misgiving as to whether that is the wisest thing to do, to follow what has been indicated as the preference of those who have the greatest responsibility with respect to this canal.

As I have intimated before in reference to this matter, I did not take the floor for the purpose of discussing it. I took the floor only to express the doubt I have and the regret I have that I can not vote as I propose to vote with greater satisfaction to myself.

REPRESENTATIVE JOHN SHARP WILLIAMS' REMARKS[1]

[The House being in the Committee of the Whole House on the state of the Union and having under consideration the bill (H. R. 12320) making appropriations to supply urgent deficiencies in the appropriations for the fiscal year.]

Mr. WILLIAMS said:

Mr. Chairman: I have no idea of occupying the time of the House for thirty minutes. I do desire, however, for five or six minutes to address myself to this proposition. It seems to me that the gentleman in charge of this bill has made a mistake in his estimate of what an estimate is. Some time ago we were faced with an emergency bill to provide sixteen and one-half millions of dollars for the prosecution of the work on the Panama Canal. The House then expressed to the Panama Commission and to the country its desire that hereafter appropriations for the construction of the Panama Canal should take the usual course. If there were any necessity for appropriating the amount of this bill,

[1] *Congr. Record*, Jan. 22, 1906.

that necessity could have been met by introducing into this House a bill duly reported from a committee, duly passed upon in a regular way, or else by a provision on a regular appropriation bill.

It seems to me that the most hopeless thing about us individually and collectively in attending to our duties in Washington as a legislative body is the contemplation of the impotency of the legislative branch of the Federal Government in connection with all sorts of matters. We are led around by the nose — with rings in our noses — by chiefs of bureaus, chiefs of divisions, and heads of departments, and whenever we give notice to the country, after voting down a part of an appropriation in an emergency bill, that we would demand the regular order, gentlemen come in later on, out of the regular order once more, this time in the phase of a deficiency bill, asking that what the House refused to do irregularly shall still be done irregularly. Now, the gentleman speaks about the estimates having been given to the committee, to the House, and to the country. No estimate, in the true sense of the word, has been given at all. In the regular routine of business an estimate means much more than what this committee brings to this House now. An estimate comes from the Department. It comes printed. It comes long in advance. It comes in time to be ready for the study and consideration of each Member of this House and for the study and consideration of the country, in order that the country may influence this House.

Mr. LITTAUER. Will the gentleman permit —

Mr. WILLIAMS. One moment. And the only thing which comes before us here now is a lot of detailed statements furnished to this committee, never furnished to this House in any proper manner, no hearings that could be followed by the country, no opportunity for the country outside of this House to consider the question before them and to influence the House. This is a popular government, or it is supposed to be. It is a government of the people, through their representatives, and not a government of committees, not a government of representatives merely, but a government of the people by the people, through their representatives and through their committees. Now I will yield to the gentleman.

Mr. LITTAUER. Does not the gentleman know that regular estimates, as full as estimates usually submitted to the House, have been forwarded by the Secretary of War, through the Secretary of the Treasury, and they are before the committee and before the House — a regular document of estimates?

Mr. WILLIAMS. I do not know that.

Mr. LITTAUER. And that the hearings were held in the usual way and that the published hearings are now to be had by anyone who asks for them?

Mr. WILLIAMS. Yes; "now to be had," but not to be had a sufficient length of time before this question was brought to the consideration of the House for the country to determine for itself the wisdom or unwisdom of this policy. I know a so-called "detailed statement" was submitted to this committee, and I do know that this committee attempted to make a detailed appropriation to this House. Let us see how detailed and how specific that appropriation is. Let me read it, Mr. Chairman: "For miscellaneous material purchased in the United States, $1,000,000." How miscellaneous? What material? What purchases? "For miscellaneous purchases on the Isthmus, $400,000." That might be held to be comparatively specific except for the language put in there later, "and miscellaneous expenditures." That will be the language of the law when it goes out. Will you tell me what possible devotion of money to any possible purpose is not covered by the language "and miscellaneous expenditures?"

PRESIDENT CLEVELAND ON THE TRANSMISSION OF OFFICIAL PAPERS

[It has often been a matter of difference of opinion as to how far executive departments are obliged to furnish information and documentary material to Congress. The Senate has made it a practice to request information of the Department of State upon matters of foreign affairs only as far as the public interests will permit the giving of such information; but in the case of the other departments more direct demands for information are made by Congress. Ordinarily the departments, of course, are ready to give a full account of their affairs for the use of Congress, but occasions have arisen when the giving of specific information was refused. An interesting controversy of this kind took place during the first administration of President Cleveland when the Senate had demanded the transmission of the papers connected with the dismissal of a certain federal official. As the Tenure of Office Act had not as yet been repealed, although it had been amended during the administration of Grant, the Senate still claimed that its consent to the dismissal of an official was necessary. The President refused to transmit the papers, and the Tenure of Office Act was shortly after repealed. The following extract is from a special message (March 1, 1886) of President Cleveland giving the reasons for his refusal to comply with the request of the Senate.]

Upon this resolution and the answer thereto the issue is thus stated by the Committee on the Judiciary at the outset of the report:

The important question, then, is whether it is within the constitutional competence of either house of Congress to have access to the official papers and documents in the various public offices of the United States created by laws enacted by themselves.

I do not suppose that the "public offices of the United States" are regulated or controlled in their relations to either house of Congress by the fact that they were "created by laws enacted by themselves." It must be that these instrumentalities were created for the benefit of the people and to answer the general purposes of government under the Constitution and the laws, and that they are unincumbered by any lien in favor of either branch of Congress growing out of their construction and unembarrassed by any obligation to the Senate as the price of their creation.

The complaint of the committee, that access to official papers in the public offices is denied the Senate, is met by the statement that at no time has it been the disposition or the intention of the President or any Department of the executive branch of the government to withhold from the Senate official documents or papers filed in any of the public offices. While it is by no means conceded that the Senate has the right, in any case, to review the act of the Executive in removing or suspending a public officer upon official documents or otherwise, it is considered that documents and papers of that nature should, because they are official, be freely transmitted to the Senate upon its demand, trusting the use of the same for proper and legitimate purposes to the good faith of that body. And though no such paper or document has been specifically upon the Departments, yet, as often as they were found in the public offices, they have been furnished in answer to such applications.

The letter of the Attorney-General in response to the resolution of the Senate, in the particular case mentioned in the committee's report, was written at my suggestion and by my direction. There have been no official papers or documents filed in this Department relating to the case, within the period specified in the resolution. The letter was intended, by its description of the papers and documents remaining in the custody of the Department, to convey the idea that they were not official; and it was as-assumed that the resolution called for information, papers, and documents of the same character as were required by the requests and demands which preceded it.

Everything that had been written or done in behalf of the Senate, from the beginning, pointed to all letters and papers of a private and unofficial nature as the objects of search, if they were to be found in the Departments, and provided that they had been presented to the Executive with a view to their consideration upon the question of suspension from office.

Against the transmission of such papers and documents I have interposed my advice and direction. This has not been done, as is suggested in the committee's report, upon the assumption on my part that the Attorney-General or any other head of a Department "is the servant of the President, and is to give or withhold copies or documents in his office according to the will of the Executive and not otherwise," but because I regard the papers and documents withheld and addressed to me, or intended for my use and action, purely unofficial and private, not infrequently confidential, and having reference to the performance of a duty exclusively mine. I consider them in no proper sense as upon the files of the Department, but as deposited there for my convenience, remaining still completely under my control. I suppose if I desired to take them into my custody, I might do so with entire propriety, and if I saw fit to destroy them, no one could complain.

Even the committee in its report appears to concede that there may be, with the President or in the Departments, papers and documents which, on account of their unofficial character, are not subject to the inspection of the Congress. A reference in the report to instances where the House of Representatives ought not to succeed in a call for the production of papers is immediately followed by this statement:

> The committee feels authorized to state, after a somewhat careful research, that within the foregoing limits there is scarcely in the history of this government, until now, any instance of a refusal by a head of a Department, or even of the President himself, to communicate official facts and information as distinguished from private and unofficial papers, motions, views, reasons, and opinions, to either house of Congress when unconditionally demanded.

DISCUSSION OF REQUESTS FOR INFORMATION [1]

MR. FORAKER. Mr. President, I desire to call up, if I am in order to do so, resolution No. 180.

The VICE-PRESIDENT. The Senator from Ohio calls up for consideration the resolution named by him, which will be read.

The Secretary read the resolution submitted by Mr. Penrose on the 3d instant, as follows:

> *Resolved,* That the President be requested to communicate to the Senate, if not incompatible with the public interests, full information bearing upon the recent order dismissing from the military service of the United States three companies of the Twenty-fifth Regiment of Infantry, United States troops (colored).

The VICE-PRESIDENT. The question is on the adoption of the resolution of the Senator from Pennsylvania.

Mr. SPOONER. Mr. President, I am opposed to the resolution offered by the Senator from Pennsylvania. My opposition to it is based entirely upon the form of it. This resolution does not, so far as the subject-matter goes, fall within the class of inquiries which the Senate has ever been accustomed to address to the President. It implies on its face, Mr. President, a doubt here which I think does not exist; as to whether the Senate is of right entitled to all the facts relating to the discharge of the

[1] *Congr. Record,* Dec. 6, 1906.

three named companies or not. Always the Senate, in passing resolutions of inquiry addressed to Cabinet officers, except the Secretary of State, make them in form of *direction*, not *request*. It rarely has happened that a request has been addressed to any Cabinet officer where foreign relations were involved. Where such a resolution has been adopted it has been addressed to the President, with the qualification that he is requested to furnish the information only so far as, in his judgment, the transmission of it is compatible with the public interest.

There are reasons for that, Mr. President. The State Department stands upon an entirely different basis as to the Congress from the other Departments. The conduct of our foreign relations is vested by the Constitution in the President. It would not be admissible at all that either House should have the power to force from the Secretary of State information connected with the negotiation of treaties, communications from foreign governments, and a variety of matters which, if made public, would result in very great harm in our foreign relations — matters so far within the control of the President that it has always been the practice, and it always will be the practice, to recognize the fact that there is of necessity information which it may not be compatible with the public interest should be transmitted to Congress — to the Senate or to the House.

There are other cases, not especially confined, Mr. President, to the State Department, or to foreign relations, where the President would be at liberty obviously to decline to transmit information to Congress or to either House of Congress. Of course, in time of war, the President being Commander in Chief of the Army and Navy, could not, and the War Department or the Navy Department could not, be required by either House to transmit plans of campaign or orders issued as to the destination of ships, or anything relating to the strategy of war, the public knowledge of which getting to the enemy would defeat the Government and its plans and enure to the benefit of an enemy.

There are still other cases. The Department of Justice would not be expected to transmit to either House the result of its investigations upon which some one had been indicted, and lay bare to the defendant the case of the Government. The confidential investigations in various departments of the Government should be, and have always been, treated by both Houses as confidential, and the President is entirely at liberty to permit by the Cabinet officer to whom the inquiry is addressed as much or as little information regarding them as he might see fit. I have no doubt the President would transmit everything upon this subject. My objection is to the form of the resolution. I think we ought to maintain the uniform practice upon the subject. I do not think, as to a matter upon which the Senate clearly has a right to be fully advised, it should depart from the usual form of directing the transmission by the Secretary of War or the Secretary of the Navy or the Secretary of the Interior, to adopt a resolution of request of the President, bearing upon its face a recognition of the fact that he is at liberty to withhold the information or to transmit such part of it as he shall see fit.

Mr. President, in time of peace as to matters relating to the organization and the administration of the Army there can be no secrecy. It is purely domestic public business, as to which the Congress has a right to know. I should be very much disappointed if in a matter of this kind the Senate should address the inquiry to the President, coupled, as it must be, with the suggestion that we doubt our right to the information. I think it is a bad precedent to establish. In such matters I think we ought to maintain the practice which, so far as I remember, hitherto has been unbroken. Therefore I am opposed to the form of the resolution of the Senator from Pennsylvania. I am in favor of the form of the resolution of the Senator from Ohio.

Mr. FORAKER. Mr. President, I desire only to say a word of the same general character as that which has been spoken by the Senator from Wisconsin [Mr. Spooner]. My objection to the resolution offered on yesterday by the Senator from Wyoming [Mr. Warren] was that under it the President would have a right to withhold information particularly called for by the resolution I had offered. Senators will observe when they come to look at that resolution that nothing is called for except only that which is specifically described, and that it is all of a character such as the Senate is clearly entitled to. No one has the right to withhold it from the knowledge of the Senate if the Senate asks for it. That was the only objection I had to having my resolution incorporated with the resolution offered by the Senator from Pennsylvania in a resolution such as was offered by the Senator from Wyoming [Mr. Warren] on yesterday. The same objection, of course, lies to the suggestion which was made, also, by the Senator from Pennsylvania that we might unite the resolutions. If the Senate sees fit to adopt it, I have no objection to the resolution offered by the Senator from Pennsylvania; but I shall insist in any contingency upon the consideration of my own resolution as calling for information we are clearly entitled to without anybody giving his judgment whether or not it is our right to have it.

Mr. LODGE. Mr. President, on the matter of precedents I have only had a moment to look back. My memory was that we had sent many inquiries to the President which did not refer to foreign relations. On looking hastily back through a book from the Secretary's desk, I find in the Fifty-ninth Congress the following resolution, offered by the Senator from Minnesota [Mr. Nelson], was adopted:

Resolved, That the President is hereby requested, if not incompatible with the public interests, to transmit to the Senate the reports of the Keep Commission on Department methods, relating to official crop statistics and the investigation of the Twelfth Census report on agriculture.

It seems nothing could be more purely domestic than that. I find another, as follows:

Resolved, That the President be requested to furnish the Senate, if not incompatible with the best interests of the service, the petition and accompanying papers of certain officers of the Army, veterans of the civil war, retired from active service for disability contracted in the line of duty, and who have not yet received the benefits of the act of April 23, 1904.

Those are two very recent ones. I thought I remembered some relating to the Philippines, and I find there are some. This book only goes back to the Fifty-eighth Congress, but I find a resolution submitted by Mr. Hoar, as follows:

Resolved, That the President be requested, if not in his opinion incompatible with the public interest, to inform the Senate whether there be any law or regulation in force in the Philippine Islands which will prevent any native of those islands who may so desire, not under arrest and against whom no charge of any offense against the United States is pending, from coming to the United States and stating his views or desires as to the interest of his people to the President or either House of Congress.

Mr. SPOONER. When was that adopted

Mr. LODGE. That was referred to the Committee on the Philippines, and printed. It was not adopted. The other two that I read were adopted. I have no doubt that others could be found. Certainly, I think that there can be no questoin that resolutions of inquiry have been addressed to the President on all possible subjects. In this case, he being Commander in Chief of the Army, it seems to me it is perfectly proper in form to address a resolution to him on a subject where he has taken direct action and about which there is a great deal of public feeling and has been a great deal of public discussion. It seems to me the proper way to get the facts before us is to make inquiry, not only of the War Department, but of the President himself, so that he may have an opportunity to state to Congress in the fullest official manner the reasons which actuated him in rendering this decision, which, of course, as we all know, is peculiarly his own.

Mr. WARREN. Mr. President, I take it for granted the President will find some way to put the Senate in possession of any information he has that he wishes to put before it. On the other hand, it seems to me entirely proper for the Senate to ask the President for such information as the Senate wants, and that he is the proper one to ask. And believing that the Senate and the country want all the information obtainable, I am willing, if I have the opportunity, to vote for both resolutions, the one proposed by the Senator from Pennsylvania [Mr. Penrose] and the one proposed by the Senator from Ohio [Mr. Foraker]. I know of no rule against such action. I know of no custom against it. I know of no reason why we should not adopt both resolutions as presented here, though by all means we should indorse the one directed to the President whether or not we adopt the other one.

Mr. TELLER. Mr. President, the precedents cited by the senior Senator from Massachusetts [Mr. Lodge] might be increased in great number. For many years past, even during the war, it was a frequent occurrence to call on the President for information. I myself have been somewhat of a stickler in reference to the form of resolutions of inquiry. We request the President, and we direct the Cabinet officers; but, after all, the whole matter of communicating information to this body by Cabinet officers is absolutely under the control of the President. If the President declines or thinks such information should not be sent, it is not sent. We request the President for information, "if not incompatible with the public interest." That is merely a courteous form of making the request. If we left out the expression "if not incompatible with the public interest," he would still have authority to withhold any information. I think it will be found that the rule among Cabinet officers, whenever requests of delicacy or importance have been presented by Congress, has been to consult the President in relation thereto.

Mr. LODGE. Will the Senator allow me to ask him a question in that connection?

The VICE-PRESIDENT. Does the Senator from Colorado yield to the Senator from Massachusetts?

Mr. TELLER. Certainly.

Mr. LODGE. My memory is that there have been cases within comparatively recent years where Cabinet officers having been directed by resolution of the Senate to send certain information to it, have withheld entirely, or withheld in part, such information by order of the President.

Mr. TELLER. Undoubtedly.

Mr. LODGE. I think it occurred under Mr. Cleveland on more than one occasion, and I think it has occurred in relation to the Department of the Interior quite recently, though I do not remember the exact date.

Mr. CARMACK. Mr. President —

The VICE-PRESIDENT. Does the Senator from Colorado yield to the Senator from Tennessee?

Mr. TELLER. Yes.

Mr. CARMACK. I think that occurred in a former session of Congress when an answer to a resolution of mine asking the Secretary of the Treasury for certain information was declined on the ground that it would be incompatible with the best interests of the public service.

Mr. TELLER. Mr. President, there are undoubtedly a large number of precedents of that kind. I had occasion some time ago to consult the precedents running back forty or fifty years, and I have a very distinct recollection of a number of cases where Presidents have declined to communicate information both to the House and to the Senate.

I do not think there is any impropriety in our asking the President in a courteous, proper manner to communicate information to the Senate. I am under the impression, Mr. President, that the better practice would be to ask the Secretary of War, the Secretary of the Treasury, or the Secretary of the Navy, whoever it might be that had the matter under control, without annoying the President and adding to his work. But, so far as I am concerned, I am willing to vote for a resolution asking the President for information, or I am willing to vote for a resolution asking the Secretary of War for information; but I do not think we ought to ask them both. It seems to me we ought to confine ourselves to one or the other. I simply express my preference for the method of asking the Secretary of War, instead of asking the President. If the President or the Secretary of War wish to communicate on the subject, they know how to do so by direct message to this body.

Mr. LODGE. Mr. President —

The VICE-PRESIDENT. Does the Senator from Colorado yield to the Senator from Massachusetts?

Mr. TELLER. Certainly.

Mr. LODGE. I was going to say that the resolution I read requesting the President for certain information in regard to veterans of the civil war was introduced by the Senator from Colorado [Mr. Teller] himself.

Mr. CARTER. Mr. President, briefly, and principally to address myself to the Senator from Wisconsin [Mr. Spooner], I think it may be taken for granted that as a matter of mere official ethics the address of the resolution of the Senator from Pennsylvania [Mr. Penrose] to the President of the United States is deferential and correct. It must not be lost sight of that the President represents the executive department, a coordinate department of the Government. The right of the President, because of his character as Chief Executive of the Nation, charged with the conduct of our foreign affairs, to be the sole judge as to the communication to Congress of matters relating to our international affairs was well stated by the Senator from Wisconsin.

The Senator further proceeded to say that in case of actual war it would be obviously improper for the Senate to call upon the Commander in Chief of the Army and Navy for plans of battles or campaigns, for drafts of fortifications or lines of defense, or for any information which, if made public, might militate against the interests of the country. But the Senator undertakes to differentiate by saying that this it a time of peace, and, therefore, the directions of the President with reference to the Army must be under a different rule as relates to the legislative department from that which would obtain in time of war. The logic of that, I think, will not be apparent to the mind of the Senator from Wisconsin when he reflects upon the particular facts in this case as made known by current information.

Mr. SPOONER. Mr. President, I desire to submit a few observations.

I agree entirely with the Senator from Colorado [Mr. Teller] that this discussion of the merits of the question is entirely premature. For one I intend to withhold any discussion of it until the incoming of a report which puts the Senate officially in possession of all the facts in relation to it.

The Senator from Colorado is mistaken in supposing that I made any point of order against the resolution offered by the Senator from Pennsylvania. I did not. I objected to the form of the resolution — that is, I objected to a resolution addressed to the President as unusual. I still adhere, Mr. President, to that objection as a matter of proper practice although there is nothing in the Constitution to prohibit it, nothing in the rules of the Senate to prohibit it. It is entirely competent for the Senate to pass it.

Mr. PENROSE. Mr. President —

The VICE-PRESIDENT. Does the Senator from Wisconsin yield to the Senator from Pennsylvania?

Mr. SPOONER. Certainly.

Mr. PENROSE. I should like to ask the Senator on that point whether he contradicts the statement made by me and the Senator from Massachusetts [Mr. Lodge] that there are numerous precedents of the Senate justifying this course. His present objection is purely theoretical and critical of a bad practice in the past as much as in the present.

Mr. SPOONER. I will get to that. Mr. President, I have not examined the precedents. I speak from my recollection as to the almost uniform practice of the Senate during a period of nearly sixteen years in which I have been a member of the body. It appears that resolutions addressed to the President have been introduced and passed — one offered by the Senator from Colorado [Mr. Teller]. I rather think it must have been inadvertently done, because it was not a subject upon which, so far as I recollect the scope of the resolution, there could have been any possibility of the Executive withholding information from the Senate. The general practice of the Senate has been — and it is a good practice, an almost universal practice, except in those cases where the nature of the subject is such as to warrant the belief that all of the information may not properly and safely be communicated to either House of Congress — not to address the resolution of inquiry to the President, but to address it to the Secretary of the appropriate Department, making it a direction instead of a request.

The precedent cited by the Senator from Massachusetts relative to a request upon the President for a copy of the report of the Keep Commission does not fall at all within the exception. The Keep Commission was not a commission authorized by law. It was a commission appointed by the President composed of officials selected from the various Departments to investigate the methods of the Executive Departments of the Government and to report to the President for his information, as I recollect it.

Mr. CARTER. Mr. President —

The VICE-PRESIDENT. Does the Senator from Wisconsin yield to the Senator from Montana?

Mr. SPOONER. Certainly.

Mr. CARTER. I should like to ask the Senator from Wisconsin if that portion of the resolution should be amended, thus calling upon the President for all the correspondence and all the facts, whether he would deem it proper to call upon the President, without qualification, to communicate to the Senate, and therefore to the public, the correspondence, if any there be, between the Department of Justice and the legally constituted authorities of the State of Texas with reference to the commission of crimes in that State by soldiers of the United States liable to punishment under State law, if such communication would militate against the ends of justice?

Mr. SPOONER. The Senator from Montana has utterly misapprehended my objection to this resolution. He insists that my objection is because of the presence in it of the words "if not incompatible with the public interests." He is quite mistaken. I know quite well that propriety demands that when a request for information is addressed to the President — and that is why I think such requests are limited, and has been in general practice, to the cases which I indicated when I first spoke — it is always qualified so far as I recollect, by these words. My preference for the resolution of the Senator from Ohio is because, being a request for detailed information, our right to which is beyond question, it is addressed to the Secretary of War, and contains no evidence that the Senate doubts its right to the information.

I do not take it to be open to debate, Mr. President, that the Senate has a right to obtain from the War Department copies of discharges, records of courts-martial — everything relating to the domestic administration of the Army not connected with plans of campaign or of war.

Mr. CARTER. Mr. President —

The VICE-PRESIDENT. Does the Senator from Wisconsin yield to the Senator from Montana?

Mr. SPOONER. I do.

Mr. CARTER. Then I wish to state that I clearly and distinctly understood the Senator from Wisconsin to object to the words "if not incompatible with the public interests" in this form of resolution.

Mr. SPOONER. Mr. President, I objected to the resolution because it requires those words and implies in the resolution itself a doubt upon the part of the Senate whether or not this information might be properly withheld from the Senate. That is my objection.

Mr. CARTER. The objection of the Senator was to the addressing of any resolution to the President on the subject.

Mr. SPOONER. For that reason. The almost universal rule of the Senate has been to address no inquiries to the President of the United States without those words; I remember no exception, where the nature of the subject of inquiry was such as to make it perfectly apparent that the Senate or the House was entitled of right to all the information covered by it, the direction, not the request, has been made as an almost universal rule upon the appropriate Cabinet officer, instead of by resolution of inquiry addressed to the President.

I said there were some exceptions, and there are. Foreign relations constitute one exception; the movement or plan of campaign of the Army or the Navy in time of war constitutes another, because even a child would know that the Commander in Chief, under our Constitution, must have the discretion in order to insure the safety of the Republic and the success of our arms, to exercise discretion and to withhold, if his judgment so dictates, information which would endanger the public interest if it were given to the public. The Senator from Montana, with a logic the like of which I have never known him to indulge in before, seemed to think that there is no distinction, and can be none, between the information which the Senate or the House is entitled to have in relation to the Army in time of war and in time of peace.

It does not at all follow, Mr. President, because certain inquiries as to the Army must be in time of war addressed to the President, and he have discretion to withhold or to transmit information, that in time of peace, upon every imaginable subject connected with the administration of the Army, it is proper, or comports with the dignity of the Senate or of the other House as legislative bodies in all cases to address inquiries to the President, qualified as courtesy requires such inquiries to be.

Mr. CARTER. Now, Mr. President —

Mr. SPOONER. I want to get through.

Mr. CARTER. I wish to address the Senator a question at that point.

Mr. SPOONER. Very well.

Mr. CARTER. It is well known that we are expending very large sums of money on our coast defenses.

Mr. SPOONER. Certainly.

Mr. CARTER. I will ask the Senator if he thinks in time of peace it is proper for the legislative department of the Government to make public all the plans of defense that are being prepared in case of war by calling on the Secretary of War or the President to disclose such information?

Mr. SPOONER. The Senator gets back to my path — that is, that the question is to be resolved with reference to the subject-matter. I admitted it, and I admit it now. I must admit that there are numerous cases in which absolute direction upon one of the Departments or upon a Cabinet officer is subject of right, I mean, to a declination by order of the President to that officer to afford the information. But that argues nothing upon a subject like this or upon the subject generally embodied in the resolution of inquiry by the Senate and by the House. We could not call upon the Attorney-General to send to the Senate copies of papers which he has acquired through investigation to be used in the trial of a gang of counterfeiters or to be used in the trial of cases prosecuted under the anti-trust law for the obvious reason, Mr. President, that it would lead possibly to the defeat of the Government's litigation. You can not put your side of the case into the hands of your opponent. If an investigation has been made by the Treasury Department with reference to the apprehension of men who are smugglers, Congress could not expect the President to permit the information to be sent to the Senate or the House, and warning thereby be given to those whom the Government seeks to apprehend.

There are many such cases. Is this a case of that kind? Congress, Mr. President, fixes the size of the Army. The Army is the Army of the people of the United States. It is created by act of Congress. The rules for its government are entirely within the jurisdiction of Congress. The grounds upon which men may be discharged is within the constitutional capacity of the Congress. Whether any man can be discharged for offense without a trial is entirely within the constitutional competency of Congress. Whether the President shall be given the right to dismiss an officer at will without trial is for Congress to say. The Army is supported by moneys appropriated by Congress. The manner of the expenditure of those moneys Congress has a right to know. I do not make any doubt whatever, Mr. President, that it is within the constitutional right of the House or of the Senate either, acting in a legislative capacity upon this subject, to direct the Secretary of War to transmit to the Senate or to the House all information within his jurisdiction upon the subject of the discharge of the three colored companies.

Now, Mr. President, the foundations of the Union will not be shaken whichever of these resolutions is adopted, or if both be adopted. I am surprised that the Senator from Wyoming [Mr. Warren] withdrew his resolution. They all three might have been adopted. The Senator from Pennsylvania thinks it improper that both should be adopted. He offered his resolution in the form which he employed addressed to the President — the form is proper if the resolution is to be addressed to the President at all — because the Senator thought it would not be within the proprieties, it having been the President's act, to address it to his subordinate, the Secretary of War.

I do not stop to discuss the question of propriety; but it is very proper, some Senators think, to pass both of the resolutions. The Senator from Massachusetts [Mr. Lodge] seems to think so; the Senator from Montana [Mr. Carter] seems to think so.

There never has been, within my knowledge, a President who is more frank with both bodies of Congress than the present Executive. The objection is based upon principle and was made because I believe it is the dignified and proper course for both bodies to pursue as to subjects upon which the House or the Senate is entitled manifestly to the information to make a direction in the usual way upon the appropriate Cabinet officer.

I think it will look rather absurd — I shall not further object to it, Mr. President — to pass the resolution calling upon the President, if not incompatible with the public interests, for full information bearing upon the subject, and also to pass the resolution of the Senator from Ohio, *directing* the Secretary of War, who has probably received most of these papers from the President, to furnish all information upon the subject on file in the War Department. But that is a matter for the Senate to determine.

Mr. TELLER. Mr. President, I do not wish to prolong this debate, but the Senator from Wisconsin [Mr. Spooner] seems to think that the resolution which I introduced some time ago must have been inadvertently introduced. I presume the files of this Senate will show a great many resolutions of mine of a similar kind. I want to say to the Senator, as a matter of history, that if he will take the trouble to go into the question of the right of the Senate and of the other House to call upon the Executive for information, he will find that in the early history of the country such requests went directly to the President. If he will take the pains to go back fifty years he will find that it was a common occurrence, and I will venture to say there has not been a President since the days of Washington who has not been called upon by the Senate and the other House for information.

During the exciting times immediately after the civil war, when Andrew Johnson was President of the United States, a great number of such resolutions from the House and the Senate were day after day directed to the President. Sometimes he furnished the information and sometimes he did not. If he did not furnish it, he would say that he did not think it was compatible with the public interests that he should do so. In such cases I believe he always courteously declined.

When we call upon the President for information, we request him; when we call upon the Secretary of War, we direct him. Suppose the Secretary of War fails to reply. Where is the power of the Senate to compel him? He is a subordinate of the President. He is the mouthpiece of the President in many ways. He becomes the mouthpiece of the President because of his special knowledge in regard to certain matters. You call upon the man who is supposed to know most about the subject concerning which information is desired. If you want to know about public lands or about pensions, you call upon the Secretary of the Interior; but if you want to know about military affairs, you call upon the Secretary of War. There is, however, no way by which you can compel the Secretary of War to reply, unless by impeachment, and we cannot institute such proceedings, for, under the Constitution, they must originate in the House of Representatives.

There is nothing unusual in the resolution of the Senator from Pennsylvania. As I said before, the resolution of the Senator from Ohio calls upon the Secretary of War for information that is not in the hands of the President, and therefore I prefer the form of his resolution. At the end of his resolution there is a request for an order issued to Major Penrose. Probably that order is not in the keeping of the President, but is in the keeping of the Secretary of War. It seems to me there is an unnecessary question of propriety raised here. I do not myself want to admit that when the Senate wants information it can not call upon the Executive for it. I do not care whether it is in one Department or another or whether it is solely under the control of the President. You may call upon him for information affecting matters of foreign diplomacy, but he is not obliged to answer; sometimes he would be derelict in duty if he did answer; but it must be fairly presumed that the Senate of the United States will never call upon the President for information which ought not to be given to the country. If he says "I do not consider it compatible with the public interests that I should give it," that is the end of the controversy.

Mr. WARREN. I want to ask the Senator a question before he takes his seat.

The VICE-PRESIDENT. Does the Senator from Colorado yield to the Senator from Wyoming?

Mr. TELLER. Certainly.

Mr. WARREN. The Senator from Colorado has been a distinguished Cabinet officer, and I want to put this question to him: In the present case the President, by the Constitution, is clearly Commander in Chief of the Army — in other words, he is the highest officer of the Army. He bears a relation to the Army and Navy that he does not bear as to other Departments. It seems to me that information regarding this particular case lies not only with the Secretary of War, but undoubtedly with the Department of Justice as well. Therefore I want to ask the Senator from Colorado if, when we make an inquiry of the President, he will not, as a matter of course, call upon the different Departments for such information as he chooses to furnish, whereas, if we call upon the Secretary of War alone, he furnishes only that which his Department has? If so, it seems to me in this case — while I am ready to vote for both resolutions — if we are to select one and vote for only one, it should be the one calling upon the President, first, because he has control over both of these Departments that may have evidence; second, he is the Commander in Chief of the Army and its highest authority, and, third, this action concerning the discharge of troops is the action of the President, in the absence from the city at the time of the Secretary of War, and therefore the President is the highest authority to appeal to and the man above all others who is able to furnish us the information we want.

Mr. TELLER. I think the Senator has answered his own question, and I think he is correct about it.

IV

THE TREATY-MAKING POWER

[The treaty-making power is shared by the President and the Senate. It is inevitable that discussions should arise as to the extent of the proper functions of each of these agents. In addition to the function of making treaties, the President holds many powers through which he can influence or determine the transaction of international business and the foreign policy of this nation. As commander in chief of the navy, he controls the action of that branch of federal service; through his power of receiving ambassadors and public ministers, he may determine the fundamental relations of our government to other States. Informal agreements have often been concluded between the Executive and foreign representatives, without reference to the Senate. For the latter see J. B. Moore's article on "Treaties and Executive Agreements" in the *Pol. Sc. Q.* 20: 385, and Reinsch, *American Legislatures*, page 94 and following. All these matters were discussed in detail most thoroughly during the sessions of 1906 and 1907, especially in connection with the San Domingo affair. The situation is briefly stated in the following extract from the point of view of the opposition; and is then discussed in detail in the debate between Senators Spooner and Bacon.]

SENATOR RAYNER ON THE TREATY-MAKING POWER [1]

I SHALL now take as the first instance where there has been a conflict between executive and legislative functions — the treaty-making power of the President and the Senate. Article second of the Constitution provides that the President shall have power by and with the advice and consent of the Senate to make treaties, provided that two-thirds of the Senators present concur. In the Santo Domingo affair the President has evidently made his own treaty. I am not discussing the proposition whether his views and purposes are right or wrong in reference to Santo Domingo. He may be right — a great many persons think that he is. He may have performed a great public service for the people of that island and for civilization and humanity in the efforts that he has made to extricate them from their difficulties and misfortunes. This is not the point at issue. The charge that I make is that he has accomplished this

---

[1] *Congr. Record*, Jan. 31, 1907.

in violation of the Constitution, and has set an example for his successors which, if followed, would abrogate the provision that gives this body
the right to be consulted in the treaty-making power.

The principal provision of the Santo Domingo treaty relates to the
collection of the revenues of the island and their distribution among its
creditors. All other parts of the treaty were subordinate to this. What
has been done? The treaty has been practically carried into effect without consulting the Senate. The appointment of an American agent as
an official of Santo Domingo to collect its customs was simply a cover
and an evasion. Under the principles of international law and the comity
of nations this Government is morally bound for the proper custody of
this fund, and would be liable in case of its waste or loss. After its collection the only act of any consequence that remained to be done was its
distribution, and even this has been practically determined upon, I understand, by settlement with her creditors.

Now, when you add to this the fact that our war ships are in the harbors of the island ostensibly for the purpose of protecting American interests, but in reality protecting the officials of the island against any
menace from without, and revolution from within, you have the establishment of a sovereignty or a protectorate without a word from Congress or the Senate sanctioning the same. This is called a *modus vivendi*,
but the phrase *modus vivendi* has no application to a condition of this
sort, and is a perfectly meaningless absurdity in this connection. What
is being done is the maintenance of a *status quo*, but a *status quo* created
by the President at the time of the negotiation of the treaty, and without
any warrant of law whatsoever. I do not believe that in all the archives
of the State Department there can be found any precedent for such a
proceeding. Any President could at that time, following this example,
make an agreement with any foreign country, uphold it by armed intervention, and then if the Senate declined to confirm his action simply announce that he proposed to maintain the *status quo* or *modus vivendi*, as
it is erroneously called, and thus practically effectuate a treaty whether
the Senate consents or not. What the President has done in reference to
Santo Domingo he can duplicate any day with respect to any of the bankrupt and revolutionary Republics of Central or South America. They
may appeal to him for help. He may negotiate a treaty and the Senate
may decline to act upon the treaty, and in the meantime he may enter
into an agreement with them to collect their customs duties, place them
on deposit in an American bank, and in the custody of an American representative, and when Congress or the Senate calls him to account he can,
with absolute defiance, announce that the work has been done, and that
it is the duty of this Government to make a proper division of the funds.

When an appeal comes to him from this quarter he can direct our war
ships to protect American interests, and incidentally the party in power
or the revolutionists friendly to our intervention, and he can assume con-

trol over their custom-houses and maintain a financial protectorate over them without a treaty and without constitutional or legislative sanction. This policy may be all right — perhaps the American people are in favor of this new doctrine; it may be a wonderful accomplishment — Central America may profit by it; it may be a great benefit to us commercially and it may be in the interest of civilization, but as a student and follower of the Constitution, I deprecate the methods that have been adopted, and I appeal to you to know whether we propose to sit silently by and by our indifference or tacit acquiescence submit to a scheme that ignores the privileges of this body; that is not authorized by statute; that does not array itself within any of the functions of the Executive; that vests the treaty-making power exclusively in the President, to whom it does not belong; that overrides the organic law of the land and that virtually proclaims to the country that while the other branches of the Government are controlled by the Constitution, the Executive is above and beyond it, and whenever his own views or policies conflict with it he will find some way to effectuate his purposes uncontrolled by its limitations.

SPEECH OF SENATOR JOHN C. SPOONER ON TREATIES [1]

Mr. SPOONER said:

Mr. President: I take the floor upon this bill, not, however, to discuss it, but to present as briefly as I may my views upon another important subject. I am impelled to do this by recent debate here, more or less critical of the conduct of our foreign relations by the President, and under circumstances which, with great deference, I can not regard as constituting in any degree wise precedent.

Matters which are being considered by the Senate as an executive body have been debated in open legislative session. Fifteen years of service here has fully confirmed in me the impression, early formed after my advent in this body, that the consideration of treaties and all questions involving our foreign relations are best, save in very exceptional cases, conducted behind closed doors. This, of course, Mr. President, not because there is anything said or done which Senators would wish withheld from our own people, but because it is inevitable that in the perfect frankness which should characterize debate involving our foreign relations many things must be said, and are always said, which, in the public interest, ought not to be said in the hearing of other nations. I am clearly of the conviction, having regard to the peculiar relations created by the Constitution between the Senate and the Executive in respect to the exercise of the treaty-making power, that it is not a healthy precedent to establish, or one much to be followed, that involves public

[1] *Congr. Record*, Jan. 23, 1906.

discussion of current foreign relations, including treaties. If indulged at all it ought to be done by a vote of the body since otherwise some feel justified in discussing phases which others feel not at liberty to debate.

* * * * * * * *

On general principles, I reiterate, after more experience in this body than the Senator has had, but not so much as he doubtless will have, my conviction that the methods of the fathers in the treatment by the Senate of our foreign relations, all things considered, is a wise one and the one best conserving the public interest of the United States.

Of course one may miss the inspiration of the larger audience, but the debates of the executive session get to be very earnest; they are very frank, they are intensely patriotic, they exhibit great research and industry, and are, in my judgment, the most interesting if not the most valuable of all discussions in the Senate.

I have heard speeches here by Senators now present, and by Senators now gone from here, some of whom are dead, which for learning, eloquence, and patriotic solicitude and forethought for the interest of the United States in foreign relations of delicacy and grave importance, are not to be surpassed, and would have received enduring admiration could they, in harmony with the interest of the people, have been given to the world. By common consent they could not, and so they live only in the memories of those who heard them.

The distinguished and patriotic Senator from Georgia [Mr. Bacon], whose friendship I greatly value, thought it wise and proper to introduce a resolution in the legislative session of the Senate calling upon the President for certain information, including the instructions given to the delegates or representatives accredited to the conference now being held at Algeciras relative to Morocco, in order that the Senate might, sitting in judgment upon the executive conduct of our foreign relations, determine whether they were being conducted in accordance with the traditions of our country or were being conducted in violation of them.

I regretted the introduction of the resolution. I justify the wisdom of the Senate in closing the doors upon its discussion. But notwithstanding, another resolution, general in its terms, dealing with the traditional policy of the United States, which no man in the United States would willingly see disregarded or departed from, opened the way for the full discussion of the subject.

Mr. President, with great respect for those who differ from me, I deprecate the course which has been pursued. I believe that it is not a proper course to be pursued by the Senate in respect of our foreign relations, save in extraordinary circumstances, if at all. The Senate has nothing whatever to do with the *negotiation* of treaties or the conduct of our foreign intercourse and relations save the exercise of the one constitutional function of advice and consent which the Constitution requires as a precedent condition to the making of a treaty. Except as to the participation in the treaty-making power the Senate, under the Constitution, has obviously neither responsibilities nor power.

From the foundation of the Government it has been conceded in practice and in theory that the Constitution vests the power of negotiation and the various phases — and they are multifarious — of the conduct of our foreign relations exclusively in the President. And, Mr. President, he does not exercise that constitutional power, nor can he be made to do it, under the tutelage or guardianship of the Senate or of the House or of the Senate and House combined.

Mr. TILLMAN. Will the Senator allow me to ask him a question?

Mr. SPOONER. Certainly.

Mr. TILLMAN. What interpretation does the Senator put upon the word "advice" in the Constitution? Can you give advice after a thing has been done?

Mr. SPOONER. Yes; you can give advice —

Mr. TILLMAN. As to whether or not a thing has been properly done, but you can not give advice after it has been done.

Mr. SPOONER. I will proceed to answer the question, if I am able.

The words "advice and consent of the Senate" are used in the Constitution with reference to the Senate's participation in the making of a treaty and are well translated by the word "ratification" popularly used in this connection. The President negotiates the treaty, to begin with. He may employ such agencies as he chooses to negotiate the proposed treaty. He may employ the ambassador, if there be one, or a minister or a chargé d'affaires, or he may use a person in private life whom he thinks by his skill or knowledge of the language or people of the country with which he is about to deal is best fitted to negotiate the treaty. He may issue to the agent chosen by him — and neither Congress nor the Senate has any concern as to whom he chooses — such instructions as seem to him wise. He may vary them from day to day. That is his concern. The Senate has no right to demand that he shall unfold to the world or to it, even in executive session, his instructions or the prospect or progress of the negotiation. I said "right." I use that word advisedly in order to illustrate what all men who have studied the subject are willing to concede — that under the Constitution the absolute power of negotiation is in the President and the means of negotiation subject wholly to his will and his judgment.

When he shall have negotiated and sent his proposed treaty to the Senate the jurisdiction of this body attaches and its power begins. It may advise and consent, or it may refuse. And in the exercise of this function it is as independent of the Executive as he is independent of it in the matter of negotiation.

I do not deny the power of the Senate either in legislative session or in executive session — that is a question of propriety — to pass a resolution expressive of its opinion as to matters of foreign policy. But if it is passed by the Senate or by the House or by both Houses, it is beyond any possible question purely advisory, and not in the slightest degree binding in law or conscience upon the President. It is easy to conceive of circumstances in which to pass in legislative session a resolution like that first introduced by my distinguished and learned friend, the Senator from Georgia [Mr. Bacon], asking the President, if in his opinion not incompatible with the public good, to transmit the correspondence in a pending negotiation to the Senate, might be productive of mischief. I think the Morocco case is perhaps one which could be productive of mischief in this, that the President's declination, which would be within his power, upon the ground that the public good required that the correspondence should not be sent to the Senate, might give rise to an inference in other countries that something with reference to one or more of the parties was being concealed from them.

Mr. President, I do not stop at this moment to cite authorities in support of the proposition, that so far as the conduct of our foreign relations is concerned, excluding only the Senate's participation in the making of treaties, the President has the absolute and uncontrolled and uncontrollable authority. Under the confederation there was felt to be great weakness in a system that made the Congress the organ of communication with foreign governments; but when the Constitution was formed, it being almost everywhere else in the world a purely executive function, it was lodged with the President. He was given the power, with all other Executive functions, "to receive ambassadors and other public ministers." His exercise of that function can not, under the Constitution, be controlled by any other body in the Government. That is a tremendous power given by the Constitution to the President — the power to receive or reject an ambassador or a public minister or any one of the representatives known to international law as it existed when the Constitution was adopted. That involves not simply the mere recognition of governments or administrations, but it involves sometimes the recognition of a new nation. It involves passing upon the question of independence. It involves decision as to the various changes which occur in the administration or government of nations — one administration or faction in power to-day, another next week, another a month later. The President decides. He was given the power to appoint "ambassadors, other public ministers, and consuls," which has been held to include diplomatic agents then known to international law and international intercourse. Those offices are not created by the Congress. The Congress controls the purse, and may not see fit to appropriate compensation for those appointed by the President, but it has been well held and is irrefutable that under the Constitution the offices are created by that instrument, and he is given his own absolute will as to when he will appoint and whom he will appoint —

Mr. TILLMAN. Mr. President —

The VICE-PRESIDENT. Does the Senator from Wisconsin yield to the Senator from South Carolina?.

Mr. SPOONER. Except as to confirmation by the Senate.

The VICE-PRESIDENT. Does the Senator from Wisconsin yield to the Senator from South Carolina?

Mr. SPOONER. Certainly.

Mr. TILLMAN. The Senator from Wisconsin having modified his statement to that extent, I will not allude to that point; but I should like to ask him, he having given us such a luminous exposition of the Constitution, what is the relation between the President and the Foreign Relations Committee of the Senate? Do those men never advise?

Mr. SPOONER. Is the Senator serious in putting to me that question?

Mr. TILLMAN. I am.

Mr. SPOONER. I will give it a serious answer.

The relation of members of the Foreign Relations Committee to the executive department of the Government in its relation to foreign relations is precisely the relation which the Senator from South Carolina and his colleagues sustain to the executive department in its relation to foreign relations. The Committee on Foreign Relations, like the other committees of this body, is not an independent entity. Its members are Senators who are designated by the body to study and report upon certain subjects, and the committee therefore is but the servant of the Senate, as all other committees are. A member of the Foreign Relations Committee, as a Senator, in his relation to the Senate and executive department is only a Senator, just as those who are not on that committee are Senators.

Of course, it will sometimes happen that members of the Foreign Relations Committee, charged by the Senate with that particular subject, will obtain information as servants of the Senate, in order to bring it to the attention of the Senate, which other Senators might not seek; but that is all.

Mr. BEVERIDGE. It is a matter of expediency.

Mr. SPOONER. It is not a matter of expediency. It is a matter of industry, and a wise attempt at least to discharge the duty which the Senate has committed to them.

Mr. BEVERIDGE. They are not compelled to do it by the Constitution.

Mr. SPOONER. Oh, no.

Mr. LODGE. Mr. President —

The VICE-PRESIDENT. Does the Senator from Wisconsin yield to the Senator from Massachusetts?

Mr. LODGE. I merely wish to remind him of a fact with which he no doubt is very familiar, that in the Administration of Mr. Madison the Senate deputed a committee to see him in regard to the appointment of a minister to Sweden, I think, and he replied that he could recognize no committee of the Senate, that his relations were exclusively with the Senate. I have no doubt the Senator intended to recall that, but as he stated the exact relations as he understood them, it seemed to bear on that point.

Mr. SPOONER. I did not recall it; I am obliged to the Senator for recalling it; but I think I covered it —

Mr. LODGE. You did, entirely.

Mr. SPOONER. By saying that members of a committee have no relations to any Department of the Government, simply being servants of the Senate, which has the relation to the Departments of the Government.

Mr. TILLMAN. If the Senator will permit me, I will explain why I asked the question.

Mr. SPOONER. Certainly.

Mr. TILLMAN. The other day I submitted some observations on the Santo Domingo business. In them I brought out a statement from the *New York Sun*, which is in the *Record* of the 17th that the present arrangement which is being carried out in Santo Domingo had the approval of the Senator from Wisconsin and the Senator from Massachusetts, both of whom are members of the Committee on Foreign Relations, or rather that those Senators having objected previously, acquiesced in it; in other words, that they advised with the President and surrendered their own convictions as to the inadvisability of his action there. The statement goes on to say that —

Mr. SPOONER. I have that here. The Senator need not worry himself about that.

Mr. TILLMAN. The Senator is not worrying himself about anything; but I was just trying to get the Senator to give us, if he will be so kind, the relationship between the Foreign Relations Committee and the President. He says they have nothing whatever to do with it, and yet the members of this committee of the Administration party are caught in the act of having something to do with it in advising and objecting and all that kind of thing, unless the Senator denies the statement. If he denies it, I am done with it.

Mr. SPOONER. I think the Senator will be done with it —

Mr. TILLMAN. I will be done with it anyway.

Mr. SPOONER. Because I will deal with that.

Mr. TILLMAN. Will the Senator pardon me for a little common-sense observation there?

Mr. SPOONER. I may wish to judge for myself as to the common sense of it.

Mr. TILLMAN. I claim it is common sense. I do not ask the Senator's indorsement of it as being common sense. I assert that it is common sense.

Mr. SPOONER. I must indorse it on that assertion.

Mr. TILLMAN. Very well. Granting the Senator's contention to be correct, and knowing, as the Senator must acknowledge, that a treaty or any agreement made by the President must be submitted to the Senate for ratification, and it is first referred to the Committee on Foreign Relations, and that committee's attitude will almost certainly decide its fate, I ask the Senator whether, as a matter of common sense, any President would not prefer to have the advice of his Senatorial friends — advice, the constitutional word " advice " — and has not the Senator given that advice in his relationship of leader in the Senate and a member of the Foreign Relations Committee and a personal friend of the President?

Mr. SPOONER. Is the Senator through?

Mr. TILLMAN. Yes; I am through for the time being.

Mr. SPOONER. I was about to say that being held down by constitutional obligations and by the rule of courtesy which prevails in the Senate, I feel bound to say that the Senator's question is a common-sense question —

Mr. TILLMAN. For which I am very deeply grateful.

Mr. SPOONER. Only as a matter of politeness.

Mr. TILLMAN. Then the Senator convicts himself of insincerity.

Mr. SPOONER. I do not.

The VICE-PRESIDENT. The Chair calls the attention of Senators to the fact that in speaking they must address the Chair. The Senator from Wisconsin will proceed.

Mr. SPOONER. Now, if the Senator from South Carolina will possess his soul in patience, I wish to hurry through.

Mr. TILLMAN. Do not be in too big a hurry lest we lose something nice.

Mr. SPOONER. I will in time reach the phase of the subject to which the Senator has been alluding.

The President is so supreme under the Constitution in the matter of treaties, excluding only the Senate's ratification, that he may negotiate a treaty, he may send it to the Senate, it may receive by way of "advice and consent" the unanimous judgment of the Senate that it is in the highest degree for the public interest, and yet the President is as free when it is sent back to the White House with resolution of ratification attached, to put it in his desk never again to see the light of day as he was free to determine in the first instance whether he would or would not negotiate it. That power is not expressly given to the President by the Constitution, but it inheres in the executive power conferred upon him to conduct our foreign relations, and it is a power which inheres in him as the sole organ under the Constitution through whom our foreign relations and diplomatic intercourse are conducted. Out of public necessity the President should be permitted to pocket a treaty, no matter if every member of the Senate thought he ought to exchange the ratification. Why? Because the President, through the ambassadors, ministers, consuls, and all of the agencies of the Government, explores sources of information everywhere, it is his business to know whether anything has occurred since the Senate acted upon the treaty which would render it for the public interest that the ratifications be not exchanged. And he is empowered to withhold exchange of ratifications, if upon later knowledge he deems it for the public interest so to do.

The conduct of our foreign relations is a function which requires quick initiative, and the Senate is often in vacation. It is a power that requires celerity. One course of action may be demanded to-night, another in the morning. It requires also secrecy; and that element is not omitted by the commentators on the Constitution as having been deemed by the framers of the most vital importance. It is too obvious to make elaboration pardonable.

We ratified the arbitration treaty unanimously, I believe. The President, in the exercise of the power which no one can dispute, pocketed it. The President may negotiate and sign a proposed treaty, and not send it to the Senate. In such case what would be thought of a resolution asking him to inform the Senate whether he had negotiated such a proposed treaty, and why he had not sent it to the Senate? Having sent a treaty to the Senate, he may withdraw it the next day.

Mr. President, the three great coordinate branches of this Government are made by the Constitution independent of each other except where the Constitution provides otherwise. We have no right to assume the exercise of any executive power save under the Constitution. We can not assume judicial functions. The President may not assume judicial functions. The President may not assume legislative functions. We as the Senate, a part of the treaty-making power, have no more right under the Constitution to invade the prerogative of the President to deal with our foreign relations, to conduct them, to negotiate treaties, and that is not all — the conduct of our foreign relations is not limited to the negotiation of treaties — we have no more right under the Constitution to invade that prerogative than he has to invade the prerogative of legislation.

Mr. MORGAN. If the Senator will allow me —

The VICE-PRESIDENT. Does the Senator from Wisconsin yield to the Senator from Alabama?

Mr. SPOONER. Certainly.

Mr. MORGAN. I wish to suggest to him that he is perhaps using the word "prerogative" in too broad a sense. I do not understand that the President has any prerogatives under the Constitution.

Mr. SPOONER. What is the power to pardon?

Mr. MORGAN. That is a power derived from the Constitution.

Mr. SPOONER. That begs the question.

Mr. MORGAN. It is not a prerogative of royalty.

Mr. SPOONER. Kings have the power of pardon, which is a prerogative of royalty. The Senator, however, is right in the last analysis. This is not a kingly government.

Mr. MORGAN. That is right.

Mr. SPOONER. In the most technical sense I cheerfully yield to him that this word is not a fit word for this atmosphere, but I have heard a thousand times talk here about the prerogatives of the Senate.

Mr. MORGAN. That was just a thousand times too many.

Mr. SPOONER. Strictly, I agree with the Senator.

The act creating the Department of State, in 1789, was an exception to the acts creating the other Departments of the Government. I will not stop to refer to the language of it or to any of the discussions in regard to it, but it is a Department that is not required to make any reports to Congress. It is a Department which from the beginning the Senate has never assumed the right to direct or control, except as to clearly defined matters relating to duty imposed by statute and not connected with the conduct of our foreign relations.

We *direct* all the other heads of Departments to transmit to the Senate designated papers or information. We do not address directions to the Secretary of State, nor do we direct requests, even, to the Secretary of State. We direct requests to the real head of that Department, the President of the United States, and, as a matter of courtesy, we add the qualifying words, "if in his judgment not incompatible with the public interest."

What does the conduct of our foreign relations involve? Does it involve simply, do Senators think, the negotiation of treaties? It involves keeping a watchful eye upon every point under the bending sky where an American interest is involved, where the American flag and citizens of the United States are to be found on sea and on land, every movement in foreign courts which might invade some American interest. It involves intercourse, oral and written, conferences, administrative agreements and understandings, not included in the generic word "treaty," as used in the Constitution. All treaties are agreements, but all international agreements and understandings are not "treaties." (See opinion Taney, C. J., in *Holmes* v. *Jennison,* 14 Peters, 570–573.)

Speaking of the power of the President under the Constitution over foreign relations, Mr. Justice McLean said (*Williams* v. *Suffolk Insurance Company,* 13 Peters, 415):

There can be no doubt that when the executive branch of the Government, *which is charged with our foreign relations,* shall in its correspondence with a foreign nation assume a fact in regard to the sovereignty of any island or country it is conclusive on the judicial department, and in this view it is not material to inquire, nor is it the province of the court to determine, whether the Executive be right or wrong. It is enough to know that in the exercise of *his constitutional functions he has decided the question.* Having done this under the responsibility which belonged to him, it is obligatory on the people and the Government of the Union. (See *Duran* v. *Hollins,* 4 Blatch., Circuit Court, 448, opinion by Mr. Justice Nelson.)

Professor Pomeroy, section 671, third edition, says:

The President is the sole organ of communication between our own and all other governments. Foreign ministers and ambassadors are accredited to him; to him they present their credentials and pay their formal official visits. The communications which they make, and the negotiations which they conduct, are, in fact, made and conducted to and with the Secretary of State, but only as that officer is the direct and personal organ of the President. All replies of the Secretary are supposed to be suggested by the Chief Magistrate, and he may, and doubtless often does, take an actual and leading part in the negotiation. Our own ministers are nominated by the President. When appointed they communicate alone with the Executive through the State Department. Instructions are sent to them, despatches forwarded, demands made, claims insisted on, principles adopted and enforced as the President deems proper. How far he will actually interfere with the Secretary of State, and how far leave that officer to the exercise of his own discretion, must depend upon his own sense of duty and propriety and the completeness of his own convictions.

SEC. 672. Over all these proceedings the Congress has absolutely no control. The correspondence and negotiations may be, and generally are, conducted secretly; and although it is customary for the President to communicate despatches to the legislature, this is never done until after their transmission, and, if necessary, they may be indefinitely withheld when the President deems that the public interests require it. Congress may pass resolves in relation to questions of an international character, but these can only have a certain moral weight; they have no legal effect; they can not bind the Executive. The necessity for this is evident. Negotiations generally require a certain degree of secrecy; one mind and will must always be more efficient in such matters than a large deliberative assembly. The President has thus intrusted to him a most momentous power, and one which he can not entirely delegate. Our foreign ministers must undoubtedly use their own judgment and discretion within narrow limits, but in all important matters hey receive definite and positive instructions from home. The magnitude of this function may be easily illustrated   The President can not declare war; Congress alone possesses this attribute. But the President may, without any possibility of hindrance from the legislature, so conduct the foreign intercourse, the diplomatic negotiations with other governments, as to force a war, as to compel another nation to take the initiative; and that step once taken, the challenge can not be refused. How easily might the Executive have plunged us into a war with Great Britain by a single despatch in answer to the demands of the British cabinet made in relation to the affair of the *Trent.* How easily might he have provoked a condition of active hostilities with France by the form and character of the reclamations made in regard to the occupation of Mexico.

I repeat that the Executive Department, by means of this branch of its power over foreign relations, holds in its keeping the safety, welfare, and even permanence of our internal and domestic institutions. And in wielding this power it is untrammeled by any other department of the Government; no other influence than a moral one can control or curb it; its acts are political, and its responsibility is only political.

SEC. 673. But the other branch of this Executive function — the treaty-making power — is even more important. The language by which this authority is conferred and described is peculiar. The President shall have power, by and with the advice and consent of the Senate, to make treaties, provided that two-thirds of the Senators present concur. All treaties made, or which shall be made, under the authority of the United States shall be the supreme law of the land. The President must, of course, take the initiative in making all treaties.

Congress, as such, has nothing to say in the matter. As a treaty is necessarily the result of negotiation, and as such negotiation is exclusively within the province of the President, the Senate having not the least authority to communicate with a foreign government, it is absolutely impossible for that body to dictate a treaty or to force the Chief Magistrate into any particular line of action. He must negotiate the treaty, make all the stipulations, determine all the subject-matter, and then submit the perfected convention to the Senate for ratification or rejection. They must take his finished work and approve or disapprove.

My friend from Georgia [Mr. Bacon] seemed to think it extraordinary and novel that the President in exercising this constitutional power to conduct our foreign relations, should send delegates or representatives to the Moroccan conference. Where can there be found any warrant for denying that right? I think the Senator did not deny the right. We have been engaged in conferences before.

Mr. BACON. Mr. President —

The VICE-PRESIDENT. Does the Senator from Wisconsin yield to the Senator from Georgia?

Mr. SPOONER. Certainly.

Mr. BACON. I do not desire to interrupt the Senator.

Mr. SPOONER. I have no objection.

Mr. BACON. I desire not to do so. I prefer to answer the Senator afterwards, if I have an opportunity, rather than to take it up by piece-meal. Therefore I only interrupt him in this instance because he suggests what he understands to be my position, and it will require some little more elaboration than to answer categorically. So I will not now interrupt the Senator, but I will endeavor, if I have the opportunity, to express as fully and as clearly as I can what is my exact position about this matter.

Mr. SPOONER. But I think I misstated the Senator's position. I must correct it. Of course, it was an inadvertence. The Senator did not deny the right of the President.

[At this point the expiration of the morning hour was announced by the Vice-President, and the unfinished business was laid aside temporarily.]

SPEECH OF SENATOR BACON [1]

MR. BACON said:

Mr. President: I have already addressed the Senate at some length upon the subject of the policy and propriety of sending delegates to the Algeciras Moroccan conference. It had not been my purpose to ask again the indulgence of the Senate upon this subject or upon questions which are nearly connected therewith. It has, however, happened that in the progress of the debate upon that subject and also on the subject of the Santo Domingo treaty certain propositions have been announced on the floor of the Senate and have been very earnestly and very ably discussed by learned and distinguished Senators, magnifying the powers of the President and minimizing the powers of the Senate, to which I can not give my assent and to which I ask the further indulgence of the Senate that I may make reply.

Before proceeding, Mr. President, I desire to say that in submitting an argument to-day on this subject I will endeavor to make it impersonal, because I consider it a very grave question, involving the relative rights and prerogatives of the President of the United States and of the Senate — a question important to be settled correctly and, if possible, without reference to partisan feeling or bias. I think I may possibly with propriety repeat what I have said upon a former occasion, that there is no justification for the statement which has been more than once made upon the floor of the Senate that the discussion of this question is in any manner an assault upon the present occupant of the executive chair. Legitimate and respectful discussion, not only of the rights and prerogatives of the Executive, but of the official acts of the Executive relating to questions of such rights and prerogatives, can not in any manner be construed into a personal assault, and it occurs to me, Mr. President, that the reiteration of the suggestion — to give it no stronger term — that such discussion is an assault upon the President — and sometimes stronger terms have been used — must imply a want of confidence in their own contention by those who seek to fortify their position by such suggestion.

The distinguished Senator from Wisconsin [Mr. Spooner] announces, as I understand him, the following proposition: That the negotiation of a proposed treaty and every phase of the work of considering and determining what shall be the subject and terms of a treaty are, up to and including the reaching of an agreement with a foreign power and until the proposed treaty is submitted to the Senate for final ratification or rejection, matters within the sole and exclusive right and power of the President; and that the jurisdiction of the Senate does not attach in any manner, and that no power or duty or right of the Senate begins until the President shall have negotiated a proposed treaty with a foreign power,

---

[1] *Congr. Record*, Feb. 6, 1906. Reported Feb. 12, 1906.

shall have agreed with the foreign power on the terms of the same, and shall have sent it to the Senate; and that for the Senate to attempt either by inquiry or suggestion to have part or lot in such work prior to the submission to the Senate, is an intrusion upon the exclusive domain and jurisdiction of the President of the United States.

As to whether or not he is correct in that construction of the powers of the President and the want of the power in the Senate, must depend upon the language of the Constitution of the United States. Fortunately, so much of the language of the Constitution as relates to that is within a very small compass; it is in one sentence. It is the second paragraph of the second section of the second article of the Constitution, and it is in these words:

He shall have Power, —

Speaking of the President of the United States —

He shall have Power by and with the Advice and Consent of the Senate to make Treaties, provided two-thirds of the Senators present concur.

That is all there is in the Constitution as to the power of the President to make treaties and as to the right and power of the Senate to participate in the work of making treaties.

Now, Mr. President, it will be seen that in that language the word "negotiate" does not occur. There is no separate, express grant of power to negotiate a treaty. It is necessarily true, however, that the power to negotiate a treaty is an implied power involved in that language; in other words, the power "to make" a treaty necessarily implies the power to negotiate a treaty. But there may be a very great difference in opinion as to what is the meaning of the word "negotiate," if we assume it and concede it to be an implied power found in that language. So far as the power to suggest a treaty to a foreign power is concerned, or to receive a suggestion from a foreign power that a certain treaty should be made, or to discuss with a foreign power the subject or the terms of a proposed treaty, undoubtedly the power to negotiate within that narrow limit is one which can only be exercised by the President, because he alone under this clause can have direct communication with the foreign power. No other officer or authority on the part of the United States can submit a proposed treaty to a foreign power. No other authority can discuss with a foreign power the terms of a proposed treaty, or come to a preliminary agreement with the foreign power regarding the same. Within this restricted sense the implied power to negotiate a proposed treaty is in the President alone.

But it is evident that the learned Senator in this discussion does not confine his understanding of the word "negotiate" to such narrow limits in defining the power of the President in the making of treaties. Evidently the Senator intends to include in the exclusive power to "negotiate" a proposed treaty, the exclusive power to do everything connected with the policy or impolicy of a treaty prior to its actual submission to the Senate for its ratification. In other words, the Senator's proposition is that under this implied power to "negotiate" everything in the way of consideration of the advantage or the disadvantage, or of the propriety or the policy of making a treaty, or of its terms, is a matter for the exclusive suggestion and deliberation and determination of the President, and that any suggestion or inquiry or advice on the part of the Senate prior to such submission is gratuitous and intrusive, and, as has been suggested, even insulting to the President. The radical and extreme position of the Senator in this regard is best understood when the fact is known that his utterance above quoted is caused by the introduction of a resolution asking information concerning the instructions given to the delegates appointed to the Algeciras conference. That resolution the Senator condemns as intrusive upon the exclusive jurisdiction of the President. According to the contention of the learned Senator, alone in the brain of the President, alone in his suggestion and deliberation, and alone in his judgment must be evolved and shaped up the policies and measures, which, if they become law, are to be the supreme law of the land.

According to that contention, the Senate has nothing to do with it — no concern, no right to consider, no right to be heard, no right to inquire, no right to advise — until the President shall have thus perfected it according to his judgment and submitted it to the Senate, to receive at its hands a perfunctory — often, I should say, a perfunctory — reply of "yes" or "no"; and according to that contention to proceed beyond that is an intrusion upon the exclusive domain and jurisdiction of the President.

Mr. President, that proposition is not sustained either by the letter or by the spirit of the Constitution or by the history of the treaty-making power as found in the history of the convention which framed the Constitution. On the contrary, they all, and the history as well of the adoption of this provision of the Constitution as found in the debates of the constitutional convention, combine to establish the proposition that in the making of treaties it is proper for the Senate to advise at all stages. Upon the very surface of it lies the oft-repeated suggestion that, if that were the case, the Constitution would limit itself to the term "consent."

Mr. Spooner. Limit itself to what?

Mr. Bacon. I say, if that were the correct construction, there is the oft-repeated suggestion that if it had been the intention of the framers of the Constitution to limit the action and function of the Senate solely to the power to ratify or to reject, the language of the Constitution would not have been "advise and consent," but the language would have been "consent," because there is no reason why the word "advise" should be given to add to or explain the meaning of the word "consent." We do not advise men after they have made up their minds and after they have acted; we advise men while they are considering, while they are deliberating, and before they have determined, and before they have acted.

As I have already said, Mr. President, there is no direct, express, separate grant of power to negotiate. The entire power is the power to make treaties; and yet the learned Senator would have us divide that power so that the term "to make" should be construed to mean, in the first place, in one division "to negotiate" and in another division "to conclude." But there is nothing in the words of the Constitution to justify any such division as that. It is one indivisible power "to make," and in the entire power "to make" the Senate is given full participation in advising and consenting.

The contention that the power of the President includes everything up to the time of the submission of the proposed treaty to the Senate might be sustained if the language of the Constitution were that "the President of the United States should have power to negotiate and, with the advice and consent of the Senate, to make treaties." Then it would indicate a separate function; then it would indicate a first division of the duty, to negotiate, the jurisdiction of which was confided entirely and solely to the President; and the second division, to make, one in which the President and the Senate together should act.

But the language of the Constitution is, "He shall have power, by and with the consent of the Senate, to make treaties," which plainly indicates not that the Senate should be limited to saying yes or no to a perfected and finished work when presented to it by the President, but rather the assistance of the Senate, the advice and coöperation of the Senate in the determination as to the propriety and policies of proposed treaties and also the terms and provisions they should contain. But the word "negotiate" is omitted before the words "to make." That is not an accidental omission. There was design in it. Aside from the fact that there is no ground upon which to predicate the suggestion that it was an accidental omission, the words used by the framers of the Constitution in the very next clause really only divided from it by a semicolon, prove that they were weighing carefully the language when they conferred the power upon the President of the United States. Separated from it only by a semicolon is this language — I will read the entire clause, part of which I have already read:

He shall have power, by and with the advice and consent of the Senate, to make treaties, provided two-thirds of the Senators present concur; —

Then follows the semicolon. Then the language proceeds:

and he shall nominate, and by and with the advice and consent of the Senate, shall appoint ambassadors, etc.

There it was the evidently distinct purpose to divide the duty and to confer in the first part of that division an exclusive function and jurisdiction upon the President of the United States:

He shall nominate, and by and with the advice and consent of the Senate, shall appoint.

Showing that the purpose was that up to the time it was submitted to the Senate, the Senate had no function in the matter of appointment; and that the function of the Senate was limited to advising and consenting to the nomination previously made by the President in the discharge of a function and of a jurisdiction exclusively confided to him.

Can it be said that the framers of the Constitution of the United States in writing a clause, or two parts of the same clause, were careless in the use of language when they were conferring the great power of treaty making; that they intended to say that the President should have the exclusive function up to the time of the submission of the treaty to the Senate, and that the duty and the power of the Senate, as the Senator from Wisconsin has said, should only begin when the President had so done, and that they used this language as found in the Constitution, leaving to be implied only the construction contended for; and then thereafter, in the less important matter of the appointing of officers, should have been critical in the use of language, leaving nothing to implication, and should have said "he shall nominate," and then added "and thereafter" — I interpolate the word "thereafter" — " and thereafter, by and with the advice and consent of the Senate, shall appoint"? Mr. President, it is incredible.

*   *   *   *   *   *   *   *

The Senator from Wisconsin in his argument said that the President was supreme — he used the word "supreme" — in the making of treaties to the extent that even after a treaty was submitted to the Senate and ratified by the Senate, the President could put it in his pocket and not promulgate it or exchange ratifications.

No doubt that is true, and in the same way when the President sends a proposed treaty to the Senate, the Senate, if it sees proper to do so, can treat it without any attention whatever and not even refer it to a committee. It would not be seemly to do so, but no more so than for a President to be likewise heedless and regardless of the views of the Senate in reference to the propriety or the policy of making a proposed treaty in a matter touching vitally the interests and the institutions of the country. It would be not less unseemly for him to reply to an inquiry or suggestion of the Senate, "Hands off."

In what particular is the power of the President thus to put a treaty ratified by the Senate in his pocket more supreme than the power of the

Senate to bury in its archives' without action a proposed treaty sent to it by the President? I am not detracting from the President or his power; I concede to him his full constitutional power; but I deny the proposition that the President has any superior power or any superior dignity in the making of a treaty over and above the Senate.

Mr. BEVERIDGE. Suppose the Constitution had been silent upon the question of the treaty-making power, where would that power have lodged? Or I will put the question in this way: Suppose the Constitution had said nothing about making treaties, would not the complete power of making treaties have been in the President, under section 1 of Article II, which lodges the executive power in the President?

Mr. BACON. I think not. I do not understand the word "executive" to mean anything of the kind.

Mr. BEVERIDGE. Does not the Senator think that in the natural division of the powers of Government into legislative, executive, and judicial the treaty-making power has always been considered an executive function, and, therefore, if the Constitution had been silent upon the subject of treaties, it would have been completely under the President's control, under that provision of the Constitution which confides in the President the executive power, and that that section concerning treaties is merely a limitation upon that universal power?

Mr. BACON. Oh, no. The Senator has gone to his favorite doctrine as to extraconstitutional power, which I will not stop to discuss with him to-day. The two continents, separated by the Atlantic Ocean, are not wider apart than the Senator and I upon the subject of the exercise of powers not found in the Constitution.

Mr. BEVERIDGE. If the Senator will permit me —

Mr. BACON. I can not discuss it to-day. It would take all my time.

Mr. BEVERIDGE. I will ask the Senator to answer this question: Since the Constitution has said nothing about —

Mr. BACON. The Senator has asked that question, and he does not let me answer before repeating it. The Senator will pardon me, but he has already asked it twice.

Mr. BEVERIDGE. I will ask this question: If the Constitution had said nothing about the treaty-making power, where would the treaty-making power have been lodged?

Mr. BACON. I have received that question from the Senator several times. I have said that I did not agree with him that it would be with the Executive.

Mr. BEVERIDGE. Where would it be?

Mr. BACON. I think, undoubtedly, in the legislative branch of the Government, for reasons which I will give.

Mr. BEVERIDGE. That is the whole question.

Mr. BACON. Here is where the sovereignty of the Government was intended to be in almost its totality — in the legislative branch of the

There it was the ꜒
confer in the first pr
diction upon the Pr꜒

He shall nominate,
shall appoint.

Showing that the
to the Senate, the S꜒
and that the functi꜒
senting to the non
discharge of a func
him.

Can it be said tha꜒
in writing a clause, ꜒
use of language wh꜒
making; that they ꜒
exclusive function u꜒
Senate, and that th꜒
from Wisconsin has
done, and that the꜒
leaving to be impli꜒
thereafter, in the l꜒
should have been cr꜒
plication, and shoul
"and thereafter" —
after, by and with t꜒
Mr. President, it is

*   *

The Senator fron
was supreme — he
treaties to the exten꜒
and ratified by the S
promulgate it or ex꜒

No doubt that is
a proposed treaty t꜒
treat it without an꜒
mittee. It would ꜒
President to be lik꜒
Senate in reference
treaty in a matter
the country. It w꜒
quiry or suggestion
In what particul꜒
ratified by the Sena

꜒ in it, recognizing the delicacy of
꜒at treaty were well understood by
꜒ by members of the Senate before
꜒ to Sir Michael Herbert.
꜒ that time? Was he carrying out
꜒n? Was he engaged in the per-
꜒vailing himself of a valuable instru-
꜒in the interchange of politeness?
꜒permit me to make an inquiry of

꜒conceive ꜒ ꜒ction between
꜒te, if b ꜒ Senators,
꜒ a bod꜒ ꜒e are
꜒ power꜒
꜒e to remark ꜒
꜒d necessarily wo꜒
꜒he Senator is sim꜒

꜒ute to my intelligen꜒
꜒onsider it a tribute t꜒
꜒directly where the S꜒
꜒he going straight in

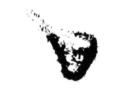

the Senate as a body, (individual Senators
dent their advice as to a)roposed negotiation,
y as a body volunteering ieir advice, especially
t to do so?

will answer the Senatordefinitely. I do not
ı, and I will tell him the :ason why.

ır the Secretary of State eher — say, the Presi-
sks a Senator what he thirs about the proposi-
ınd such a treaty, and wht he thinks as to the
corporated in that treaty, e does not ask that
as he asks Mr. Jones or Ir. Smith, whom he
' '·ɔnue, in order thatɪe may have the ad-
˜ ɔ man ɑ whose intellectual
heasks him because of
: makes the Senator
nselor in the mak-

nt, if that is truᴖ,   ʰing which
:lusively within his cɔ.   ·ʳ which
ich he alone can get thᴖ   ¹ɔes
ᴄonstitutional provisio ɯ.   ʹ
ᴅenefit?
ɪ₦ʷʰᵎˡᴑ ᵎ· ·   Sₑₙ

hat wɪᴎᴖ | ★
ɳate would appɪᴖ   ₦.
vance, of what it ᴅᴇ|ᴖ.
Can it be proper for t!
ıt as to the policy or i.
ɪe improper to ask for :¹·
: counsel? Where is thᴖ ʲ
it be proper to advise thᴖ ʲ
negotiating a treaty where ı.
to and where the suggestion oɪ.

Government, and the vast array of powers in the first article of the Constitution prove it; and, further than that, the Constitution of the United States was intended to take the place of and to supersede the Articles of Confederation, under which articles the power to make treaties did lodge in Congress alone; and it was not to be presumed when the Constitution was formed, in the absence of some special and particular designation, that it was the intention to confer it upon the Executive. The presumption would be the other way.

I was about to say, however, at the time of the interrogatory propounded to me by the learned Senator, in concluding what I had to say on the history of this matter, that President Washington in one of his messages casts a very strong light upon the question as to what was the estimate which this convention had of the treaty-making power and of the duty and function which the Senate should exercise in the treaty-making power. In a famous message, which the Senator from Wisconsin cited and which has been cited frequently and with which we are all familiar, where President Washington refused to send certain papers to the House of Representatives upon its demand, upon the ground that the House of Representatives had nothing to do with treaties, and that the Senate alone was the body with which he was to deal, the Senate alone was the body which had the right to ask of him information, the Senate alone was the body which had the right to share with him the secrets connected with foreign affairs, stated this fact:

It is found in his message. He said not only was the treaty-making power confided in part to the Senate, but, speaking as he did and as he said, as a member of the convention and familiar with what had been done and said there, he added that there was a very strong effort made not only to require that two-thirds of the Senate present should agree to a treaty, but that two-thirds of the entire Senate, whether present of not, should be required before a treaty could be put into effect. There could scarcely be stronger evidence than is found in this historical fact of the supreme estimate which was placed by the convention on the importance that the Senate should be the controlling influence in determining whether or not any given treaties should be made with foreign countries.

Mr. President, we have often had cited the fact that Washington during his Administration met personally with the Senate to advise as to the making of treaties. He had been present during all the deliberations of that Convention; he was president of the Convention which made the Constitution; he had heard all the deliberations; he had doubtless in personal interviews canvassed this matter and discussed it with members of the Convention, and the fact that he met personally with the Senate, the fact that he conferred personally with the Senate as to the propriety of making treaties before attempting to negotiate them, show what he understood to be the intention of the Convention — that the Senate should be not simply the body to say yes or no to the President when he proposed a treaty, but that the Senate should be the adviser of the President whether he should attempt to negotiate a treaty. What possible doubt can there be under such circumstances as to what was his understanding of the purpose and intention of those who framed the Constitution? And what possible doubt can there be that his understanding was correct?

Mr. President, it is true that that practice has been abandoned, so far as concerns the President coming in person to sit in a chair on the right of the presiding officer to confer with members of the Senate, as our rules still provide he shall do should he come here personally, showing we recognize the propriety of his coming and his right to come. But nevertheless during my official term it has been the practice of Presidents and Secretaries of State to confer with Senators as to the propriety of negotiating or attempting to negotiate a treaty.

I know in my own experience that it was the frequent practice of Secretary Hay, not simply after a proposed treaty had been negotiated, but before he had ever conferred with the representatives of the foreign power, to seek to have conferences with Senators to know what they thought of such and such a proposition; and, if the subject-matter was a proper matter for negotiation, what Senators thought as to certain provisions; and he advised with them as to what provisions should be incorporated.

I recollect two treaties in particular. One is the general arbitration treaty. I do not know whether he conferred with all Senators, but I think he did. I think he conferred with every Senator in this Chamber, either in writing or in person, as to the general arbitration treaty. He certainly conferred with me.

Mr. SPOONER. Who did?

Mr. BACON. Mr. Hay. He certainly conferred with me, not only once but several times, and I presume he did the same with other Senators, not simply as to the question whether a treaty should be negotiated, but as to what provisions should be incorporated in it. I am sorry to say that while agreeing with the purpose in view I could not agree with some of the provisions incorporated in that particular treaty, and he went on and the treaty was formulated with which in all particulars I did not agree. But I am simply speaking of the fact that he conferred with Senators before he formulated a treaty, not simply before the President sent it here, not simply before it was negotiated with Sir Mortimer Durand and the ambassadors of other countries, but before it had been formulated.

Then, as to another, I recollect distinctly the Alaskan treaty. Time after time and time after time Mr. Hay, then Secretary of State, conferred with Senators, and, I presume, with all the Senators, as to the propriety of endeavoring to make that treaty and as to the various pro-

visions which should be incorporated in it, recognizing the delicacy of
the situation, and the provisions of that treaty were well understood by
members of the Senate and approved by members of the Senate before
it was ever formulated and submitted to Sir Michael Herbert.

But what was Mr. Hay doing in all that time? Was he carrying out
the contemplation of the Constitution? Was he engaged in the performance of a high duty? Was he availing himself of a valuable instrumentality, or was he simply engaged in the interchange of politeness?

Mr. SPOONER. Will the Senator permit me to make an inquiry of
him?

Mr. BACON. With pleasure.

Mr. SPOONER. Does the Senator conceive of no distinction between
consultation by the Secretary of State, if he so wills it, with Senators,
and the participation of the Senate, as a body, the thing of which we are
speaking, as a part of the negotiating power?

Mr. BACON. The Senator leads me to remark what I said to a Senator yesterday, that the Senator's mind necessarily works more rapidly
than another man's tongue can. The Senator is simply anticipating
what I was coming to on that point.

Mr. SPOONER. That is a high tribute to my intelligence.

Mr. BACON. On the contrary, I consider it a tribute to me, that the
logical sequence of the question is directly where the Senator put it,
and that I had been so fortunate as to be going straight in that direction.
So I can take it as a compliment to myself.

I will, however, now take the subject which I was about to discuss
otherwise, just in the form in which the Senator puts it, because it is
practically the same as that which I had intended.

The Senator asked me this question: Do I draw no distinction between the voluntary action of the Secretary of State endeavoring to get
the opinion of the Senator or of myself and the act of the Senate seeking — I do not know whether I am correctly quoting him; if not, the
Senator can correct me — to proffer to the State Department or to the
President advice unasked? Is that the question?

Mr. SPOONER. Well, yes; substantially —

Mr. BACON. That is the way I understood it.

Mr. SPOONER. Although I want the Senator to understand that I
have not questioned the right of the Senate —

Mr. BACON. I know; but the Senator asked me a question. Let us
discuss that afterwards.

· Mr. SPOONER. To offer its advice, either in public or in private.

Mr. BACON. I do not understand the Senator's question.

Mr. SPOONER. The question I put to the Senator was this: If he
did not recognize a distinction, from the standpoint of the matter of constitutional power, between the President — leave out the Secretary of
State — asking individual Senators their judgment as to a proposed

treaty, and his inviting the Senate as a body, or individual Senators volunteering to the President their advice as to a proposed negotiation, and the action of the body as a body volunteering their advice, especially if they asserted the right to do so?

Mr. BACON. Well, I will answer the Senator definitely. I do not recognize the distinction, and I will tell him the reason why.

When the President or the Secretary of State either — say, the President, to simplify it — asks a Senator what he thinks about the proposition to negotiate such and such a treaty, and what he thinks as to the specific terms to be incorporated in that treaty, he does not ask that Senator that question as he asks Mr. Jones or Mr. Smith, whom he happens to meet upon the Avenue, in order that he may have the advantage of advice and assistance from a man in whose intellectual processes and capacity he has confidence, but he asks him because of the fact that the Constitution of the United States makes the Senator his adviser, his constitutional, official adviser and counselor in the making of treaties.

Now, Mr. President, if that is true, is that advice something which the President has exclusively within his control? Is it something which he can ask, and which he alone can get the benefit of in case he does ask, or is it a great constitutional provision which makes it a reciprocal right for a common benefit?

Can it be said that while it is proper for Senators or the Senate to respond when advice is asked, it is improper, under the constitutional provision, to volunteer such advice? It is undoubtedly true that the President alone determines whether he will approve and act upon the advice of the Senate, just as the Senate determines whether it will or will not approve a proposed treaty. But can it be contended that the Senate, although the constitutional adviser of the President, can only give advice when asked for it, and that it is an intrusion to proffer it when thus not asked for it? Where is the warrant in the Constitution for such contention? That it has not been so recognized by the President or by the Senate is shown by the fact that it has frequently happened that resolutions have frequently been passed by the Senate informing the President that the Senate would approve a treaty for a given purpose. Can it be said that while proper to thus notify the President, in advance, of what the Senate would approve in a treaty, it is improper to notify him also, in advance, of what it deprecates, if it is proposed to embody it in a treaty? Can it be proper for the Senate to offer advice or counsel to the President as to the policy or impolicy of a proposed treaty, and at the same time improper to ask for the information upon which to base such advice or counsel? Where is the logic or such a contention?

Again, can it be proper to advise the President as to the desirability and policy of negotiating a treaty where he has not taken any action relative thereto and where the suggestion originates with the Senate, and on the other hand be improper to advise him of the undesirability and impolicy, in the opinion of the Senate, in a case where it is reliably learned through other sources that he has begun to take or has taken action relative thereto? Where does the Senate get power to amend a treaty if its authority is limited to consenting to what the President has done? When the Senate has amended a proposed treaty and the President thereafter submits the amendment to the foreign power for its consideration, has not the Senate taken part in the negotiation of that treaty?

If the contention is correct that the jurisdiction and power of the Senate do not begin until the proposed treaty is sent to the Senate, then none of these things are proper, and to make an inquiry of the President relative to a proposed treaty is an intrusion upon his exclusive jurisdiction. If the contention is correct, it matters not what may be the well-understood purpose of an Executive in negotiating a treaty or in sending delegates to a conference, the Senate is dumb until it receives a proposed treaty. It may be, as forcefully suggested by the Senator from Maine [Mr. Hale] a few days ago, that the proceeding tends inevitably to war, and yet it will be an intrusion for the Senate to even make an inquiry of the Executive concerning the same.

Again, the Executive may, without ever sending any proposed treaty to the Senate, continue to send delegates to European international political conferences, and in time practically destroy our recognition of the long-established doctrine of non-entanglement by us in such disputes. After having taken an active part by our delegates in the Algeciras conference, no proposed treaty may be submitted to the Senate. Nor is that all in sight. We are told in the press despatches that European questions concerning the Balkan States are again becoming acute; that there is great tension, and that another European war cloud is gathering in the East. Doubtless there will be another conference to deal with that situation and determine the relative rights and powers of the war lords of Europe. To that, according to the new doctrine, it will again be in order to send delegates from the United States. And after having taken an active part in the deliberations of the conference, again no proposed treaty may be sent to the Senate. And although in attending each of these conferences by our delegates tremendous strides will have been taken in establishing precedents and in destroying the doctrine of an hundred years against entanglements in European international disputes, still in the absence of any proposed treaty submitted, the Senate must be dumb, and it is an intrusion to even make an inquiry of the President in the interest of the preservation of the cherished policies of our country. Mr. President, I can not subscribe to such a doctrine.

It seems to be somewhat remarkable that there should be such extreme sensitiveness about the Senate assuming to advise as to the "negotiation" of a treaty, when it seems to be entirely proper for "advice" to be given by the President to Senators as to how they should vote on the question of the ratification of a treaty.

Mr. SPOONER. If the Senator will permit me, does he think if the President asked a Senator's advice as to whether a treaty should be negotiated or not, the Senator is under any constitutional duty to give it, or would be committing a breach of Senatorial duty if he declined to advise in advance?

Mr. BACON. If the Senator declined?

Mr. SPOONER. If the Senator declined. The Senator speaks of reciprocal rights. He says the President has the right to ask a Senator for his advice as to whether any foreign policy shall or shall not be pursued in the matter of negotiating a treaty. To test that, does the Senator think if the President has a right to ask it —

Mr. BACON. Ask the question now.

Mr. SPOONER. The Senator, I should think, ought to have a reciprocal duty to answer.

Mr. BACON. I think so, undoubtedly.

Mr. SPOONER. Does the Senator think the Senator is obliged to answer?

Mr. BACON. Undoubtedly he may not be able to give it. He may say, "I have not the information; I have not made up my mind." But for the Senator to say, "I have an opinion, but I will not give it to you," would, in my opinion, be a contravention of his constitutional duty. There is but one possible ground upon which a Senator could base any such refusal, and that is, if he were to say (and I do not think he would be correct in that), "I recognize that this is an act which should be performed by the Senate as an organized body and not by myself in my official individual capacity, and therefore I decline to give any individual opinion." That is the only ground upon which he could put it, and I do not think that would be a correct ground.

Mr. SPOONER. Would it not be an eminently proper and wise ground for the Senator to take that the people were entitled to his independent judgment on the question as to whether a treaty should be ratified or not by the Senate after it had been negotiated and submitted to the Senate?

Mr. BACON. I ask the Senator to please repeat his question.

Mr. SPOONER. Would it not be entirely proper and wise and almost a duty for a Senator to say, "I decline to commit myself as a Senator in advance to a proposed treaty. I prefer to wait until the power of negotiation, which the Constitution lodges in the President, shall have been put forth and the Senate is in possession of the instrument, so that I can read it, study it, have the advantage of debate upon it among my associates, and then give to it the independent judgment to which the people are entitled from every Senator?"

I doubt myself, and I have had some experience, the wisdom of a Senator committing himself blindly to a foreign policy, to end in the negotiation of a treaty, to find himself later, when the negotiation is ended and the document is laid before the Senate, halfway (which with an honorable man means a great way) committed, and committed too early and too hastily.

Mr. BACON. The Senator asks me the abstract question whether or not I consider it to be the constitutional duty of a Senator to give advice to the President as to the propriety of the making of a treaty before it has been sent to the Senate. I answer in the affirmative. The Senator goes on to say that no Senator ought to give blindly his advice. I quite agree with him, as I have intimated before. A Senator may decline to give the advice upon the ground that he has not had the proper time for making up his mind satisfactorily to himself, or for other good reason.

But, Mr. President, advice means also counsel. Advice means more than giving simply the statement of what the Senator thinks ought to be done. It means counsel; and, therefore, while the Senator might say to the President, "I am not in a position to make up my mind definitely as to what ought to be done," the President would then proceed to counsel with him and suggest such and such a condition of affairs and such and such remedies which might be applied, with a view to arriving at a conclusion as to what would be the proper thing to do. Then, I say if the Senator would turn his back on the President and say, "I decline to counsel with you or to hear your suggestion or to confer with you as to what is the proper thing to be done," while, of course, it would be a matter of conscience for each Senator, from my point of view the Senator would be derelict in so doing.

Now, Mr. President, I am not certain whether I had fully answered the inquiry of the Senator from Wisconsin [Mr. Spooner] or not. He is present, and if I have not, I hope he will call my attention to it. My attention has been so diverted I am really not certain whether I completely replied to his interrogatory. But before leaving it I wish to say in a general way that according to my view of the treaty-making power, of the duty of the President, and of the duty of the Senate, it is a reciprocal and a common duty, one in which each has the advantage of the services of the other, one in which there is, perhaps, no compulsion, one in which each can defeat the work of the other, one in which the coöperation and combination of the two from the inception to the end is necessary in order to fully comply with the intention and design of the Constitution makers in this regard.

The Senator from Wisconsin, in order to accentuate and emphasize the fact that the President of the United States sat away up on a pedestal above us in all matters which related to treaty making, except the simple matter, as he himself expressed it, of "ratification," because he translates the words "advice and consent" as meaning in the common parlance "ratification," the Senator, I say, in order to emphasize that fact, goes further, and in the clauses of his speech which I have already read he puts up as the supreme power, the supreme controller in all foreign affairs, the President of the United States. The President, according to the Senator from Wisconsin, in all of our foreign affairs is supreme. And, Mr. President, he lays down the proposition with much emphasis, and says that that is — I am not quoting the words now, but the substance — practically conceded by every man who has ever studied the Constitution. He asserts this so broadly and so emphatically that for one to assert the contrary is to recognize in advance that in so doing he, according to the Senator, puts himself out of the pale and class of reputable lawyers. Yet, Mr. President, at the risk of being thus debarred, I want to analyze a little bit the powers conferred by the Constitution with reference to foreign affairs, and see whether they rest with the President alone or whether, in the main, they rest with Congress, and with the Senate in conjunction with the President.

It is true, Mr. President, that in the countries antedating our Government the executive, who was almost universally a king — I believe little Switzerland was the only exception at that time, and I am not sure that it was at that time, because it has had varying fortunes, and I have forgotten whether at that particular time it was a republic or not — but almost universally the executive of a nation was a king, and he did have, among other kingly powers, all control over foreign affairs. But, Mr. President, when our Constitution came to be framed there was particularly and definitely withheld from the executive every important foreign function, according to my view of it. I know in one particular the Senator differs from me, but in all others he will agree. It took away from the Executive, with the exception of the treaty-making power, all power over foreign affairs. It made him, in the language the Senator used the other day, the organ of intercommunication with foreign nations. It made him the spokesman for the Government. It made him the person to discuss with foreign governments, to make demands, if you please, on foreign governments, to guard so far as watchfulness goes, the interest of our country and of our citizens in foreign lands. But when it came to action, when it came to the power to do anything, that power was expressly conferred upon Congress, or upon the President in conjunction with the Senate.

What is the most important of all foreign relations? Why, the most important of all foreign relations is the relation of peace and war. Can the President declare war? Can the President prevent a declaration of war? The President not only can not declare war, and it is not only conferred in terms upon Congress, but even if the President should be opposed to a proposed war, two-thirds of each Branch can declare war. It would not require his approval. There is the most important of all foreign relations. It does not belong to the President. Nor can the

President alone make peace. He can only do so with the cooperation of the Senate.

The question of commerce is certainly an important matter of relation between two countries, and yet the President has no power over commerce with foreign nations. The power to regulate commerce is not simply withheld from the President, but it is expressly conferred upon Congress; and the subsidiary question as to what shall be the terms upon which the merchandise of a foreign country shall come to this country is a question largely important in foreign relations, and is one over which the President of the United States has no power. It belongs, under the Constitution, to the lawmaking power; and that lawmaking power can be exercised by Congress not only without the consent of the President, but over his objection.

The terms upon which foreign ships shall be allowed to enter our ports or do business with us is an important one in our foreign relations, but the power to fix and determine them is altogether with Congress.

The question as to whether or not citizens of another country shall be allowed to come to this country, and if so, upon what terms, is an important question of foreign relations; and yet the President has no power to control it. It is a question exclusively within the lawmaking power. The question whether this country will permit any of a certain nationality to come at all to this country is a question not with the President, but a question with the lawmaking power.

Nay, sir, the question whether this Government will hold any relations with a foreign country is a question with Congress. It is entirely within the competency of Congress to pass a law that no citizen of a given country shall come to this country, that no goods shall be received from it, that no merchandise shall go from this country to it, that no letters shall come from it, that there shall be no intercommunication of any kind whatever. Who doubts the power of Congress to do so?

In other words, it is within the power of Congress to absolutely sunder the relations between this country and any given foreign country. When that is said the whole thing is said; when that is said the whole argument is exhausted as to where rests the supreme power in foreign affairs, because the whole must include every part. If it is within the power of Congress to absolutely sunder all relations of every kind, commercial, social, political, diplomatic, and of every other nature, it is certainly within the power of Congress to regulate and control every question subsidiary to that and included within it. Congress and not the President is supreme under the Constitution in the control of our foreign affairs.

Now, Mr. President, there is but one question about which there is even any controversy as to the power of the President over foreign relations, and that is the one about which the Senator and myself have differed for years, and about which I presume we will continue to differ. It is as to the right of the President of the United States to finally recognize or finally refuse to recognize the independence of a revolutionary or rebellious country.

Of course, time does not permit me now to discuss that question at length. I have heretofore discussed it in the Senate, and while I am not very fond of labor, if the time shall ever come when that question is *per se* discussed, I shall endeavor to take my part in it, for it is a most interesting and important question. It is a matter to me of the strongest and most absolute conviction as a legal proposition. Of course, I do not question at all that where it is a question as to what is the *de facto* government in a fully independent country, that is a question which is practically determined by the President of the United States in the recognition of diplomatic relations, but where a country is in a condition of rebellion, which has asserted its independence and is endeavoring to establish its independence, and where the parent country is denying its independence and is by the force of arms endeavoring to put down the rebellion or the insurrection, to say that the President of the United States solely and alone can determine finally that question for this country, and that Congress has no power over it, is a matter to me absolutely without the domain of logic. I say in every act of that kind, the supreme power, the final power of decision, is with Congress, the lawmaking power, and whatever is done by the executive department in that regard is necessarily subject to the revision and control and reversal of the lawmaking power.

Why, Mr. President, we have seen in the papers that a province of Russia some month or two ago rebelled and set up an independent government, or, rather, professed to do so. We have heard nothing of it lately. I presume it has been suppressed. Suppose in a case of that kind, not this President, but any President, had taken upon himself to say, "I recognize that province as an independent government." To claim that that would have been a final, conclusive act on the part of the Government of the United States, and that Congress would in such case have no right or power to reverse the decision and save the country from war with Russia, is something to me, I say, beyond the possibility of comprehension. But I will not go into that argument now, because I know I would necessarily enter upon a field which in itself would be larger really, or as large, as the main one upon which I am now engaged in this discussion.

Mr. SPOONER. Will the Senator allow me to ask him a question?

The PRESIDING OFFICER (Mr. McCumber in the chair). Does the Senator from Georgia yield to the Senator from Wisconsin?

Mr. BACON. Certainly.

Mr. SPOONER. The Constitution gives to the President the power to receive ambassadors and ministers. Does the Senator think that the action of the President in the exercise of that function is subject to the control of Congress?

Mr. BACON. I have not the slightest doubt in the world that Congress, in such a case as I have just mentioned, could pass a law and send that ambassador back to the country from which he came.

Mr. SPOONER. What sort of a law would that be? I am not talking now about declaring war or severing diplomatic relations.

Mr. BACON. It can be done that way.

Mr. SPOONER. What sort of an act would be that instruction to the President to send the ambassador back?

Mr. BACON. I do not suppose that the President would need any instruction more than the law.

Mr. SPOONER. But what law?

Mr. BACON. The act —

Mr. SPOONER. What form of law?

Mr. BACON. The act which should be passed by Congress.

Mr. SPOONER. What would be the form of such a law in a general way?

Mr. BACON. Simply to say we would not have an ambassador at all from that country, because we did not recognize it as an independent country. That is the act of Congress I have in mind when I say it would control the President and reverse his decision recognizing that province as an independent nation.

Now, as to whether or not Congress should say to the President of the United States, You must not receive John Jones, or William Smith, or any other particular man from any particular country. Of course nobody contends Congress could do that. That is not the question at all. It is the question whether in the case where a country, or part of a country in rebellion to the mother country sets up a professed or pretended independent government and sends an ambassador to this country, the reception by the President of the United States of that ambassador is a conclusive and final determination on the part of the Government of the United States that henceforth there shall be no question but what that is an independent country so far as the recognition of this country is concerned. My reply to the Senator is that if such an ambassador were sent, Congress would have it within its power to pass a law that it would not recognize that country as an independent country, and that it would continue as in the past to recognize it as a part of Russia, for instance, and when that law was passed it would be the duty of the President to give that ambassador his passports and no longer recognize him or any other as an ambassador from that pretended government.

* * * * * * * *

Mr. BACON. Compared to this great array of sovereign powers granted to Congress, those conferred upon the President present a most striking contrast. He is clothed with the great power and responsibility of the execution of the laws, but beyond this the only prerogative of sovereignty with which he is exclusively invested is the pardoning power, and even that is denied to him in cases of impeachment by the House and conviction by the Senate.

We have passed by more than two hundred years the period in the history of our race when one man could assume and exercise the power to determine, independently of the legislative department, what should be, even in part, the laws of the Government. The framers of the Constitution stood nearer by a hundred years than we do to the time when a King sought to rule without Parliament and in defiance of Parliament; when he sought to take to himself all the powers of government and set at naught the laws of the country's constitutional legislators. The great and wise men who framed our fundamental law stood in the century next removed from that which had witnessed the culmination of that great struggle from the events of which they gathered the lesson that the material interests and the liberties of a people are safest when the great powers of government are lodged not in the control of one man, of whatever title or office, but in the hands of their elected representatives.

They had learned from it that one man invested with such powers was quick to consider his own fortunes and the fortunes of his favorites of more consequence than the prosperity of the whole people. They were taught by that history to fear that one so girt with power would grow great in his own conceit; that he would attempt to draw to himself all the authority of Government, and that not only one born to the kingly office, but also one who held but temporarily the elective office of President, might come to think himself compassed with —

The divinity that doth hedge a king.

While they hoped that only good and wise men would be chosen to that high office, they forgot not the frailties of the weak nor the grasping ambitions of the strong. They guarded against the worst. They designed that in the hands of a weak Executive the Government should not fail, and that in the hands of one strong, self-willed, and ambitious there should not be imperiled the free institutions which they sought to establish. Therefore, while they created a great and noble office, one within its legitimate sphere the greatest and noblest of all the earth, they designed that its greatness and nobility should not consist in the arbitrary powers of the kingly office.

The greatness of the Presidential office does not consist in his will being the law to 80,000,000 people, but in the fact that the President in himself personifies the will of a great and free people as that will is expressed by them through another department of the Government. No man can shut his eyes to the fact that to that end, while they invested the President with all the great dignity and power of the Executive office, they carefully withheld from him the grant of the powers of sovereignty. Every power given to him was most carefully restricted and guarded.

While they gave him the power of the veto, they gave the Congress the power to override his veto by a two-thirds vote of each House.

While they gave him the power to make treaties with foreign nations, by and with the advice of the Senate, they refused to him the power to make such treaties without their sanction.

They gave him power to pardon those convicted of crime, but denied to him the power to pardon in cases of impeachment.

They gave him the power to appoint all civil officers, but except temporarily, when Congress is not in session, such appointments are of no validity until confirmed by the Senate.

They made him Commander in Chief of the Army and Navy, but they left it to Congress to determine what should be the size and constitution of the Army and Navy, and whether there should be any Army and Navy. They denied him the power to appoint a single officer of either the Army or the Navy, from the commanding officers to the lowest subalterns, unless each of such appointments should receive the confirmation of the Senate. They gave him no power to equip and maintain either Army or Navy for a day. They gave him no power to make war, nor can he of himself conclude peace. The power to make rules for the government and regulation of the Army and Navy is denied to him and is expressly conferred upon Congress. It is evident that as Commander in Chief of the Army and Navy he is but the Executive arm, and that in that capacity he is himself, in every detail and particular, subject to the commands of the lawmaking power.

Finally, they made the Chief Executive, as well as every other civil officer, from the head of the Cabinet to the most obscure civil official, subject to trial and removal from office, without appeal, upon impeachment by the House and conviction by the Senate — a power, in much conservatism and wisdom, but seldom exercised, but nevertheless a power, resting as it does, without defined limits as to what shall be deemed a high crime or misdemeanor, almost exclusively in the discretion of the House and Senate, which is the great safeguard against encroachment and official misconduct.

Mr. President, the fact is not to be disguised that the actual exercise of power by the executive branch of the Government in this day far exceeds the bounds originally contemplated for it by the Constitution. The correspondence in relative position of a president in a republic, and of a king in a monarchy; the glamour of a great office in which one man among 80,000,000 is chosen as the sole head of a great department of the Government, while in the other departments the honors are divided among many; the gigantic measure of patronage and removal, where he seems to have unlimited power to bestow, or to withhold, or to take away —⋅ these and other influences combine to elevate in the popular mind the prerogatives of the President far above the point designed for them in the Constitution.

It is a remarkable fact that in England, a monarchy, the constant progress has been toward restraint of executive power and the enlargement of the power of the legislative branch of the Government, until now practically all political power is in the control of the elected representatives of the people. It is a fact still more remarkable that in the United States, designed distinctively as a representative republic, there has been a no less steady progress in the direction of the absorption of power by the Executive and of its practical surrender by Congress.

Mr. President, Senators are concerned and solicitous about the alleged encroachment of the legislative branch, or of the Senate in its executive capacity, upon the powers of the Executive; but it seems to me there is very much more reason why they should be concerned about the invasion by the executive department of the power conferred in the very first sentence of the Constitution of the United States. What is that first sentence, found in Article I, section 1?

All legislative powers herein granted shall be vested in a Congress of the United States, which shall consist of a Senate and House of Representatives.

Mr. BEVERIDGE. Will the Senator permit me to interrupt him right there?

The VICE-PRESIDENT. Does the Senator from Georgia yield to the Senator from Indiana?

Mr. BACON. I will yield; but I want to comment upon what I have just read.

Mr. BEVERIDGE. It is merely to call the attention of the Senator to the first section of Article 2 of the Constitution, which says that —

The executive power shall be vested in a President of the United States of America.

Mr. BACON. Who doubts that?

Mr. BEVERIDGE. Nobody doubts it; but the Senator is arguing against it.

Mr. BACON. No; I am not.

Mr. BEVERIDGE. The Senator said the President had no other power than a limited treaty-making power and the power to see that the laws were faithfully executed.

Mr. BACON. I consider that latter an executive power.

Mr. BEVERIDGE. Certainly it is one of the executive powers; but does the Senator say it is all of the executive power?

Mr. BACON. I say that is the generic meaning of the word "executive." The Senator has diverted me from what I was saying. I want to go back. I will say to the honorable Senator that, when I have finished, if he desires to revert to that branch of the argument, I will return to it with pleasure, provided the Senate has the patience and can be induced to listen to it.

Mr. BEVERIDGE. I regret that I diverted the Senator. I merely wanted to place immediately parallel with his statement about the legislative powers being vested in Congress, which nobody denies, the statement that the executive power is vested in the President of the United States, which nobody denies; and that "executive" powers include the power to make treaties, so that anything said in the Constitution about the making of treaties is not so much the conferring of power as the limitation of power. If nothing had been said about treaties in the Constitution the power to make them, absolute and unlimited, would have been in the President under the grant to him of "executive" powers, would it not?

Mr. BACON. I will not stop to discuss that matter now. I confess that I can not see the pertinency of the Senator's suggestion. If he will permit me to proceed I will simply say to him that the word "executive" comes from the verb "to execute," and it means one who is to execute the laws of the government. He is an executive officer and not a legislative officer. I have just read this section of the Constitution, and I read it again after the interruption in order that it may be in proper connection.

All legislative powers herein granted shall be vested in a Congress of the United States, which shall consist of a Senate and House of Representatives.

Is that the law to-day? It is the law on the book, but who will say that the legislative power of this Government is exercised in the two branches of Congress? Who does not know that the most influential part of the legislative power of the Government is at the other end of the Avenue — in the White House? I am not speaking only of the present occupant, although I think he is doing his full share of it; but it has been so in all Administrations in greater or less degree within a generation. The Executive has encroached continuously upon the legislative branch of the Government, and it has never been more pronounced in its encroachment than it is to-day.

Why, the time was when one who desired legislation by Congress came to Congress, and with proper or improper means, if you please — certainly with proper means — endeavored to influence Congress in the enactment of certain legislation. How is it to-day? Who is it that wants legislation who comes to the House of Representatives or to the Senate? We see every day in the newspapers accounts of pilgrimages to the White House for the purpose of securing legislation; we see every day in the newspapers forecasts as to whether or not such and such legislation will be passed or can not be passed, according as it may be announced that it will receive the support or the active opposition of the Executive.

Absolutely, Mr. President, I saw within the past few days an explanation given that the stock market had gone up or down — I have forgotten which — in consequence of the announcement of the position of the Executive as to a proposed piece of legislation which would affect prices. And I have seen statements in the papers that Members of Congress had gone to the White House to solicit the aid of the President to secure the passage of certain desired legislation. More 's the pity!

Well, Mr. President, as I say, it is not only this President, nor the last one, nor the one before, but it has been going on and increasing for more than a generation. It is better that Senators and Representatives should concern themselves about the question as to whether or not their own prerogatives and rights and powers are being encroached upon rather than be supersensitive as to whether or not in the assertion of our own powers we may be overstepping the mark. Of course, we ought not to transgress the limits set to our powers by Constitution, not by a hair's breadth, but our particular and special duty is to preserve and protect against encroachment our own rights and our own powers in this matter.

Mr. President, the time will come, if this thing continues and increases, when the question of the attitude of Senators and Representatives with reference to any proposed legislation will not be an important matter, and when it will be well understood that such and such legislation is to be enacted or defeated, as the case may be, regardless of the personal views of Senators and Representatives. When that time comes members of each House will cease to discuss measures, because of the absolute uselessness of it. Only "Administration measures" will be enacted, and none others will be attempted from very hopelessness.

* * * * * * * *

So, Mr. President, if things continue to progress, it may happen — I think, though, it will be a long time before it does, because our disposition is different from theirs, and such subjection and such servility it is impossible to conceive will ever come to the American people — but in practical result it will be so that the question of what this Congress shall do, in any important matter will be a question not decided by their own judgment or the judgment of a majority, but decided by other influences. It is largely so now. More and more the idea will be that, excepting "Administration measures," the only business of Congress is to pass appropriation bills and then disperse. It is notorious right now that most important subjects of legislation, such, for instance, as the revision of the tariff, are receiving no attention, and the question whether Congress will or will not legislate on them depends solely on whether they will or will not be made "Administration measures." That is openly and undisguisedly now recognized in the case of the question of the revision of the tariff.

There can be no condition more dangerous to the maintenance of free government than is found in the concentration in the hands of one man at the same time of both the executive power and practically the power to make the laws he is to execute. Whatever may be the form of government, when these two powers are thus concentrated in the hands of one man the government where that condition exists is an autocracy pure and simple. It makes no difference in practical effect whether that one man himself decrees the laws or whether they are enacted in obedience to his dictation.

Mr. BACON. I am opposed to the United States Government attending conferences which are in essence and in fact political conferences as to European international matters and where the other pretended interests are mere devices and shams for the purpose of disguising the fact of our presence there.

Mr. SPOONER. Well, Mr. President, that is the Senator's view, and he is entitled to it. He frankly states it. I am in favor of a proposition which goes beyond that. I am in favor of the United States attending any conference to which it is invited by European nations which involves in any degree our interests — first, to look after our interests, and, second, to use the kindly offices and the influence and power of the United States to prevent war between foreign governments at friendship with us. I am not afraid, as the Senator seems to be; I am not distrustful of the present President of the United States ——

Mr. BACON. Now, Mr. President ——

Mr. SPOONER. Nor am I distrustful, Mr. President, of anyone who is to succeed the present President. Taking our history from the beginning to this day, we have had Presidents of exceptional prudence and skill in the conduct of our foreign relations; we have had Secretaries of State admirably fitted, with here and there possibly an exception, for the discharge of the delicate functions involved in the discharge of the duties of their office. I think the Presidents hereafter and the Secretaries of State hereafter will know quite as well as the Senator from Georgia or any who are to follow us here whether the interests of the United States demand our representation at a foreign conference and how far we may go as a nation, our interests having been conserved, in the employment of our power and influence and friendship to prevent war between other nations. I put but one limitation, Mr. President, upon the exercise of the constitutional power of a President in that respect, and that is that we shall not attend any conference, for full participation in it, which would involve us to the extent of war or the incurring of international hostility; and I believe I speak in this respect the sentiments of our people. They are not afraid to go abroad; they are not afraid to sit in foreign assemblages, to participate in foreign conferences, not under the limitations put by the Senator from Georgia, which eliminates all such conferences, but on the broader ground and with the larger limitation which I put upon them. So much for that.

Mr. President, I admit — to come back to what I wanted to say to the Senator — his contention that the Senate may in open session, so far as the power goes, adopt a resolution such as he introduced. I challenge its propriety. I admit, as he contends, that it is entirely within the constitutional capacity of the Senate to adopt in executive session a resolution asking the President to inform the Senate whether he is negotiating a treaty, if you please, with Great Britain or with Germany, to advise the Senate upon what subject and with what view he is carrying on the negotiation, to advise the Senate as to its progress — I grant all that. · That is not in controversy at all. But what I assert is, that it in no wise binds the President. He may give the information or he may refuse to transmit it. He may refuse to transmit it upon the ground that its transmission would be to the detriment of the public interest ——

Mr. BACON. Will the Senator pardon me right there?

Mr. SPOONER. Wait a moment until I finish the sentence.

Mr. BACON. Very well.

Mr. SPOONER. Or he may refuse to transmit it, and may give no reason, if he shall so choose, for his declination. In other words —

Mr. BACON. Mr. President —

The VICE-PRESIDENT. Does the Senator from Wisconsin yield to the Senator from Georgia?

Mr. BACON. I will wait until the Senator finishes his sentence.

Mr. SPOONER. Mr. President, what I contended, and what the Senator, I think, has not at all weakened is that, as a matter of power, it is entirely in the hands of the President, uncontrolled and uncontrollable, either by the Senate or by both Houses of Congress.

Mr. BACON. Now, Mr. President, if the Senator will pardon me just a moment, I want to say that when we come to talk about a question of power, we mean that we are discussing constitutional powers — the exercise of constitutional powers — we are not talking about physical power or actual power; we are talking about the legal right when we are talking about power.

Mr. SPOONER. Legal right?

Mr. BACON. Legal right, or legal duty, if it is not a legal right.

Mr. SPOONER. Call it that.

Mr. BACON. But what I rose to say to the Senator was this: The Senator will read again, as I know he has read heretofore, the message, to which I alluded in the remarks which I submitted this morning, of President Washington to the House of Representatives, where he declined to furnish them with certain information which they called for. I am not speaking now as to what the President can do, but what he ought to do, and what is recognized in him as proper to do. President Washington said, that while he refused to communicate it to the House, and gave as a reason that such things ought frequently to be kept secret, yet in that case he said it should be communicated to the Senate. He recognized the Senate. He did not say that it should be withheld, but he said the secret should be shared by the Senate with the President.

Of course I recognize the fact that the question of the President's sending or refusing to send any communication to the Senate is a matter not to be judged by legal right, but a question which has always been recognized as one of courtesy between the President and this body, and which the Senate — except, perhaps, in the case in which the Senator took a very notable part and to which I have had occasion heretofore to allude — has always yielded to the judgment of the President in the matter and has never made an issue with him about it.

Mr. SPOONER. I go beyond that.

Mr. BACON. But any resolution which I have introduced could have been easily answered by the President to the effect that, in his opinion, it was not compatible with the public interest; but the Senator and those who thought with him never allowed it to get to him.

Mr. SPOONER. If we had adopted the Senator's resolution, introduced in public, cabled to every court in Europe, coming from a distinguished member of the Committee on Foreign Relations of this body, which is a part of the treaty-making power, and the President had communicated to the Senate in secret session, how would the matter have stood abroad? If we had been honorable men and observed the obligation of secrecy, the communication of the President would have been confined to members of this body; outside there would have been this implied arraignment of the President, or disgust of the President, either as to his power or as to his wisdom, *with no reply whatever from the President.*

Mr. BACON. As it happened in this case, though, the State Department gave it out that there was no cause for secrecy and that anybody who went there could see it.

Mr. SPOONER. That is not what I am talking about.

Mr. BACON. A good many have gone there and have seen it. I have not.

Mr. SPOONER. I am talking upon the principle. The Senator says "legal right" or "legal duty." I admit that we have a right to pass resolutions calling for any information from the President; but does the Senator say it is the legal duty of the President to send it?

Mr. BACON. I do not dispute the fact that there may be occasions when the President would not.

Mr. SPOONER. Who is the judge?

Mr. BACON. The President, undoubtedly. Nobody has ever controverted that; and the very resolution concerning which the Senator is animadverting was expressly conditioned upon the President viewing the transmission of the information requested as being compatible with the public interest.

Mr. SPOONER. Mr. President, it all comes to an entire corroboration by the Senator of the proposition which I made the other day, and which I supposed he had spent some time in attacking, that in the last analysis, so far as the question of constitutional power and constitutional duty is concerned, it is absolutely in the President. He is the sole organ of communication by this Government with foreign governments. At his option he may consult the Senate in advance or he may not. At his option he may send information requested or he may not.

The Senator is mistaken when he says that all there is upon that subject in the Constitution is that line of the sentence which gives the President the power, by and with the advice and consent of the Senate, to make treaties. That is not all there is in the Constitution upon which I rely to sustain the proposition that under our system the President is the sole organ of negotiation and of communication between this country and foreign governments. Under the Confederation the Congress was the sole organ; the Congress negotiated treaties and ratified treaties; the Congress received ambassadors and ministers, and the Congress practically sent ambassadors and ministers.

That was all changed when the Constitution was adopted. It was not changed for any idle reason. It was changed because it was found to be an inherent, elemental, and terrific weakness in the Confederation; and so, Mr. President, when the Constitution was formed they gave to the President, by and with the advice and consent of the Senate, the power to make treaties. That is not all. They vested in the President alone the power to receive ambassadors, ministers, and other diplomatic agents. That is not all. They vested in him the power to appoint, subject to the advice and consent of the Senate as to the person only, ambassadors, ministers, etc.

A foreign minister or ambassador comes to this country. We have no function to perform in relation to his reception. He presents his credentials to the President. The President receives him or not as he may decide. Can Congress compel his reception or prevent his being received by the President? I never heard that contended until the Senator intimated it this afternoon.

Mr. BACON. Mr. President, on the contrary, I said exactly the reverse. I said this ——

Mr. SPOONER. The Senator said they could be sent away by order of Congress.

Mr. BACON. The Senator pressed me on that and asked me how it was done. I said the Congress could sunder the diplomatic relations between this country and another, and that that would be the law; but I expressly said that where relations were existing between the countries, so far as the recognition of a particular ambassador was concerned, or another ambassador, that was in the power of the President. If the Senator will notice the stenographic report, he will find that is exactly what I said.

Mr. SPOONER. Could the framers of the Constitution any more clearly have made the President the sole organ of communication between this Government and foreign governments than they did? Of course, the power to receive an ambassador or a foreign minister implies necessarily the power to determine whether the government or country from which he comes is independent and entitled to send an ambassador or a minister. So the President is authorized to determine, and he must determine, when he sends an ambassador or a minister to some other country, whether that country is an independent country, a member of the family of nations, entitled to be represented by an ambassador or minister here and entitled to receive an accredited ambassador or minister from this country. When the ambassador or the minister has any communication to make in relation to foreign affairs, he does not make it to the Senate. If it be in the negotiation of a treaty — and most treaties are negotiated here — he has no communication with the Senate. We will not tolerate that ambassadors or ministers or diplomatic agents from other countries shall communicate in any way with the Senate or with the committees of the Senate.

Mr. BACON. The Senator says that with very great earnestness. Does the Senator understand that anybody has ever suggested such a proposition?

Mr. SPOONER. The Senator implies that almost of necessity ——

Mr. BACON. Oh, no.

Mr. SPOONER. When he argues that under the Constitution the Senate as an executive body is as much a factor in the negotiation of treaties as is the President or is any factor at all in negotiation.

Mr. BACON. Yes; with its own peculiar functions to perform. That does not imply that —

Mr. SPOONER. If the Senator does not mean that, then the Senator does not mean anything by his proposition.

Mr. BACON. The Senator is mistaken; the Senator is not justified in that statement.

Mr. SPOONER. Because to say that the Senate is as much a factor under the Constitution in negotiating treaties as the President —

Mr. BACON. I did not say that.

Mr. SPOONER. Then I misunderstood the Senator.

Mr. BACON. I said in the making of treaties, and I distinctly denied that the making of treaties was confined to the function which would succeed the transmission of that treaty to the Senate.

Mr. SPOONER. Mr. President, I certainly am not mistaken. The whole point of the speech, which I had the honor of making the other day, and which the Senator has attacked — was my contention that in the *negotiation* of treaties the President is absolutely supreme and independent of the Senate.

Mr. SPOONER rose.

Mr. BACON. Pardon me a moment. But that if the Senator meant to include in the term "negotiation" not only that, but everything which related to the framing of the treaty the determination of its terms, and everything else up to the time when it was sent to the Senate, then his definition of the term "negotiation" was too broad, and I denied that the President had exclusive right in it; but so far as the term "negotiation" could be limited to its being the organ of communication and of discussion and of original suggestion, if you please, to the foreign power, I granted the Senator's position.

Mr. SPOONER. What does the Senator understand by the negotiation of a treaty as contradistinguished from the making of a treaty; dividing the negotiation of the treaty from the point of jurisdiction of the Senate over the treaty?

Mr. TILLMAN rose.

Mr. SPOONER. If you please, one at a time.

Mr. BACON. I said that the Senator's position was that "negotiation" included everything up to the time the treaty was sent to the Senate; I said that "negotiation" was a term which was implied under the term "make"; that the making of a treaty included the entire operation by which a treaty was conceived and framed and brought to its conclusion, and as to all such matters, even before it was submitted to a foreign power, while it was under consideration as to whether there should be a treaty and what its terms should be — that that was a part of the making of a treaty and not a part of what technically the Senator calls the "negotiation of a treaty."

Mr. SPOONER. It would be nonsense, Mr. President, to talk of the President *negotiating* a treaty and yet of his not having the absolute power to reduce to writing the terms agreed upon at the end of his negotiation. He must have something to lay before the Senate. Is the signing of the treaty a matter that the Senate has anything to do with? Until the President is through the Senate's function does not begin.

I admit that the Senate may ask to be informed as to the state of the negotiation. The Senate may ask to be informed whether the treaty has been reduced to writing or not. The Senate may ask the President to inform it as to its terms. It may request him to send a copy in order that it may advise him, if it wants to do it, that it should be signed or not, or whether it should be amended before being signed. But the President has the same right to refuse to do it that the Senate has to request it.

Mr. BACON. Yes.

Mr. SPOONER. That has been the practice since the State Department was created by the first Congress under the Constitution.

Mr. BACON. That does not change the fact.

Mr. SPOONER. What can the Senate do in the way of negotiating a treaty or reducing it to writing or signing it? Will the Senator tell me?

Mr. BACON. That is the smallest splitting of small hairs.

Mr. SPOONER. I can not split it so fine that the Senator cannot see it.

Mr. BACON. The question is not as to matters of detail; as to whether every "t" is crossed and every "i" is dotted ——

Mr. SPOONER. I did not say that.

Mr. BACON. Or even as to the drafting of it. The question is whether the President has in the Senate advisers whom he can bring to his assistance before he submits a treaty to the Senate, or whether the Senate is in a position where, in a case in which it thinks there is a public interest requiring its intervention, it has the right to suggest to him and to advise with him voluntarily, without his request, or whether, as the Senator says in the speech from which I have read to-day, that no right of the Senate attaches and no duty of the Senate begins until the President sends in his message. There is a vast difference between the two.

Mr. SPOONER. Will the Senator tell me what power the Senate has to intervene in the negotiation of a treaty by the President up to the time of its signing?

Mr. BACON. That is the very point I was trying to bring to the attention of the Senator when I tried to differentiate between power, in the sense of a man who can go and compel a thing, and a legal right, as contemplated by the law. The law contemplates that the Senate shall be the adviser of the President, not simply after he has sent us a treaty, but at any time, either at the instance of the President or at the will of the Senate, in no instance having the power to compel the President to formulate, as they see fit to suggest, in the same way that the President has no power to compel the Senate to consent to it. Each of them is supreme in their respective functions.

Mr. SPOONER. If the framers of the Constitution had intended to make the Senate a potential factor in the negotiation of treaties, they would have done it.

Mr. BACON. I think they have done it.

Mr. SPOONER. They would not have left the President entirely at liberty to refuse the Senate any participation, even to the extent of informing the Senate, in response to a courteous request, of the state of the negotiations or the subject-matter of a proposed treaty. They would have given the Senate the right to *demand*, not to request. They would have made it the duty, not compellable by mandamus — no, no; they would have made it the sworn duty of the President to respond to the request for information. They did neither, Mr. President. It would have been a breach of constitutional duty for the President to refuse information which under the Constitution the Senate had a right to demand, and the President would have been answerable on the complaint of the other House. Had they intended not to invest the President with the absolute power of the negotiation of treaties, they would have made the Senate's power efficient. They would not have made it a mere question of "If you please, Mr. President, the Senate would like to be informed of the status of the negotiation, if any exists, between this country and Great Britain." They never would have left it in that way.

Mr. BACON. The Senator forgets that the only power to negotiate is a power implied by the power to make, and that the Constitution, in conferring the power to make, confers it upon two and not upon one.

Mr. SPOONER. But implied powers are as perfect as expressed powers.

Mr. BACON. If the Senator will permit me, he might as well say, as to the failure of the Constitution to give the power of compulsion upon the President, that there was equal failure in the omission to give the President power to compel the Senate to ratify. The one is as logical as the other.

Mr. SPOONER. Not at all. The Senator asserts a relation under the Constitution between the Senate and the President in respect to the negotiation of treaties which he can not sustain, or he imputes a purpose to the framers of the Constitution which they have not expressed, and which they have not in anywise, even by inference, made apparent.

Mr. BACON. There is where we differ. I think it is very evident that the Senator and I are not going to agree.

Mr. SPOONER. In one clause of the Constitution — and the Senator remarked upon that — the *nomination* of a person for office is separated from the "advice and consent of the Senate." It could not have been otherwise. It would have been quite absurd for the framers of the Constitution to have said that the President and the Senate might "appoint" officers. That would have left it open to debate as to who should take the initiative. It would have been unenforceable for its looseness and its stupidity. Some one must select the official. That, of course, being an executive function, was given to the President. That had to be done before the Senate could "advise and consent" to the appointment. That in the very nature of things was a condition precedent. How does the other differ? The Senator saw a difference in the language of the two provisions, in that in the one case they drew the line between the nomination and confirmation; in the other they did not.

The Senator forgot that negotiation is of necessity antecedent to the making of a treaty, as completely as the nomination of an officer is precedent to his confirmation or final appointment. It is clear as the sunlight that the framers of the Constitution intended the President should negotiate the treaty, for he is the organ of communication with foreign governments. They gave that power to no one else, and the Senate could not advise and consent to the treaty *until it had been negotiated and signed and laid before it.* Somebody must do that preliminary work. If it is not given to the President, it is given to no one. It was given to the President. He has done it from the foundation of the Government. No one has ever challenged it. The Senate, to my knowledge, never has demanded a right to participate in the *negotiation* of treaties. Whenever the President has consulted the Senate it has been entirely in the exercise of an option which the Constitution gives him. He may exercise it or not. He keeps his oath to support and defend the Constitution as faithfully in the one case as in the other. The great sage of Democracy, Mr. Jefferson, did not agree with the Senator from Georgia or the Senator from South Carolina ——

Mr. TILLMAN. Will not the Senator allow me to quote him?

Mr. SPOONER. I hope the Senator from South Carolina will please not interrupt me at this point.

Mr. TILLMAN. I have the words of the sage right here, and I want to give you some of his utterances.

Mr. SPOONER. Have you? Read them.

Mr. TILLMAN. Thank you. I have been waiting half an hour here endeavoring to give some light to my friend the Senator from Wisconsin, and, perhaps, the Senator from Massachusetts.

Mr. SPOONER. I can get light from Thomas Jefferson on this question.

Mr. TILLMAN. You did not think I had this book here, over a hundred years old, and was going to give my own views?

Mr. SPOONER. I thought it was a new edition of the Constitution, revised, amended, and annotated by BENJAMIN R. TILLMAN, of South Carolina.

Mr. TILLMAN. BENJAMIN R. TILLMAN knows some little about it. He has learned it from his friend the Senator from Wisconsin. I read:

[Mr. Jefferson, Secretary of State, to Mr. Morris, minister plenipotentiary from the United States to France.]

PHILADELPHIA, August 23, 1793.

DEAR SIR: The letter of the 16th instant, with its documents accompanying this, will sufficiently inform you of the transactions which have taken place between Mr. Genet, the minister of France, and the Government here, and of the painful necessity they have brought on of desiring his recall. The letter has been prepared in the view of being itself, with its documents, laid before the executive of the French Government. You will, therefore, be pleased to lay it before them, doing everything which can be done on your part to procure it a friendly and dispassionate reception and consideration. The President would, indeed, think it greatly unfortunate were they to take it in any other light, and therefore charges you, very particularly, with the care of presenting this proceeding in the most soothing view, and as a result of an unavoidable necessity on his part.

Mr. SPOONER. Is that all?

Mr. TILLMAN. Oh, no.

Mr. SPOONER. Will the Senator give me some idea as to how long he will take?

Mr. TILLMAN. Just long enough to give you some light; that is all.

Mr. Genet, soon after his arrival, communicated the decree of the National Convention of February 15, 1793, authorizing their Executive to propose a treaty with us on liberal principles, such as might strengthen the bonds of good will which unite the two nations; and informed us in a letter of May 23 that he was authorized to treat accordingly.

This, you see, was written in August.

The Senate being then in recess —

Now listen, please —

The Senate being then in recess and not to meet again till the fall, I apprised Mr. Genet that the participation in matters of treaty, given by the Constitution to that branch of our Government —

That is, the Senate — .

would, of course, delay any definitive answer to his friendly proposition. As he was sensible of this circumstance, the matter has been understood to lie over till the meeting of Senate. You will be pleased, therefore, to explain to the Executive of France this delay, which has prevented as yet our formal accession to their proposition to treat; to assure them that the President will meet them, with the most friendly dispositions, on the grounds of treaty proposed by the national convention, as soon as he can do it in the forms of the Constitution; and you will, of course, suggest for this purpose that the powers of Mr. Genet be renewed to his successor.

Now, just one comment and I will let you off.

Mr. SPOONER.   I have the light the Senator intended to give me.

Mr. TILLMAN.   I am very glad he got it, but the point I wanted to illustrate is this: Jefferson, who was certainly familiar with the opinion of the makers of the Constitution — more so than the Senator from Wisconsin — and who was Washington's Secretary of State, recognizes here the principle that the Senate is such an important part of the treaty-making power that he does not feel willing even to enter upon negotiation with the minister from France until the Senate reconvenes.

Mr. SPOONER.   That all shows that Mr. Jefferson was a very skillful, adroit, and accomplished diplomat.   •

Mr. TILLMAN.   Just like my friend the Senator from Wisconsin.

Mr. SPOONER.   That was a paper which Mr. Jefferson wrote for the eye of the French Government as to a proposed treaty which Mr. Jefferson then did not desire to enter into and which Mr. Jefferson never did enter into.

But I have a few sentences here from Mr. Jefferson. I do not know whether it will be any "light" to the Senator from South Carolina, but in Mr. Jefferson's Opinion on the Powers of the Senate, a very celebrated document, which he gave at the request of the President, this language was used:

The transaction of business with foreign nations is *executive altogether*. It belongs, then, to the head of that department, except as to such portions of it as are especially submitted to the Senate. *Exceptions are to be construed strictly.*

That is what Mr. Jefferson said on this precise question in a carefully prepared opinion for the guidance of the President, whose Cabinet officer he was. To give the opinion was a part of his official duty under the Constitution. I put that against that adroit, diplomatic letter for the *eye of the French Government*.

He says another thing on the subject of the powers of the Senate:

The Senate is not supposed, by the Constitution, to be acquainted with the concerns of the executive department. *It was not intended that these should be communicated to them.*

SENATOR HOAR ON DIPLOMATIC APPOINTMENTS[1]

[The following selection from Senator Hoar's autobiography deals with the practice, sometimes resorted to, of appointing Senators to important though temporary diplomatic positions.]

THE President has repeatedly, within the last six years, appointed members of the Senate and House to be Commissioners to negotiate and conclude, as far as can be done by diplomatic agencies, treaties and other arrangements with foreign Governments, of the gravest importance. These include the arrangement of a standard of value by international agreement; making the Treaty of Peace, at the end of the War with Spain; arranging a Treaty of Commerce between the United States and Great Britain; making a treaty to settle the Behring Sea Controversy; and now more lately to establish the boundary line between Canada and Alaska.

President McKinley also appointed a Commission, including Senators and Representatives, to visit Hawaii, and to report upon the needs of legislation there. This last was as clearly the proper duty and function of a committee, to be appointed by one or the other branch of Congress, as anything that could be conceived.

The question has been raised whether these functions were offices, within the Constitutional sense. It was stoutly contended, and I believe held by nearly all the Republican Senators at the time when President Cleveland appointed Mr. Blount to visit Hawaii, and required that the diplomatic action of our Minister there should be subject to his approval, that he was appointing a diplomatic officer, and that he had no right so to commission Mr. Blount, without the advice and consent of the Senate. President McKinley seemed to accept this view when he sent in for confirmation the names of two Senators, who were appointed on the Commission to visit Hawaii. The Senate declined to take action upon these nominations. The very pertinent question was put by an

[1] From the Autobiography of Senator Hoar, II, 48–51; published by Scribner's Sons, N. Y., 1905.

eminent member of the Senate; if these gentlemen are to be officers, how can the President appoint them under the Constitution, the office being created during their term? Or, how can they hold office and still keep their seats in this body? If, on the other hand, they are not officers, under what Constitutional provision does the President ask the advice and consent of the Senate to their appointment?

But the suggestion that these gentlemen are not officers seems to me the merest cavil. They exercise an authority, and are clothed with a dignity equal to that of the highest and most important diplomatic officer, and far superior to that of most of the civil officers of the country. To say that the President can not appoint a Senator or Representative postmaster in a country village, where the perquisites do not amount to a hundred dollars a year, where perhaps no other person can be found to do the duties, because that would put an improper temptation in the way of the legislator to induce him to become the tool of the Executive will, and then permit the President to send him abroad; to enable him to maintain the distinction and enjoy the pleasure of a season at a foreign capital as the representative of the United States, with all his expenses paid, and a large compensation added, determined solely by the Executive will; and to hold that the framers of the Constitution would for a moment have tolerated that, seems to me utterly preposterous.

Beside, it places the Senator so selected in a position where he can not properly perform his duties as a Senator. He is bound to meet his associates at the great National Council Board as an equal, to hear their reasons as well as to impart his own. How can he discharge that duty, if he had already not only formed an opinion, but acted upon the matter under the control and direction of another department of Government?

The Senate was exceedingly sensitive about this question when it first arose. But the gentlemen selected by the Executive for these services were, in general, specially competent for the duty. Their associates were naturally quite unwilling to take any action that should seem to involve a reproof to them. The matter did not, however, pass without remonstrance. It was hoped that it would not be repeated. At the time of the appointment of the Silver Commission, I myself called attention to the matter in the Senate. Later, as I have said, the Senate declined to take action on the Commission appointed to visit Hawaii. But there was considerable discussion. Several bills and resolutions were introduced which were intended to prohibit such appointments in the future. The matter was referred to the Commission on the Judiciary. It turned out that three members of that Committee had been appointed by President McKinley on the Canadian Commission. One of them, however, said he had accepted the appointment without due reflection, and he was quite satisfied that the practice was wrong. The Committee disliked exceedingly to make a report which might be construed as a

censure of their associates. So I was introduced to call upon President
McKinley and say to him in behalf of the Committee that they hoped
the practice would not be continued. The task I discharged. President
McKinley said he was aware of the objections; that he had come to feel
the evil very strongly; and while he did not say in terms that he would not
make another appointment of the kind, he conveyed to me, as I am very
sure he intended to do the assurance that it would not occur again. He
said, however, that it was not in general understood how few people
there were in this country, out of the Senate and House of Representatives, qualified for important diplomatic service of that kind, especially
when we had to contend with the trained diplomatists of Europe, who
had studied such subjects all their lives. He told me some of the difficulties he had encountered in making selections of Ministers abroad,
where important matters were to be dealt with, our diplomatic representatives, having, as a rule, to be taken from   ly different pursuits
and employments.

That Congress in the past has thought it   and rather than
restrict this prohibition is shown by the statu   bids, under
severe penalty, members of either House of Co   represen
the Government as counsel.

`HE SENATE

'A voluminous ... ~en produced in rent ... the United
~s Senate. T ... s been largely crital ... the temper
~tion of this ... tive body. The ... ~rticles here
ced will gi ... ' the discussion. ... ~resentative
~ritten by ... nd importance ... ~osition to
e Senate ... 'on. The read ... ~ form his
of the ... r of senatori ... the many
Senate ... ~ this colle

T. ... ' TH ... N OU ... 1ENT '

... EN ... D W

... th ... George
~COR ... vas the
~gtoi ... poured
~o w. ... ramers
me. ... to be
... ~ging,
... ~lieve
... Sen-
... re-
... ost
... ~n
... ~-

censure of their associates. So I was introduced to call upon President McKinley and say to him in behalf of the Committee that they hoped the practice would not be continued. The task I discharged. President McKinley said he was aware of the objections; that he had come to feel the evil very strongly; and while he did not say in terms that he would not make another appointment of the kind, he conveyed to me, as I am very sure he intended to do, the assurance that it would not occur again. He said, however, that it was not in general understood how few people there were in this country, out of the Senate and House of Representatives, qualified for important diplomatic service of that kind, especially when we had to contend with the trained diplomatists of Europe, who had studied such subjects all their lives. He told me some of the difficulties he had encountered in making selections of Ministers abroad, where important matters were to be dealt with, our diplomatic representatives, having, as a rule, to be taken from entirely different pursuits and employments.

That Congress in the past has thought it best to extend rather than restrict this prohibition is shown by the statute which forbids, under a severe penalty, members of either House of Congress from representing the Government as counsel.

V

THE SENATE

[A voluminous literature has been produced in recent years upon the United States Senate. This literature has been largely critical, censuring the temper and action of this important legislative body. The three general articles here reproduced will give a good idea of the discussion. They are representative articles written by men of standing and importance, men also in a position to judge of the Senate by direct observation. The reader will be able to form his own opinion of the quality and temper of senatorial action from the many extracts from Senate debates contained in this collection.]

THE PLACE OF THE SENATE IN OUR GOVERNMENT [1]

By Henry Litchfield West

ACCORDING to a tradition, more or less authenticated, it was George Washington who remarked that the Senate of the United States was the saucer into which the hot tea of the House of Representatives was poured to cool. Some idea of this kind was certainly in the minds of the framers of the Constitution. Madison suggested that the Senate ought to be so constituted as to protect the opulent minority against the changing, irresponsible, and turbulent majority. Hamilton, who did not believe that the voice of the people was the voice of God, would have had Senators appointed for life. More than one of the Constitution-makers referred to the Senate as the Privy Council of the President; and, almost without exception, they regarded it as the brake of conservatism upon the wheels of national legislation. They found its model in the confederation of Grecian States, "where each city, however different in wealth, strength, or other circumstances, had the same number of deputies and an equal voice in everything that related to the concerns of Greece." The States of the United Netherlands, the Confederated Cantons of Switzerland, and, in some degree at least, the British House of Lords were all replete with suggestion for the constructive statesmen who

[1] *The Forum*, June, 1901. Reproduced by permission. Copyright.

created the American Senate. And yet, while this is true, the fact remains, as Fisher points out in his "Evolution of the Constitution," that the Senate is really the outgrowth of our own experience. It is the gradual development from the Governor's Council of colonial times. As early as 1769 the members of the Council of Massachusetts were chosen to represent certain localities or great districts, a function still preserved in the representation of each State by two Senators, irrespective of area, wealth, or population.

Within the last few years the Senate of the United States has assumed so dominant a part in national legislation that it becomes interesting and instructive to consider how far the original idea of its establishment has been maintained in the evolution of our government. Washington's quaint and expressive phrase still has some meaning and significance. The Senate is still the conservative branch of the Congress. Its members, elected for six years by State Legislatures, decide national questions with minds less perturbed by fear of popular clamor than the Representatives, whose reëlection, after a brief term of two years, is dependent upon the suffrage of a proverbially fickle public. The Senatorial view is of a wider horizon. It is less subservient to prevailing sentiment, but, it is worth while to note, the register of its judgment has generally been accurate.

Take, for instance, the famous struggle over the so-called Force Bill, a measure passed by a partisan House of Representatives in the first flush of political victory. The contest waged by a skilfully led and determined minority in the Senate resulted in the defeat of the proposed law. The wisdom of that outcome will not, I take it, be seriously questioned to-day. The enactment of the Force Bill would have solidified the South politically, and would have retarded for several decades the material development which has blessed that section. The pouring and cooling process which resulted in its defeat was undoubtedly for the country's good.

Not content, however, with merely refusing to coöperate with the House in the enactment of proposed legislation, or with revising and editing so to speak, the bills which come to it from the lower body, the Senate of the United States has been responsible, in late years, for numerous measures of great importance. The Wilson Tariff Bill, as framed in the House of Representatives, was discarded by the Senate and a new measure substituted; the latter being accepted by the House with scarcely a whisper of opposition. Identically the same experience befell the resolutions passed by the House declaring that Spain's rule in Cuba was intolerable and not to be endured; while, still more recently, we have seen the Senate originate two of the most important measures ever enacted by Congress — the amendments to the Army Appropriation Bill, one of which bestowed upon the President absolute authority to govern the Philippines, while the other outlined the conditions precedent to the withdrawal of the American troops from Cuba. These amendments, fraught with consequences of the most far-reaching character, were adopted bodily by the House of Representatives after the briefest possible consideration. From the moment that the Senate engrafted these amendments upon the Army Bill, it was a foregone conclusion that the House would swallow them without the dotting of an "i" or the crossing of a "t."

It must not be supposed that the Representatives themselves are either ignorant of or indifferent to this condition of affairs. On the contrary, one of the most emphatic, not to say passionate, speeches in the closing hours of the last Congress was a protest by Representative Cannon, Chairman of the Committee on Appropriations, against the arrogance of the Senate in assuming to dictate to the House in the matter of legislation. And yet the House is, in itself, largely responsible for the very situation against which it rebels. When, under Mr. Reed, rules were enacted which made the Speaker of the House the autocrat of Congress the decadence of the House began. The members, individually and collectively, surrendered themselves into the keeping of one man, who wields a despotism as complete as that of the proverbial Czar. It is the Speaker who appoints the committees, arranging their personnel so as to secure harmony with his own views; it is the Speaker who, as the deciding member of the Committee on Rules, determines whether the House shall or shall not consider certain measures; and, finally, it is the Speaker to whom each Representative must appeal for recognition upon the floor of the House. The individual member, unless he be the favored appointee to some prominent committee chairmanship, is rarely a factor in the proceedings of the House. The concentration of power in the Speaker's hands has practically destroyed all personality. Indignant constituencies have sent back to private life for apparent inefficiency members who were never accorded an opportunity to prove their worth. Their political existence has been crushed out beneath the Juggernaut of despotic rules. The Washington correspondents, who are trained to observe the trend of national events, fully realize the change which has come over the House. There was a time, years ago, when every newspaper representative in the National Capital appreciated the necessity of acquainting himself with the temper of the House upon every important proposition. To-day the labor is unnecessary. If the correspondent knows the attitude of the Speaker the problem is at once solved.

It is worth while to understand this situation thoroughly, because, it seems to me, it explains the loss of prestige which the House has sustained and the importance which the Senate has assumed. In the Senate the individual is supreme. Any Senator may address the presiding officer and secure recognition at any time when the floor is not occupied by a colleague. He can offer a resolution upon any subject, and, through admirable rules, can place the Senate upon record as to its disposition. If the majority of the Senate desires to send the resolution to some committee crypt, where it shall remain buried until the campaign, for instance, is safely over, the reference is secured only after a yea-and-nay vote. If the resolution goes upon the calendar, any Senator can at any time move that the Senate proceed to its consideration — a question which must be determined without debate. This again places the Senate upon record, and is a proceeding absolutely unknown in the House. Thus, in the closing hours of the last Congress, Senator Jones, of Arkansas, the leader of the Democratic minority, proved a thorn in the side of the Republican party by demanding consideration of his resolution discharging the Committee on the Judiciary from further consideration of the Anti-Trust Bill. The effort was not successful, the Republican majority voting solidly in the negative; but Senator Jones had placed the responsibility where it belonged. Almost every day the record is made up in the Senate upon some test question, because the right of the individual is not abridged or restricted.

This preëminence of the individual in the Senate of the United States goes to a remarkable and much-criticised extent. As long as any Senator desires to speak upon any bill under consideration, just so long must hearing be accorded and a vote postponed. This is what is popularly known as unlimited debate. It is the one thing which makes the Senate absolutely unique in legislative bodies. Only recently the River and Harbor Appropriation Bill failed to reach a final vote, because a Senator occupied the floor during the last thirteen hours of the session, ostensibly criticising the measure, but, in reality, talking against time, with the knowledge that when the hands of the clock reached the hour of noon, Congress would expire by limitation, and the bill would die. This performance, extremely irritating to Senators who were interested in the generous appropriations of the bill, has led to a renewal of previous efforts to amend the rules of the Senate, so as to provide for closure, under certain conditions.

These endeavors have failed in the past, and there is no reason to anticipate success in the future. They ought to fail. Under no circumstances ought there to be limitation of debate in the Senate of the United States. It is the only forum where great and grave public questions can be thoroughly and exhaustively discussed. This high position, once held by the House, has been abdicated by that body. We have seen a bill which proposed a complete revision of the tariff considered in the House for a few days and then passed, when only a score of pages, out of two or three hundred, had received attention. Crude, ill-digested, and lacking all sense of proportion, the measure has been hastily sent to the Senate with all its imperfections upon its head. Provisions which were of questionable propriety escaped criticism, because they were buried in the pages which were not reached; and, for the same reason, important amendments, upon which the House was anxious to vote, remained unoffered upon the members' desks.

Very different was the course pursued in the Senate, where a rule arbitrarily fixing a day and an hour when a vote must be taken is a thing unknown. Conscious that it could not be hampered, the minority at once prepared to assert itself. It proceeded deliberately to question the Chairman of the Finance Committee as to the reasons which influenced the figures of each schedule, and the answer was necessarily forthcoming. If the reply was not satisfactory or convincing, there was a possibility that the error might be remedied; or, if no alteration was allowed by the majority, the explanation and the action went upon the record, to be read and judged by all men. In the case of the McKinley Bill the Democrats were the inquisitors; while, when the Wilson tariff measure was under consideration, the Republicans assumed the offensive. In both instances several weeks were occupied in the discussion — a period during which there was much criticism of the deliberation of the Senate. The result, however, in each case, proved the wisdom of delay, for the proposed law was vastly improved before its final enactment. The tariff measures which bear the names of McKinley, Wilson, and Dingley, were largely framed in the Senate, while the same is true of the law recently passed to reduce the taxation imposed during the war with Spain.

The value of unlimited debate in the Senate has been so completely established in innumerable instances that it hardly seems worth while to continue an argument in its favor. On the other hand, it will be urged, and with truth, that many measures have been prevented from reaching a final vote because their opponents have talked them to death. It is equally true, however, that no measure ever failed of enactment which had behind it a persistent, earnest majority, supported by public opinion. The defeat of the Force Bill is often cited as a thwarting of the will of the majority of the Senate; but the fact is that, during the long struggle over that measure, the minority became a majority, and the Force Bill was finally displaced by a proposition looking to the free coinage of silver. In the last Congress the Ship Subsidy Bill failed to reach a vote; but there never was, at any time, a solid Republican support for that measure. Some Republican Senators openly opposed it; others gave it only a half-hearted assistance; and many others encouraged the Democrats who planned and executed the campaign of debate. The discussion exposed many of the inequalities, injustices, and iniquities of the measure; so that when the subject is considered at the next session of Congress a more satisfactory bill will be enacted.

And this brings to mind another fact. All the great issues of recent political campaigns have been formulated through Senatorial debates. This is especially true of the silver question, which leaped into national prominence through the three-months' struggle over the repeal of the Sherman Silver-Purchasing Law. In those three months the financial problem was debated as it never had been, and never could be, in the House; and it is worth while emphasizing the fact that if the bill had been brought to a vote immediately after being reported to the Senate, it would have been defeated. The prolongation of the debate secured the majority necessary for its passage. In the Senate, and in the Senate alone, has the Philippine question received that thoroughness of examination to which it is entitled; and the same might be said of every other important issue before the country.

The power of the individual is still further demonstrated in the Senate of the United States through the fact that nearly all minor legislation is enacted by unanimous consent; the objection of a single Senator being generally fatal to the passage of any bill. This is a tremendous power to lodge in an individual even though he be a Senator of the United States; but it is to the credit of the members of the Senate that the privilege is rarely, if ever, abused. Objections are, of course, not infrequent; but when they are met by amendments or satisfactory explanations, they are almost invariably withdrawn. In the closing days of a session unanimous consent is absolutely essential to the consideration of any measure. While this may result in the failure of some laudable propositions, the statute books are also protected against the imposition of much unwise and hasty legislation. The Senator who objects does so publicly, and is answerable to his own conscience and to his constituency for his action. If he thus records his opposition, it is safe to assume that he believes himself to be acting wisely; and experience proves that Senators are restrained from undue objection by a wholesome regard for the sentiments of their colleagues. It would have been in the power of Senator Tillman, for instance, to have blocked all legislation as soon as he had learned that his much-desired appropriation of $250,000 for the Charleston exposition had been sacrificed. But, as a matter of fact, he did nothing of the kind. He could not have stood up against the torrent of indignation which would have been poured out upon him. Senator Carter, it is true, did defeat the River and Harbor Bill; but he was fully aware that in so doing he was acting in harmony with the sentiment of many of his colleagues, who regarded the bill as extravagant and harmful. If it had not been for the existence of this feeling, Mr. Carter never would have dared to take his stand in opposition, even though he was about to retire to private life.

In its own way, the Senate accomplishes more work — that is, it enacts more bills — than the House of Representatives. No Senator objects for the mere sake of objecting; because he is aware that if he is captious, he will himself encounter innumerable stumbling-blocks when he seeks the passage of measures in which he is interested. He is only one of ninety Senators, any one of whom has every privilege which he enjoys. It is the fact that each Senator is a power unto himself that gives the Senate its peculiar place in our system of government. When a vote upon a treaty or an important measure is to be convassed, it is necessary to know the individual view of each Senator, a task frequently surrounded with some difficulty. There is more independence of thought and action in the Senate than in the House. Instances where two Senators of the same political party from the same State vote upon opposite sides of the same question are by no means rare, and, of late years, have become quite common. Party leaders, therefore, take occasion, during the days occupied in a prolonged debate, to investigate the condition of their own ranks, and strengthen, by such pressure as may be most effective, any weakness they may discover. The very necessity for this preliminary canvass emphasizes the individuality of each Senator, and makes him a power to be courted or feared.

The right of any Senator to speak at any time, upon any subject, and at any length, develops orators and debaters. No man who possesses a talent in this direction need lack for opportunity to prove his capacity. If he is really a great orator, if he actually demonstrates his logical and thoughtful mind, he forges to the front, and must be reckoned with by those who assume leadership. If, on the other hand, he is dull and slow-witted, lacking both strength of thought and forcefulness of expression, he will sink by his own weight. The right to speak cannot be denied him, but he will not command an audience; and very promptly will he recognize that he has ceased to be a factor of importance. In olden times, a new Senator maintained silence for a year or two before affording his colleagues an opportunity to judge of his capacity. He familiarized himself with his surroundings; he felt the ground securely under his feet, so to speak, before he essayed to venture into public notice. The début of a Senator was in those days a noteworthy event. It was his crucial test; and it was not without some fear and trembling that he invited the verdict of his colleagues. Nowadays, however, in the haste and rush of modern legislation, few Senators undergo the term of probation which was formerly customary. They plunge at once into the vortex of debate. Sometimes they emerge safely and creditably; but more frequently they are carried underneath the surface, and in subsequent obscurity pay the penalty of their rashness.

Within the last few years some rich men have secured seats in the Senate, with comparative ease, through the manipulation of State politics; and their presence has given that body the nickname of "The Millionaires' Club." As a matter of fact, a large majority of the Senators are poor men. This is especially true of those who represent Southern States, who are proverbially lacking in plenitude of this world's goods. The millionaires in the Senate can be counted upon the fingers. Some of them are notoriously rich, like Clark, of Montana, while large fortunes are undoubtedly possessed by Hanna, of Ohio; McMillan, of Michigan; Elkins, of West Virginia; Kearns, of Utah; Proctor, of Vermont; Aldrich, of Rhode Island; Turner, of Washington; Platt and Depew, of New York; and Wetmore, of Rhode Island. To two-thirds of the Senators the annual salary of $5,000 is a consideration not to be despised.

There are few perquisites to eke out this comparatively meagre compensation — none, in fact, worth mentioning. The Government provides one or two clerks to attend to the Senator's correspondence, which is always heavy; it allows a minimum of free stationery; and it returns some of his travelling expenses.

There is opportunity, of course, to make money through speculation; and some Senators avail themselves of it. One Senator, who was a large holder of Washington real estate, increased its value very materially by steering legislation for street improvements in its direction; while every manipulation of tariff schedules and of internal revenue taxation, affecting steel and iron, tobacco, whiskey, and sugar, reveals the close connection between the Senate of the United States and Wall Street. But this acquisitiveness, to call it by no harsher name, is, after all, confined to the few Senators who are noted for their commercial instincts. The majority of Senators do not speculate. They content themselves with their modest salary; and how they manage to live upon it is a daily wonder. The demands upon the Senatorial purse are incessant. Every Senator is persistently approached by stranded constituents, who expect, and generally receive, financial assistance. Unless he elects to live in absolute retirement, it is also incumbent upon him to maintain some social position. Occasionally a Senator will come to Washington with the idea that he can be something or somebody upon $5,000 a year. It does not take many months to show him the futility of the effort. In fact, it is impossible for a Senator to save anything from his salary, unless he hides in a back street, burying himself like a hermit, neither entertaining nor being entertained. In the diplomatic service, the leading ambassadorial positions are bestowed upon men whose *entourage* can be maintained by their private fortunes; and the time does not seem to be far distant when the Senate of the United States will be composed in large degree of rich men, simply because a poor man can not afford to accept the position.

It is to the credit of the Senate that wealth is not yet the standard by which its members judge each other. There are millionaires in the Senate who occupy insignificant places, who are never consulted by their colleagues, and who simply follow where others lead. On the other hand, men who possess brains are consequential factors in determining legislation, although in material wealth they may be as poor as church mice. A man can not rise to eminence in the Senate by wealth alone. Herein, it seems to me, is much basis for felicitation. Until this condition changes, the Senate will continue to be, what it is to-day, the greatest legislative body in the world. Of course, the time may come when the sordid influences which measure a man by the size of his bank account may control the Senate. Let us, at least, be thankful that this time has not yet arrived; and let us hope, for the sake of the Republic, that it will never come.

THE POWER OF THE SENATE [1]

By S. W. McCall, Member of Congress from Massachusetts

SHORTLY before daybreak, in the closing night of the session of the Congress which came to an end on the 4th of last March, Mr. Cannon made a remarkable speech. One of the great appropriation bills of vital importance to the government was in conference between the two Houses. Unless it should pass before twelve o'clock on that day it would be necessary to have an extra session, or the wheels of some of the great governmental departments would be stopped. A Senator had delivered an ultimatum that an ancient claim of his state should be fastened upon the bill, or, as an alternative, he would talk until the end of the session and defeat the measure. Under the rules of the Senate it was clearly in the power of one Senator to carry on, as long as his physical strength would last, the appearance of debate, which would in no fair sense be debate at all, but simply a forcible stopping of the legislative machine. Mr. Cannon very unwillingly consented to pay the price demanded, but he declared with emphasis that the Senate should change its procedure, or that another body, "backed up by the people, will compel that change, else this body, close to the people, shall become a mere tender, a mere bender of the pregnant hinges of the knee to submit to what any one member of another body may demand of this body as a price for legislation."

Such instances of the effect of the rules of the Senate are by no means rare. Perhaps one more strikingly illustrating not merely the tendency to efface the House as a legislative body but also the overthrow of the rule of the majority in the Senate itself, was seen two years ago. The River and Harbor Bill, after a protracted consideration on the part of both Houses and of their committees, and after passing both Houses in its substantial form, had reached its last stage in the report of the conference committee within less than twenty hours of the final adjournment of the Congress. An unsuccessful attempt had been made to attach to the bill, to which it bore no relation, an irrigation scheme involving scores of millions of dollars. A Senator who had the irrigation project much at heart determined to defeat the bill. It did not appeal to him that the measure had received the careful attention and approval of both Houses. The rules of the Senate permitted him, under the guise of debate, to consume all the remaining time of the session. He took the floor against the measure. To talk against time for twenty hours demands qualities which few, if any, of the greatest parliamentary orators have possessed. The "debate" which followed afforded a rare display of physical endu-

[1] From *The Atlantic Monthly*, Oct., 1903. Reproduced with the consent of the Publisher and Author. Copyright.

rance. The Senator demonstrated his capacity to defeat the bill, and, to save the little time that was left to the Senate for the transaction of other urgent public business, the supporters of the bill surrendered and withdrew it from consideration.

It is scarcely a conclusive answer to indulge in the time-honored epithet and say that the measure in question was a "River and Harbor steal." Very little public money is expended with greater benefit to the people of the country at large than the money which is spent to deepen the rivers and improve the harbors along the oceans and the Great Lakes. Some portion of it doubtless is mere waste, and never should be appropriated at all. A large proportion of that waste is due to the fact that some Senators, like the one to whom I have just referred, with small states behind them, but with the same power as Senators from the great taxpaying states, are careful that their localities shall receive their share of the public money, and their ingenuity expends itself in finding other objects for public bounty in default of oceans and navigable rivers. I shall subsequently refer, more fully, however, to the unequal character of the constitution of the Senate. I am only referring here to the effect of the Senate rules.

The House of Representatives may devote its time to the perfecting of a great measure which also receives the approval of a majority of the Senate, and then the measure is to be overthrown, and the labors of the House brought to naught unless consent is given to engraft upon it the pet scheme of some individual Senator to which the great majority of both bodies may be opposed. As much can be said for the freedom of debate which exists in the Senate as for the summary procedure which often prevails in the House, under which a vote is taken upon most important measures with practically no debate at all. But unless a change of the Senate rule is made, as applied to new matters sought to be put upon bills which have received in substance the approval of both Houses, the House of Representatives will be compelled to submit to the demands of individual Senators, and accept the principle of government by unanimous consent instead of by majorities, or see necessary legislation fail of passage.

From the time of the adoption of the Constitution to the present day there have been frequent protests against the large measure of power possessed by the Senate, especially in view of the very unequal and very unrepresentative principle upon which that body is constituted, but its power appears to have fattened upon these protests, and to have been, on the whole, increasing. If, in spite of the constitution of the Senate, its power has been employed as a rule for the general good, it must be remembered that something can be said in favor of the most unequal system of government that has ever existed. The purest despotisms and the most exclusive oligarchies have frequently been responsive to popular opinion, and have often sheltered order and sometimes individual freedom. I shall take for granted, however, that the democratic idea, which our nation is supposed to represent, will be accepted without argument as applied to North America. Caution compels me to say "as applied to North America," for the government of the American people has decreed that the "consent-of-the-governed" declaration of our forefathers was either not a declaration of a principle at all, or had only a local application and did not possess vitality across the seas.

The great and growing power of the Senate is not more odious on account of any degeneracy in its personnel. The lament of the degeneracy of the present as compared with the past is one of the oldest things one can find in history. There always have been, and there probably always will be, people in the world who disparage the times in which they live, — people who, as Macaulay said, are always painting a golden age which never existed save in their imaginations. I am not one of those who think that the talent in public life has declined. I believe it is true that, on the whole, even the national Congress for the last ten years will compare very favorably with the national Congress of any other time in our history. Some exceptionally great figure may depart from one House or the other and be greatly missed for a time, but the average of membership maintains itself very fairly. If I were dealing with the House of Representatives, I could cite many names from the last decade of its history that would show the strength of its membership, — statesmen like Reed and Dingley and Wilson, orators like Cockran and Dalzell and Bryan, debaters like Turner, Cannon, Hepburn, and Crisp. But I am dealing with the Senate. It contains in its present membership one, whose name will readily occur to all, who will pass into history as among the three or four greatest statesmen who ever had a place in that body. When has it had, since the days of Douglas certainly, a more accomplished debater than Spooner, or a more pungent and brilliant speaker than Vest; or when has it ever had more tactful and discerning leaders than Allison and Aldrich? And the list of striking figures might easily be made longer.

The striking circumstance in connection with the power of the Senate is that it holds the commanding place at the center of the government. It brings to mind the condition of things in Europe under the feudal system, where the nobles had the position between the king and the people, and gradually encroached upon both until they were able to oppress both, — a condition which continued until a union was effected between the people and the sovereign, and the feudal system was finally overthrown. The Senate shares the powers of legislation with the House and some of the most important executive functions with the President. The latter is unable to appoint a collector or a postmaster, or even a member of his own official household, without the Senate's consent. Such important powers, exercised at the center of the state, would naturally increase by encroachment upon both extremes, and they certainly would not diminish.

The course of the Revolution made it almost inevitable that in the Continental Congress, and in the Congress under the Articles of Confederation, the states should vote as a unit and exercise an equal authority; but when the time came to formulate the Constitution, the most enlightened of our statesmen were strongly impressed with the idea that there could not be such a thing as a permanent free government established upon so unequal a principle. The question of the relative power of the large and small states in the new government became a pressing one. That was the rock upon which the Convention was more than once very nearly destroyed. In the long contest which ensued it must be admitted that the representatives of the small states played the better game and won upon almost all points. Their most effective resource was found in the ardent desire of the leading statesmen from the larger states to substitute a real national government for the mere shadow of a government that then existed, and they made the larger states pay a high price to obtain it. They secured an equal representation in the Senate, and they exaggerated the powers of the body by conferring upon it a great variety of important functions.

The large states made a determined stand upon the question of taxation. They insisted that the people and not the states paid the taxes, and that, as the larger states would yield more taxes than the smaller states, the representatives of the people, chosen substantially upon the basis of population, should have a peculiar control over revenue bills. Mr. Gerry well stated the prevailing idea of the time with reference to taxation when he said, "Taxation and representation are strongly associated in the minds of the people, and they will not agree that any but their immediate representatives shall meddle with their purses."

Although the representatives of the smaller states insisted upon an equal power even over revenue bills, they did not lack in thrift when it came to guarding themselves against liability to pay an equal share of the expenses of the government, and the Constitution accordingly provided that representation and direct taxes should be apportioned among the states according to population.

An apparent concession, however, was finally made by the small states with regard to revenue bills, and I shall refer to it more fully hereafter, because it is the one point where I think the Senate, not satisfied with the great powers conferred upon it, has directly encroached upon the prerogatives of the House. Having secured the great grant of power in the Constitution, the smaller states then demanded a provision that that instrument should never be amended so as to take away the equal representation of the states in the Senate without the consent of every state, — something which obviously it would be impossible to obtain, and which was equivalent to providing that the Constitution, in that particular, should never be amended at all.

The constitution of the Senate was recognized, at the time of its establishment, as a violation of the democratic principle, but a violation which the peculiar conditions seemed to require, and I think it was never imagined that the inequality would not be limited to that which existed, or might grow out of the states at first forming the Union. While the Senate's constitutional powers have not changed, the course of events has greatly intensified their undemocratic character. The practical inequality originally was sufficiently bad, but, by the admission of so many new and small states, it has become almost intolerable. The original inequality bore heavily upon three states, yet was not essentially glaring with reference to the others; but to-day it is possible to select fifteen states having together in round numbers five millions of people, or about two-thirds of the population of the state of New York. The senatorial representatives of those five millions would lack only a single vote of the number necessary to defeat some great treaty which the Senators of the other seventy millions might support. States having less than one-sixth of the population choose a majority of the entire Senate, while more than five-sixths of the people of the country are represented by a minority in that body. The state of Nevada, under the last census, had less than forty-three thousand people. If New York were permitted to have the same proportional representation in the Senate, it would have some three hundred and fifty Senators. There are many things in the constitution of the Senate which are admirable. Such a conservative body is to-day of vital importance. The length of the term, the different method of choice from that of the Representatives, and the very gradual change in membership, are highly valuable features. But none of its good features grows out of the great inequality of its constitution, giving one man in one section of the country the power of a hundred equally good men in another.

This exaggerated inequality, so utterly subversive of the American dogma of government, is undoubtedly the great fault in the constitution of the Senate. There is none of the common traditional attributes of aristocracy that enters into this situation. The theory of government which treats sovereignty as a mere possession, passing from father to son like any other species of property, at least has something human in it. But even the human element disappears entirely when a capricious bestowal of power is made upon a mere incorporation. If the owners of land and other property, the mercantile interests, and the workingmen are treated as classes and permitted to choose their representatives in the governing body, there is at least a representation of the diversity of interests with which legislation deals. And the proposition is not entirely lacking in force that individuals, separated from property or class interests, are affected in much the same way by legislation, and have a substantial identity of interests. In other words, that the touch of nature will affect legislators when they pass laws concerning life and liberty to which they themselves will be subject; and that they are representatives in a stronger sense than if they exercised a mere delegated authority; but that when property and class rights are dealt with, the rapacity of one class should be held in check by the rapacity of another, and that there should be such a balance in the assembly that those broad interests which are weak in mere numbers should not be devoured by those that are strong. But what conceivable thing is there in the state of Nevada, estimable as her people doubtless are, to entitle one individual there to a hundred times as much weight in governing the country as is possessed by a man residing in New York or Pennsylvania or Illinois, or indeed to a particle greater weight? On any rational theory of government such inequality is unthinkable, unless, indeed, it be true that those having a particular occupation should exercise a special and almost potent control in governing the myriads of other occupations.

We have had recent illustrations that this system of inequality does not merely violate our ideals, but that it has serious practical results. Ten years ago, in consequence of concessions to the silver mining interests, the country had reached the verge of the precipice, and our financial system was at last almost at the point of falling upon the silver standard. Under the law requiring the government to purchase 4,500,000 ounces of silver bullion every month, gold was rapidly leaving the treasury, while its vaults were groaning under the great mass of silver. The spectacle was then witnessed of Senators from states, containing mining camps but comparatively few people, almost holding the balance of power, and, having an equal voice with that of the populous commercial states of the Union, struggling desperately to continue the fatal policy of the government purchase of silver. It was only by the inflexible and heroic conduct of the President, supported, as he chanced to be, by the great body of the party in opposition to him, that the most vital commercial interests of the great majority of the people and the financial honor of the nation as well were not sacrificed.

Other illustrations might be given, but they would only tend to prove what is axiomatic — that the Senators from the small states, as well as the Senators from the large states, will, as a rule, vote for those measures furthering the special interests of the states they represent. They would, I think, be accused of betraying their trust if they did less.

The great practical encroachment of the power of the Senate beyond its fair constitutional limits is seen in connection with bills relating to taxation. The chief concession in the formation of the Constitution was that by which the large states were given at least the appearance of a special power over taxation in proportion to their population as a set-off against the great proportional powers given the small states through their equal representation in the Senate. The small states, however, on the basis of population, would possess entire equality with the large states, and it would certainly be no good ground for complaint that they should not be accorded the right to impose taxes for other people to pay.

This compensating power is found in that clause of the Constitution providing that all bills for raising revenue shall originate in the House of Representatives, reserving to the Senate the right to propose or concur with amendments as on other bills. Unless a substantial power was intended to be conferred by this clause, the contemporary construction put upon it by the Federalist, in a paper written either by Madison or Hamilton, was strikingly erroneous. "Admitting, however," says the author of this paper, "that they should all be insufficient to subdue the unjust policy of the smaller states, or their predominating influence in the councils of the Senate, a constitutional and infallible recourse still remains with the larger states by which they will be able at all times to accomplish their just purposes. The House of Representatives can not only refuse, but they alone can propose the supplies requisite for the support of government. They, in a word, hold the purse, — that powerful instrument by which we behold, in the history of the British Constitution, an infant and humble representative of the people gradually enlarging the sphere of its activity and importance, and finally reducing, so far as it seems to have wished, all the overgrown prerogatives of the other branches of the government. This power of the purse may, in fact, be regarded as the most complete and effectual weapon with which any constitution can arm the immediate representatives of the people for obtaining a redress of every grievance, and for carrying into effect every just and salutary measure."

. But what would this power amount to if the imposition of a tax upon a single article would confer upon the Senate the right to go over the whole range of taxes and construct any sort of a bill it desired? By giving such an interpretation to the meaning of the exception the great power itself is practically destroyed. At the time of the framing of the Constitution there was no such thing known as amendment by complete substitution, and the fair construction of that clause, having reference to the conditions surrounding its adoption, is that if the House should send a bill to the Senate imposing a tax upon an article, the Senate might amend by raising or diminishing the proposed tax as it saw fit. It was such an abuse of the right of amendment as to destroy the power to originate taxation laws, when the Senate, as it did in 1872, substituted for a House bill relating to a tax on coffee a general revision of the tariff. The Senate's action at that time called out a protest from Garfield, who had deeply studied this subject, and who contributed to it one of the most notable efforts of his career in Congress. Garfield held that the action of the Senate in the case cited was an abuse, and that its action should be confined substantially to the subjects in the House bill. He declared that the action of the Senate invaded "a right which can not be surrendered without inflicting a fatal wound upon the integrity of our whole system of government." No hard and fast rule can be set up in such a case, but it is a question of prerogative, and each body should respect the constitutional prerogatives of the other. Surely the body representing the people should struggle for its own.

The great Senators have almost uniformly contended for a broad construction of the prerogative of the House. Webster held that it was purely a question of privilege, and that the decision of it belonged to the House. Benton, who belonged to the opposite political party, in the same debate declared that "in all cases of doubtful jurisdiction between the Houses my rule is to solve the doubt in favor of the House, which, by the Constitution, is charged with the general subject. Taxation and representation go together. The burdens of the people and the representation of the people are put together. An important and full representation of the people is in the House of Representatives." Sumner, Wilson, Seward, and Hoar have also declared in the Senate for a broad construction of the prerogative of the House.

It has been said that the Senate will construct a better tariff than the House. The framers of the Constitution, and especially its great interpreter, Hamilton, did not foresee in its full force the influence of special great interests in framing tariff laws. It is for the benefit of those interests, sometimes pressing for governmental protection and sometimes for governmental indifference, to have tariffs constructed by a few men, responsible practically to no great body of public opinion, as many of them as possible with small constituencies, so that after having protected the interests of those they particularly represent, they might be unattached and without special electoral responsibility. A scrutiny of. the recent bills relating to taxation will show that the House bills have usually been drawn upon more popular lines. Take the repeal of some of the war revenue taxes two years ago, when the House of Representatives sent to the Senate a bill, the chief feature of which was the removal of nearly all the troublesome and vexatious stamp taxes which had been imposed upon almost all the instrumentalities of trade. The tax upon bank checks, insurance policies, real estate conveyances, and similar taxes of a wide application were removed by the House bill. The Senate, under the guise of its power to amend, struck out all after the enacting clause of the House bill, and substituted a measure of its own. The distinguishing feature of the Senate bill was an extension of the amount of the reduction of the tax on beer and tobacco by about twelve millions, and to enable this to be done, it retained many of the stamp taxes which the House bill removed, and especially the stamp tax upon checks. The tax upon checks was a direct tax upon hundreds of thousands of people, and was not of sufficient importance to any individual, vexatious though it might be, to lead him to make any special effort for its repeal. On the other hand, the millions which were remitted upon beer went to a very small class who had so much at stake as to warrant an extraordinary effort. The House repeal was in favor of the great number, and the Senate repeal was in favor of the few.

It does not require a close study of the tariff laws of the last twenty years to lead to the conclusion that, although special interests have fully as much consideration shown them in the House of Representatives as they should have, yet the Senate has been the citadel of those interests. The representatives are reached directly by the people who pay the taxes and can be visited with public indignation, while the Senators in some instances at least are for all practical purposes irresponsible to the taxpayer.

The question primarily is not one of wise or unwise laws, or whether small states do not often have strong Senators, while large states have weak ones. It involves a principle which is not disregarded even in a constitutional monarchy like Germany. It involves the principle of one set of men imposing taxes for another set of men to pay, and if the House of Representatives would insist, as some of its greatest members have advised, upon a broad and fair construction of its prerogatives, we should be upon a platform more consistent with the principles of sound government. We should, I am sure, have laws of taxation formulated upon more popular lines. The masses would suffer less for the benefit of the great special interests, and there would be some compensation to the large states, and to the people who are directly represented, for the extraordinary powers conferred upon the Senate.

By a sort of attraction of gravitation the great powers of the Senate increase by drawing other powers to them, and this species of expansion is especially seen in the tendency to confer special official functions upon the Senators individually. Take the negotiation of the treaty of peace with Spain in 1898, which was, in effect, a treaty of war rather than of peace, and which embarked us upon a policy nobody contemplated when we entered upon the war for the liberation of Cuba. Of the five commissioners who were appointed to negotiate that treaty, three were Senators. That is not an exceptional instance, but it is becoming the rule. A more recent illustration is found in the appointment of the commission, soon to meet, to decide the Alaskan boundary dispute, a tribunal which, under the agreement, was to be composed of impartial jurists of repute. Two of the three American members of the commission were chosen from the Senate. We may concede to those two Senators the utmost their warmest friends could claim for them, and yet there is no danger in the assertion that there are plenty of other jurists in the country as impartial and of as high repute. If there were a paucity of American talent, or if the great part of it were concentrated in the Senate, then it might be desirable to fill such places, which, for all essential purposes, are offices, from the membership of the Senate. But there is certainly no such lack of talent in private life as to call for a duplication of parts in the play, or for imposing on Senators important public functions in addition to those belonging to their own office. Mr. Hay had not been conspicuous as a public man before the first election of Mr. McKinley.

The public career of Mr. Richard Olney had been limited to a term in the Massachusetts legislature before he rendered his notable service in the Cabinet of President Cleveland. I think neither Mr. Gage nor Mr. Root nor yet Mr. Knox had ever held important public office before he entered President McKinley's Cabinet. Scores of instances can be found where men of little or no experience in the public service have been selected to fill the most important offices, and have infused new strength and energy into the government.

In a government which is a republic in anything but name the offices should be as widely distributed as is consistent with good administration, and the rich red blood which the country possesses in abundance should course through the channels of office. Even if the country were so poor in talent as to make it desirable to appoint Senators to such places, even if there were no impropriety in their negotiating treaties upon which they were to pass judgment as Senators, such appointments come perilously near being an infraction of the Constitution. A Senator is disqualified from holding any other office under the United States, and if it is not a most important office of government to determine in the first instance the great question of peace and war, or to settle a disputed boundary with another nation, then the term has an exceedingly narrow meaning.

The expansion of the power of the Senate in an undemocratic as well as an unconstitutional direction is also seen in the growing tendency to pass laws, and especially taxation laws, by treaty. Treaties are high contracts between nations, and it can hardly be believed that it was within the contemplation of the framers of the Constitution so elaborately to construct a legislative machine and at the same time to throw the whole mechanism out of gear by a single clause regarding treaties, providing that the President and Senate might call in a foreign potentate and might make laws for the internal government of the United States. Treaties have the force of law, but they should obviously be within the fair scope of the treaty-making power. At any rate, it would scarcely be reasonable to claim that they set aside the Constitution, and if we are to regard the Senate as a part of two legislative machines, it can not, as a part of either, do the things prohibited by the Constitution. Under that instrument revenue bills must originate in the House. How, then, can they originate by treaty? It would, indeed, be a curious spectacle, that of the Senate, composed in the way it is, sitting behind closed doors, and deciding in secret what taxes the American people are to pay.

The four years' term of the presidency is too short for a struggle with the Senate, and its part in executive transactions is so great that any such struggle would expose an administration to failure. The period of life of the House of Representatives is still shorter, and its term would be likely to come to an end before a contest between the two Houses would acquire any great momentum. The custom under which Representatives are expected to secure offices for their constituents, and thus to ask for senatorial favors, makes a contest between the two Houses less apt to occur. As I have said, an amendment to the Constitution depriving states of their equal membership in the Senate is not within the range of possibilities, as such an amendment would require the unanimous consent of all the states. It would be possible to pass an amendment in the ordinary way, reducing the powers of the Senate, but the friction of the amending machinery is so great that it would involve an intense and long continued pressure of public opinion to set it in motion. The only practical hope of even a partial remedy lies in the jealous insistence by the House upon its constitutional prerogatives. If it should do that, it would be more likely to realize the advantage of its position in a nation imbued with the democratic idea. The doubtful powers of government would gravitate toward the House, our laws would become more popular in character, and would respond to broad and general needs in the community, while the character of the Senate as a conservative body would be unimpaired.

But things have drifted long enough. Nothing can be clearer than that in the long lapse of time institutions of government may be corrupted and become vastly different from their original character. Venice began her national career as a republic in fact, and for centuries was governed by elected rulers responsible to a popular assembly, but, while maintaining the name of republic, she came to have, in the Council of Ten, sitting in secret, or, as it might be called to-day, "in executive session," as despotic and cruel an oligarchy as ever existed. It might be said that we have the restraints of a written Constitution, and a Supreme Court to enforce them, but already we have heard made, not entirely without effect, that appeal to an utterly false national pride, "Is not the American government able to do anything that any other government can do?" as if that which has been accounted our glory, as if the restrictions in favor of freedom and against tyranny, even by the government itself, were a defect and a badge of weakness. And in view of the tendency of recent decisions, how long may we expect the Supreme Court to remain the austere guardian of the Constitution against the encroachments of executive or congressional power? That court may not always be composed of Marshalls and Storys and Harlans, and what will become of the limitations of the Constitution if ever the high aery, about which the eagles of our jurisprudence once hovered, shall be held by the twittering judicial tomtit? At any rate, the preservation of our institutions in their purity requires that each branch of the political department of the government shall be the guardian of its own powers, and, without encroaching upon any other branch, shall stand firmly for its own prerogatives. Any determined conflict will be settled, not by mere popular clamor, but by public opinion. Popular clamor is often stirred up by an ardent cultivation of the galleries, and the sensation of yesterday is thrust aside and forgotten for the sensation of to-day. But the settled and potent public opinion, which is the product of patient discussion, and of the persistent education of the people, usually leads to policies in quite an opposite direction. When that shall be appealed to in any determined contest between the two Houses, it can scarcely be doubted that the decision will be in favor of those great principles of popular government which underlie the American Commonwealth.

THE OLIGARCHY OF THE SENATE [1]

By A. Maurice Low

Over the doors of the Senate of the United States might well be inscribed the motto, "*Do ut des,*" for it expresses the principle which governs the members of the Senate, especially the inner circle that really controls the Upper House of Congress, that is, in fact, the government of the United States. Bismarck translated this maxim and used it in the sense of "I give in order that you may give;" Mr. Goschen rendered it into English as "the exchange of friendly offices, based on the avowed self-interest of the parties." Whether the Bismarckian or the Goschen version be accepted, the result is the same.

Basing the Federal Constitution on the British system, *mutatis mutandis,* the framers of the Constitution might well regard the House as having higher authority than the Senate, because it had the sole power to originate money bills. While that is technically correct, the power of the Senate over money bills is, in some respects, even greater than that of the House, since it is able to amend any bill which the House may send to it for concurrent action. This was the very thing feared by Mason, of Virginia, and pointed out by him; and the right of the Senate to originate, by the power of amendment, bills raising revenue and making appropriations has been confirmed by judicial approval. Technically, such bills have not originated, or rather have not been initiated, in the Senate. But when the Senate takes, for example, a tariff bill, strikes out all except the enacting clause, writes in and returns to the House a new bill, which that body is compelled to accept, it may be asked whether that particular law providing for the collection of revenue has not been created, that is to say, originated, by the Senate, in defiance of the seventh section of the first article of the Constitution, despite the permission given to the Senate to propose amendments. That which is *res adjudicata* is no longer open to question. But one may safely hazard the opinion that none of the framers of the Constitution in discussing this

The *North American Review*, February, 1902. Reproduced in part, by permission. Copyright.

clause of that instrument anticipated a day when a tariff bill framed by the House would be treated with contemptuous indifference by the Senate, and a tariff bill framed by the Senate would become the law of the land. But the fact is greater than the opinion. By the power of the Senate to amend, the preponderating control supposed to have been secured to the House by endowing it with the sole right to originate money bills, has been effaced. "They, in a word, hold the purse," Hamilton said of the House; but to-day the House holds the purse while the Senate dips into it.

The Senate and the House, therefore, stand on an equal footing, so far as the control of the public purse is concerned, the House having lost the ability to coerce the Senate by withholding supplies because the Senate by "amendment" can defy the House. But the Senate always has the advantage of the House in any contest, because of the fact that it is a small and well-disciplined body, and because of the feeling of superiority which belongs to the Senatorial estate. Objections have been frequently urged against the common use of the term "Upper House" as descriptive of the Senate, on the ground that, the Senate having coördinate and not greater privileges than the House, it is a mistake to give it an appellation that would signify superior authority. Technically, it is true that there is no distinction in the delegated powers, and yet the Constitution itself makes a distinction between the membership of the two Houses, requiring that the Senator shall be possessed of the wisdom that follows from greater age, and the more thorough comprehension of the spirit of the country proceeding from longer citizenship, if of alien birth.

The legislative surrender of the House of Representatives to the Senate began with the election of Mr. Reed to the Speakership of the Fifty-first Congress. Mr. Reed found himself confronted by a state of affairs which needed a drastic remedy. It is only necessary here to refer incidentally to the practice which prevailed in the House of Representatives before Mr. Reed's election to the Speakership, as the conditions are too well known to the student of current parliamentary history to require more than passing mention. The rules of the House were too feeble to permit the transaction of business unless by unanimous consent or a test of endurance. The minority always had the majority at a disadvantage. It was always possible for the minority to prevent a vote being reached simply by offering dilatory motions, or by breaking a quorum; in the one case time was consumed in calling the roll, in the other nothing could be done until the sergeant-at-arms secured the attendance of a quorum, and it often required several weary hours for the sergeant-at-arms to round up his quarry. Mr. Reed, when he came to the chair, must have had very distinct, and very unpleasant, memories of the bitter contest over the Direct Tax Bill, when for twenty-six consecutive hours the doors of the chamber were kept locked because a call of the House was in progress. If the majority were to be held responsible for legislation, it was only proper that they should have power.

Mr. Reed had the courage and the ability to frame a code of rules that made it possible for the House to conduct business in an orderly and expeditious manner. How absolutely necessary his code was is shown from the fact that his Democratic successor substantially made the Reed rules his own; and, still later, when the swing of the pendulum once more placed the House in control of the Republicans, the Republican majority saw no good reason why any change should be made in the rules. A code that has stood the test of time, that could have been easily altered but was not, that has been approved by political opponents, must possess merit. Mr. Reed's parliamentary services entitle him to the highest gratitude of the country.

Unfortunately, Mr. Reed was a revolutionist; he accomplished with one bold stroke and in a few days what, under other circumstances, would only have been brought about very gradually and after long years of discussion. The danger of a revolution is that it is apt to run to extremes; that instead of moving slowly and naturally along the line of least resistance it takes a short cut to its objective point by employing cataclysmic methods.

But further, not only did Mr. Reed feel it his duty to put an end to interminable and frivolous debate, he also regarded it as incumbent upon him to check the rapidly rising tide of extravagant expenditure. Those were the days when the taunt of "a billion dollar Congress" made men turn pale. A billion dollar budget no longer affrights us.

Two important things followed from the new dispensation. One was that even vital measures were disposed of without proper consideration. When the time arrived for taking a vote the gavel fell, often in the midst of a sentence, and all debate ceased. The other was that members of the House who were unable, because of the Speaker's rigid ideas of economy, to secure appropriations in House bills, accomplished their purpose by inducing Senators to offer for them bills in the Senate in the form of amendments. Senators were not averse to doing this, as it placed Representatives under obligations to them, it increased their prestige in their States, and it added still more to the growing power of the Senate. To such an extent has the practice grown that it is now recognized, as a matter of course, that the Senate will "take care" of routine legislation to which the House is opposed or on which it is not safe to risk the chance of possible defeat in the House. Appropriations for the construction of a revenue cutter, a lighthouse tender, public buildings, and other things were made by the Senate at the request of Representatives who knew the impossibility of securing favorable action by the House if the bills originated in the latter body. To preserve its own reputation for economy, the House will wink at the extravagance of the Senate. The Senate, not being so close to the people as the House, is less frightened by the charge of extravagance.

There is no way in which debate in the Senate can be abridged or terminated except by unanimous consent. The state of affairs which existed in the House prior to the election of Mr. Reed to the Speakership exists to-day in the Senate. The majority governs only by the will of the minority. It is true that it does not always suit the purpose of the minority to exercise its power, but the power is latent and not surrendered. We have seen tariff bills "amended" by the Senate so that their framers did not recognize them; we have seen a single Senator compelling a majority to come to terms with him because he threatened to make a speech which it would take six weeks to deliver; we have seen a single Senator defeat a bill carrying an appropriation of some $70,000,000 — a bill passed by the House and having a majority in its favor in the Senate — because it suited his purpose so to do.

It is because business in the Senate can only proceed by "unanimous consent" that the principle of "*Do ut des*" governs. A Senator who wants to secure an appropriation must not be too particular about some other Senator's little raid into the Treasury. Even great party measures can be brought to vote only by agreement. That is the reason why, during the course of a session, the *Congressional Record* has frequent mention of these agreements; that is why the announcement is repeatedly made that a vote will be considered as ordered on a certain bill on a definite day and hour, "if there be no objection," and no objection is ever made. A pact once made in the Senate is not broken. It is an agreement between gentlemen.

It has been shown that the Senate has equal power with the House over the control of appropriations; that it can create a tariff bill by the right of amendment; that it can prevent the enactment of any bill passed by the House; that it encourages members of the House to look for legislation in the Senate rather than in the House, where it rightfully belongs. One has never heard of Senators asking favors from Representatives.

To say that the House has been reduced to a negligible quantity in legislation would be an overstatement of the case; it is no exaggeration to say that it has become an insignificant factor. In further support of this assertion let it be said — and no greater practical proof of its correctness could be offered — that the correspondents who represent in Washington the leading newspapers of the country no longer think it necessary to consult members of the House regarding legislation; they confine their attention almost exclusively to the Senate. Time was, not many years ago, when important questions were pending, when the opinions of leaders in the House were as eagerly sought by these correspondents as were the opinions of leaders in the Senate, but to-day the mastery of the Senate is so clearly recognized that it would be a waste of time to seek for information elsewhere. When the important "Platt amendment " was under discussion last spring, scarcely a word was said, either in the newspapers or at the Capitol, about the attitude of the House. The same indifference as to the position of the House was displayed while the question was being argued whether the Philippines were to be governed by Congress or were for the time being to be left in the hands of the President.

Legislation, therefore, in Washington is represented by the Senate. Does the Senate dominate the President?

There is no more striking example of the encroachment of the Senate than the way in which the Senate deals with appointments and its interference in the conduct of foreign relations. Hamilton dismissed as idle the suggestion that the President's nominations would be overruled, or that the Senate could coerce the President into nominating a particular individual; but Hamilton could not foresee a senatorial oligarchy. Presidential nominations have been frequently rejected; no President now dares to make a nomination unless the Senators from the State in which the nominee resides have given their approval. Fitness, merit, talents are not the conclusive consideration. A man nominated to be a Justice of the Supreme Court of the United States was rejected because he and the Senator from his State, although of the same political faith, had been opposed to each other; the nomination of a man seeking a commission as a paymaster in the army was prevented because this man had written certain things in criticism of a Senator. No nomination is too important or too unimportant to escape this scrutiny. Here again the principle of "*Do ut des*" prevails under the euphonious guise of "senatorial courtesy." A nominee personally distasteful to a Senator must be rejected, because the time may come when some other Senator will ask a similar favor at the hands of his associates.

This is mischievous and, at times, humiliating to the President; but it is seldom dangerous. The interference of the Senate in the conduct of foreign relations and its meddling with diplomatic negotiations are fraught with serious consequences. The Constitution gives the President the power "to make treaties, provided two-thirds of the Senators present concur," which has been interpreted by some expounders of the Constitution to mean that the Senate may ratify or reject a treaty as it sees fit, but it has not power to amend. This, however, is not the judicial interpretation, and the Supreme Court has decided (*Haver* v. *Yaker*, 9 Wall. 35) that the Senate is not required to adopt or reject a treaty as a whole, but may modify or amend it. But the Senate has assumed an even more advanced position. It now chooses to regard a treaty as simply "a project." In a letter which Senator Lodge wrote to the Boston *Transcript*, December 29th, 1900, in which he defended the position of the Senate, he used these words: "The Senate is part of the treaty-making power, and treaties sent to it for ratification are not strictly treaties, but projects for treaties; they are still inchoate." This statement, Mr. Lodge observes, is a "constitutional truism." It is in the sense that Mr. Lodge is simply paraphrasing the Constitution when he declares that the Senate is part of the treaty-making power, and he is absolutely correct in declaring that a treaty negotiated by the President is not a consummated compact until ratified by the Senate, but whether the Senate has not encroached upon executive prerogatives can not be so lightly answered.

As showing the assumption of the Senate, notice the remarkable change made in the wording of a recent treaty. Last year the Senate ratified a treaty with Great Britain (The Tenure and Disposition of Real and Personal Property), providing for the Disposition of real estate and giving any British colony the right to adhere to the convention on notice from the British Ambassador at Washington to the Secretary of State; and, similarly, any possessions of the United States beyond the seas were to be included in the compact upon notice "being given by the representative of the United States at London, by direction of the President." The Senate amended this to read "by direction of the treaty-making power of the United States." Thus, by the addition of a few words, the Senate assumed to itself the right to conduct foreign relations, an assumption for which no warrant can be found in the Constitution.

Presidents who were more jealous of their prerogatives than Mr. McKinley have read Congress a sharp lecture for attempting to interfere in foreign affairs. Jackson vetoed an act [1] because "in my judgment inconsistent with the division of powers in the Constitution of the United States, as it is obviously founded on the assumption that an act of Congress can give power to the Executive or to the head of one of the Departments to negotiate with a foreign government. . . . The Executive has competent authority to negotiate . . . with a foreign government — an authority Congress can not constitutionally abridge or increase." Would Jackson have permitted the Senate to amend the Property Treaty as McKinley did? Certainly not, as we may infer from the stinging language used in the memorable "Protest" of April 15th, 1834, in which he said:

"The resolution of the Senate presupposes a right in that body to interfere with this exercise of Executive power. If the principle be once admitted . . . the constitutional independence of the Executive Department would be as effectually destroyed and its powers as effectually transferred to the Senate as if that end had been accomplished by an amendment to the Constitution."

Grant was equally jealous that the line of demarcation between the legislative and the executive should not be overstepped. In returning

[1] An "act to authorize the Secretary of the Treasury to compromise the claims allowed by the commissioners under the treaty with the King of the Two Sicilies, concluded Oct. 14, 1832."

to the House of Representatives a "joint resolution relating to congratulations from the Argentine Republic," which directed the Secretary of State to acknowledge a dispatch of congratulation, Grant said:

"I cannot escape the conviction that their adoption has inadvertently involved the exercise of a power which infringes upon the constitutional rights of the Executive. . . . The Constitution of the United States, following the established usages of nations, has indicated the President as the agent to represent the national sovereignty in its intercourse with foreign powers and in all official communications from them."

After quoting from the act establishing the Department of State, Grant continued:

"This law, which remains substantially unchanged, confirms the view that the whole correspondence of the government with and from foreign states is intrusted to the President; that the Secretary of State conducts such correspondence exclusively under the orders and instruction of the President."

Cleveland had no scruples about making Congress understand that it must not interfere with the conduct of foreign affairs, and that the recognition of an independent state was an executive act purely, and not one with which the legislative branch could concern itself.

Having advanced the doctrine that treaties negotiated by the President are merely "projects for treaties; they are still inchoate," the Senate has now still further encroached on the Executive by claiming to know the details of a treaty while in process of negotiation and before the treaty is submitted to it for ratification. Minos must be admitted to the secrets of Jove. That, virtually, is what the Senate compelled President McKinley and Secretary Hay to do when it so amended the Hay-Pauncefote canal treaty as to make its acceptance by the British Government impossible. Mr. Hay, instructed by the President to reopen negotiations in the endeavor to secure the assent of the British Government to a new convention, deemed it not only politic but absolutely indispensable that he should consult with leading Senators; that he should inform them of the lines on which he proposed to negotiate the new treaty, and ascertain from them if the suggested stipulations met with their approval. This he did by the direct instruction of President McKinley; not only did he advise with Senators but also with the Vice-President, who is not a member of the Senate and can not vote on a treaty.

That "perfect *secrecy* and *immediate* dispatch" which Jay held to be "sometimes requisite" are impossible if the Senate must be consulted in advance of negotiations. Jay, who was wise enough to see that there were persons "who would rely on the secrecy of the President, but who would not confide in that of the Senate," thought that the constitutional convention had done well in providing "that although the President must, in forming them [treaties], act by the advice and consent of the Senate, yet he will be able to manage the business of intelligence in such a manner as prudence may suggest." This is antiquated doctrine. The modern doctrine makes the President merely the agent of the Senate in framing a treaty.

"The State Department in its negotiations with foreign governments has one hand tied behind its back and a ball and chain about its leg," was the remark made to the writer by a man who has had a long experience in American diplomacy. Jay voiced the fear entertained at the time of the adoption of the Constitution "that two-thirds [of the Senate] will oppress the remaining third," but to-day it is always the one-third that has the power to oppress the remaining two-thirds and the Executive as well. A treaty is always sure to meet with political opposition, the opposition, that is, of the party antagonistic to the President; or opposition originating in prejudice, self-interest, or ignorance. As instances may be cited the defeat of the Olney-Pauncefote general treaty of arbitration (the defeat of which was caused by dislike of Mr. Cleveland and Mr. Olney, and by the general prejudice then existing against the negotiation of a treaty of that character with England); the failure to act affirmatively on the French reciprocity treaty, because it was believed it might injure certain manufacturing interests; the amendments to the Hay-Pauncefote canal treaty, inserted because certain similar amendments were found in the convention on which the new treaty was based, which were perfectly proper in the one and had no place in the other; and also because certain Senators were honest enough to say that they feared the construction of the canal would seriously injure the transcontinental railroads. Every treaty will meet with opposition from one or all of these sources, which explains the extreme difficulty of securing the ratification of a treaty in these days, and why it is so much easier for the one-third to prevent ratification than it is for the two-thirds to secure it. Lest it be said that this is a criticism of the Constitution, it may be frankly answered that it is nothing of the kind; but it is a criticism of the assumption of the Senate, and it justifies the statement that the State Department is always hampered by the ball and chain of the Senate.

The desire of the Senate to leave its impress upon all treaties is shown by trivial and absurd amendments, "the customary disfigurement at the hands of the United States Senate," to use Mr. Cleveland's vigorous language in discussing the Venezuelan settlement. Illustrative of what amounts almost to a mania, in recent years, on the part of the Senate to amend treaties, is the convention of 1896 with Great Britain for the settlement of claims arising out of the unlawful seizure by the United States of British vessels in Behring Sea. The convention as negotiated and signed by the plenipotentiaries of the contracting powers provided that "the commission may sit at San Francisco, California, as well as Victoria, provided it shall determine in any case that the interests of justice so require, due regard being had to the necessary expense and to all other considerations involved." The Senate, to make the language conform to its own ideas, changed the article to read: "The Committee shall also sit in San Francisco, California, as well as Victoria, provided that either Commissioner shall so request, if he shall be of the opinion that interests of justice shall so require, for reasons to be recorded on the minutes."

In 1883, a treaty was submitted to the Senate extending the life of a previously concluded convention with France for the adjustment of claims between the two countries. Defining the practice to be observed, the negotiators used these words: "If the proceedings of the Commission shall be interrupted by the death or incapacity of any one of the Commissioners," etc., which the Senate amended to read: "If the proceedings of the Commission shall be interrupted by the death, incapacity, retirement, or cessation of the functions of any one of the Commissioners," etc.

An examination made by me of original treaties in the archives of the Department of State shows that, in the early days, the Senate exercised the right of amendment very sparingly and with great discretion, but of recent years, especially during the last decade, it has exerted its power with the greatest freedom, until now the treaty that is ratified without amendment is the exception.

What enables the oligarchs of the Senate to exercise their dominant power, to reduce the House to a legislative nonentity and to keep the President in subjection, is the peculiar code of the Senate, the unwritten code which is more powerful than the printed rules. The fear expressed by Hamilton, that a few of the members of the House by long experience and a mastery of public affairs would dominate their associates, finds its realization in the Senate. An *imperium in imperio* exists there. Despite the fact that all Senators are free and equal, that one man may be able to block business, and that "government by agreement" eliminates friction, all real authority is centered in a few hands; at the present time not more than half a dozen Senators have reached censorian dignity. The *Congressional Directory* of November 27th, 1900, a recent edition, gave the biographies of eighty-five Senators, there being five vacancies at that time. Of the total number, forty-eight were then serving their first term, nineteen their second, six their third, eight their fourth, and four their fifth; but even these figures are misleading, as some of the men credited with two terms have not seen six years of service; they were appointed to fill vacancies and then elected for a full term. But taking the figures as they stand, nearly eighty per cent of the Senate has served less than twelve years and twenty per cent more.

In the Senate authority comes with length of service. A new Senator is placed at the foot of unimportant committees, no matter how long his experience in public life or his standing in the House of Representatives or elsewhere (Mr. Carlisle was one of the rare exceptions), and he can only reach a chairmanship of a leading committee by the retirement of Senators who outrank him. The system is so automatic that it is almost military in its operation. No matter how brilliant the attainments of a captain, he must bow to the superior wisdom of a colonel or a general. A Webster entering the Senate to-day would perforce sit at the foot of the table and find it futile to try and oppose the chairman; and a Webster would find himself on a committee of minor importance, while men his intellectual inferiors and his juniors in years, but his seniors in service, would be members of great committees. By this method power always centers in the hands of a few men, the half dozen or so Senators who are at the head of the few really important committees. No legislation can be enacted, no policy can be put into execution, unless these men are first consulted and give their consent. They are, in effect, the Senate of the United States.

. At the beginning of this article was used one of Bismarck's favorite maxims. Perhaps it may not be inappropriate to close with the remark made by the Iron Chancellor when discussing the terms of peace with France, an observation that the Senate might remember with profit: *"La patrie veut être servie, et non pas dominée."* [1]

SENATE PROCEDURE. OBSTRUCTION ON THE CURRENCY BILL, 1908 [2]

[The procedure of the Senate has been characterized by its flexibility and the absence from it of any general rules limiting debate. According to the traditions of the Senate there should not be any hindrance to free and full debate in that chamber. The closure or previous question has never been used in the Senate, nor has a limit been fixed to debate by a special vote. In every respect the procedure of the Senate has been in diametrical opposition to that in the other branch of the federal legislature. Repeatedly this freedom of debate has been used by individual Senators for the purpose of blocking legislation to which they were opposed, especially toward the end of a short session which expires by limitation on the 4th of March. Thus Senator Carter defeated the River and Harbor Bill, Senator Quay conducted a lengthy filibuster on the Statehood Bill, and Senator Tillman insisted upon an appropriation for a claim in favor of his state which had been repeatedly disallowed. On May 30, 1908, Senator La Follette assisted by several other Senators, used obstructive tactics against the passage of the conference report on the Currency Bill. Every technicality was utilized for the purpose of consuming time. The question of "no quorum" was raised thirty-six times within a few hours, necessitating the calling of the roll at brief intervals. The session, beginning at noon on May 29, lasted on

[1] An answer to the above article, by William H. Moody. member of Congress, now Justice of the Supreme Court was published in the *North American Review*, March, 1902.

[2] *Congr. Record*, May 30.

through the night until late in the afternoon of the following day. As the official term of Congress would not have come to an end for nearly a year, the process of obstruction might have gone on indefinitely had not an entirely new turn been given to Senate procedure. Between midnight and 6 o'clock of May 30, three very important precedents were established which may in the future materially interfere with the traditional liberty of unlimited discussion in the Senate. The precedents may be summarized as follows: First, The vice-president announced that it was within the providence of the chair to count a quorum and that a roll call would not be ordered if a quorum was actually present. This decision gives the vice-president practically the same power with respect to a quorum that is enjoyed by the speaker of the House. Second, The Senate determined that the question of "no quorum" could not be raised if a previous roll call had disclosed the presence of a quorum, and if no business had intervened. It was held that debate was not such intervening business. Third, A rule of the Senate which in practice has always lain dormant was invoked, prohibiting a Senator from addressing the Senate upon any question more than twice in any one day.

The great importance of these precedents as well as the interest of the proceeding in itself warrant a study of the occasion upon which the precedents were applied. The manner in which this conference report on the Currency Bill was brought about will be illustrated later. See page 210 *et seq.*]

THE VICE-PRESIDENT. Fifty Senators have answered to their names. A quorum of the Senate is present. The Senator from Texas will proceed.

Mr. LA FOLLETTE. I rise to a question of parliamentary inquiry.

The VICE-PRESIDENT. Does the Senator from Texas yield to the Senator from Wisconsin?

Mr. CULBERSON. I prefer ——

Mr. LA FOLLETTE. It is not necessary for the Senator from Texas to yield to the Senator from Wisconsin when the Senator from Wisconsin rises to a parliamentary inquiry.

The VICE-PRESIDENT. The Senator from Wisconsin will kindly state his parliamentary inquiry.

Mr. LA FOLLETTE. It is this, Mr. President: That if at any time during the daily sessions of the Senate a question shall be raised by any Senator ——

Mr. NELSON. Mr. President, I rise to a point of order.

Mr. LA FOLLETTE (continuing). As to the presence of a quorum ——

Mr. NELSON. I rise to a point of order, Mr. President.

Mr. LA FOLLETTE (continuing). The presiding officer shall forthwith direct ——

The VICE-PRESIDENT. The Senator from Wisconsin is stating a point of order.

Mr. NELSON. I rise to a point of order, Mr. President.

Mr. LA FOLLETTE. I decline to yield, Mr. President.

The VICE-PRESIDENT. The Senator from Wisconsin will state his point of order.

Mr. LA FOLLETTE. I desire to bring Rule V to the attention of the President of the Senate. Rule V, subdivision 2, provides —

2. If, at any time during the daily sessions of the Senate, a question shall be raised by any Senator as to the presence of a quorum, the presiding officer shall forthwith direct the Secretary to call the roll and shall announce the result, and these proceedings shall be without debate.

I have been a member of this Senate, Mr. President, but a brief time, but I have on numerous occasions, without any Senator yielding the floor, noted the fact that the attention of the presiding officer, under subdivision 2 of Rule V, had been called to the fact of the absence of a quorum, and that thereupon, without the consent of any Senator, either the presence of a quorum was demonstrated or its absence demonstrated by the calling of the roll; and I call the attention of the presiding officer to the fact that no quorum is present.

Mr. NELSON. Mr. President, I desire to make a point of order.

The VICE-PRESIDENT. The Senator will state his point of order.

Mr. NELSON. Mr. President, a parliamentary inquiry is not a point of order under our procedure in the Senate. That is a practice that has grown up in the other House of Members applying to the Chair and asking to make a parliamentary inquiry. Our rules know nothing of the kind. There is no point of order in it. I make the point of order that the Chair is not obliged to respond to any parliamentary inquiry.

Mr. ALDRICH. I make the further point of order that in order to make a parliamentary inquiry a Senator must be in possession of the floor, and that he can not take the floor by asking to make a parliamentary inquiry and then make any motion.

The VICE-PRESIDENT. The Chair ——

Mr. LA FOLLETTE. If I may be permitted a suggestion, Mr. President, I had the attention of the presiding officer of the Senate. I brought to his attention the fact that there was no quorum present; and under subdivision 2 of Rule V it seems to me that there is but one proceeding open, and that is to ascertain by a roll call, under the direction of the presiding officer of the Senate, as to whether or not there is a quorum present.

Mr. GALLINGER. Regular order, Mr. President.

The VICE-PRESIDENT. The Chair is of opinion that the Senator from Texas [Mr. Culberson] had the floor, and that he declined to yield to the Senator from Wisconsin [Mr. La Follette]. The Chair, therefore, sustains the point of order.

Mr. LA FOLLETTE. I am very reluctant to have to appeal from that decision.

The VICE-PRESIDENT. The Senator from Wisconsin appeals from the decision of the Chair. The question is, Shall the decision of the Chair stand as the judgment of the Senate?

Mr. LA FOLLETTE. I suppose I am entitled to a hearing upon that appeal. I do not propose to trust to myself in discussing that question. I simply propose to read into the RECORD of this Senate the rules of the Senate, and to take the ruling of the Senate upon that proposition.

Mr. GALLINGER. We are ready to give it.

Mr. LA FOLLETTE. Having obtained the floor, I called the attention of the Presiding Officer of this body to the fact that no quorum was present. Under Rule V, subdivision 2, I find the following:

2. If, at any time during the daily sessions of the Senate, a question shall be raised by any Senator as to the presence of a quorum, the Presiding Officer shall forthwith direct the Secretary to call the roll.

Mr. President, I submit that the proceedings of this Senate and the integrity of its proceedings can never be protected unless that rule be enforced, and enforced rigidly. You are about to make a precedent here, which may return to plague you some time, because, under a certain leadership, you have set your faces to enact certain legislation. I submit to you that you may go to that extent that you will find yourselves embarrassed greatly in the future. Is it possible that important proceedings in the Senate, if one man can get the floor, may be conducted here for an unlimited period of time in the presence of the Presiding Officer and one single Senator, he declining to yield the floor? It might be possible for him to incorporate into the proceedings of this Senate the most outrageous matters, because there is an organization here that resists whenever an effort is made upon this floor for the great body of the people of this country. Let me say to you Senators who are yet free, that you may go to such an extent as to completely commit yourselves for the future.

Now, I want to read the balance of that rule to this body:

The Presiding Officer shall forthwith —

I am reading from Rule V, subdivision 2 —

If, at any time during the daily sessions of the Senate, a question shall be raised by any Senator —

I will undertake to say, Mr. President, that a hundred times in the two years that I have been a member of this body I have seen Senators rise on this floor, call upon the presiding officer, and, without any assent upon the part of the Senator who had the floor, raise the question that no quorum was present. I will undertake to say that an examination of the records of this Senate will show that that has occurred during the present session possibly a hundred times.

If, at any time during the daily sessions of the Senate, a question shall be raised by any Senator as to the presence of a quorum, the presiding officer shall forthwith direct the Secretary to call the roll and shall announce the result —

Now, I submit that neither the presiding officer nor this body ought to let the decision of that question turn upon the proposition of who raises it —

And these proceedings shall be without debate.

The third subdivision of Rule V is as follows:

3. Whenever upon such roll call it shall be ascertained that a quorum is not present, a majority of the Senators present may direct the Sergeant-at-Arms to request, and, when necessary, to compel the attendance of the absent Senators, which order shall be determined without debate; and pending its execution, and until a quorum shall be present no debate nor motion, except to adjourn, shall be in order.

See, Mr. President and Senators, how carefully the maker of those rules guarded this important question of the presence of a quorum during all the deliberations of this body.

Mr. ALDRICH. Mr. President, it is very evident that a question of this kind can not be raised under the provisions of the rule unless the Senator raising the question has the floor, and I therefore move that the appeal taken by the Senator from Wisconsin be laid upon the table.

Mr. CULBERSON. I hope the Senator will not make that motion now.

Mr. ALDRICH. I think I must make it now.

Mr. CULBERSON. I desire to make a statement.

Mr. ALDRICH. I withhold the motion for the purpose of allowing the Senator to make a statement.

Mr. CULBERSON. Mr. President, in my judgment the decision of the Chair is erroneous. I believe that the question of the existence of a quorum can be raised at any time, even without the consent of the Senator who may at the time hold the floor in debate. The notes of the stenographer will show that, being asked by the Chair if I yielded to the Senator from Wisconsin, I stated that I preferred not to; and that is true. I preferred, as I have stated once or twice, to go on with the financial statement I have to make to the Senate and to the country about the extravagance of the Administration of President Roosevelt and be through with it; but I do not believe — and it has not been my purpose in anything I have said or anything I have done to make such a suggestion — that by asking not to be interrupted I could cut off any Senator from making the point that there was no quorum.

Mr. ALDRICH. I ask for a vote on my motion.

The VICE-PRESIDENT. The Chair will state that Rule XIX provides that —

No Senator shall interrupt another Senator in debate without his consent.

The Chair certainly construed the language of the Senator from Texas [Mr. Culberson] to mean that he did not yield to the interruption of the Senator from Wisconsin [Mr. La Follette]. The Senator from Rhode Island [Mr. Aldrich] moves that the motion be laid upon the table. All in favor of that motion will say "aye" ——

Mr. LA FOLLETTE. Mr. President, upon that question I demand the yeas and nays.

The VICE-PRESIDENT. The Senator from Wisconsin demands the yeas and nays. Is the demand seconded? [Putting the question.] One-fifth of the Senators present have not joined in the demand.

Mr. LA FOLLETTE. I ask for a division.

The VICE-PRESIDENT. A division is demanded. Those in favor of the motion will rise and stand until counted.

The question being put, there were, on a division — ayes 32, noes 14.

Mr. BACON. Mr. President, I desire to state ——

Mr. GORE. Mr. President ——

Mr. BACON. I have the floor, I think.

The VICE-PRESIDENT. The Senator from Georgia [Mr. Bacon] is entitled to the floor.

Mr. BACON. As I did not have the opportunity to express myself before the vote, and as the motion to lay the appeal upon the table did not permit of an expression, I desire to say that in voting not to lay the appeal on the table I was not unmindful of the old adage that "hard cases make bad law," and I was unwilling to establish a precedent.

Mr. ALDRICH. Mr. President ——

Mr. BACON. I hope the Senator will not interrupt me; I will occupy but a minute. I just want to say that, while I voted that way, I do not wish to be construed as being in sympathy in any particular with any obstructive proceedings to-day in regard to the pending matter. I voted that way because I thought that was the correct rule. So far as I am concerned, I prefer that the proceedings of the Senate should go on in the ordinary and usual manner.

Mr. GORE. Mr. President, I submit that the division discloses that there is not the presence of a quorum.

Mr. KEAN. Let us have the regular order, Mr. President.

The VICE-PRESIDENT. The division disclosed the existence of a quorum.

Mr. GORE. It takes forty-seven to constitute a quorum.

Mr. KEAN. Let us have the regular order.

The VICE-PRESIDENT. The Chair is of the opinion that a quorum is present.

Mr. GORE. I should like to say that there are ninety-two members of this body. Half of that number is forty-six. A division disclosed the presence of forty-six. As I understand, it takes one more than half to constitute a quorum.

The VICE-PRESIDENT. There was present a Senator who did not vote. A quorum is present, in the opinion of the Chair.

Mr. CULBERSON. Mr. President ——

The VICE-PRESIDENT. The Senator from Texas is recognized.

Mr. LA FOLLETTE. Mr. President, may I make a parliamentary inquiry?

The VICE-PRESIDENT. The Senator from Wisconsin rises to a parliamentary inquiry.

Mr. LA FOLLETTE. It is this: Whether the decision of the President of the Senate at this time establishes the precedent in this body of counting a quorum when the vote discloses that no quorum is present.

The VICE-PRESIDENT. The Chair will read from the decision of the President pro tempore of the Senate on June 19, 1879. The Chair understands that the occupant of the chair at that time was Allen G. Thurman, then a Senator from Ohio. A roll call was ordered and had, whereupon the following occurred:

The PRESIDENT pro tempore. No quorum has voted. The Chair has counted the Senate. There is a quorum present, but no quorum voting.

Mr. HOUSTON. Mr. President, as I understand the construction of Rule No. 2, by the Presiding Officer, whenever it is disclosed on a vote that there is no quorum he may have the roll called.

The PRESIDENT pro tempore. The Chair has usually taken the fact of there being no quorum voting as evidence that there was no quorum present; but the Chair has not decided that it is not possible to ascertain otherwise whether there is a quorum. The Chair does not think the fact that a quorum has not voted is conclusive evidence that a quorum is not present. On the contrary, in the opinion of the Chair, he has a right to count the Senate. He has counted the Senate and found that a quorum is in attendance, but a quorum has not voted.

In the present instance the Chair has counted the Senate, and there is a quorum present.

Mr. KEAN. Regular order, Mr. President.

The VICE-PRESIDENT. The Senator from Texas [Mr. Culberson] has the floor.

Mr. CULBERSON. Mr. President, as I have the floor, there will either have to be order on the floor, or I will call for a quorum. I do not suppose there will be any question about that.

The VICE-PRESIDENT. The Senate will be in order.

Mr. Culberson resumed his speech. After having spoken about ten minutes.

Mr. HOPKINS. Mr. President ——

Mr. CULBERSON. I decline to yield, Mr. President.

The VICE-PRESIDENT. The Senator from Texas declines to yield.

Mr. CULBERSON. I do so with the utmost respect to the Senator from Illinois, inasmuch as I declined to yield to others. I want to get through with this statement.

The VICE-PRESIDENT. The Senator from Texas declines to yield.

[Mr. Culberson resumed and concluded his speech.]

The VICE-PRESIDENT. The question is on agreeing to the report of the committee of conference.

Mr. LA FOLLETTE. What is the question?

Mr. KEAN. Let us have the question.

*   *   *   *   *   *   *   *

Mr. LA FOLLETTE. Mr. President, if I am at liberty to proceed, I am very glad. I was afraid I was going to be interrupted for some time, while the Senate sent for absentees. I did not understand the proceeding exactly, and I do not like to be off the floor a moment longer than is absolutely necessary to get the attendance of a quorum. And now may I make a parliamentary inquiry before starting in? Suppose it should develop on top of this situation that there is not a quorum present, can I raise the point of no quorum?

Mr. HALE. Clearly the Senator can not raise that point while we are proceeding under the previous call to secure the attendance of Senators by the Sergeant-at-Arms. When the Sergeant-at-Arms reports and that proceeding is ended, then if there is no quorum another call may be made, but it can not be made until those proceedings are completed.

Mr. LA FOLLETTE. Mr. President, I want to remind Senators that you are making precedents now. I have been informed that there is going to be a rule sprung on me before I get through that a Senator, in a single legislative day, can speak only twice upon a question.

Mr. GALLINGER. That is the rule.

Mr. LA FOLLETTE. That is the rule. It has never been enforced since I have been a member of this body.

Mr. FORAKER. The rule is that he can not speak more than twice ——

The PRESIDING OFFICER. Does the Senator from Wisconsin yield to the Senator from Ohio?

Mr. LA FOLLETTE. Surely.

Mr. FORAKER. As I understand it, a Senator can not speak more than twice during the same legislative day on the same subject except by unanimous consent.

Mr. LA FOLLETTE. Yes; and I hardly expect to obtain unanimous consent, if I should yield the floor at any time.

Mr. CULBERSON. Mr. President ——

The PRESIDING OFFICER. Does the Senator from Wisconsin yield to the Senator from Texas?

Mr. LA FOLLETTE. I am not sure whether I have a right to the floor or not.

Mr. CULBERSON. I call the attention of the Senator from Ohio to the exact wording of the rule.

The PRESIDING OFFICER. Does the Senator from Wisconsin yield?

Mr. LA FOLLETTE. If I have the floor, I yield to this interruption from the Senator from Texas.

Mr. CULBERSON. I simply wanted to call the attention of the Senator from Ohio to the exact wording of the rule. It is that —

No Senator shall speak more than twice upon any one question in debate on the same day without leave of the Senate.

Mr. FORAKER. I was in error in saying "by unanimous consent." I understand very well, of course, that that is the language of the rule. I want to suggest to the Senator that when he gets to that point he ask the leave of the Senate.

Mr. LA FOLLETTE. Mr. President, of course I understand perfectly well that the Senate would deny me leave to proceed.

Mr. FORAKER. Oh, Mr. President, I do not think the Senator should assume anything of the kind in view of what has occurred to-day. I think the Senate will allow the Senator anything he may ask.

Mr. LA FOLLETTE. . The Senator says "in view of what occurred to-day." I do not think that I was given any indulgence to-day at all. I think that I was entirely within my right. And I do not expect any indulgence from the Senate. I never have had any since I have been a member of it.

Mr. FORAKER. The Senator surely was entirely within his right. I was not making any complaint of the Senator, and I am not complaining of anybody, but I was referring to the vote of the Senate on the occasion the Senator has in mind.

Mr. OVERMAN. Mr. President, I rise to a parliamentary inquiry. Can the Senator from Wisconsin proceed until the Sergeant-at-Arms reports?

Mr. HOPKINS. There is a quorum present.

The PRESIDING OFFICER. There is a quorum present, and the Chair is of opinion that the Senator from Wisconsin has the floor and may proceed.

Mr. OVERMAN. The question I raise is whether it has been established that a quorum is present.

The PRESIDING OFFICER. A quorum is present.

Mr. OVERMAN. And at any time can the point of a quorum be raised if there is no quorum?

Mr. GALLINGER and others. Regular order!

The PRESIDING OFFICER. The Senator from Wisconsin is entitled to the floor.

Mr. LA FOLLETTE. I should like to know the Chair's ruling upon that point.

The PRESIDING OFFICER. The Chair is of opinion that the Senator from Wisconsin has the floor and may proceed.

Mr. LA FOLLETTE. That was not the parliamentary inquiry. I would present the parliamentary inquiry to the Chair just presented by the Senator from North Carolina.

The PRESIDING OFFICER. The Chair will determine that question when it arises.

Mr. LA FOLLETTE. Then I will raise the question now — that there is not any quorum present.

The PRESIDING OFFICER. The Chair is of opinion that ——

Mr. LA FOLLETTE. It is not a question of the opinion of the Chair.

The PRESIDING OFFICER. There is a quorum present.

Mr. LA FOLLETTE. Mr. President, I submit that when the question is raised it is not for the Chair to state that there is a quorum present.

The PRESIDING OFFICER. The Chair will read clause 3 of Rule V:

> 3. Whenever upon such roll call it shall be ascertained that a quorum is not present, a majority of the Senators present may direct the Sergeant-at-Arms to request, and, when necessary, to compel the attendance of the absent Senators, which order shall be determined without debate; and pending its execution, and until a quorum shall be present, no debate nor motion, except to adjourn, shall be in order.

This implies, of course, that when a quorum is present the business of the Senate shall proceed. The Senator from Wisconsin has the floor.

Mr. LA FOLLETTE. That was not the parliamentary inquiry presented by the Senator from North Carolina. If it was, I want to present another, and that is this: It having developed that a quorum is present and that the regular legislative business of the Senate may be resumed, I ask, if the question is raised, under subdivision 2 of Rule V, that there is no quorum present, whether it does not then become necessary to ascertain by a roll call whether there is a quorum present. That is my parliamentary inquiry.

Mr. TELLER. Mr. President, I understand the rule to be that when a quorum is found to exist and it is announced business may then proceed, and no Senator can call for a quorum until after some business, at least, has been transacted.

Mr. LA FOLLETTE. I think that is true, Mr. President.

The PRESIDING OFFICER. The Chair is of the opinion that after a quorum is announced the business of the Senate must proceed until there has been some transaction of business.

Mr. LA FOLLETTE. Yes; I think that is true, and I was, perhaps, anticipating somewhat in raising this parliamentary inquiry. But it came up at the suggestion of the Senator from North Carolina, and being a rather interesting question ——

Mr. OVERMAN. It came from the Senator from Maine.

Mr. LA FOLLETTE. That is true.

Mr. OVERMAN. I differed with him on the question, and that is the reason why I made the inquiry of the Chair.

Mr. ALDRICH. Mr. President, I rise to a question of order. The suggestion of the Senator from Wisconsin is not in order. We have had 32 roll calls within a comparatively short time, all disclosing the presence of a quorum. Manifestly a quorum is in the building. If repeated suggestions of the want of a quorum can be made without intervening business, the whole business of the Senate is put in the hands of one man, who can insist upon continuous calls of the roll upon the question of a quorum. My question of order is that, without the intervention of business, a quorum having been disclosed by a vote or by a call of the roll, no further calls are in order until some business has intervened. I should be glad if the Vice-President would submit that question of order to the Senate.

I call the attention of the Chair to a decision in a case, which is on all fours with this, made on March 3, 1897, when this precise question was raised by the then Senator from New York, Mr. Hill, who sustained it by the same argument which I am now calling the attention of the Chair to; and the point made by the Senator from New York was sustained. It is found on page 2737 of volume 29, part 3, of the *Record*, second session, Fifty-fourth Congress. The language was —

MR. HILL. My point is, that the presence of a quorum was determined by the last roll call, and that a Senator can not immediately thereafter suggest the absence of a quorum.
The PRESIDING OFFICER. Does the Senator mean to embrace the feature that no business has intervened?
Mr. HILL. Yes; that no business has intervened.
The PRESIDING OFFICER. The Chair sustains the point of order.

The VICE-PRESIDENT. Will the Senator from Rhode Island kindly restate his point of order.
Mr. ALDRICH. It is that the roll of the Senate having disclosed the presence of a quorum and no business having intervened, the suggestion of the absence of a quorum is not in order.
The VICE-PRESIDENT. The Chair submits to the Senate the question of order raised by the Senator from Rhode Island.
Mr. LA FOLLETTE. Mr. President, I just wish to suggest, in order that it may appear upon the RECORD that debate has intervened since the last roll call.
Mr. ALDRICH. That is not business.
Mr. LA FOLLETTE. I just wish that to appear upon the *Record*.
Mr. ALDRICH. My suggestion was that debate was not business.
Mr. LA FOLLETTE. And I want to remind Senators here to-night, before this vote is taken, that every precedent you establish to-night will be brought home to you hereafter.
Mr. GALLINGER. Mr. President, I simply desire to add to what has been said, that if the entire business of the Senate can be put in

the hands of one man, that one man could destroy the Government; he could prevent appropriations being made to carry on the governmental machinery, and it is absurd to suppose that it was ever so intended.

Mr. CULBERSON.   Mr. President, I understood the Senator from Rhode Island to read from subdivision 2 of Rule V.

Mr. ALDRICH.   I did not read any rule.   I make the point upon the ordinary parliamentary law, which governs this body in the absence of rules, that the Senate itself has decided this precise point upon, I think, two or three occasions.   I have one precedent before me, which is exactly on all fours with the present situation.

Mr. CULBERSON.   The Senator then read from a decision on the question?

Mr. ALDRICH.   Yes; I called attention to a case which appears in the *Record*.

Mr. CULBERSON.   Mr. President, that refers to a particular proceeding of the Senate.   I simply want to read the rule, which provides:

2. If, at any time during the daily sessions of the Senate, a question shall be raised by any Senator as to the presence of a quorum, the Presiding Officer shall forthwith direct the Secretary to call the roll and shall announce the result, and these proceedings shall be without debate.

It not only provides that it shall be done at any time during the daily sessions, but provides that the proceedings shall be had without debate.

The VICE-PRESIDENT.   The question is on the point of order submitted by the Senator from Rhode Island [Mr. Aldrich].

[The roll call was concluded.]

The result was announced — yeas 35, nays 5.

The VICE-PRESIDENT.   A quorum has not voted.

Mr. FORAKER.   Mr. President, I ask if it is not a rule of the Senate that all Senators in the Chamber when the roll is called shall vote unless they be excused by the Senate?   I noticed quite a number of Senators in the Chamber who were in the Chamber when the roll was called who did not answer in any way to their names.

The VICE-PRESIDENT.   Rule XII covers the question raised by the Senator from Ohio.   It reads in part as follows:

1. When the yeas and nays are ordered, the names of Senators shall be called alphabetically; and each Senator shall, without debate, declare his assent or dissent to the question, unless excused by the Senate.

Mr. HOPKINS.   I ask that the Secretary call the names of the Senators present who have not answered, so as to give them an opportunity to answer.

The VICE-PRESIDENT. The Secretary will call the names of those Senators who have not voted.

The Secretary called the name of Messrs. Allison, Bacon, Bailey, Bankhead, Beveridge, Borah, Bourne, Bulkeley, Burnham, Clarke of Arkansas, Clay ——

Mr. CLAY (when his name was called). "Here." I have already announced my pair with the senior Senator from Massachusetts [Mr. Lodge].

Mr. HOPKINS. The Senator votes "present."

The Secretary called the names of Messrs. Crane, Culberson ——

Mr. HOPKINS. I observe the Senator from Texas [Mr. Culberson] is present, and I should like to have a record of that fact made. The Senator from Texas is present in the Chamber.

Mr. GALLINGER. You would prefer to have him vote, would you not?

The VICE-PRESIDENT. For the information of the Senate, the Chair will read section 2 of Rule XII. It is as follows:

2. When a Senator declines to vote on call of his name, he shall be required to assign his reasons therefor, and having assigned them, the Presiding Officer shall submit the question to the Senate: "Shall the Senator, for the reasons assigned by him, be excused from voting?" which shall be decided without debate; and these proceedings shall be had after the roll call and before the result is announced; and any further proceedings in reference thereto shall be after such announcement.

The Secretary will continue to call the roll of absent Senators.

[The Secretary called the remaining names. . . .]

The VICE-PRESIDENT. Thirty-five Senators have voted in the affirmative and eight in the negative. There is a quorum present, the roll call having disclosed that fact.

*   *   *   *   *   *   *   *

Mr. LA FOLLETTE. What I said was, that I had seen it announced in the morning papers that the leaders were going to permit us to enact a Government employees' liability bill; and when I said "leaders" I looked at the Senator from Indiana, and he nodded his head [laughter]; and I thought he had been informed.

Mr. BEVERIDGE. Mr. President ——

Mr. LA FOLLETTE. Wait just one moment. Mr. President, I thought probably the Senator had been encouraged by the gentlemen who have been opposing his strenuous efforts to get this legislation. I refer to the older leadership of the Senate, who have by calling for the reading of the Journal, prevented his getting the floor to urge this legislation. He started early enough, so that he should, with a fair chance, have gotten through a good proposition which he announced that he would offer as a substitute for this makeshift bill.

But we have had the reading of the Journal, as well as the reading of messages that came over from the House. In this way a good deal of time has been used here to prevent action upon this Government employees' bill, which was being urged by the Senator from Indiana.

I do hope that the leaders have decided to let us have that legislation. That is the only way we can get it; at least that was the way the morning papers presented it. I am not very experienced here; I have not been in this body very long; but it has rather seemed to me that, some way or other, unless it met the approval of a very limited number of men in this body, whatever a Senator introduced was referred to some committee and pigeonholed. In that way, I suppose, it falls within the power of a very limited number of men, who are the leaders, to be in control of legislation. It has rather seemed to me, Mr. President, that this was not exactly the sort of government that our fathers planned for us. It has always been my idea — it was before I came down here, you know — that the States were represented here; that there was an equality of representation; that the Senator from Missouri and the Senator from Rhode Island were on a plane of equality with respect to legislation. I had had only a limited service over in the House. It was not then just as it is now, and all the while I have labored under a sort of impression that if any Senator came here with an absolutely good proposition; if he stuck to it and was loyal to it and hammered away at it, it would get consideration just the same as if it was introduced by somebody else. But a couple of years here brings me quite a bit of enlightenment on that subject.

I attended a caucus at the beginning of this Congress. I happened to look at my watch when we went into that caucus. We were in session three minutes and a half. Do you know what happened? Well, I will tell you. A motion was made that somebody preside. Then a motion was made that whoever presided should appoint a committee on committees; and a motion was then made that we adjourn. [Laughter.] Nobody said anything but the Senator who made the motion. Then and there the fate of all the legislation of this session was decided.

The Senator from Indiana [Mr. Beveridge], in an able speech which he made in advocacy of the creation of a tariff commission here, turned a little light upon the legislative methods of this body. In speaking of the impossibility of the Finance Committee taking up the great tariff question and giving to it the study necessary to make a thorough investigation upon scientific and economic lines, establishing a just basis for a tariff, one under which the business interests of the country can thrive and rest in security, one which will be stable, one which will be unassailable, one which will be honest to the manufacturers and honest as well to the consumers, the Senator pointed out the facts and called attention to the number of places that the members of the Committee on Finance had upon the other important committees of this body and to the tax which that made upon their time and upon their service. It was unanswerable;

but it was more than that. I want to carry the thing a step further than the Senator from Indiana did. He cited the fact and applied it to this particular piece of legislation; but, Mr. President, if you will scan the committees of this Senate, you will find that a little handful of men are in domination and control of the great legislative committees of this body and that they are a very limited number.

I have heard this talk about seniority and all the like explanations, but I want to tell you, Senators, that this is a representative Government. California and Wisconsin and Maine are entitled to equal representation here; and the hour will come when this system which you have inaugurated to lodge the power of legislation in the hands of a dozen men in this body can no longer be maintained; and it ought not to be maintained. It is not democratic; it is not republican; it is not right. It places upon those members burdens which they are unable to carry, if they take proper care of the great interests committed to those committees. If that be not so, then you may as well dispense with two-thirds, practically, of the membership of this body.

* * * * * * * *

Mr. GORE. Now, Mr. President, I submit that gentlemen on the other side have not only changed their convictions with reference to this measure, but they are, as I understand, changing, if not the rules, at least the practices and customs of this body. A suggestion was made during the early hours of the morning that there was no quorum present. That suggestion was overruled or held out of order. An appeal was taken to the Senate, and the Chair was sustained. When I reported here this morning, not altogether upon my own motion, a different Senator, to my surprise, I may say, was holding the floor and entertaining the Senate. In the meantime this action had been taken and this business transacted by the Senate — an order, sir, that when this measure shall be voted upon it shall be by the yeas and nays.

During the speech of the Senator from Missouri [Mr. Stone] I made the suggestion of no quorum. That suggestion was held to be out of order on the ground that no intervening business had transpired. Then, sir, I appealed from the decision of the Chair, and the distinguished Senator from Rhode Island [Mr. Aldrich], with an ingenuity that added luster to his renown, interposed with the statement that a suggestion that was out of order could not be appealed from.

Mr. President, I am a new man in the Senate, but I shall have to change my decision if I ever appeal from a suggestion or from a ruling of the Chair that is made in my favor. It will be only those rulings which are adverse to my views and my convictions that I shall challenge, and that was the reason why I appealed from the decision of the Chair.

I make these observations in order to show, Mr. President, the revolutionary methods which are being employed to aid in the passage of this measure through the Senate. The majority of the Senate have changed not only their convictions, but changed the practices of a century, sir.

It has been the pride of the American Senate, and I may say of the American people, that there was at least one forum where free discussion forever prevailed. The Senate may not always have stood as high in the esteem of the public as it deserved to stand, and modesty forbids me to say that since my accession to the body its reputation ought to be enhanced in public favor, but, sir, it has been the pride of the American people that free discussion prevailed in the United States Senate. There was one forum where the truth could be elicited, where the merits and demerits of every measure could be discussed and illuminated without limitation or without hindrance, and I hope the day will never come when that tradition and that precedent shall be permanently abandoned.

I do not know what irresistible power is impelling the passage of this measure that Senators should resort to what seem to be such revolutionary tactics. It strikes me — perhaps born of inexperience and perhaps born of fear — that this proceeding is but the shadow of another scepter. I trust the time will never come when a measure can be passed through this Senate — a financial measure, a tariff measure, or any other measure of public concern — with a limitation of debate to one hour, to two hours, or even to three hours upon the side. I hope if that time ever comes there will be another branch of this Government, impelled by a regard for the Constitution, which will say that no measure can pass that body, which did not pass this body under constitutional methods and practices.

To illustrate, if a public buildings bill were pending in the Senate and a currency measure were pending in the House, I should never be willing for the Senate to insist that unless the currency measure passed the House the public buildings measure would be murdered in the Senate. I hope it will never come to that pass, and I am sorry that the parliamentary regulations forbid me to speak with even greater plainness.

I desire to ask the parliamentary status of the conference report. As I understand, no amendment can be offered to the pending report; not one letter can be stricken out or added to it; it must be accepted as a whole or it must be rejected as a whole.. Am I correct?

The VICE-PRESIDENT. The Senator from Oklahoma is correct. The only question is on agreeing to the report of the committee of conference.

Mr. GORE. I desired an explicit ruling on that point in order that the American people who are not experts in parliamentary law and usage might understand why the minority party did not offer salutary amendments to the pending report.

*   *   *   *   *   *   *   *

Mr. BACON. I was endeavoring to state that several things had occurred during the progress of the debate upon this question which I am unwilling should pass by as having met with general recognition, through acquiescence, by the Senate, because of the fact that in the Senate a precedent is a matter of gravity and importance, and occasions may arise hereafter where these questions may be of very much more vital importance than they have been while the pending question has been under discussion.

Of course, Mr. President, I recognize the fact that, in the heat of controversy, Senators, as well as others, will do and say things which will be conducive to the particular end which they then have in view, which, from a more conservative standpoint and under other circumstances they would neither say nor approve.

One precedent was made last night to which I wish to enter my dissent. That precedent was made by a vote of the Senate. It was to the effect that after a roll call had been had upon the suggestion of the want of a quorum, and after the roll call had disclosed the presence of a quorum, it was out of order, when nothing else had transpired but debate, to again suggest the absence of a quorum and again having a roll call for the purpose of determining whether or not a quorum was present. In other words, the Senate determined, by a vote, that a continuance of debate after a roll call did not amount to the intervention of other business, and that no business having intervened — debate not being recognized as business — regardless of the time which had elapsed, or regardless of the fact that there were, perhaps, only ten Senators present, there could be no suggestion of the absence of a quorum, and that the Senate must proceed with the ascertained fact that there had been a quorum, and without power to inquire whether or not there was then a quorum.

Mr. President, I did not vote upon that question when it was submitted to the Senate for this simple reason: The Senator from Rhode Island [Mr. Aldrich] had read what he alleged was a precedent in that matter, and had read from the *Congressional Record* a ruling which had been made by the Chair on March 3, 1897, which the Senator from Rhode Island contended established that proposition. It so happened, although the fact was not known, I think, to the Senator from Rhode Island at the time that he cited the precedent, that I was the Senator temporarily occupying the chair on the 3d of March, 1897, who made the ruling which was cited by the Senator from Rhode Island last night. I was unwilling to cast a vote last night which might appear to be in antagonism to that ruling, as there would then be no opportunity for me to show that the vote thus cast would not have been in contravention of that ruling made by myself when in the chair.

I recollect the incident well out of which the ruling grew. It occurred during a night session, and the then senior Senator from Pennsylvania, Mr. Quay, was the Senator who demanded the roll call upon the suggestion of the lack of a quorum. He had previously demanded several such roll calls. The point had been made between the two previous successive roll calls that no business had intervened and that therefore the second roll call was not in order. The Chair ruled that business had intervened, from the fact that in the interval the bill then under consideration had been reported from the Committee of the Whole to the Senate. Immediately after that roll call, which was then authorized by the decision of the Chair, the Senator from Pennsylvania, without waiting for any debate or any other action on the part of the Senate, immediately again suggested the absence of a quorum. That matter was taken up at once by the then senior Senator from Massachusetts, Mr. Hoar, and by the then Senator from New York, Mr. Hill, and the question was finally reduced to this point — whether or not business had intervened.

The Chair ruled that business had not intervened, and that therefore the second roll call was not in order. There had been no debate after the roll call, and there was no suggestion that debate was not the intervention of business. There was no question raised that the debate following a roll call did not constitute business which had intervened after the roll call. There was no question whether debate did or did not constitute business.

The question last night was whether debate constituted business. There confessedly had been debate last night after the roll call, and the question decided by the Senate last night was that the occurrence of debate did not constitute business.

Mr. President, I deemed it due to myself to state why I did not vote on the question, because I do not avoid any vote that comes along; but I wished to call the attention of the Senate to the fact that the precedent cited last night by the Senator from Rhode Island was not a controlling precedent upon the question raised by him, because in one case there was no question whether debate constituted business, and in the case last night the sole question was whether debate constituted business.

I desired, Mr. President, to say this much, because I was unwilling that what occurred last night should pass as an unchallenged precedent. I regard it as a revolutionary precedent, and, if so considered by the Senate, I am willing for it to pass as one adopted under the heat of contest for the purpose of effecting a particular end; but it will be a most grievous mistake, in my opinion, if that rule should be adopted as the rule or precedent to hereafter govern the action of the Senate. In fact, frequently here, in cases of protracted contests, for days and days there is nothing practically but debate. It is true we have the morning hour, and some measures may be considered; but so far as the main body of the work of the Senate during the whole day is concerned, frequently there is nothing but debate. To say that it having once been disclosed that there is a quorum there can be thereafter no challenge of the question as to whether or not there is a quorum, it seems to me, must be a very grave mistake.

THE COMMITTEE WORK OF SENATORS[1]

[Senator Hoar in his autobiography remarks that the Committee on Claims alone required of him more individual work than is performed in a year by any judge of a state court, and the amounts dealt with were greater than those involved in the annual litigation before any state supreme court. Though state judges may dissent from this estimate, at any rate it indicates the impression which the drudgery of committee work made upon Mr. Hoar. The nature of this work is illustrated by the following extracts.]

MR. BAILEY. Mr. President, of course the labor to be performed by the Senator himself and therefore the labor to be performed by the clerk or his assistant grows greater every year. The Government is touching the people at so many new places, I regret to say, that the correspondence of a Senator to-day is perhaps five times what it was in the days to which the Senator from Maine refers.

The truth of it is the correspondence of a Senator has become the burden of a Senator's life, and the task of writing thirty or forty and sometimes fifty letters is an almost daily one with us. Writing those letters for a thousand years would not add a cubit to a man's intellectual stature. It is purely a burden, but it is one which must be performed. When a Senator's constituent writes him on any subject, that constituent is entitled to a prompt and a respectful answer, and if the Senator does not allow the constituent to hear from him the Senator is very apt to hear from the constituent at the proper time; and I share the resentment which a constituent feels toward a Senator who ignores his communication.

This correspondence, growing from year to year, has become such a great burden that it would be utterly impossible for a Senator to perform his duties without clerical assistance. As for my part I am willing to give all that is necessary, but I am not willing to spend one dollar of public money to provide patronage for anybody. If the work of a Senator's committee or the work of a Senator requires three, let him have them. But I will not vote one dollar of public money merely to provide somebody a place. Patronage is not a very wholesome thing for a Senator to cultivate, and certainly it is not a very wholesome thing for the Senate to provide places merely that Senators may fill them.

But, Mr. President, that was not the purpose for which I rose. I rose to protest against the inequality which offends against the rule of justice. Either some clerks are paid too much or other clerks are paid too little. My own opinion is that some clerks are paid too much. But if Senators do not agree with me in that, they must agree with me that men who perform the same services should receive the same pay.

[1] *Congr. Record*, January 4, 1906.

I beg to say that I do not mean this in the nature of a complaint against the Senator from New Jersey or the committee over which he presides; I do not mean it as a complaint against any committee or as against the Senate, because I recognize that it has grown up from time to time, as suggested by the Senator from Maine [Mr. Hale], but I do insist that it is an inequality which ought to be corrected.

Mr. DANIEL. Mr. President, I am not one of those Senators who are suffering from any incumbrance of patronage, but every Senator has to deal with a great many people who have very mistaken notions as to his power to exercise patronage. I do not think that any Senator here, on either side of the House, wishes to increase the clerical force of the Senate with any view to patronage. It is purely a matter of public business and the prompt despatch thereof.

I observe in a detailed statement of the clerical and other committee force now employed and paid out of the contingent fund of the Senate that a great many committees have three or four employees, some of them perhaps more. Amongst the committees that have three or more I will enumerate the following: First, the Committee on Printing Records. I do not see the name of a Committee on Printing Records in the list of committees, and I did not know there was one. I presume it refers to the Joint Committee on Printing. Probably it may be otherwise named in this statement. The Committee on Appropriations has four; the Committee on Finance four; the Committee on Claims four; the Committee on Commerce three; the Committee on Pensions five; the Committee on the Judiciary three; the Committee on Military Affairs four; the Committee on Post-Offices and Post-Roads four; the Committee on the District of Columbia three; the Committee on Foreign Relations three; the Committee on Agriculture and Forestry three; the Committee on Territories three; the Committee on Interstate Commerce three; the Committee on Privileges and Elections three; the Committee on Pacific Islands and Porto Rico three; the Committee on the Philippines three; the Committee on Immigration three.

Mr. President, I am chairman of a very modest committee and which has a very modest establishment in what is sometimes called the "catacombs." I have no right to complain in any respect. It is the best the situation admits of. In addition to that, those committees which have as many as three employees having already been stated, there was a motion to give the Committee on National Banks a messenger. The Committee on National Banks is not one of the great committees of the Senate, like Appropriations or Finance, and it seemed that if we were going to give a messenger to a committee which had a single topic of treatment, and that a minor one as compared to the great and constant affairs of Government, other committees of like order ought to have them.

Now, in respect to committee chairmanships held by minority members, this observation seems appropriate: Few of those committees have much business. For the most part they have little or no business. The committee of which I am chairman has at present no business of general public concern. The committee rooms are used by the Senators as offices, especially the small committees. They are indispensable to the conduct of their public business. The committees vary as to their business. A particular incident happens in our Government by which a committee is overwhelmed for the time being with business and then, after a freshet, again there is a drought. You can not in the nature of things tell when a particular committee is going to have much business. Our Committee on Privileges and Elections, for instance, has had very heavy business and many hearings for a year or two. The time will soon come perhaps when they will not have a case or any matter of importance referred to them. We can not measure the necessities of a committee by the particular business which may be upon them at a particular moment.

I had presumed, and I believe such is the case, that the minority Senators were allowed this service because of their multifarious connections with the Government, rather than in the view that they would need these appurtenances and this aid for mere committee work.

Mr. President, I am told by the chairman of the committee which reported this resolution, and doubtless it is true, that in addition to these employees who are paid out of the contingent fund of the Senate the Senators who at this time represent the majority of the Senate have numerous other employees who assist in their work. There is no impropriety whatsoever in that if it is indispensable or appropriate to their efficient work.

The view I have of this question is simply this: It is to the interest of the Senate as a body that every Senator should be sustained by such appropriate help as is desirable for his efficient discharge of his Senatorial duties. A day may come at any time when his committee will have a good deal of work, although at that particular day it has none. Whether that day comes or not, his office in the Capitol, or as near thereto as accommodations will permit, has to be attended by his clerical force and by those who are ready to wait upon him and to help him in the execution of his office.

The Senate, Mr. President, like every other department of our Government, is congested. Our Calendars are congested with bills. There is not a bureau of the Government that is not congested. We must remember that we have added an empire to this Republic, call it by whatever name you will; and I am not adverting to it for the purpose of the slightest censorious observation. We have to take things as we find them. But the truth is that the American Republic at home is a republic, and the truth is also that from the far Orient to out in the Atlantic it is an empire. The men who are elected here as Senators of the United States are the legislators of a great empire, as well as of a republic, whether they will or no. That has come about in the destiny of this nation, and I am not discussing it at all save to call attention to the fact. We had brought up before the Senate this morning railroads in the Philippine Islands, 7,000 miles from where we are. What Senator knows anything about the subject, and how is he to inform himself? In order to the efficient discharge of the Senatorial duty here, the Senator ought to be sustained and have every employee in his service who is necessary or desirable to write his correspondence, to visit the Departments, and to meet those who wish to see him on public business.

*   *   *   *   *   *   *   *

Mr. GALLINGER.   Mr. President, a single word.

The first two years I had service in this body I had the honor of being chairman of the Committee on Transportation Routes to the Seaboard, a committee that did not hold a meeting during those two years and has not held a meeting since. The committee had a clerk, I think at $1,500, and we got along very comfortably. I was promoted from that position to that of chairman of the Committee on Pensions, and I need not more than suggest to the Senate that more service was required there of a clerical nature than was required for the committee I had formerly served as chairman. From that committee I was either promoted or demoted, I do not know which, to the chairmanship of the Committee on the District of Columbia. That committee is trying to legislate for about 300,000 people who are denied the right of suffrage, and I think it is safe to say that at least 200,000 of them are constitutional kickers. We have a procession in that committee room constantly. We have to deal with sewers, with lamp-posts, with electric lights, street railways, steam railways, telephones, telegraphs, gas, and almost every other conceivable subject. That committee has one clerk, an assistant clerk, and a messenger. It ought really to have more clerical assistance, but we manage by hard work to get along.

The proposition embodied in the resolution which was adopted a few days ago, and which I did not understand fully, was to give the Committee on Woman Suffrage, as an illustration, the Committee on Ventilation and Acoustics, the Committee on Standards, Weights, and Measures, the Committee on National Banks, and the Committee to Investigate Trespassers upon Indian Lands ——

Mr. KEAN.   The Committee on Ventilation and Acoustics no longer exists.

Mr. GALLINGER.   The Senator from New Jersey says the Committee on Ventilation and Acoustics no longer exists. If necessary, it will be revived. The proposition was to give those committees two clerks and a messenger, precisely the number that the Committee on the District of Columbia has.

Now, Mr. President, it would not be fair to have an adjustment of that kind made, and I submit to the Senate, without desiring to make any further suggestion about my own committee, that if each of these minor committees gets a clerk and an assistant clerk, or a clerk and a messenger it will be a very liberal disposition, and we ought all to be satisfied with it. I am very glad to know that the Senator from Idaho, after thinking the matter over, has concluded that it is a proper thing for us to adopt the resolution as amended.

Mr. BACON. Mr. President, I desire to say simply one word in order that what has just been said by the Senator from New Hampshire may not be misunderstood, either here or by the public in regard to the clerks of committees that do no work.

We all know the fact that there are committees, some of which have been mentioned by him, which are merely nominal committees. But it is a mistake, Mr. President, to have the impression that the clerk of that committee has no duty to perform by reason of the fact that the committee itself does no work. The fact is that every Senator, whether he is chairman of a committee or not, has a secretary, and when a Senator is chairman of a committee he has not a secretary in addition to the clerk of the committee. His own secretary becomes ex officio clerk of that committee, or, vice versa, the clerk of that committee is ex officio his clerk or secretary.

So, when it is said that the clerk of the committee is the officer of a committee which is never called together, it will certainly produce a very wrong impression if it is understood from that that the clerk of that committee has absolutely no duties to perform. He has just the same duties that the clerk or secretary of every other Senator has in the performance of the clerical duty required by that Senator, and the only effect of being the clerk of one of these nominal committees is that he gets a little more salary than he would get if he were not named as the clerk of a committee. He is in fact in such a case but the private secretary of the Senator and in no manner differs from any other private secretary of a Senator except in the fact that he gets an additional amount of salary.

The Senator from Florida [Mr. Mallory] asks me about the assistant clerk. It is true also in that case that the clerk of a committee, who is ex officio the clerk or secretary of a Senator, and the assistant clerk are both of them in such cases simply employed in the work of the Senator.

I may speak for myself as the chairman of one of the so-called nominal committees (Woman Suffrage), having only occasionally some very interesting audiences from a very interesting and charming portion of the public. Outside of that particular duty which devolves upon the clerk of the committee and the assistant, who is detailed from the Sergeant-at-Arms' office, the official work which those two officers have to do, in addition to the committee work, is more than can be reasonably required of them without other clerical assistance. As stated by the Senator from Idaho ever since I have been a member of this body, with rare exceptions, it has been necessary for me to have additional clerical force to that which is supplied to me by the Senate. To all, except those of us who have had experience in this matter, it is difficult to realize the vast amount of office clerical work and departmental work devolving upon even those of us who belong to the minority, and how utterly impossible it is for any one man as the clerk of a Senator to do the clerical work of that Senator. Two are required for every Senator, and I believe for an average of the Senators more than two are necessary to properly discharge the duties.

A Senator represents the constituency of a whole State. My State, Mr. President, is not the largest by any means. It occupies about the same relation to the other States now that it did when the Government was formed. It is about the thirteenth State. It was one of the original thirteen and the smallest of the original thirteen in population, unless Delaware or Rhode Island. I do not know what their population was at that time. It was the youngest of the colonies. My State at the time of the adoption of the Constitution was the youngest colony which became a State. It was the thirteenth in its relation to the other States. It is still about the thirteenth.

Yet, Mr. President, there are in Georgia two million and a half of people and it is the usual thing when a man in my State has any business of particular importance in Washington about which he writes to his Representative that he also writes to one of the Senators and most frequently to both of them. This involves not only the correspondence, but the work to which that correspondence relates. I presume the same is true of all other Senators.

Now, Mr. President, considering for a moment Georgia as an average, if you please, what must be the immense mass of business which devolves upon a Senator, even if you confine it to the routine business, with a vast constituency behind it, with even a fraction of 1 per cent of them having something to attend to in Washington?

Mr. President, I do not think it becomes this Government (and I know I speak not only my sentiment but the sentiment of the public at large) that one of its officials shall be required to go down into his own pocket to pay for the clerical help which should be paid for by the Government.

I do not know what the status of this resolution is. I unfortunately reached the city on a delayed train and was not here when the discussion opened. I do not propose in anything I say to impede the course of such procedure as those who have been here all the time and have participated from the beginning in this debate see proper or best to be done. But I thought it was proper that I should say this in connection with what had been said by the Senator from New Hampshire, and also, in addition, to say what I have said in justification of what may seem from this debate, or from certain things which others have said in this debate, to be extravagance on the part of the Senate in the provision it makes for the clerical force assisting a Senator in the discharge of his labors.

SENATE SECRET SESSIONS [1]

DEAR old Senator Morgan's "well simulated fury" over the breaking of the inviolability which is supposed to guard the secret sessions of the Senate has been the one gay patch in the inconclusive ending of a drab winter. It is to be suspected that Mr. Morgan gladly availed himself of the report of his San Domingo plot, as published, to introduce in the Senate in open session and give the widest publicity to his resolution instructing the Foreign Relations Committee to examine into all of our recent relations with San Domingo, including the preliminary correspondence leading to the present comatose protocol.

Whatever the fathers may have intended, the executive sessions of the Senate have come to be mere farces. They are always reported, and even more fully than the open debates. No senator would think of taking the floor in a closed session and saying things that he did not care to have printed broadcast, or that he would not say with the doors of the Senate chamber open and the galleries filled.

Had Senator Morgan that "easy grasp of the obvious," which an English journal has credited to President Roosevelt and Emperor William, he would not wonder how the reports of the secret proceedings of the Senate were secured. They are not obtained from Senator Morgan or any of the "old line" senators. Nor were they to be had from Senators Hoar, Cockrell, or Benjamin Harrison. Mr. Morgan retains the "high manner" of the old days. His account of how he repelled an unsophisticated correspondent who came to him for information is in his best style:

"Yesterday I was kept on the floor for a long time, as senators remember, by a current discussion of matters, a mere current discussion among senators, and I was prevented by that from really completing the speech I intended to make. I had not left my desk, I had not more than taken my seat, when a person who is accustomed to being about the lobbies of the Capitol here, a reporter, rushed up to my desk and asked me to give him a statement about the great imbroglio that had been sprung, or something of that sort. I said to him, 'Sir, you have no right to ask me a word about what occurred in the Senate. You will get no information from me.' I repelled his advance. That ought to have sufficed. A man who will then do that to a senator ought to be expelled from that gallery, and never permitted to take a seat there again, and his paper ought not to be permitted to be represented in that gallery."

[1] The above article, a special correspondence of the *New York Evening Post*, March 18, 1905, gives an interesting account, of course by an outsider, of Senate secret sessions in which executive matters, *i. e.*, treaties and appointments are discussed.

An Incident of 1871

The Alabama senator softened the force of his blow by his declaration that he was not "in the slightest degree interrupted, or offended, or distraught" by anything that had been printed. Few senators are. His plaint did not have even the slight merit of novelty. Just thirty-four years ago a colloquy took place on the floor of the Senate that, with a mere change of names, might almost have served as a report of yesterday's proceedings. It came about this way:

The Senate was called in extra session in May, 1871, to ratify the so-called "Washington treaty" between this country and Great Britain. While the treaty was still under consideration correspondents of a New York newspaper secured a copy and printed it. The disclosure made a great furore. A special committee was appointed to investigate, the correspondents were arrested and imprisoned, and many senators and Senate employees were questioned. How the correspondents got the treaty was not learned. When they were brought to the bar of the Senate a long debate ensued in which all the leaders in the chamber took part. It was in the course of that discussion that Senator Chandler of Michigan said:

"It is well known that for years there has been scarcely an utterance on this floor that has not been reported the next day in the New York newspapers. It is utterly impossible for these gentlemen to be in a position where they can hear the debates, and yet with wonderful accuracy those debates have been spread upon the pages of newspapers the next morning. There must be a culprit in this body, and I hope this committee will continue its investigations until the culprit is found out and brought to condign punishment, I care not who he is. Let the culprit be expelled from this body, for he has no business here."

Senator Wilson of Massachusetts accused Chandler himself of telling things to the correspondents. Chandler jumped to his feet and cried hotly, "I deny it."

Then Mr. Wilson said: "The senator denies it. I know it to be true. I know it to have been so over and over again. I will explain what I mean. I have been here over sixteen years. The proceedings of this body in executive session have found their way into the press all this time. It was so before I came here. These accounts published of executive sessions have been more or less accurate. How did they get into the newspapers? The leading papers of the country employ gentlemen to come here and obtain news. They are men of capacity, of character. They are men who know the proceedings of this Government as well as we here in the Senate know them. They understand what the Executive is doing; what the departments are doing. They know something of the history of the country. Their business is to get the news, even ahead of time, and let the people know what is to happen.

"How do they get it? We are here doing business. Various things come up here in executive session, nominations, treaties, debates, talks. Does it all end here? The senator from Michigan knows it does not. He knows that in the presence of other parties, he and all senators talk about what is said and done. They do so in their rooms, in this chamber, in their committee rooms, in the street, and especially in the F Street cars. Every senator knows this is true. It is no use for us to assume this virtue here and pretend to be what we are not. The truth is we have talked too much. We have all done our full share of giving information, and the man who protests the most that he has not done it has probably done more than any other member."

Whereupon, adds the unimaginative chronicler in the *Congressional Globe*, the senators burst into laughter, recognizing the truth of the picture the Massachusetts senator had drawn. His words are as true to-day as they were in 1871. As showing how the temper of the Senate has changed towards these disclosures of its mysteries, the excitement caused by the premature publication of the "Washington Treaty" and the publication of the San Domingo protocol in the *Evening Post* last week may be fairly contrasted. Thirty years ago it was a great piece of enterprise to print a treaty while it was being considered in secret session; to-day it might almost be considered a part of a correspondent's routine duty from the calm way in which it is received.

The Expulsion of Secretary Young

In the debate following Mr. Morgan's anachronistic plea for protection, Mr. Teller declared that the Senate would never be able to stop these publications, and referred to the expulsion of an executive secretary for divulging what went on behind the closed doors of the Senate Chamber. He had in mind James Rankin Young of Philadelphia, a brother of John Russell Young, formerly Librarian of Congress. Mr. Young, as executive clerk of the Senate, for many years attended the secret sessions and kept the record of the proceedings. A committee of the Senate was appointed in 1892, with the late Joseph Dolph of Oregon as chairman, to determine the responsibility for the leakage of secrets. This body, popularly known as the "smelling committee," examined many newspaper men and learned nothing, but decided that somebody must be guilty, and the Senate expelled Mr. Young.

He was generally regarded as innocent; in fact, those whose business it was to find out for the newspapers what the Senate did in secret session knew that he was. Mr. Young went back to Philadelphia, and before long was elected to Congress. He is now superintendent of the dead letter office.

SENATOR HOAR'S INDIGNATION

The late Senator Hoar, like Mr. Morgan, was a great stickler for the traditions of the Senate, and carefully observed its rules. He almost exploded with fury one day, and justifiably, when a breezy youth accosted him in a corridor, and, slapping him on the shoulder familiarly, said: "Say, Senator, what are you old fellows doing in there to-day?"

"Young man," was the choleric response, "if it befitted my age and the dignity of my position, I should take you by the scruff of the neck, haul you out on those steps, and chastise you as you deserve to be."

At another time when some of the old senators were restive because of unusually full reports which were being printed on some important matter then under consideration in secret session, Senator Clapp of Minnesota introduced one day, when the doors were closed, a humorous resolution setting forth that, whereas the reports of the executive proceedings of the Senate in the newspapers were not as full as they might be, and whereas the newspaper men were put to the expense of some time and trouble in securing their information, therefore be it resolved, etc., that in future reporters be invited to attend closed sessions, so that they might get their accounts at first hand. Mr. Hoar took the resolution in all seriousness, and the next day, while Mr. Morgan was indulging in some singularly frank comments on Nicaragua, the senior Massachusetts senator sought out Clapp and said: "Now, Senator, you see the good of executive sessions. If what Morgan is saying was reported, Nicaragua would be ablaze to-day."

"Well, Senator," was the Westerner's response, "do you think this country would come to any harm if Nicaragua blazed until she became charcoal?"

One day while the Senate was in secret session a group of correspondents were awaiting in the lobby near the marble room for their friends to come out, when Senator Tillman came along. He saw the waiting group and began banteringly: "We are attending to you men now. You will never get any more reports of our secret proceedings. Some of the old fellows in there are giving you Hail Columbia, and they are going to get up a scheme so that you will not be able to find out anything else that we do."

Presently he was followed by Jones of Arkansas, like Morgan and Hoar a strong defender of senatorial privileges. He thought the time ripe for a jibe, and remarked, "I suppose you gentlemen are fully informed as to what is going on inside?"

"Yes," said the spokesman of the correspondents, who told him what they had all learned from Tillman, omitting, of course, any reference to the source of his information. Mr. Jones was aghast. He hurried back into the Senate, and quickly secured recognition from the chair. "Mr.

President," he said, "it's no use trying to do anything. Things are worse than I suspected. I stepped out of the chamber a few moments ago, and met a number of correspondents. They know everything that we are doing in here. They know what we are saying, and what we are trying to do. We might as well give up hope of trying to stop them from learning our secrets."

SENTIMENT FOR ABOLISHING THE CLOSED SESSION

A growing sentiment to do away with the closed session except in the confirmation of Presidential appointees, is making itself felt among the younger men in the Senate. These secrets are always faithfully kept, or given in confidence to the newspaper men, because they often involve questions touching men's characters and private lives. No real pretence is made of keeping any other Senate business from the public. The effort to have the debates on the Dominican protocol made public was significant, as showing the changed attitude of the more progressive among the members of the upper chamber.

.

SENATORIAL MAIDEN SPEECHES [1]

A TRADITION has grown up about the snubs and sarcasms which await the Senator who addresses the Senate before he has a term or so of unobtrusive service behind him. We do not hear so much about what such an iconoclast gains. Senatorial dignity was shocked profoundly, no doubt, last Wednesday, when the new Senator from Arkansas took the floor for a long speech on his anti-Trust bill. Yet the impartial Associated Press records that "all of the Senators, both Republicans and Democrats, were in their seats and gave strict attention to his remarks." The speech, to be sure, was balderdash. A Southern auditor is said to have remarked that the new Senator had omitted the only thing he had ever said that was worth while — namely, that he was no relation to Jefferson Davis. But it got at least twice as much publicity as if its author had waited till he himself had ceased to be a novelty at Washington.

Moreover, when one refers in these days to the immemorial tradition that new Senators should be seen and not heard, he must recognize that a notable line of contrary precedents has also been laid down. Davis is not the first Senator, but the fourth, within a little more than ten years, who "refused to wait until his hair had turned gray before taking up his work actively." He was, to be sure, the most impatient, for he held back his eloquence for only nine days after the beginning of his first session,

[1] Editorial from the *New York Evening Post*, 1907.

whereas Beveridge restrained himself for 36 days, Tillman for 58, and La Follette for 109. In spite of Tillman's reputation for bluntness, it may be recalled that he took more time than any of the others in justifying himself for speaking at all before taking up his speech proper. This was the beginning of his "pitchfork" speech:

I shall make no apology for doing what is my right here, to exercise the functions of a Senator, and discuss the issues presented to the Senate. I know, sir, that custom has made it a rule that new members of this body should listen rather than be heard, and my brief experience — and while in the city I have been very attentive upon the sessions of the Senate— has shown me that the custom is a wise one, because new men who come in here, especially those who, like myself, have had little, in fact, no, legislative experience, realize very soon that what they do not know about the affairs of this great government is far more than they do know or can hope to learn without much labor.

Of course, the novelty of a farmer pretending to talk finance, or to understand the question, is so great that most of my colleagues are doing me the honor, I believe for the first time this session, to sit here and listen to me. I thank you, gentlemen, that you have not adjourned and gone off.

Beveridge, as might be expected, did not speak because he wanted to, but only to perform a public service. .These were the words of his introduction:

Mr. President, I address the Senate at this time because Senators and mem-bers of the House on both sides have asked that I give to Congress and the country my observations in the Philippines and the Far East, and the conclusions which those observations compel; and because of hurtful resolutions introduced and utterances made in the Senate, every word of which will cost, and is costing, the lives of American soldiers.

La Follette made no exordium at all. He had spoken the equivalent of eight columns in the *Congressional Record* before he made any allusion to his auditors. Then:

I pause in my remarks to say this: I cannot be wholly indifferent to the fact that Senators, by their absence at this time, indicate their want of interest in what I may have to say upon this subject. The public is interested. Unless this important question is rightly settled seats now temporarily vacant may be permanently vacated by those who have the right to occupy them at this time. [Applause in the galleries.]

Different as were and are these four contemners of tradition in other respects, they all could claim credit for having something to say. It is only on men of this type that the Senatorial tradition bears hard. What is the proper course for the man who sincerely believes that he has something to say which needs to be said but which no one else will say if he keeps silence? His dilemma is not new. When Charles Sumner was elected to the Senate his constituents and the anti-slavery people of the country generally expected him to make things lively for the slaveholders' ring at Washington. He believed in biding his time, and spoke on land grants, foreign postage, and various routine matters before he so much as mentioned slavery. As Moorfield Storey says in his life of Sumner, "he felt it wise to become familiar with his colleagues and his surroundings, with the rules and atmosphere of the Senate, and to show that he was not 'a man of one idea' — a fanatic at once unreasonable and unpractical." In spite of misconstruction of his silence by both friends and opponents, he waited ·till May 26, one hundred and seventy-seven days after the opening of the session, before giving notice of a slavery speech, and this he did not actually secure the chance to deliver until the end of August.

Aside from the activities of men with something special to say, the traditions of the Senate are not and never have been in the slightest danger. The average of new Senators take their places amiably on the back seat. Our own Senator Depew, though accustomed to being bound up with Demosthenes and Patrick Henry, was quite content to make his Senatorial *début* with one of the conventional Sunday eulogies on deceased members.

Yet we are of the opinion that length of service is counting for rather less than formerly in making up the sum of Senatorial influence. Disregarding the orators with outside reputations, first-term men have been pretty prominent in the Senate for some time. Those Senators promoted from the House, like Dolliver and Hemenway, Bailey and Newlands, have not had to wait long for a chance to be more than auditors. Crane, without previous legislative experience, is named among Senate leaders. Thus no sooner does the outside public become duly impressed with the awful tradition that only graybeards count in the Senate than it begins to break down.

PRINTING SPEECHES IN THE RECORD [1]

THE VICE-PRESIDENT. The request is that the Senator from Missouri, being ill, may be permitted to print the residue of his speech in the *Record*, together with such additions and extensions as he may desire.

Mr. BACON. I think that would be a very unfortunate precedent. I have never known such a request to be made in the Senate. We know that in the other House it is the common practice and the recognized practice, but I think it would be very unfortunate for us to set a precedent of that kind here to print speeches which are not delivered. I hope it will not be done.

[1] *Congr. Record*, Apr. 29, 1908.

I am perfectly willing that every indulgence possible may be given to the Senator from Missouri, but if this be done once, where will be the end of it? I know it is generally supposed throughout the country — I say generally — possibly that is probably too broad a term, but it is thought by many that the practice which obtains in one House obtains also in the other. But it has never obtained here. There is great liberality as to publishing without being read exhibits or papers which are used in a speech. They are allowed to be inserted in the *Record;* but this is the first time I have heard during my limited term of service here a request made that a speech which has not been delivered should be printed in the *Record.*

I would say this, Mr. President: If it were near the close of the session and the Senator from Missouri had been prevented by illness from delivering his speech, that would be a providential matter which might be recognized as a sufficient ground upon which to base exceptional action on the part of the Senate. But we have no reason to doubt the fact, I presume, that the Senator will have the opportunity before the session closes to conclude his remarks. While I have every disposition to concede everything which circumstances may demand, I do not think that the present circumstances demand that we should make such a wide departure from the practice of the Senate and inaugurate a precedent which certainly would be followed in the future in other instances.

Mr. LODGE. I am, of course, entirely aware of the rule of the Senate against extending speeches in the *Record.* I think it is an extremely wise rule and I hope it will never be changed. In this particular case the Senator who has given the notice that he would complete his speech to-day is ill. He may be several days absent from the Senate and it may be some time longer before he will be able to complete the delivery of his speech. He sent a message to me desiring to express to the Senate the hope that he might be permitted to print his speech as it stands, most of it having already been delivered. It contains a large number of extracts from testimony which could be perfectly well embodied and which permission is constantly given.

I have no desire to infringe any rule, nor would he have any such desire. I am as strongly in favor of the practice and rule of the Senate in this respect as anyone can be. I thought this was an exceptional case in which this relief might be given to a Senator who was ill.

I certainly shall not insist on the request if there is any objection to it. I merely desired to say that the Senator from Missouri could not go on to-day and it is uncertain when he will be able to complete the delivery of his speech.

Mr. TELLER. Mr. President, I understand that if at any time a Senator is unable to read a speech which he has prepared, it has been the custom here for some time, I know, that he may ask some Senator to read it for him. It may be read for him, but it must be either read by him or some one else before it goes into the *Record*.

Mr. LODGE. If the Senator from Missouri desires to have the remainder of his speech read to the Senate and to complete it in that way, I am sure I should be very glad to assist him, and I have no doubt others would be, in arranging it in that manner and relieve him from the delivery of the remainder of his speech.

I thought it well, however, to make the statement at this time that he would not be here to-day to carry out the notice which appears on the Calendar, and which would leave the day clear, if the Senator from New Hampshire desires, as I hope he does, to take up the child-labor bill this morning, because I understand the agricultural appropriation bill will not be taken up until to-morrow.

VI

SENATE AND HOUSE CONFERENCE COMMITTEES

[Conference committees composed of members of both Houses constitute a most essential part of the legislative machinery. Many questions and controversies have arisen with respect to them. In the first place, the conference committee has often been used as an instrument by which the Senate has made its will prevail over the House. Towards the end of the session, when little or no time remains for action in either House, the conference committees meet. The representatives of the Senate, a body which is ordinarily quite sure of its purposes, have frequently used the general freedom of debate in the Senate as a cudgel to force the House of Representatives to yield its position. It is argued on such occasions that unless the view of the Senate is adopted no legislation can be secured, because any other alternative will be talked to death by individual Senators. Action of this kind led to Mr. Cannon's remonstrance, which is given below. Matter which under the rules of the House can not be introduced in a general appropriation bill will frequently be put in as a Senate amendment and will come back to the House as a part of the conference report.

But it is especially the procedure of the House which makes the conference committee so powerful. When the Senate amendments are returned to the House no debate is allowed by the Speaker; the regular practice is to disagree to the amendments in bulk and appoint a conference committee by which the details of legislation will be settled. The discussion of the conference report on the Rate Bill will illustrate this procedure. Certain of the amendments proposed by the Senate would have been sure of adoption in the House, had the Speaker permitted a separate vote on such amendments; but as will be seen from the debate on this matter, the House was not permitted to express itself upon the amendments. It has been suggested that these amendments were allowed to pass in the Senate because it felt sure that the House would not be permitted to vote on them, but would disagree, and that they might then be disposed of in the conference committee. About this matter the reader will be able to form his own opinion from the documents. The action of the conference committee on the Currency Bill in 1908 was also especially significant. In this case the committee on currency in the House had been divested of its jurisdiction through the action of a party caucus. The House bill resulting from this action was thrown into conference together with the Senate bill, and only most limited debate was allowed at any time during the proceedings. We have already seen the result of this action upon the procedure in the Senate.

The following extracts deal with: 1. The conference committee on the Railway Rate Bill of 1906. 2. The Army Appropriation Bill of 1902. 3. The Naval Appropriation Bill of 1908. 4. The Currency Bill of 1908.]

REPORT ON THE RAILWAY RATE BILL [1]

MR. DALZELL. Mr. Speaker, I submit the following privileged report from the Committee on Rules, which I send to the desk and ask to have read.

The Clerk read as follows:

The Committee on Rules, to whom was referred House resolution 534, have had the same under consideration, and herewith report the following in lieu thereof:

"*Resolved*, That the bill (H. R. 12987) to amend an act entitled 'An act to regulate commerce,' approved February 4, 1887, and all acts amendatory thereof, and to enlarge the powers of the Interstate Commerce Commission, be, and hereby is, taken from the Speaker's table with Senate amendments thereto, to the end that the said amendments be, and hereby are, disagreed to, and a conference be, and hereby is asked with the Senate on the disagreeing votes upon the said amendments; and the Speaker shall immediately appoint the conferees without intervening motion."

Mr. DALZELL. Mr. Speaker, on that I demand the previous question.
The SPEAKER. The question is on ordering the previous question.
While the House was dividing Mr. Williams demanded a division.
Mr. DALZELL. Mr. Speaker, I demand the yeas and nays.
The yeas and nays were ordered.
The question was taken; and there were — yeas 155, nays 83, answered "present" 15, not voting 128.
The SPEAKER. The previous question is ordered, and the gentleman from Pennsylvania is entitled to twenty minutes and the gentleman from Mississippi to twenty minutes.
Mr. DALZELL. Mr. Speaker, the bill referred to in the resolution which has just been read is what is popularly known as "the rate bill." It is a matter of common knowledge that it passed the House almost unanimously and went to the Senate some seven or eight weeks ago. It comes back now with fifty Senate amendments and is on the Speaker's table. The purpose of this rule, if adopted, is to take that bill from the Speaker's table, nonconcur in all the Senate amendments, and send the bill to conference. That is all there is in the rule. I reserve the balance of my time.
Mr. PALMER. Suppose a man wants to vote to concur in some of the amendments and to nonconcur in others?
Mr. DALZELL. This rule prevents that.

[1] *Congr. Record*, May 25, 1906.

Mr. PALMER. You have got to take the whole dose?

Mr. DALZELL. In the absence of this rule there would be of course a possibility of debate on fifty amendments. The House will of course have an opportunity to pass upon the question of the amendments on the report of the conferees.

Mr. PALMER. There will be some opportunity somehow or other to debate the amendments?

Mr. DALZELL. Undoubtedly. This has no reference to anything in connection with the bill except the present procedure.

Mr. PALMER. When the report of the conference committee comes in, suppose you introduce another rule of a similar character to cut off all debate in the same way you are doing now, how about that?

Mr. DALZELL. I can of course only speak for myself, but, in the first place, a rule amounts to nothing unless the House adopts it, and, in the second place, I do not believe there is a disposition on the part of anybody to do any such thing.

Mr. BARTLETT. I would like to ask the gentleman a question.

Mr. NORRIS. I would like to ask the gentleman with a view of getting the parliamentary situation as it would be before us in the conference report. Suppose now, to illustrate, that the amendment which I understand the Senate has added to the bill providing for including within the terms of the bill express companies — an amendment which very many of us voted for when the bill was here — suppose, now, the conferees bring in a report in which the Senate amendment placing express companies in the bill is eliminated? What opportunity then would we have after they have made that sort of a recommendation to vote in favor of including in the bill express companies?

Mr. DALZELL. Why, the House, of course, can disagree to the conference report and can instruct its conferees.

Mr. WILSON. It would defeat the entire bill if we were to disagree to the conference report.

Mr. DALZELL. Not at all.

Mr. NORRIS. Would not this rule, if the gentleman will permit a further interruption, be regarded by the conferees, and ought they not in fact regard this vote, if we adopt this procedure, as an instruction to the conferees that the House is opposed to all of the Senate amendments?

Mr. DALZELL. By no manner of means. Speaking for one of the Committee on Rules, there are some of these amendments that personally I should vote to concur in right now.

Mr. NORRIS. I would like to vote to concur in some of them.

Mr. DALZELL. It is a mere question of procedure to facilitate the public business. Has the gentleman, or any other gentleman in this House, any idea that we are going to adjourn until the rate bill is disposed of?

Mr. NORRIS. Oh, no. I want to reach a parliamentary situation that will give us all an opportunity to vote for any of these amendments that we favor.

Mr. DALZELL. I think the gentleman will have that opportunity under the rules of the House.

Mr. BARTLETT. May I ask the gentleman from Pennsylvania if, under the rules, no matter what the conferees agree to or disagree to, the House will not be called to vote up or vote down the report as a whole and will not be permitted to vote for any separate amendment? In other words, under the rules of the House, as they have been construed, we will be compelled to vote for the report as a whole?

Mr. DALZELL. The House can vote down the conferees' report and instruct the conferees as to anything in the report.

Mr. BARTLETT. I understand that. The House will not get an opportunity, if we adopt these rules, to vote for any one of these amendments separately. If we had them before us now, we could say whether we are in favor or opposed to them.

Mr. DALZELL. The gentleman knows that under the rules of the House the House will have an opportunity to pass on every amendment the Senate has suggested.

Mr. COOPER of Wisconsin. The gentleman from Pennsylvania [Mr. Dalzell] says that we could instruct the conferees later. What earthly objection is there to giving the House an opportunity to instruct the conferees now? [Applause.] Why not vote now on the express-company amendment, that every man in this House who wants regulation of transportation desires?

Mr. DALZELL. We can not very well allow any particular amendment to be voted on at this time, and unless we do follow the mode of procedure that is suggested, we will run into a discussion of fifty amendments right away. I have no idea that any gentleman will be disappointed as to having a vote on any particular amendment he wants at the proper time. I think it is not customary to instruct conferees in advance of a full and free conference.

Mr. COOPER of Wisconsin. Will the gentleman permit me to make one statement?

Mr. DALZELL. Certainly.

Mr. COOPER of Wisconsin. I have to say this, that I have been informed by a gentleman in whose word I place implicit confidence that gentlemen — I am not saying whether members of the Senate or of the House — who will, under the rules that obtain in the respective bodies, be upon the conference, have in conversation said that in so far as they have the power the express-company amendment shall go out — that they were heard to say so.

Mr. DALZELL. I know nothing about that, but I do not take much stock in the expression of what a single Member of the House is going to do. The House is in control of the bill at all times.

Mr. Cooper of Wisconsin. Let me suggest to the gentleman from Pennsylvania that the House is in a hurry to adjourn. Suppose the conferees hold this up two or three weeks, until tacitly we have agreed that we will adjourn on the 15th or 20th of June. There will be then no opportunity for debate, because everybody will be in a hurry to get home.

Mr. Dalzell. There will be an opportunity for debate.

Mr. Hepburn. Will the gentleman from Pennsylvania [Mr. Dalzell] permit me for a moment to ask the gentleman from Wisconsin to state the persons that have thus declared themselves?

Mr. Cooper of Wisconsin. I do not wish to offend especially the feelings of the gentleman from Iowa, and ——

Mr. Hepburn. You will not offend my feelings, sir, by answering that question.

Mr. Cooper of Wisconsin. I will then say to the gentleman from Iowa ——

Mr. Hepburn. Name them out.

Mr. Cooper of Wisconsin. I am not going to name a man who came to me and told that story. The gentleman from Iowa is one of the men who was said to have remarked in conversation that the express amendment will go out.

Mr. Hepburn. I say that any man who has told the gentleman that statement stated a falsehood [applause], and I am inclined to believe that, until the name of that individual is given, the gentleman may be drawing upon his imagination. [Applause.]

Mr. Williams. Mr. Speaker, I call the gentleman from Iowa to order.

Mr. Hepburn. Mr. Speaker, I withdraw the language that is offensive to the distinguished gentleman from Mississippi.

Mr. Williams. It is not offensive to the "gentleman from Mississippi" at all; it is offensive to the House.

The Speaker. The language is withdrawn. The gentleman from Pennsylvania has the floor.

Mr. Cooper of Wisconsin. Will the gentleman yield?

Mr. Dalzell. I yield to the gentleman from Wisconsin.

Mr. Cooper of Wisconsin. Just one minute to reply to the gentleman from Iowa. I wish to say, Mr. Speaker, to the gentleman from Iowa, that I am not the only person to whom that statement has been made. There are other members of the House to whom that statement has been made. There is no object, can be no specific purpose on my part, to deliberately misstate that ——

Mr. Hepburn. Will the gentleman permit me ——

Mr. Cooper of Wisconsin. One moment; you have no right to interrupt me at this point.

Mr. Williams. A point of order, Mr. Speaker.

Mr. Heprurn. In veiw of the fact ——

Mr. Williams. I make the point of order, Mr. Speaker.

The SPEAKER. The gentleman from Mississippi makes the point of order.

Mr. WILLIAMS. The gentleman has not yielded.

The SPEAKER. That the gentleman has not yielded. The House will be in order.

Mr. COOPER of Wisconsin. I can not understand how the gentleman from Iowa ever propounded that question, unless he had heard that this statement was going around. He put me in a very embarrassing position. But I told him what was told to me; I told exactly the truth as told to me; and this is the first time that any man, anywhere, ever accused me of deliberately telling a falsehood. This is a thing which was said to me in confidence in a conversation I had with a gentleman who said: "I would not like my name mentioned in this connection."

The SPEAKER. The time of the gentleman has expired.

Mr. MURPHY. Will the gentleman allow me to ask him a question?

Mr. DALZELL. I yield to the gentleman.

Mr. MURPHY. Is not this the fact: "It is manifest, therefore, that if we are to have speedy legislation and adjustment of the differences between the two Houses the bill must be at once sent to conference, and that is the purpose of the rule I have introduced?"

Mr. DALZELL. Undoubtedly.

Mr. MURPHY. I am reading from the remarks of the gentleman from Pennsylvania, as found on page 4224 of the *Congressional Record*, on the rule sending the statehood bill to conference.

Mr. DALZELL. Well, now, Mr. Speaker, I say that this is a very simple matter. That bill is now on the Speaker's table with fifty amendments. There is a great diversity of opinion as to whether a number of these amendments should be accepted or should be rejected, but whether they shall be accepted or whether they shall be rejected we have to meet this question. With the gentleman from Mississippi in the saddle, and with his idea of statesmanship, under which the gentleman ties up the House by opposition, we could have separate votes on each of these fifty amendments to the bill. It is entirely within the power of the House to vote upon the conferees' report and refuse to accept the conference report, and then the whole matter will be open and within the control of the membership of this House to amend the bill until it is in just such shape as the majority of the House desire to have it.

The SPEAKER. The gentleman has six minutes of his time remaining.

Mr. DALZELL. I reserve the balance of my time.

Mr. WILSON. Will the gentleman yield to a question?

Mr. PAYNE. The gentleman reserves his time.

The SPEAKER. The gentleman from Mississippi.

Mr. WILLIAMS. Mr. Speaker, I had not intended just at this moment to say anything, but the gentleman from Pennsylvania has rendered it necessary that I should before I yield to anybody else. As I understood him, he tried to gather partisan strength upon that side by asking the question "What condition this bill would be in if the gentleman from Mississippi, with his revolutionary methods," I believe was the language ——

Mr. DALZELL. I did not say "revolutionary methods." I said "with his ideas of statesmanship."

Mr. WILLIAMS. "Ideas of statesmanship," then. I want to quote the gentleman exactly right — "if the gentleman from Mississippi, with his ideas of statesmanship, were put in the saddle by voting down this special rule?" Why, the gentleman from Pennsylvania is not such a child as to imagine that giving the House a right to vote a motion to concur in one or more of these Senate amendments would "place the gentleman from Mississippi in the saddle." He knows that it would simply place the House of Representatives in the saddle. [Applause on the Democratic side.] And the gentleman from Pennsylvania, moreover, knew from what had occurred in the Committee on Rules that the gentleman from Mississippi was perfectly willing, if only there were an opportunity furnished to the House to vote to concur upon Senate amendments, 2, 6, 31, 47, and 48, that all the balance of the Senate amendments might, without objection, go to the conference as amendments nonconcurred in. Gentlemen, do not let that sort of thing fool you, whatever else fools you ——

Mr. DALZELL. The gentleman from Mississippi certainly does not claim that the House is to be bound by his particular wishes. Other gentlemen have a right to their opinions as well as he.

Mr. WILLIAMS. The gentleman from Mississippi does not claim that the House would be bound, but the gentleman from Mississippi claims that, so far as his position is concerned, he would be bound, and that therefore there was no reason in fact or in truth for the statement made by the gentleman from Pennsylvania to the effect that the gentleman from Mississippi would be put in the saddle. The House would be put in the saddle, and that is what the gentleman and men in this Hall who are opposed to the Senate amendment putting express companies in the bill as common carriers and to some other amendments of the Senate, in which this House upon a free vote would concur at once; that is what they are trying to avoid. You want the Committee on Rules and the conferees to be in the saddle to ride the House bitted and spurred. You do not want the House to be in the saddle. If I consented right now that every single Democrat should leave this Hall, and that no point of "no quorum" should be made, you dare not put even that side of the House in the saddle for a day. [Applause on the Democratic side.]

Now, Mr. Speaker, I yield five minutes to the gentleman from Missouri [Mr. De Armond]. [Applause on the Democratic side.]

Mr. DE ARMOND. Mr. Speaker, the question before the House is at once a very simple and a very important one. It is the question whether the House will pass upon some of these amendments itself or whether it will commit then to the uncertainties of a conference. That is the plain, simple question.

The importance of this legislation or of the subject with which this legislation deals can hardly be overstated.

In the other end of this Capitol weeks and months were spent in discussion and consideration of this measure. A number of amendments were added to it. Some of them, I am sure, should meet with the hearty concurrence and approval and indorsement of every man in this House, and of every man out of this House who wishes effective railroad rate legislation. As has already been suggested by the gentleman from Mississippi [Mr. Williams], my colleague on the Committee on Rules, so far as we upon this side are concerned, I believe that with a vote now upon two or three or four or five of these amendments, it would be satisfactory to us to let the others go to conference, if that be insisted upon. What are they? They are very easily understood. One is amendment No. 2, that the term "common carrier" shall include express companies and sleeping-car companies. [Applause.] Now, a man ought to know whether he is for that or against it. We are for it. I believe the House is for it. If so, why send it to conference? Why take the chance or the risk of what may be done in conference concerning it? The man who votes against giving himself the opportunity to vote upon that amendment here in the House now, for the time being votes against it and takes the chance of having or not having the opportunity to vote for it later, if he really wishes to vote for it at all.

Now, take amendment No. 6. That provides that common carriers shall furnish switch facilities. Who is in favor of that, and who is against it? We are in favor of it. I believe the House is in favor of it. Why not let us determine by vote here? Why send it to a conference committee, with its hazards and its chances, in the closing days of a session to determine whether or not that wholesome and just amendment shall remain in the bill and become a part of the law?

Take amendment No. 31. It strikes out the words "fairly remunerative"; a catch trap those words are, making room for litigation, room for uncertainty, room for thwarting, if possible, the will of the people with respect to this bill. Why not vote upon that? We are in favor of the amendment which strikes those words out.

No. 47 provides that there shall not be incorporated in the receipt or bill of lading any words, however carefully chosen or however skillfully covered, which will exempt the railroad company from its ordinary common-law liability. [Applause.] Who is in favor of that, and who is against it? We are in favor of that amendment. It is not onerous on the railroads, it is not unjust, it is not rash; it is decent and fair and corrective and improving in this bill. We are in favor of it. I believe the House is in favor of it. Why commit to the chances and hazard of this committee performance that amendment?

Then there is an amendment, No. 48, which strikes out the section in the bill when it went from this House, unnecessarily providing that each of the Interstate Commerce Commissioners shall receive $10,000 a year instead of $7,500, and that there shall be seven instead of five Commissioners. I would like to see a vote upon that, and would like to vote for it.

But are you willing to give us a vote upon anything? Are you willing yourselves to vote upon anything? Or are you in favor of turning over every amendment, no matter how important, to the hazard, and juggling, and chances, and uncertainty, and the influence that may prevail against fair consideration, in this committee of conference? That is the question, and nothing can take us away from it. A vote upon the one side is a vote to give this House an opportunity to do what it chooses to do, and a vote upon the other side is to deny it. [Applause on the Democratic side.]

The SPEAKER. The gentleman's time has expired.

Mr. KLEPPER. Mr. Speaker, I ask unanimous consent that the gentleman's time be extended one minute that I may ask him a question.

Mr. DE ARMOND. That is perfectly satisfactory to me.

The SPEAKER. The gentleman from Missouri asks that his colleague's time be extended one minute.

Mr. WILLIAMS. That is in addition to the usual forty minutes?

The SPEAKER. Yes; is there objection?

Mr. PAYNE. What is the question, Mr. Speaker?

The SPEAKER. The gentleman from Missouri asks that his colleague's time be extended one minute to answer a question.

Mr. PAYNE. That is in addition to the forty minutes?

The SPEAKER. Yes.

Mr. OLMSTED. Then, one minute ought to be added to the time for debate on this side.

The SPEAKER. The Chair hears no objection.

Mr. KLEPPER. I want to ask my colleague if it is not a fact that quite a number of the minority, including the leader of the minority, did not vote to exclude express companies on the passage of the bill in the House, and if that be true, why they are agonizing over this subject and objecting to its going to conference?

Mr. DE ARMOND. Mr. Speaker, I am asked a question as to what somebody else did, and somebody else thought, and about what somebody else thinks now. That kind of a question I can not answer, but I will say to the gentleman that when he or any other man votes to send this to conference without an opportunity to vote upon it, he votes for excluding from this classification the express companies and the car companies.

Mr. KLEPPER. I will say to the gentleman that I voted to include express companies, and if I remember correctly the minority leader voted to exclude express companies. I for one am willing to submit the matter to the conferees, believing that they will recommend that which is just and proper.

The SPEAKER. The time of the gentleman has expired.

Mr. DE ARMOND. I hope I will have an opportunity to answer the gentleman.

Mr. WILLIAMS. I will yield to the gentleman from Alabama [Mr. Underwood] three minutes.

Mr. UNDERWOOD. Mr. Speaker, the condition of this proposition under the rule is this: The rate bill is on the table, and the rules of this House provide that House bills with Senate amendments, which do not require to be considered in Committee of the Whole, may be at once disposed of as the House may determine. It is now in the power of the gentleman from Iowa [Mr. Hepburn] to call the rate bill from the table, and the House to consider each of these amendments without a special rule, where the House will be able to vote up or down each of the amendments, as it deems best in its judgment. The effect of this special rule is to take that power away from the membership of the House, put it in the hands of the conferees, composed of three members of the House and three members of the Senate, sitting behind closed doors, where nobody in this House or nobody in the United States can know what is being done, and when they come back with their report, if it is a full and complete report, such as they will bring to this House, the membership of the House will be confronted with the question, Will you accept the bill as it is reported from the committee of conference or not? We will have to swallow their report whole, good or bad, or be put in the attitude of voting against a rate bill, and if the majority passes it in that shape, there will be no explanation. When this matter was before the House of Representatives I moved in the House to include express companies within the terms of the bill. The gentleman from Iowa [Mr. Hepburn], the chairman of the committee, and the chairman of the conference committee of this House when it is appointed, fought that proposition and said the Hepburn bill did not include express companies and he was not in favor of putting them in the bill. [Applause on the Democratic side.] I say to this House, if you are honestly and earnestly in favor of putting these express companies within the terms of the bill, are you going to put that in the hands of the gentleman from Iowa [Mr. Hepburn], who openly and aboveboard has told you on the floor of this House, when this bill was last before it, that he was not in favor of the proposition? Can you justify yourselves before your constituents in such circumstances.

The SPEAKER. The time of the gentleman has expired.

Mr. WILLIAMS. Mr. Speaker, I would ask the gentleman from Pennsylvania if he proposes to use the balance of his time in one speech?

The SPEAKER. The gentleman from Mississippi has eight minutes remaining and the gentleman from Pennsylvania has six minutes remaining.

Mr. WILLIAMS. Of the eight minutes, I yield two minutes to the gentleman from Wisconsin [Mr. Cooper].

Mr. COOPER of Wisconsin. Mr. Speaker, in line with what the gentleman from Alabama [Mr. Underwood] has just said, I would also beg to remind the House that while the original bill was pending here an amendment was offered by the gentleman from Alabama [Mr. Underwood] and one or two others — there were two or three amendments — putting express companies within the purview of this bill. The gentleman from Iowa [Mr. Hepburn] had said to the House that express companies were not included in the bill. The gentleman from Michigan [Mr. Townsend] thought they were, as did also my colleague [Mr. Esch], the gentleman from Wisconsin. In my remarks I called attention to the fact that the phraseology of the bill did not include express companies, unless the original act included them, and that the Interstate Commerce Commission had always held that express companies were not included under the original act. I called attention also to the fact that a member of the Interstate Commerce Commission, with whom I had had a conversation on that day, told me that there was no question that express companies were not included under the terms of the then pending bill. When the amendment to include express companies came up, the gentleman from Iowa [Mr. Hepburn] voted against it, in line with the remarks which he made, as just narrated by the gentleman from Alabama [Mr. Underwood]. Now, why should any gentleman who wants express companies included and who wants to stop the infamous discriminations which they now practice, vote to turn the whole question over to conferees to bring in such a report as they please? Gentlemen are not obliged to do this. The rules do not require it. How can any gentleman who honestly does not wish to have express companies omitted from the law vote to send this proposition to a conference that may be hostile to his views? When are you to get the report — in two weeks, three weeks, four weeks? What will it contain?

The SPEAKER. The time of the gentleman has expired.

Mr. WILLIAMS. Mr. Speaker, the gentleman from Missouri [Mr. De Armond] has already outlined what amendments 2, 6, 31, 47, and 48 are. These are the amendments which we as minority members of the Committee on Rules asked that the House should have a right to vote upon in a motion to concur. We still insist on that right. We therefore oppose this rule. It is very true that I did vote against amendments like this, some of them almost identical with them, upon the floor, but it was because — and the gentleman from Iowa [Mr. Hepburn] will bear me out in that statement — for tactical and strategic purposes we had thought it important to send this rate bill, with all the weight and influence of this House, like a catapult against the other side of this Capitol, so that the utmost influence might be had to bring forth a bill. It was not because there was ever a minute of my life when I or a majority of the Democrats on this side were not in favor of these propositions embodied in the Senate amendments. I will answer the question the gentleman from Missouri [Mr. Klepper] asked his colleague [Mr. De Armond]. The gentleman from Mississippi voted against all amendments to the Hepburn-Davey House rate bill because he was in honor bound to stand by the bill as it had been agreed upon and to vote against all amendments, and on that day I and a majority of us over here voted against half a dozen amendments that we were in favor of, as everybody knew. It may probably be difficult for the gentleman to understand, but not difficult for a Democrat to understand, that a man may do that which he otherwise does not want to do in order to keep faith and in order to keep honor, and the six Democratic members of the committee and I did exactly that thing. What was the result? We did bring the weight of this House like a catapult to bear, with the President and public opinion behind that catapult, as well as ourselves, and Senators fell over themselves in order to out-Herod Herod in giving us what we and what the people wanted and what we had feared that a majority of the Senate did not want. There was no mistake made when for tactical purposes we came together in a nonpartisan bill, and the Republicans adopted in the bill several things which they did not want, and we left out of the bill several things which we did want, and keeping faith with one another as men of honor should, we stood by the bill, I and the six Democratic members of the Committee on Interstate and Foreign Commerce. Mr. Speaker, this has come back a better bill than it went out, and we want to keep it good. It has been said — I know not with how much truth — that when these amendments were being adopted it was whispered at the other end of the Capitol, "Oh, that is all right; let it go; the conferees will take care of that."

Now, I do not want the conferees to take care of it. Voting down this rule is the first, perhaps the only, opportunity to concur upon these five propositions, 2, 6, 31, 47, and 48, and to drive a nail through the plank and clinch it on the other side. Gentlemen say they want something in conference "to trade upon." Well, I do not want them to trade about either one of those five amendments; neither does this House of Representatives want them to do it. They all say so. There are many who say they would vote to concur; if so, why not do it now? I may be excused for not being able to understand a man who says he is in favor of a proposition and then, when the opportunity is offered to him to make that proposition irrevocably good upon the statute books, refuses the opportunity. The gentleman from Pennsylvania says that the House will have "an opportunity" later on "to vote." Will the House have it? Who knows it? Will or will there not be another rule to gag the House? Why, you know there will be another rule, provided only that the gentleman from Iowa [Mr. Hepburn] and the Committee on Rules desire to have another rule. It is true the House might at that time vote down the second rule, but the House might at this time vote down this rule; and if in blind partisanship it will avoid the first opportunity to do what it says it wants to do, what reason have we to believe it would avail itself of it in the second case? This is your first chance; take advantage of it. The next chance will be the Aldrich chance. Now, there are only two possible reasons why the House shall not be given an opportunity to vote to concur upon the five Senate amendments, the character of which has been outlined by the gentleman from Missouri. One is that somebody may want to imitate the game that was played at the other end of the Capitol. At the last moment, after having used patriotic Representatives as a lever to procure the desired legislation — to keep the fight alive — they at the last moment attempted to put the stamp of partisanship upon a great measure, which was advocated first by the Democrats, and which is more earnestly favored by them now than by any other people. That may be one reason, and the next reason would be to leave the final moulding of a bill to the uncertainty and secrecy of conferees, through whom these amendments might be killed, scotched, or emasculated.

The SPEAKER. The time of the gentleman has expired.

Mr. GROSVENOR. I yield one minute to the gentleman from Iowa.

Mr. DALZELL. I yield the balance of my time to my colleague [Mr. Grosvenor].

Mr. HEPBURN. Mr. Speaker, I simply desire to say, for a moment, that I agree entirely with the gentleman from Mississippi in the suggestion that the vote upon any one of these amendments that were offered in this House to the bill when it was under consideration does not indicate the views that the individual voting might have upon the subject. It will be remembered that it was the effort of the Committee on Interstate and Foreign Commerce to report to the House a bill that would embody the recommendations of the President and place them into law — that much and nothing more. Everything else beyond that was opposed by the committee. There was an agreement of the entire eighteen members of the committee that they would oppose any amendment and strive to secure the bill as reported. The gentleman from Mississippi, patriotic in his anxiety to get such a bill as the President had asked for, united with us in that purpose, and in accordance with the plan every one of the amendments was voted down, without regard to the individual views of us who voted against them. [Applause.]

The SPEAKER. The time of the gentleman has expired.

Mr. WILLIAMS. Mr. Speaker ——

The SPEAKER. For what purpose does the gentleman rise?

Mr. WILLIAMS. For the purpose of calling the attention of the House to the fact the gentleman from Pennsylvania said he would close in one speech.

Mr. DALZELL. I yielded my time to the gentleman from Ohio and I assumed that he would use the time.

Mr. WILLIAMS. You also yielded to the gentleman from Iowa.

Mr. DALZELL. No, sir; the gentleman from Ohio yielded to the gentleman from Iowa.

Mr. WILLIAMS. I just want the record to show the occurrence.

Mr. GROSVENOR. Mr. Speaker, I think it is rather unbecoming of the gentleman to quibble about a minute's time being yielded to the gentleman from Iowa, who has been so bitterly assailed here on the floor, to explain his position. Now, Mr. Speaker, the situation is practically this: The organization of this House is responsible for the progress and despatch of business. We have a bill here with fifty-one amendments. We have a gentleman on the other side who is supreme in the minority, with power enough to demand the yeas and nays upon every question, who can take this bill and upon these fifty-one amendments could occupy the time of the House for six days and a half by the call of the roll. And he has not for a long time failed to demand a call of the roll whenever he has had an opportunity. Now, I respectfully submit to gentlemen on this side if it is not about time that the Republican majority of this House should take possession of the House and transact its business on its own hook and in its own way, or is it wise to turn over to a faction, full of the idea of filibustering as a remedy for its minority, the future of this important legislation?

Mr. WILLIAMS. Will the gentleman permit an interruption?

Mr. GROSVENOR. I do not know what for. I do not intend that the gentleman shall make any more speeches.

Mr. WILLIAMS. I do not intend to make a speech. May I ask the gentleman a question?

Mr. GROSVENOR. Ask it.

Mr. WILLIAMS. Would the gentleman consent to permit these six amendments to be voted upon by the House if I repeated here what I had offered to do in the Committee on Rules, to wit, to give unanimous consent that the balance should be nonconcurred in and go to conference?

Mr. GROSVENOR. I am not willing that the Republican majority of this House shall waive their prerogative and turn it over to the gentleman from Mississippi. [Applause on the Republican side.] We have had enough of that. If we are coming out of this session of Congress with any self-respect, let alone the respect of the country, it is time we attempted to do business ourselves and not permit other gentlemen to dictate to us. And then — just think of it, gentlemen. Here is the minority, representing about 125 votes, and the gentleman from Mississippi stands up calmly and deliberately and picks out the amendments he wants to vote upon, and demands that his dictation shall be heard by the House, and when it is not heard, then he pours out the vials of his wrath here. Now, let us proceed in an orderly way, just as we have done a hundred times in the memory of many of us — disagree to all of the amendments and send the bill to conference.

The gentleman from Wisconsin [Mr. Cooper] is certainly seeking a point of attack. This House has the power to bring back the members of that committee at any time it sees fit to do so. We are not in the hands either of the Democratic minority or in the hands of a conference committee. Is there any man here who by his vote will doubt that that conference committee will at a very early date report this important bill back? And let me make a statement, Mr. Speaker, and I ask the House to hear what I say and measure my language — when that conference report comes back there will be a chance to vote on every amendment the House desires to vote upon, and there will be debate, and for once in my life I think I occupy a position where I can enforce the suggestion which I have made. But I desire to disclaim on the part of the majority of the Committee on Rules the slightest intention of gagging the bill through this House. Many of us are strongly in favor of the very amendments that the gentleman from Mississippi [Mr. Williams] has spoken about, and you have all heard the explanation made by the gentleman himself that entirely exonerates the gentleman from Iowa [Mr. Hepburn] from having placed himself in a position of hostility to the particular amendment which the gentleman has seen fit to point out. He voted against any amendment, and I can go a little further and say that he appealed to me not to offer an amendment that I had prepared, and which would have made this bill, in my humble judgment, far better than it was when it left the House, and I refrained from offering it simply and solely for the purpose of aiding the passage of the bill and getting it into the hands ultimately of the committee of conference.

The committee may go out and agree or disagree on certain points and come back again. I recollect very well that on a certain night here we voted down a conference report five times, and stayed here until nearly morning, and ultimately, upon the demand made by the House, we saved the Government of the United States from the disgrace of having to report for duty to a vagabond crowd in the island of Cuba. I hope the committee will be sustained in this report.

The SPEAKER. The question is on agreeing to the resolution.

THE ARMY APPROPRIATION BILL, 1902 [1]

Mr. CANNON. Mr. Speaker, in the five minutes' time I can only refer to one or two matters that my attention has been directed to. This appropriation for barracks and quarters makes $2,000,000, and $250,000 in addition, immediately available in the Philippines, and contains some other immediately available provisions. In other words, between two and three million dollars — nearer three millions than

[1] *Congr. Record*, XXXVI, 2347.

two millions — are made immediately available. This is an appropriation bill for the coming year and a deficiency bill for this year. How much more may be in this bill, how much more in other bills I do not know; but I do know that this practice of going from committee to committee under the rules of the House has jurisdiction, and then, before the matter has been investigated, by the aid of a willing Senate, failing in one place, rushing to another that has not jurisdiction, and sticking in amendments here and there and yonder ought to be done away with. Appropriation for the next year, appropriation for ·this year, legislation here, legislation there. If action is continued along these lines it will demoralize the matter of appropriation and bring scandal and criticism — deserved criticism — from the people of the country.

Now, touching this retirement matter, I do not know whether it is right or not. I want to treat the Army liberally. This provision had no place in the House bill; it is legislation pure and simple, on a large scale, by Senate amendment. How does it come here? In a conference agreement, by the grace of the Senate — wholesale. I should be glad if every member here who thinks he understands this provision would stand up. These matters ought to be treated of upon their merits. If I vote for this conference report on this great bill to supply the public service, I am compelled to vote for a bill that supplies that service for the next year as well as for this year, a bill that amends the law and introduces a new policy touching the retired list. It may be justifiable; I do not know. I have got to take it upon trust. In this body, close to the people, we proceed under rules. In another body — and I think I can say it within parliamentary lines — legislation is by unanimous consent. And when I say that, gentlemen understand what it means. [Applause.]

Mr. RICHARDSON of Tennessee. Mr. Speaker, the House is put at a very great disadvantage when we come to vote upon a conference report if we are not satisfied in the House with amendments that have been put upon the bill by the Senate. It seems that in this case the Senate put upon this bill certain amendments which are obnoxious to our rules. As has been stated by the gentleman from Illinois [Mr. Cannon], the legislative provisions that they have put upon this bill would have no standing under our rules if proposed here. Now, when that has been done and the bill comes back to us from the Senate, we ought to have the right to vote as an independent matter upon every such proposition presented to us, and should not be required to vote upon various propositions as a whole in a conference report.

Now, we have not that permission, we have not that privilege. And why? I undertake to say of the statement of the gentleman from Iowa [Mr. Hull], whether he meant to do it or not, he has misled the House of Representatives. I do not believe the gentleman from Iowa would intentionally mislead the House, but that is the effect of the action that we are now taking. And why do I say it? Because when this bill came from the Senate with Senate amendments the gentleman from Iowa, the chairman of the Military Committee, as it was his duty to do, asked of the House unanimous consent to nonconcur in the Senate amendments. He could not have nonconcurred and sent the bill to conference without unanimous consent of this House, and he was held up, as we all know, on that request upon a promise, almost expressed, certainly implied, that we should have the right to vote upon the Senate amendments. We are denied that right unless we vote down the conference report.[1]

MR. CANNON'S REMONSTRANCE, 1903 [2]

[In connection with the South Carolina claim forced upon the Senate by Senator Tillman.]

GENTLEMEN know that under the practice of the House and under the rules of the Senate the great money bills can contain nothing but appropriations in pursuance of existing law, unless by consent of both bodies. If any one of these bills contains legislation, it must be by the unanimous consent of the two bodies; and the uniform practice has been, so far as I know, the invariable practice has been, with the exception of one amendment upon this bill, that when one body objected to legislation proposed by the other upon an appropriation bill, the body proposing the legislation has receded. . . .

The House conferees objected, and the whole delay has been over that one item. In the House of Representatives, without criticizing either side or any individual member, we have rules, sometimes invoked by our Democratic friends and sometimes by ourselves — each responsible to the people after all said and done — by which a majority, right or wrong, mistaken of otherwise, can legislate.

In another body there are no such rules. In another body legislation is had by unanimous consent. In another body an individual member of that body can rise in his place and talk for one hour, two hours, ten hours, twelve hours. . . .

. . . Your conferees were unable to get the Senate to recede upon this gift from the treasury against the law, to the state of North Carolina. By unanimous consent another body legislates, and in the expiring hours of the session we are powerless without that unanimous consent. . . .

---

[1] It may be noted that it is quite common for committee chairmen to state that there will be a chance for the discussion of individual amendments later, but that chance rarely comes.

[2] *Congr. Record*, March 3, 1903.

Gentlemen, I have made my protest. I do it in sorrow and in humiliation, but there it is; and in my opinion another body under these methods must change its methods of procedure, or our body, backed up by the people, will compel that change, else this body, close to the people, shall become a mere tender, a mere bender of the pregnant hinges of the knee, to submit to what any one member of another body may demand of this body as a price for legislation.

THE CURRENCY BILL OF 1908[1]

THE SPEAKER. There is a motion before the House to suspend the rules, and the Clerk will read.

The Clerk read as follows:

Resolved, That after the adoption hereof the Committee on Banking and Currency shall be discharged and the House shall proceed to the consideration of H. R. 21871, "A bill to amend the national banking laws;" debate thereon shall be concluded at not later than 5 o'clock P. M. to-day, the time to be equally divided between the friends and the opponents of the bill, to be controlled on one side by Mr. VREELAND and on the other by Mr. WILLIAMS. It shall be in order to offer in lieu of the bill H. R. 21871 a substitute, namely, H. R. 16730, "A bill to further protect depositors in banks, to secure a safe and elastic emergency currency, and to amend the national-bank act and previous amendments thereto." On the conclusion of the debate as herein provided, a vote shall be taken without delay or intervening motion, first on the question of substituting H. R. 16730, if said bill shall have been offered, and then upon the passage of the bill, or the substitute bill in lieu thereof as the case may be.

General leave to print remarks on the bill is hereby granted for five legislative days.

* * * * * * * *

Mr. PRINCE. Mr. Speaker, there is now presented to this House, a very strange rule of adoption. In the *Record* of yesterday, that is now on the desk of every Member, under date of May 13, page 6508 of public bills, resolutions, and memorials introduced, is one by Mr. Vreeland, a bill (H. R. 21871) to amend the national bank laws, referred to the Committee on Banking and Currency.

That is the bill that the House is now asked to take up. Hardly a Member has the bill before him now; it is only within the last ten minutes that it has been printed and brought to the House. That committee is to be discharged from the consideration of a bill referred to them by the Speaker of the House. The committee has not had time to consider it, and a rule is brought in here to discharge a committee of this House. Why set the sixty-four committees of this House aside? I submit that the House is called upon to insult a committee of this

---

[1] *Congr. Record*, May 14, 1908.

House, without its having an opportunity to pass upon the bill, and say that it shall be discharged. [Applause on the Democratic side.] If our heads go first, yours may follow. Members of this House — 223 of us — if our heads are to be put upon the block now, whose heads are to follow in the desire to carry out the purposes of the leaders on this side when they want to consider any particular business? I say to you that the Committee on Banking and Currency stand ready to meet this afternoon and report this bill to this House, so that it may proceed in an orderly, regular manner before the country and before the committee of this House. Is there any justification for this proceeding?

Will the country justify such action as this? Will the country justify us in saying that a handful of Democrats in the minority can force legislation through this House, where there are 233 Republicans and 166 Democrats, or sixty-seven Republican majority? How much of a majority do we need on this side of the House to transact business under the rules? How can we of this branch, that represents the voice of the American electorate, go before our constituents and say that we have subordinated ourselves, say that we have denied to ourselves the right to proceed according to the rules of the House to have committees report, and that committees shall be discharged, because, forsooth, for political exigencies and none other, a bill must be presented to this House and to the country? Who is asking for it? Men on this floor have received thousands of letters asking their vote for or against putting wood pulp and print paper on the free list. Thousands of letters have come here asking us to do something on the anti-injunction bill, to do something on the eight-hour bill, to do something that the people want. I pass the platter around to my colleagues and ask you, who has asked you to do this act? Political exigency! Throw to the business people of the United States a bone when they ask you for something that is good. When they ask you for bread, throw them a stone! Can you proceed in this line? You say, perhaps, that I am speaking outside of my party. No, no! I am speaking, and I have authority to speak, by the very party to which I belong. When we met in conference May 5, 1908, I offered the following resolution which was unanimously adopted ——

The SPEAKER pro tempore. The time of the gentleman has expired.

Mr. PRINCE. I ask time to read this resolution.

Mr. WILLIAMS. Will two minutes longer be sufficient?

Mr. PRINCE. A minute and a half will do.

Mr. WILLIAMS. I yield three minutes more to the gentleman, or so much thereof as he may desire.

Mr. PRINCE. This resolution was unanimously adopted:

Resolved, That this meeting, or any adjournment thereof, is only a conference and not a caucus, and shall not have the binding effect of a caucus; and that those who participate in its deliberations shall be absolutely free hereafter to act in accordance with their own judgment with reference to all matters considered before it.

My fellow-Members, put the yoke upon you, if you will. Walk under the yoke, "under buck," as the expression was in the time of the yoke of oxen. Now, the yoke may be easy and the burden light, but I want to say to you I will not put on the yoke; I will not assume the burden and go before my constituents and say that I am in favor of makeshift legislation; that I am in favor of discharging committees of this House; that I am in favor of overriding the wishes of the people; that I am to be a mere tobacco sign, to be moved hither and thither, a mere pawn upon the chessboard! I am here to represent my people. That resolution permits me to represent them, and I shall vote against such resolutions as this, and I ask other men who will have to go before their constituents to consider well, because no one of you can say, as they tried to say when the crime of 1873 was committed, "We did not know anything about it." You all know. You have your eyes open. You walk intelligently and knowingly, and if you vote for this resolution, remember that the next time your committee does not see fit to do what some people want you to do, your heads will be laid upon the block, they will be cut off, and the whole legislation for 90,000,000 of people is to roll around three men. [Applause on the Democratic side.] Three men! And I say here and now, to the House and the country, the do-nothing Congress has been here long enough. If it were not for the bright, brainy, forceful character at the other end of the Avenue, I doubt whether we would have done anything except pass a few appropriation bills; but, thank God, there is somewhere in this country, at the other end of the Avenue, a man whose ears are to the ground, a man whose heart is in sympathy with the people, and he is insisting upon legislation, and what little we get is through him. It is through him and his special messages that we accomplish anything in the first session of the Sixtieth Congress for the benefit of the 90,000,000 of people that we represent here on this floor. [Applause.]

Mr. WILLIAMS. How much time have I remaining, Mr. Speaker?

The SPEAKER. The gentleman has twelve minutes.

Mr. WILLIAMS. I will ask the gentleman from New York whether he expects to conclude and use all of his time with one speech, or expects to have more than one speech?

Mr. VREELAND. We will use the remainder of our time with one speech.

Mr. WILLIAMS. Mr. Speaker, there is nothing hitherto evolved out of the history of the human race quite as kaleidoscopic as the Republican party. Some time ago we upon this side of the Chamber were informed by the gentleman from New York [Mr. Payne], the majority floor leader, and by the Speaker's "Rules Deputy," the gentleman from

Pennsylvania [Mr. Dalzell], and by the other member of that committee, the gentleman from New York [Mr. Sherman] that no legislation having a Democratic initiative would be so much as considered by the majority of this House. You announced to the country that we were legislatively disbarred and that there was no use in our burning our lights over legislative study.

This morning one of the same gentlemen comes to us — I started to say, with a carefully concocted rule, but I am afraid the Speaker has got so that he is afraid even of the Committee on Rules — but with a carefully concocted motion to suspend the rules, in words in which, I think, I find the fine hand of the gentleman from Pennsylvania not only proposing that the Democrats shall initiate legislation, but undertaking to designate just precisely what legislation they shall initiate. [Applause on the Democratic side.] And it is done upon the ground that that legislation bears my name. He does not even permit this side to amend the bill H. R. 16730 to suit itself in as far as it desires to amend it. The rule does not even permit me to amend it in so far as I desire to amend it, especially in one essential part of it, where a typewriter's carelessness in section 7 exists in the bill that was introduced on the 7th of February, 1908.

It is an old adage "Beware of the Greeks bearing gifts"; and if in the old time men were to beware of Greeks bearing gifts, my heaven! how much more ought we to beware, in these latter days of improved ingenuity, of Illinois, Pennsylvania, and New York Republicans bearing gifts. [Laughter and applause on the Democratic side.]

The Banking and Currency Committee considered a bill, and they reported the bill and recommended it to this House. I am opposed to it. I believe everybody, or nearly everybody, on this side is opposed to it, but there is a chance, at any rate theoretically if not practically, that it would receive serious consideration. Indeed, there are those who believe that in a fair fight with the Vreeland bill it might win. There is not a man of you that would propose to give a moment's serious consideration to the Williams currency bill. It is a Democratic bill. If it was the best bill on banking and currency ever introduced in the world, there is not one of you that would dare privately to express an opinion favorable to it without having previously seen the Speaker and explained why you were going to do it and received his permission to do it. [Laughter and applause on the Democratic side.]

You have virtually served notice on us that we are disbarred legislatively, and then you select a bill for us and say, "Play to the gallery, you Democrats," by voting for or against it. It is a better bill than yours and we are for it, but we will not let you obscure the real issue which is the abominability of your bill, by putting ours in front. You are inviting us to commit a tactical error offending those few conscientious, honest, nonpartisan Republicans that are opposed to this infamy of the Vreeland bill by substituting ourselves in point of consideration for them and their views. [Applause on the Democratic side.] We decline to be "deposited in that cavity." [Laughter and applause on the Democratic side.]

Now, Mr. Speaker, what have you done? You are going to introduce a bill to reform the currency that goes to the very commercial vitalization of 80,000,000 of people, and you are going to give four hours of debate! Four weeks would not have been sufficient. The gentleman from New York [Mr. Vreeland] says we will oppose his bill "because it is a Republican bill." Why, bless your hearts, we are not in the habit of opposing things because they have a Republican origin, and you know it. [Derisive laughter on the Republican side.]

There is not one of you laughing that does not know it, and you know that your laugh is not sincere, but hypocritical. Upon this side for the last three years there has not been a good measure recommended by a Republican President or a Republican committee — good in our opinion, I mean, of course — that we have not advocated and that we have not helped through. It has been our boast that it is no longer a maxim that "the duty of an opposition was to oppose," but that the duty of the opposition is to oppose wrong things and advocate right things, no matter whence they come. [Applause on the Democratic side.] The history of the party in the rate bill, the history of the party in connection with the anti-injunction recommendations of the President, the history of the party in connection with the employers' liability bill, all prove that what I state is true, and proves your recently attempted vaudeville laugh is a pretense and hypocrisy.

Who stands for this Vreeland bill? Nobody but the Republican machine in this House. The gentleman from Pennsylvania, Mr. Rothermel, telegraphed all the banks within his district and got answers this morning from nineteen of them, and only three of them did not reply, advising him to beat the Vreeland bill. They regard it as worse than nothing. The people are not demanding it; the business men, farmers, and the banks are not demanding it. Nobody is demanding it. You, even, that Republican machine over there, are not demanding it because you want it. You are demanding it merely to be able to go before the people and say: "We passed something in the shape of an emergency-currency bill." You are passing it simply to get something into conference, and in a secret conference committee to hatch plutocratic mischief. There is not one of you that does not know that it is an abomination and a miserable makeshift. It ought to be called a bill of "authorization for clearance-house associations of national banks which have violated the law," or a "bill of indemnity for Secretaries of the Treasury who have suspended the operation of the law in behalf of the national banks and clearance-house associations." [Applause on the Democratic side.]

Conference Report on the Currency Bill [1]

Mr. Vreeland. Mr. Speaker, I move to suspend the rules and adopt the conference report which I present.

The Speaker. The gentleman from New York moves to suspend the rules and agree to the conference report which he presents.

The conference report was read, as follows:

The committee of conference on the disagreeing votes of the two Houses on the amendment of the Senate to the bill (H. R. 21871) to amend the national banking laws, having met, after full and free conference have agreed to recommend and do recommend to their respective Houses as follows:

That the House recede from its disagreement to the amendment of the Senate, and agree to the same with an amendment as follows: Strike out all of the matter inserted by said Senate amendment and insert in lieu thereof the following:

"That national banking associations, each having an unimpaired capital and a surplus of not less than 20 per cent, not less than ten in number, having an aggregate capital and surplus of at least $5,000,000, may form voluntary associations to be designated as national currency associations. The banks uniting to form such association shall, by their presidents or vice-presidents, acting under authority from the board of directors, make and file with the Secretary of the Treasury a certificate setting forth the names of the banks composing the association, the principal place of business of the association, and the name of the association, which name shall be subject to the approval of the Secretary of the Treasury. Upon the filing of such certificate the associated banks therein named shall become a body corporate, and by the name so designated and approved may sue and be sued and exercise the powers of a body corporate for the purposes hereinafter mentioned: *Provided,* That not more than one such national currency association shall be formed in any city: *Provided further,* That the several members of such national currency association shall be taken, as nearly as conveniently may be, from a territory composed of a State or part of a State, or contiguous parts of one or more States: *And provided further,* That any national bank in such city or territory, having the qualifications herein prescribed for membership in such national currency association, shall, upon its application to and upon the approval of the Secretary of the Treasury, be admitted to membership in a national currency association for that city or territory, and upon such admission shall be deemed and held a part of the body corporate, and as such entitled to all the rights and privileges and subject to all the liabilities of an original member: *And provided further,* That each national currency association shall be composed exclusively of banks not members of any other national currency association.

"The dissolution, voluntary or otherwise, of any bank in such association shall not affect the corporate existence of the association unless there shall then remain less than the minimum number of ten banks: *Provided, however,* That the reduction of the number of said banks below the minimum of ten shall not affect the existence of the corporation with respect to the assertion of all rights in favor of or against such association. The affairs of the association shall be managed by a board consisting of one representative from each bank. By-laws for the

[1] *Congr. Record,* May 27, 1908.

government of the association shall be made by the board, subject to the approval of the Secretary of the Treasury. A president, vice-president, secretary, treasurer, and an executive committee of not less than five members shall be elected by the board. The powers of such board, except in the election of officers and making of by-laws, may be exercised through its executive committee.

"The national currency association herein provided for shall have and exercise any and all powers necessary to carry out the purposes of this section, namely, to render available, under the direction and control of the Secretary of the Treasury, as a basis for additional circulation any securities, including commercial paper, held by a national banking association. For the purpose of obtaining such additional circulation, any bank belonging to any national currency association, having circulating notes outstanding secured by the deposit of bonds of the United States to an amount not less than forty per centum of its capital stock, and which has its capital unimpaired and a surplus of not less than twenty per centum, may deposit with and transfer to the association, in trust for the United States, for the purpose hereinafter provided, such of the securities above mentioned as may be satisfactory to the board of the association. The officers of the association may thereupon, in behalf of such bank, make application to the Comptroller of the Currency for an issue of additional circulating notes to an amount not exceeding seventy-five per centum of the cash value of the securities or commercial paper so deposited. The Comptroller of the Currency shall immediately transmit such application to the Secretary of the Treasury with such recommendation as he thinks proper, and if, in the judgment of the Secretary of the Treasury, business conditions in the locality demand additional circulation, and if he be satisfied with the character and value of the securities proposed and that a lien in favor of the United States on the securities so deposited and on the assets of the banks composing the association will be amply sufficient for the protection of the United States, he may direct an issue of additional circulating notes to the association, on behalf of such bank, to an amount in his discretion, not, however, exceeding seventy-five per centum of the cash value of the securities so deposited: *Provided*, That upon the deposit of any of the State, city, town, county, or other municipal bonds, of a character described in section 3 of this act, circulating notes may be issued to the extent of not exceeding ninety per centum of the market value of such bonds so deposited: *And provided further*, That no national banking association shall be authorized in any event to issue circulating notes based on commercial paper in excess of thirty per centum of its unimpaired capital and surplus. The term "commercial paper" shall be held to include only notes representing actual commercial transactions, which when accepted by the association shall bear the names of at least two responsible parties and have not exceeding four months to run, etc. [There followed numerous specific regulations.]

And the Senate agree to the same.

Managers on the part of the House. { EDWARD B. VREELAND, THEODORE E. BURTON, JOHN W. WEEKS,

Managers on the part of the Senate. { NELSON W. ALDRICH, W. B. ALLISON, EUGENE HALE.

The Speaker. Is a second demanded?

Mr. Pujo. Mr. Speaker, I demand a second.

The Speaker. A second is ordered, under the rule.

Mr. Pujo. I ask the gentleman from New York, in the interest of the orderly enactment of legislation, that we be allowed an hour on a side, at least, of debate, the gentleman from New York to control one half of the time and the ranking Member on the committee on this side to control the other half of the time. It is known to all Members that the bill has just reached the desks about two minutes ago, and there is not a Member, not even the conferees, who have had an opportunity to make themselves familiar in the slightest degree with the provisions of this bill; and I ask the gentleman, in the interest of orderly legislation ——

Mr. Vreeland. I want to make a parliamentary inquiry. Does this come out of anybody's time?

The Speaker. No; the gentleman made a parliamentary inquiry somewhat extended, but the Chair does not take it out of the time of either gentleman. The gentleman from New York is entitled to twenty minutes and the gentleman from Louisiana is entitled to twenty minutes.

Mr. Pujo. Now, Mr. Speaker, I ask unanimous consent of this House that debate on the conference report upon what is known as the "national currency" legislation, proposed a few moments ago, be extended so as to allow one hour for each side, the time to be controlled by the gentleman from New York and the ranking Member on this side.

The Speaker. Is there objection?

Mr. Vreeland. I regret to say that I shall have to object, for the reason —— [Cries of "No, no!"]

The Speaker. Objection is heard.

Mr. Vreeland. I want to say in explanation that a great many gentlemen have told me —— [Cries of "Regular order!" on the Democratic side].

The Speaker. The gentleman is in regular order. The gentleman has twenty minutes.

Mr. Clark of Missouri. Are you taking it out of his time?

The Speaker. The Chair is keeping the time.

Mr. Cockran. Would it be in order to ask an extension to half an hour?

·The Speaker. The gentleman from New York asks unanimous consent for an extension of the time to thirty minutes on a side instead of twenty minutes on a side.

Mr. Vreeland. I consent to that.

The Speaker. The Chair hears no objection. The gentleman from New York is entitled to thirty minutes and the gentleman from Louisiana is entitled to thirty minutes.

Mr. Pujo. Mr. Speaker, I will ask the Chair to inform me when I have used three minutes.

This is a composite bill. It incorporates the Aldrich bill and the Vreeland bill, and as presented is a composite measure here. It authorizes the issuance of five hundred millions of our circulating currency, should the bill be passed, to be based upon United States bonds, State bonds, county bonds, municipal bonds, all with a taxing power behind them. So far those are the main features of the Aldrich bill. Each political autonomy is vested with the power to levy a tax to proteet the notes should the issuing bank fail to retire it when presented and the bonds deposited as security fail to realize a sufficient sum when disposed of. The other features of the bill are novel, and I am surprised and amazed to witness their adoption for the first time by the Republican party — an asset currency pure and simple, a subtreasury scheme practically.

I call attention to the language on page 4 of the bill. When uniting banks with a minimum capital of $5,000,000 form an association, they can have money issued by dispositing certain securities with the Treasurer of the United States. Now, what is the character and what is the class of securities required to be deposited? I read, beginning on page 3:

The national currency association herein provided for shall have and exercise any and all powers necessary to carry out the purposes of the section, namely, to render available, under the direction and control of the Secretary of the Treasury, as a basis for additional circulation, any securities, including commercial paper, held by a national banking association.

A warehouse receipt issued for any agricultural product, an elevator receipt for wheat, for corn, for oats, held by a bank can be used for deposit with this association, and in turn with the Secretary of the Treasury, as the basis for circulation.

[Here the hammer fell.]

I will use two minutes more of my time, Mr. Speaker.

The ninety-day draft of a merchant in Kansas City who would ship hay to New York, or a ninety-day draft of a merchant in Kansas City who would ship a carload of mules to Louisiana, drawn by him, accepted by the buyer, and discounted at the bank, becomes commercial paper, with two names on it, a legal subsisting basis for this currency.

I want to congratulate the Republican party, being a sound-money party (purely in a Pickwickian sense), for advocating a scheme like this. Evidently the political emergency must be great, otherwise they would not in a moment, without giving an opportunity to discuss the measure, try to force such a currency upon the American people.

Mr. VREELAND. I regret that I felt obliged to object to an extension of time for debate upon this bill, but quite a number of gentlemen on this side who wish to get away on afternoon trains have informed me that if the extension is granted they will be unable to remain until a vote is taken.

Mr. Speaker, the motion which I have made to agree to the conference report means that the Republican conferees on the part of this Republican House and the conferees on the part of the Republican Senate have agreed upon a financial bill, have brought it in here with a unanimous report, and hope that it will be adopted by this Republican House.

Mr. Speaker, we believe that the Republican party has not ceased to be a great constructive party. We believe that it is still the great business party of the country. We believe that this conference report now before us is evidence that the Republican party is still a great cohesive body, with power tò get together and place upon the statute books legislation which will prevent the recurrence of such a disaster as befel the American people last October.

Mr. Speaker, the concessions that have been made between the House and the Senate in the preparation of this conference report are honorable concessions, such as might properly be made. The financial bill which we have brought in here today is the bill passed by this House with amendments to which the House conferees have consented. We believe that it is a good bill and one which this House may place upon the statute books, satisfied that it will carry out the purpose for which it is enacted. The bill which we have brought in here with amendments is substantially the House bill in all its essential features that was adopted by the Republican conference, drawn by a committee appointed by that conference, and passed through the House of Representatives.

Amendments to the House Bill

I desire, first, to refer to the amendments which have been made to the House bill. We have added to our bill a portion of the Senate bill. I suppose the minority upon this floor will ring all the changes and use their keenest sarcasm and invective in charging that we have adopted the Aldrich bill. But, Mr. Speaker, although the leader of the minority · may run his dagger through the cloak of the Aldrich bill he will find that the body has been removed from the inside of it. What were the objections to the Aldrich bill? What were the criticisms made upon this side of the Chamber or by Republican Members of this House when the Aldrich bill came over from the Senate? We all understand the objections which were made to section 8 of that bill, changing the law applying to the reserves of banks, and section 11, with its restrictions upon the directorate and officers of banks. There are many who believe that these provisions might be changed so that they would be useful as a part of our banking laws. But it was thought that they might better be left to be considered by the commission provided in this bill. But there was further objection to the Senate bill as it came to the House by many upon this side of the Chamber. What is the purpose of this law? It is to provide a great reservoir of currency, to be drawn upon only in case of need. It is not intended to provide for the ordinary needs of business. It is to provide against a currency famine such as we had last•October. It is to give a feeling of confidence to the bankers of the country and to the depositors of the banks. It is· to assure them against fright and panic which, for some unexpected reason, may take possession of the people. It is to provide that $500,000,000 shall be printed and ready for use, held as a reserve, to come out only with the consent of the Secretary of the Treasury and upon his certificate that it is needed.

Mr. McHENRY. ·The House of Congress, Mr. Speaker, is supposed to be both a deliberative and a representative body, but in this action which you now propose the people are to learn that this legislative body is governed not by deliberation, but by party passion; controlled not by the people, but by one man. You can pass this iniquitous measure if you choose, because you have the power; but there is one thing you can not do — you can not compel the people to accept the provisions of a law which they do not approve.

For six long, tedious months the Committee on Banking and Currency have given faithful study and consideration to this vitally important question. The committee was unanimous in a desire to frame a non-partisan measure which would work to the good of all the people and not for the special interest of a favored few. There were some basic principles upon which we disagreed, but the disagreement was an honest and nonpolitical one. But the gentleman from New York, Mr. Vree-land, who seems to have become the spokesman for the Republican managers in the House, appeared before our committee at the public hearings, literally whipping the Republican members into line, injecting a discordant partisan element in our deliberation. We have been frankly told that a panic was on and another one coming, and that it was necessary, in order to secure the election of a Republican President, that some sort of financial legislation be placed upon the statute books. No matter what, only so it was something. We accept the challenge, Mr. Speaker. But while we of the minority are fighting with every ounce of strength we have to prevent the passage of this bill, we feel that it is a hopeless fight; that the orders from Wall street and Republican party bosses are more powerful in this Congress than the appeals or the needs of the people.

*　　*　　*　　*　　*　　*　　*　　*

I am anxious, Mr. Speaker, that proper currency legislation shall be enacted, but I am not willing that the people shall be fooled and that the sovereign right of the Government to issue money shall be taken from it and delegated to Wall street gamblers. Rather than have a bill of this kind, it would be infinitely better for the country to have no legislation at all at this session.

Under the rule by which this bill is brought up for action practically all debate is shut off and no amendments permitted. If you will give us two days' debate, Mr. Speaker, the bill can probably be so amended that it will be a workable measure and fair to all parts of the country alike and to all people, but this is not a part of your plan — the Wall street plan demands that the bill shall go through just as it was, without any changes. It has just come from the conference report and we are to vote on it immediately, and I will venture the assertion that nine out of ten Members of the House have not had time to read the bill — do not know what they are voting upon, and are simply obeying the order of the party — Wall street bosses. Why this haste? If the measure is an honest one, it will bear the light of investigation and intelligent discussion. Is it the part of a deliberative body to rush a conference report here and demand that we shall speak and vote aganist the measure without even having had time to read the bill? It is now just twelve minutes since the printed conference report has been delivered, and without any study or preparation whatever we are called upon to register our protest against the bill. This represents the most important legislation that Congress has had before it since the civil war. To now vote upon it, without a full knowledge of the bill and without any privilege to amend, do you suppose, sir, that the American people can view our action with favor?

If you will give us reasonable time for debate, I have sufficient confidence in the intelligence and integrity of the individual Members of the House to believe that the bill will either be honestly amended or killed outright, which, for the country's sake and for the Republican party's sake, too, would be the better plan.

The bill provides that ten banks with a total capitalization of $5,000,000 may go together and form themselves into a so-called "clearance-house association," with the power delegated to them by the Government to issue currency to the extent of $500,000,000. At the present time, Mr. Speaker, the currency of our country is on what is termed a gold and United States bond basis. That is, every dollar of currency except our present outstanding national-bank notes is guaranteed by the actual gold or silver coin in the United States Treasury and is redeemable in gold or silver on demand. In the establishment of the national banking system, it was agreed that a national bank could, to the extent of its capital, issue money against the United States bonds. The United States Government, through this medium, merely divides up the bonds, which represent the people's obligation, into small denominations in order that they may be used in circulation to meet the demands of trade. So successful has been the practical working of this plan that to-day no man thinks of looking at a note to see whether it is a national-bank note, a United States Treasury note, a gold certificate, or a silver certificate. The people have absolute confidence in their currency at the present time. If anything is needed, it is a bill which will unify our currency system and not make it more diverse, as this does. As I have already told you,in my previous address, the country is now suffering more from lack of confidence than lack of money, and that any legislative action upon this question should be with the idea of restoring confidence, not of creating further doubt or distrust in the minds of the people as to the character or value of the money which they are to receive in exchange for the sale of their labor or the products of their labor. This bill is the entering wedge for a radical and violent change in the currency of our country. It means the retirement of the present United States bond-secured note as rapidly as it can be done under the law, and to replace the national bond security with whatever railroad or other bonds or notes which a bank issuing currency may have.

I will not go into the economic side of this question or burden you with statistics, but will discuss the practical workings of the bill and prove to your satisfaction, if you are open to conviction, that the bill is impractical; that its use will be confined entirely to Wall street banks; that it will not stop panics, but, on the contrary, will precipitate them; that it will absolutely insure the monopoly of the people's money by predatory interests. In brief, sir, I will prove to you that it is a Wall street measure pure and simple; that it is a measure against the honest business interests and producers of all classes, and to enact it into a law will be a crime against the people which they will resent at the polls in November. [Applause.]

BRIEF SUMMARY OF THE BILL

I do not want to burden the *Record* by offering the entire bill, but will briefly outline its essential features.

First. It provides for an association of not less than ten banks, with a total capitalization of not less than $5,000,000 for the purpose of issuing money. Each bank in said association to have one vote, and to choose a board of five managers, of which three shall constitute a quorum for the transaction of business.

Second. It provides that the total issue shall not exceed $5,000,000.

Third. That the issue shall be based upon national, State, county, or municipal bonds, railroad stock, or bonds and notes or any security which a bank may own or hold as collateral.

Fourth. It provides that the rate of tax on said circulation shall be 5 per cent per annum for the first month and 1 per cent per annum for each additional month until a maximum tax of 10 per cent is reached.

Fifth. It provides an interest rate of 1 per cent per annum on Government deposits — perhaps.

The Wall street interests have become alarmed at the attitude of the people in their demand for banking and currency reform. Realizing that all such demands are eventually enacted into law, they have decided, while they have the power, to fool the people under threat of another panic, and enact a law which will continue their present control of the currency of the country. That is, if a supplemental issue of currency is to be authorized, it must not be allowed to pass beyond the control of the large banking syndicates, so the underlying principles of this forced measure may be found in two definite objects.

First, to enable them to control and regulate panics at will and to stop panics when it suits their purposes to have them stopped.

Second, to provide a permanent fund for the Wall street gambler's use.

Mr. WILLIAMS. Mr. Speaker, you were never so highly honored in all your life as you have been to-day. This bill ought to be entitled the "Cannon-Aldrich political emergency bill." [Applause on the Democratic side.] Your influence over this House was never so vastly shown as to-day. But the other day the House said, "the Aldrich bill is altogether wicked," and it would have none of it. It was not good enough for the House. But the other day the Republican Senate said that the Vreeland bill was altogether iniquitous and destructive of the best interests of the country, and it would have none of it. Nobody so poor in the House as to do reverence to the Aldrich bill; nobody so poor in the Senate as to do reverence to the Vreeland bill. But to-day the great discovery — two iniquities compose a perfect good. Neither bill was good enough for either House, but to-day both bills combined are good enough for both Houses. [Applause on the Democratic side.] Why, this comes in response to the sincere prayer of the Speaker, because he does pray. [Laughter.] It has not been long since his prayer began to bear this refrain: "Anything, O God, anything; it makes no difference what, even if it be really nothing, just so that I can call it something; anything before the House adjourns." [Applause on the Democratic side.]

"It will not do for the Republican party to go to the country with absolutely nothing. It must have something that can be called something by somebody somewhere." And in response to that prayer, directed not to the Almighty, but to the members of the House here present, and with the conference report on public buildings held back, those who were lions to thwart the pathway of the Aldrich bill are now lambs. I find on page 6635 of the *Congressional Record* these words of the gentleman from Ohio [Mr. Burton] referring to the Aldrich bill:

If it passes this House, it will be without my vote and without my support.

Now you bring back the Aldrich bill. [Applause on Democratic side.]

I said the other day, because sometimes I am accidentally a prophet, that "nobody here wanted the miserable makeshift that passed the House, but that you merely wanted to get into conference so that you could go back with the Aldrich bill," and that was the reply that was received from that side of the House, as worded by the gentleman from Ohio.

The gentleman from New York [Mr. Cockran] says that there is no such thing as an emergency currency. The gentleman is mistaken. Emergency Republican currency is absolutely necessary to Republican political emergencies, and necessary right now. [Loud applause on Democratic side.]

The SPEAKER. The time of the gentleman has expired.

Mr. VREELAND. Mr. Speaker, has the other side used up all of its time?

The SPEAKER. Yes.

Mr. VREELAND. I yield to the gentleman from Ohio [Mr. Burton] the remaining time on this side. [Applause on the Republican side.]

Mr. BURTON of Ohio. Mr. Speaker, the incompetency of the Democratic party to rule this people was never more emphatically displayed than by their course on this currency legislation. [Applause on the Republican side.] Last autumn there was a frightful panic. The mightiest financial institutions tottered as if they would fall, the wheels of commerce and industry were clogged, hundreds of thousands were thrown out of employment. Men who had walked with head erect and proud were compelled to beg in the streets for bread, and much of the cause of this distressful condition was the rigidity and insufficiency of our currency system.

The Republicans of this House came here determined, in spite of barren theories, in spite of selfish interests, and against the solid opposition of the Democratic party, to do something for this country, so that such a calamity might not occur again. [Applause on the Republican side.]

If you gentlemen had been in power and had gone home, having done nothing, you might better have called on the rocks and the hills to fall on you because of your inability to take care of this most urgent problem. And yet you fill the air with cries that this measure is prompted only by a political emergency, that it is partisan. Gentlemen, if there is any question which should be approached dispassionately, if there is any question wherein we should seek to grasp the real situation and solve it it is this which relates to the money supply of the country.

The gentleman from New York [Mr. Cockran] wants to know what is an emergency. If he had been in New York, or even in any small manufacturing town last October or November, he would have gotten a lesson as to what is an emergency that would have sunk deep, and which he never would have forgotten.

You say we have a composite bill, made up of the Aldrich and the Vreeland provisions. The Aldrich measure, with its iniquities, you say is brought in here. Why is it, gentlemen, that you have not said one word about this fact, that the basic principle of your bill — the Williams bill — was identical with that of the Aldrich bill — the issuance of currency based upon municipal or public bonds? [Applause on the Republican side.] Not only did you make municipal and State bonds the basis for currency, but you would have allowed them to constitute half of your reserves. You out-Aldriched Aldrich in your bill. [Applause on the Republican side.]

I trust we will not hear from you in this next campaign about the Aldrich bill unless you explain that fact. Why, it looks as if Senator Aldrich had imitated you in drawing his measure. [Laughter.]

The gentleman from Mississippi has quoted at length some remarks of mine. I want to congratulate him, or gentlemen on either side, who read my remarks; it is an evidence they are very thorough students and that they will be thoroughly posted. He quoted a statement of mine that I would not vote for the Aldrich bill. I have not, and am not going to [derisive cries on the Democratic side], because that bill gave the right to issue emergency currency exclusively to banks which had State, county, and municipal bonds. I do not believe in that on principle. I do not believe that you ought to compel banks to carry a stock of bonds as a requisite for the issuance of currency.

But this bill throws open to any national bank of the country the opportunity to become a member of an association of banks, each of which may issue currency upon its resources — that is, upon commercial paper or securities approved by the association.

There must be at least ten banks associated, having a capital and surplus of not less than $5,000,000. But if any single banking association having public bonds wishes to issue currency under the method embodied in the Aldrich bill, it may do so.

On this side we have had the courage to bring forward a measure for the relief of the country and to meet the fear of panic and distress; on the other side you have fled from your own measure. [Laughter on the Republican side.] And now you accuse others because they introduce a bill for the purpose of meeting the existing situation, containing a principle to which even you can not make objection.

FROM THE SENATE DEBATE ON THE CURRENCY BILL[1]

MR. LA FOLLETTE. Consider for one moment the proceedings which have led up to this present situation! Here we have thrust in upon the closing hours of this session legislation, the most far-reaching in its consequences to the American people of any which Congress has considered for many years. It has been held in conference for many weeks, while the session has been permitted to drag along. Appropriation bills have been gotten out of the way. Bills which found favor with those who con-

[1] *Congr. Record*, May 29, 1908. See other parts of this debate, *supra*, p. 156 *et seq.*

trol have been allowed to pass. For days and days we have been held here in idleness, while many urgent public measures have been denied consideration. Efforts have been made from day to day to take up important public measures only to encounter the opposition of the leaders who control the proceedings of the Senate. Day after day has been wasted in filibustering, demanding the reading of the *Journal*, at length making dilatory motions, interposing bills of private and local interest, and all of the many ways known to those who seek to delay legislation have been practiced by those who assume here to direct and control in legislation. Members of both Houses have grown restive and eager to return to their homes, and still this currency legislation was held in conference. From time to time we have been told that there would be no legislation upon this subject; that no conference report would be made. One other measure, the public building bill, has likewise been held back. Finally, when the decks are all cleared, to the surprise of everybody, the conference report is brought forward in its present form, forced through one branch of Congress with thirty minutes debate on a side, and brought into the Senate, subject to no possible change under the rules, to be swallowed or rejected whole. And, yet, this is called the "greatest deliberative body in the world!"

Is this fair legislative procedure? Is it just to the American people? If it were a good measure in the public interest, would it have been necessary to take this course to pass it? Why have the very best provisions been stricken out? Why has the amendment strengthening and protecting the bank reserves been dropped? Why has the penalty clause to prevent reckless inflation and contraction been omitted? Why was the section to prevent the investment of bank funds in the stocks and bonds of other corporations promoted and controlled by bank directors suppressed? Why is it made possible for a banking association to use bonds as a basis for currency issue without respect to their par value? Why is the railroad bond provision again thrust in under different phraseology? And, sir, why is all this done at a time and in a form that admits of neither deliberate consideration nor amendment to meet these wrongful changes?

Mr. President, I can not expect, single-handed and alone, to defeat this measure, whatever its character. If it were possible, I should be fully warranted in obstructing its passage in any parliamentary way to secure its everlasting defeat. I can not hope to do this alone. But, sir, I can and do hope — if the proposition which I shall hereafter submit is rejected — to so husband my resources as to hold this measure up to public view long enough to arouse the country and bring public opinion to my support. This course is open to me under the rules, and this course I shall, in the discharge of what I believe to be a public service, pursue to the limit of my impaired physical strength.

Mr. President, I have for the most part confined myself to a discussion of the one phrase to which I sought the attention of the chairman of the

The CLERK.
to their names;
for Speaker.

Mr. HEPBURN. I
the Republican Mem
Cannon, a Represen
candidate for Speake
continued applause or
Mr. CLAYTON. Mr
~ ·· ·ntatives of th
·····

of Penns,
[The quest.
votes; for Mr. \
Mr. Cannon, hav.
Speaker of the Sixtieth
Mr. Williams of Mississi
Mr. Ollie M. James, of K
elect to the Chair. [Applause.
[When Mr. Cannon apeared
Members of the House, sing in
general applause, which ws renewed
Mr. WILLIAMS. Fellow Representati
office in the United State and therefore
Speaker of the Amerian House of
Representatives.
I have the honor, for th third time in my h
present, to a House of Representatives of the
States the Hon. Joseph G. Cannon, of Illinois, as
applause.]
The SPEAKER. Gentlnen of the House of R
to-day organizing the Sixeth Congress, marking
eighteenth milestone in te history of government
the Constitution. Our pedecessors in the years th
to us an example of wisom, moderation, and cou
failed to preserve the ides and the interests of republ
many crises, whether of peace or war, adversity or p
Each generation of stasmen has had its own pecu

arrassments. N problems of government ever
spects, and themay never be treated in exactly
las of actionn one exigency may never be
overnment,o far as it relates to courses of
ts; and ncveneration for those who have
'n in apprrching live problems with pur-
ped by the mitations of the past. But the
governmet are eternal and unchanging,
bility of te people, and are put in action
scientiou and fearless representatives of
nly instution under our Constitution
pe expissed with a fair approximation

ernrmt have lofty and important
'long the peculiar, the delicate, and
·etiz and putting in definite form
nu. perform ourselves. The prin-
'n of showing us the points of the
end on our own wisdom, our
own fidelity to duty.
ouse shall devolve upon me, I
vay to justify the confidence
the great purposes for which
· rest not alone on myself.
n your integrity, wisdom,
as on mine. I have a
'neration will be your
ise of my efforts to

Mr. Bingha
was named by
elect; and the

he House,
Speaker-

The SPEAKER.
and Members and Delegates, as a
forward to the area in front of the
oath of office.

Finance Committee and of the Senate at the very outset of my remarks. I want to say that I questioned him with the hope and expectation of being able to arrive at an early understanding of the scope and meaning of this bill as interpreted by him in so far as it relates to railroad securities. I have been able to gather from the statements made by the Senator, as found in the *Record*, upon this question just what his views were with respect to railroad bonds and their relation to this proposed legislation.

But I felt that as a foundation and preliminary to a proposition which I had to submit to the Senator from Rhode Island I wanted right in the *Record* of this day a definition of that particular phrase. I was unfortunate, perhaps. I am not able now to say why, but I did not succeed in getting it and was forced to go to the *Congressional Record* to obtain the best definition that I could from the chairman of the Finance Committee.

I am awfully sorry, Mr. President, to be obliged to call your attention to the fact that there is not a quorum present.

The PRESIDING OFFICER (Mr. Bacon in the chair). The suggestion being made that a quorum is not present, the Secretary will call the roll.

*   *   *   *   *   *   *   *

VII

ORGANIZATION AND RULES OF THE HOUSE

THE PROCEDURE OF ORGANIZING THE HOUSE [1]

[An account of the formalities involved in the organization of the House of Representatives is given in the following extract from the *Record*. It will be noted that the clerk of the preceding Congress makes out the roll of membership, a function which at times might become of great importance. The candidates for the speakership and for other offices are, of course, determined by party caucuses preceding the session of the House, so that the election is merely formal. The rules of the preceding Congress are ordinarily adopted without much objection. The last general revision took place in 1890. Should any member attack the rules, this continuity of their enforcement is always insisted upon. Effectual opposition to the system of rules at this time would be possible only if a speaker had been elected who was in favor of such a change, because otherwise his entire influence would be exerted against such a change. At this time the entire committee organization is as yet potential in the Speaker's mind, and he can exercise a great influence over the members of the House through appointments to important positions. See in this connection Wilson, Congressional Government, and Reinsch, American Legislatures, chap. 2. It will be noted that on this occasion, even before the rules had been adopted, only one man was recognized, — the mover of the resolution, — and that all other speakers were obliged to get their recognition through him; also that he moved the previous question before finally yielding the floor.]

THIS day, in compliance with the provisions of the Constitution, the Members-elect of the House of Representatives of the Sixtieth Congress assembled in their Hall and were called to order by Mr. Alexander McDowell, the Clerk of the last House.

The CLERK. Prayer will be offered by the Chaplain of the last House.

Prayer was offered by the Rev. Henry N. Couden, D.D., Chaplain of the last House.

The CLERK. The clerk will call the roll by States to ascertain if a quorum of the Sixtieth Congress is present.

The roll, as made by the Clerk, was then called, when the following members answered present:

[Here follows a list of the members.]

[1] *Congr. Record*, Dec. 2, 1907.

The CLERK. Three hundred and sixty-nine Members have answered to their names; a quorum is present. We are now ready for nominations for Speaker.

ELECTION OF SPEAKER

Mr. HEPBURN. Mr. Clerk, I am directed by the unanimous vote of the Republican Members of this House to present the Hon. Joseph G. Cannon, a Representative-elect from the State of Illinois, as their candidate for Speaker of this Sixtieth Congress. [Loud and long-continued applause on the Republican side.]

Mr. CLAYTON. Mr. Clerk, I nominate for Speaker of the House of Representatives of the Sixtieth Congress of the United States the Hon. John Sharp Williams, a Representative-elect from the State of Mississippi. [Loud and long-continued applause on the Democratic side.]

The CLERK. Are there any other nominations? If not, the nominations are closed. The following tellers will please take their places at the desk: Mr. Heflin of Alabama, Mr. Rucker of Missouri, Mr. Wheeler of Pennsylvania, and Mr. Murdock of Kansas.

[The question was taken; and there were — for Mr. Cannon, 207 votes; for Mr. Williams, 159 votes; not voting, 24.]

Mr. Cannon, having received a majority of all the votes cast, is elected Speaker of the Sixtieth Congress. [Applause.] The Clerk will appoint Mr. Williams of Mississippi, Mr. Sulloway of New Hampshire, and Mr. Ollie M. James, of Kentucky, as a committee to escort the Speaker-elect to the Chair. [Applause.]

[When Mr. Cannon appeared with the committee designated, the Members of the House, rising in a body, greeted him with loud and general applause, which was renewed as he ascended to the chair.]

Mr. WILLIAMS. Fellow-Representatives, the second to the highest office in the United States, and therefore in the world, is the office of Speaker of the American House of Commons, the House of Representatives.

I have the honor, for the third time in my life, not to introduce, but to present, to a House of Representatives of the Congress of the United States the Hon. Joseph G. Cannon, of Illinois, as its Speaker. [Prolonged applause.]

The SPEAKER. Gentlemen of the House of Representatives, we are to-day organizing the Sixtieth Congress, marking the one hundred and eighteenth milestone in the history of government by the people under the Constitution. Our predecessors in the years that are past have left to us an example of wisdom, moderation, and courage that has never failed to preserve the ideals and the interests of republican government in many crises, whether of peace or war, adversity or prosperity.

Each generation of statesmen has had its own peculiar problems and its own particular embarrassments.   No problems of government ever recur in exactly the same aspects, and they may never be treated in exactly the same way.   The formulas of action in one exigency may never be applied safely in another.   Government, so far as it relates to courses of action, has no fixed precedents; and no veneration for those who have gone before justifies living men in approaching live problems with purpose or with vision circumscribed by the limitations of the past.   But the fundamental principles of free government are eternal and unchanging, resting on the will and responsibility of the people, and are put in action through the deliberations of conscientious and fearless representatives of that will.   This House is the only institution under our Constitution where that will of the people may be expressed with a fair approximation to scientific accuracy. [Applause.]

Other departments of the Government have lofty and important functions, but to this House alone belongs the peculiar, the delicate, and the all-surpassing function of interpreting and putting in definite form the will of the people.   This duty we must perform ourselves.   The principles of the past may help us to the extent of showing us the points of the compass; but beyond that we must depend on our own wisdom, our own constancy, our own industry, and our own fidelity to duty.

So far as the duty of organizing this House shall devolve upon me, I shall endeavor to perform the duty in a way to justify the confidence which your selection implies and to promote the great purposes for which we are assembled; but the duties of the hour rest not alone on myself. They rest on each one of you individually; and on your integrity, wisdom, and conservatism the people are relying as well as on mine.   I have a right to expect your coöperation, because such coöperation will be your duty.   I hope also that as we go on I may have it because of my efforts to merit your confidence and good will. [Applause.]

I am now ready for the oath.

Swearing in the Speaker

Mr. Bingham, the Member longest in continuous service in the House, was named by the Clerk to administer the oath of office to the Speaker-elect; and the oath was accordingly administered.

Swearing in of Members and Delegates

The Speaker.   The Clerk will call the roll by States and Territories, and Members and Delegates, as their names are called, will please come forward to the area in front of the Clerk's desk and take the prescribed oath of office.

The Speaker then administered the oath of office to the Members and Delegates presenting themselves.

Mr. Butler and Mr. Cocks of New York qualified by affirmation.

[Then followed the election of the officers of the House, on nomination by the two great political parties, those of the opposition being of course rejected. The officers so elected came to the bar of the House and the oath was administered to them by the Speaker. Resolutions of the notification to the President of the United States and to the Senate of the readiness of the House to do business or receive communications were made. This notification is effected by message to the Senate and by a committee composed of the committees appointed by the Senate and House of Representatives respectively. A resolution to provide for the distribution of rooms in the House office building and Capitol completed the necessary introductory measures to be taken for getting the House into working order. Then follows the all-important matter of the question of adoption and amendment of the Rules. The traditional protest against the concentration of power in the Speaker's hands, and the repression of individual initiative is in evidence.]

Rules of the Sixtieth Congress

Mr. Dalzell. Mr. Speaker, I offer the following resolution.
The Clerk read as follows:

Resolved, That the rules of the House of Representatives of the Fifty-ninth Congress be adopted as the rules of the House of Representatives of the Sixtieth Congress, including the standing orders of March 8 and March 14, 1900 (relating to consideration of pension and claim bills on Fridays), which are hereby continued in force during the Sixtieth Congress.

Mr. Williams. Mr. Speaker ——
The Speaker. Does the gentleman from Pennsylvania yield to the gentleman from Mississippi?
Mr. Dalzell. I will yield to the gentleman from Mississippi five minutes.
Mr. Williams. Mr. Speaker, of course I have no desire to make a useless play to the galleries. I know, of course, that the resolution is going to pass, but I do not consider it consistent with the past record of this side of the House to permit it to pass without a protest. We are of the opinion, and have been for a long time, that entirely too much power is concentrated in the hands of the Speaker of the House, and without any party spirit at all, speaking only what I think is best for the country at large, believing if my party were in the majority I would still take that same view, I want to protest against the adoption of the rules in their present drastic form, without any opportunity to the Members of the House to propose amendments and without any opportunity for the

House itself to pass upon proposed amendments. We will of course, vote against the resolution.

Mr. Cooper of Wisconsin rose.

Mr. DALZELL. How much time does the gentleman from Wisconsin want?

Mr. COOPER of Wisconsin. Five minutes.

Mr. DALZELL. I will yield five minutes to the gentleman from Wisconsin.

Mr. COOPER of Wisconsin. Mr. Speaker, like the gentleman from Mississippi, I have no desire to consume the time of the House in an argument against the adoption of these rules. It was impossible for me to be present at the caucus on Saturday night. I did not arrive in the city until that evening. If I had been at the caucus I would have opposed the adoption of this rule.

I agree with the gentleman from Mississippi that there is altogether too much power concentrated in the Speaker of the House of Representatives. [Applause on the Democratic side.] It is more power, gentlemen, than ought to be given to any man in any government that pretends to be republican in form and democratic in spirit. [Applause on the Democratic side.]

Now, in saying this I do not wish to be understood as uttering a word by way of criticism of the very distinguished and honorable gentleman who has discharged the duties of Speaker of the past two Congresses with such great success. But, as the gentleman from Mississippi has just said he would oppose this if the House were Democratic, I oppose it not because it is a Republican House, but because the power given to the Speaker under these rules is unrepublican and undemocratic. [Applause on the Democratic side.]

To show that that is true, I call the attention of the House and candid listeners and readers everywhere to these facts: That the Speaker of the House of Representatives has the sole power of recognition of those who rise on the floor; he appoints all the committees, including all the chairmen; he appoints the Committee on Rules, which, in conjunction with the other rules, practically enables the Committee on Rules to dictate what legislation shall come before the House; he is himself ex officio the chairman of the Committee on Rules, and ever since I have been here there has never been a Speaker but who appointed two men with him of the majority party constituting the majority of the committee, who are with him in everything that comes before that committee.

Therefore the Speaker becomes practically the Committee on Rules. [Laughter on the Democratic side.] That was so in a Democratic House, gentlemen, when Mr. Speaker Crisp was here. [Laughter on the Republican side.] That has been so in a Republican House ever since.

Now, when the Committee on Rules reports a proposition, every man on the floor knows that the Speaker wants it adopted nine times out of ten, where it is of any importance, and we all know his power, which compels us to go into his room if we wish to ask to be recognized for unanimous consent. [Applause on the Democratic side.] We all know that we can not get a bill passed — every man on the floor does, Republican or Democratic — by unanimous consent unless the Member presenting it first goes to the private chamber of the Speaker and asks to be recognized. The Speaker does not have to give his reasons before the House for any objections he may have. He does not rise upon the floor but in his private chamber he objects. I wish to say that the present Speaker of the House has always treated me with the utmost courtesy and kindness. A former Speaker of this House compelled me to go to his room at one time. I went there to present a bill which provided simply for the changing of the material which was to go into a public building and which had been recommended to him in a letter from the office of the Supervising Architect. I did not know that that letter had been written to him; I did not ask that it should be written to him. It was a voluntary letter and a voluntary suggestion upon the part of the Architect. I went to the Speaker's chamber. I had refused on a former occasion to do his bidding. When I went to his room he said, "I will see about that; come in again." I went in again. He did not ask me to sit down. He said, "I do not think I can do that; I do not want to do that; I can not allow that to come up." Not only that, but he compelled me to stand there, and when a perfect stranger came in, he sat him down in his seat and turned his back upon me. [Laughter.]

A very important rule had previously come before the House of Representatives. That same Speaker had stopped me at the entrance there and put his hand upon my breast and said, "Mr. Cooper, you will oblige me very much by not opposing this rule." That rule related to the Pacific Railroad funding bill. I did oppose it. I was the only Republican of the minority of the committee that reported against the bill; the rule was modified, and for the first time in thirty years the Pacific Railroad people lost their bill.

That same Speaker refused practically to recognize me for four or five years for any purpose, and never when he could help it.

The SPEAKER. The time of the gentleman has expired.

Mr. COOPER of Wisconsin. May I have three minutes more?

Mr. BURLESON. Mr. Speaker, I ask unanimous consent that the time of the gentleman be extended.

The SPEAKER. The gentleman from Pennsylvania [Mr. Dalzell] has charge of the time.

Mr. DALZELL. Mr. Speaker, I yield three minutes more to the gentleman from Wisconsin.

Mr. COOPER of Wisconsin. Mr. Speaker, one more thing. That this is too much power ever to give to one man in the House of Representatives is demonstrated by this fact: If the Vice-President of the United

States had a similar power, then the Vice-President would appoint all of the committees of the Senate. He would appoint the Committee on Rules of that body and have the sole power of recognition. So that the Speaker of the House of Representatives and the Vice-President of the United States together could agree practically to allow or not to allow legislation to come up before either Chamber.

Of course it is said that the House can at any time bring up legislation, but gentlemen know that they have repeatedly heard said on this floor, not alone in the last Congress, but in other Congresses, "I do not like this proposition, but the Speaker wants it."

My position is this: That the leader of this House should be on the floor and not in the chair. I say as a matter of practical experience that the very distinguished and very able gentleman who has the chair could render his country greater service leading the Republicans upon the floor than he renders them as the Speaker of the House. I think if the distinguished gentleman from Maine, the parliamentary clerk, who now stands at the right hand of the Speaker, were elected Speaker to sit there simply as a presiding officer after the manner of the speaker of the House of Commons, and the distinguished gentleman from Illinois [Mr. Cannon] who is now the Speaker of this House, were upon this floor leading us under a system of rules which would enable the House itself to elect a Committee on Rules, at the head of which would be the distinguished gentleman from Illinois [Mr. Cannon], much better business would be done in the way of legislation on this floor.

I think it is also unfair to adopt the pending resolution, because there are about 100 new Members, and they have not seen the working of the rules and know little about them. But of course the caucus having adopted what it did adopt the other night, it does not become me to vote against the resolution. I may say that I can not consistently as a Republican — for I understand that the Republicans of the House by unanimous vote adopted this rule in caucus, and that the caucus was properly called, although I did not know it — I can not, as I say, consistently vote against the adoption of the resolution.

Mr. De Armond rose.

The SPEAKER. Does the gentleman from Pennsylvania yield to the gentleman from Missouri?

Mr. DALZELL. How much time does the gentleman want?

Mr. DE ARMOND. Mr. Speaker, I would like to know if I can not be recognized in my own right as a Member of the House of Representatives? [Applause on the Democratic side.]

The SPEAKER. The gentleman from Missouri is informed by the Chair that the gentleman from Pennsylvania [Mr. Dalzell] is entitled to the floor, and at this time the gentleman from Pennsylvania is privileged to yield if the gentleman sees proper to do so and the gentleman from Missouri sees proper to accept the time.

Mr. Dalzell. I am willing to yield to the gentleman. How much time does the gentleman desire?

Mr. De Armond. About twenty minutes.

Mr. Dalzell. Oh, I cannot yield that much.

Mr. De Armond. Mr. Speaker, I would be glad ——

Mr. Dalzell. I yield ten minutes to the gentleman.

Mr. De Armond. Mr. Speaker, I would be glad to ask the gentleman from Pennsylvania to inform me and also inform the House what is there pressing that he can not spare that much time now?

Mr. Dalzell. I will yield the gentleman twenty minutes. [Applause on the Democratic side.]

Mr. De Armond. Mr. Speaker, I listened a very short time ago, as I have no doubt the other Members of the House did, to the carefully worded and blandly sounding address from the Speaker-elect, in which, among other things, the Members of the House and the people of the country were told that here in this House is lodged the power of the people to make known their wishes and to execute their will. It sounded well; it was expressed handsomely. But a few minutes have elapsed since that performance, and now here, with time so precious that only a few minutes can be conceded to anybody to express an opinion upon the subject, it is proposed to tie and shackle the House by rules about which a good many know nothing, and about which a good many others know a great deal. Talk about the people having here representation and about here the will and wish of the American people being executed, when here, at once, out of hand, blindly, without consideration, without reading the code of rules, designed, cunningly designed, to put the Representatives in this House, the membership of it, and the mighty interests of the people of this nation in the sacred keeping of the Speaker! What is the occasion for hurry? You are determined to adopt these rules. Why not at least have the grace and decency to permit a little discussion and give a little time for their consideration; for the work predestined, cut and dried, to be put through? Why not? [Applause on the Democratic side.] The greatest reform needed in this land is required here. The crying abuse of all abuses, against which the citizenship of this Republic protests and long has protested in vain, is the subversion of the rights of the individual Members of this body. [Applause on the Democratic side.] Here we stand under the Constitution as equals, each one of us commissioned by the sovereign citizens of his district to come here and represent that district and its interests, and as a patriotic American citizen, a Member of the Congress of the United States, to represent and to voice as best he can the interests and rights and promote as far as he can the welfare of the whole people of these United States, and yet the first formal act is to throttle and gag and bind the membership of this House — to make it subservient in fact, whether in deed some of you realize it or not, to the autocratic will of the Speaker.

Now, we have no rules. Here is a moment, here is a brief space of time — would to God it could be prolonged and enlarged — when there is some semblance of freedom, when there is something like equality upon this floor, and yet even in this hour within which this Congress has been assembled and organized, the period of sixty minutes, a man can not speak in opposition to this legislative outrage except by permission. He can not be recognized in his own right as an American citizen. He can not be recognized as a chosen Representative, charged with the duties and freighted with the responsibility of his position, unless it be with the permission of some other Member, who possesses no rights superior to his own. [Applause on the Democratic side.] For one, representing an independent constitutency of unshackled men, men neither upon whose limbs nor spirits are the gyves of tyranny, I avail myself of even this poor permission, which I ought not to be forced to ask, and but for the necessities of the situation would not accept, to express my protest. I know it is vain now and here, but I have faith in the God who rules over the nation, and I have faith and confidence in the patriotism and manhood of American citizenship upon which to base the hope that the time is not far distant when such protests as this will cease to be necessary because the evils against which they are raised will have passed away. [Applause on the Democratic side.]

Why the hurry for the adoption of this code of rules? Why do you wish to enslave yourselves and enslave us? Are you proposing to go back to your constituencies, as manly as they are independent American citizens, and when they ask you why you did not do this or why you suffered the doing of that, do you propose, as cowards and cravens, to defend yourselves and apologize upon the mere, miserable, mean pretext that these rules hampered you and controlled you and that you could not do anything else?

You can do something now. Now is the time of times for the American Representative to stand up proudly in the power and glory of his high office. [Applause on the Democratic side.] It is a high office. Upon the average, we represent there, or ought to be permitted to represent, if the Constitution were enforced and observed, and would then represent, on the average, about 200,000 American citizens. Not one, not an iota of the rights of the citizenship which I represent, of the citizenship of any district in this Union, North or South, East or West, Republican or Democratic, shall be cut away or frittered away or bargained away, in what amounts in effect, however you may gloss it and veneer it, to absolute surrender into abject slavery, without at least a feeble protest from me.

Why not refer the rules which you propose to a committee? Why not give opportunity for the consideration of proposed amendments? Why hasten pellmell into slavery? You will find these bonds galling. You will find the time coming when your manhood may long to break the shackles for the time being and intuitively assert itself when chafing under the bonds which you put upon it. Behold the spectacle! There are no rules here at all. And yet in this membership of three hundred and ninety-one, the gentleman from Pennsylvania, the right hand of the Speaker — the man standing next to him upon the Committee on Rules, echoing his every wish, voicing his every sentiment, and voting to carry out his every purpose — is recognized here upon this floor, and no man is to be given permission even to say a solitary word in criticism or in opposition unless the gentleman from Pennsylvania kindly and generously concedes to him a little modicum of time! [Applause on the Democratic side.] I know well that if the gentleman from Pennsylvania pursues the course which I presume he will pursue, and which has been followed heretofore, he will avail himself of the opportunity to move the previous question, cutting off all debate.

But for that I would scorn, under these circumstances and at this stage of proceedings, to accept a minute or second of time within his control, but would insist upon my right to time as a Representative from the Sixth district of Missouri. [Applause on the Democratic side.] I know full well that the gentleman from Pennsylvania [Mr. Dalzell] before an hour shall have expired may be expected to move the previous question, and if we are to judge of what is to happen by what has happened repeatedly in the House, a partisan majority behind him will sustain that resolution to cut off debate and come to an immediate vote, so that the man who says anything — and it must be said hurriedly and under adverse circumstances — must say it by reason of the gracious permission accorded to him under the kind ministration of the Speaker by the gentleman from Pennsylvania [Mr. Dalzell].

Adopt your rules, if you will, but note this, and have warning of it now, that there are some here who will not be tamely tied and who in the days to come, who in the legislative history of this Congress, will avail themselves, as occasion may offer — and it is not to offer very frequently — of the little opportunity that it is beyond your power to take from them, and that we shall appeal beyond this tyrannous decision, beyond this surrender, this humiliating surrender, of the rights of the American Representative. We shall appeal over your head, shall appeal through your rules, shall appeal in the mighty right of the American Representative of the mighty sovereign, the American citizen. And we shall hope that the time is not far distant when those who are chosen to represent free men in the greatest legislative body, as we frequently hear, upon the face of the earth shall stand forth panoplied in the glory of a noble trust, possessed of the powers of the real Representative, not by permission of anybody, responsible alone to his God above him and to his constituents behind him. [Loud applause on the Democratic side.]

Mr. DALZELL. Mr. Speaker, I can not conceive of anything more unnecessary than a discussion of the rules that are now offered for adoption at this day. They have been discussed time and again in this House and elsewhere — in the magazines, in the newspapers — and they have been vindicated by their results. Prior to the Fifty-first Congress the rules of the House of Representatives had remained for a great number of years unchanged. These, our rules, are an evolution. Rule after rule has gone upon the book in answer to some present emergency. The rules that prevailed prior to the Fifty-first Congress were so constructed as to place all the power of the House in the hands of the minority. In that Congress, which was presided over by that great Speaker and illustrious statesman, Thomas B. Reed [loud applause on the Republican side], the rules were amended by a committee consisting of William McKinley, Joseph G. Cannon, and J. G. Carlisle. [Applause.] Of the rules then on the book but a very few met with any change. The only substantial changes that were made were those with respect to counting a quorum, which placed in the hands of the majority — where it belongs — the power of this body, those that related to the order of business, and that rule which provided that 100 should constitute a quorum in the Committee of the Whole. With these exceptions the rules that you are asked to adopt are substantially the rules that have been in force, with their additions from time to time, since the foundation of the Government.

Now, these rules are not only the rules of the Fifty-ninth Congress; they are not only the rules of the Fifty-first Congress, both of which were Republican Congresses, but they are substantially the rules of the Fifty-second and Fifty-third Congresses — Democratic Congresses, presided over by a Democratic Speaker. [Applause on the Republican side.]

So far as the power of the Committee on Rules is concerned, it received its impetus and the power it now possesses under the régime of your Democratic Speaker, Mr. Charles Crisp. So far as the power of the Speaker is concerned, it is to-day as it has been for a hundred years. It has been his power for a hundred years to recognize or to fail to give recognition. It has been his power for a hundred years to appoint the committees of this House; and it is nothing new now to find some Member who has been disappointed in his recognition by the Speaker for the purpose of passing some measure that the Speaker thought ought not to pass to get up on this floor and denounce the power of the Speaker.

Now, Mr. Speaker, this side of the House, the majority, is charged with the responsibility for legislation. This side, thus charged with the responsibility, has the right to prescribe the rules under which legislation shall be had. It is no secret at all that in the caucus of the Republican Members of the House these rules were directed to be adopted, as they have been in every Congress since the Fifty-first; and as I said a few moments ago, in the outset, they are vindicated and their wisdom has been proved by some of the best legislation in the history of the Republic now on the statute books, put there by virtue of these rules, and some of the best legislation in the future is likely to be put on the statute books by virtue of these same rules. Lest my friend from Missouri should be disappointed, I now ask the previous question. [Laughter.]

The SPEAKER. Will the gentleman from Pennsylvania for a moment withhold the demand for the previous question?

Mr. DALZELL. Certainly.

The SPEAKER. The Chair desires to add that the rules as yet have not been adopted, and we are proceeding under general parliamentary usage, the gentleman from Pennsylvania having the floor. When the gentleman from Pennsylvania yields the floor, if he does yield it, then any other gentleman is entitled to the floor. Holding the floor, the gentleman indicated that he would yield twenty minutes to the gentleman from Missouri. The Chair took that to be in substance notice to the gentleman from Missouri that, yielding to him, he still holds the floor, that he might move the previous question on resuming the floor. That is the effect, as the Chair understands it, of the gentleman yielding to the gentleman from Wisconsin, and also to the gentleman from Missouri, under general parliamentary usages.

Now, the Chair may be indulged one minute further. The Chair, the Speaker of the House, is a Member of the House the same as any other Member. Unanimous consent being asked, it would not be granted should any Member object. The usage in many Congresses in the past was that the Chair would submit the request to the House; and it is an open secret to gentlemen who have served in some of the former Congresses that the Chair, keeping track of the business of the House, as the Speaker and at the same time exercising his right as a Member, would often indicate to some Member upon the floor, by messenger or otherwise, that he desired an objection to be made. The Chair has seen that frequently occur under both Democratic and Republican Speakers. The present occupant of the chair, ever since he has occupied that position, has thought the better way and the more manly and fairer way was to exercise his right as a Member to object to a request for unanimous consent. Therefore the practice has grown up that gentlemen see the Speaker, and if he has objections then he invariably says that it is useless to recognize the Member for unanimous consent, because if nobody else objected the Chair in his capacity as a Member of the House would object. [Applause on the Republican side.]

Under the rules, if adopted, the Chair begs to call the attention of the gentlemen to the fact that the right of a Member to be recognized can in most instances not be denied by the Chair. There are a large number of motions which are privileged in their nature, and a question of privilege, first, and a privileged motion, second, halts all business before the House, and the Chair has no discretion. Gentlemen who have had service in the House will recollect that those motions are many.

The Chair desires to state again that the Speaker of the House is the servant of the House, and it is in the power of the House of Representatives as a question of the highest privilege to at any time elect a successor to any Member of that body who may be holding this place. One further observation. When special orders or special rules are suggested, as they have been under all administrations, Democratic and Republican, at least for twenty years, those orders or rules can not be vitalized until a majority of the House has adopted them under the Constitution and the Rules of the House.

The question is on the motion of the gentleman from Pennsylvania that the previous question be ordered.

Mr. DE ARMOND. Mr. Speaker, I would submit a parliamentary inquiry, if I may be indulged.

The SPEAKER. The gentleman will state it.

Mr. DE ARMOND. That is, whether or not the Speaker will permit the House to act upon propositions and dispose of measures when a majority of the House requests him to do so.

The SPEAKER. When the majority acts under the Constitution and the laws no Speaker would dare to fail to obey the will of the majority. [Applause on the Republican side.]

Mr. DE ARMOND. Mr. Speaker ——

The SPEAKER. For what purpose does the gentleman rise?

Mr. DE ARMOND. The gentleman rises for the purpose of getting an answer to his parliamentary inquiry, and for the purpose of putting another question.

The SPEAKER. If the gentleman is not answered, it is the misfortune of the Chair or the misfortune of the peculiar state of mind of the gentleman. The gentleman from Pennsylvania moves the previous question.

Mr. DE ARMOND. But, Mr. Speaker, I would like to submit this parliamentary inquiry.

The SPEAKER. The gentleman will state it.

Mr. DE ARMOND. I wish to state that it is not the misfortune of any peculiar state of mind on the part of the gentleman from Missouri who submitted the inquiry. In times past a majority have made a request for the consideration of this or that measure, and consideration has been denied. What I am asking now is whether or not if a majority of the membership of the House requests the Speaker to permit action upon a particular matter, he will or will not do it — and it is not necessary to refer to the Constitution in making the answer. [Applause on the Democratic side.]

The SPEAKER. The Chair, so far as the Chair knows or has any knowledge, desires to say to the gentleman from Missouri [Mr. De Armond] that in the knowledge and belief of the Chair the gentleman is mistaken. The will of the majority always, for thirty-four years to my knowledge, has been law unto the Speaker.

Mr. Williams rose.

Mr. DALZELL. I can not yield any further, Mr. Speaker. I demand the previous question.

The SPEAKER. The question is on ordering the previous question.

The question was taken.

Mr. WILLIAMS. Mr. Speaker, I think we better have the yeas and nays. I demand the yeas and nays.

The yeas and nays were ordered.

The question was taken, and there were — yeas 199, nays 163, answering "present" 3, not voting 23.

DEFENSE OF THE RULES [1]

[The frequent criticism passed upon the rules of the House of Representatives led Mr. Dalzell to make the following defense of them. Whenever the authority of the Speaker or the leaders is attacked, they, as is done in this case, always advance the argument that they are simply representing the majority and that their power stands and falls with the will of the majority in the House.]

MR. DALZELL. There are few subjects of public discussion about which there is more unjust criticism — I might, without exaggeration say, unjust abuse — than the rules of the National House of Representatives. The criticism and abuse come largely from Members of the House when in the minority, and from newspapers and magazine writers, and some others of whom, without unfairness, it may be said that they have very little knowledge or intelligent conception of what they are writing or talking about. Indeed, I think it may be truly said that there are comparatively few Members of the House itself, much less outsiders, who have any real knowledge of the rules. The rules are simple enough and entirely logical, but to the majority of Members of the House who have no special ambition to familiarize themselves with them they seem complicated.

There is nothing new in this protest against the rules. It is human nature to be uneasy under restraint, and in all Congresses, even among the first, when the membership was small and the rules were simple, complaint was heard as now from those who could not have their own way.

The rules of the National House of Representatives are not the conception of any one man or set of men; they are not the product of any one Congress or of any combination of Congresses; they are an evolution, the outgrowth of the parliamentary experience, necessities and exigencies of all the hundred years and more of our Congressional life. The book of rules contains no rule that had not a reasonable necessity for its adoption in the first instance and has not a like necessity for its continuance now. As a whole the rules are so made as to render possible

[1] *Congr. Record*, March 18, 1906. (Reported March 23.)

the most expeditious accomplishment in the wisest way of the legislative business of our ninety millions of American people.

An impartial examination of them will show that the power of recognition popularly attributed to the Speaker as autocratic is grossly exaggerated; that that power, in point of fact, so far as the rules are concerned, is limited; and that the apparent restrictions upon individual initiative, so far as they exist at all, are due not to the rules, but to the character of the House as now constituted, and to the exigencies of the public business.

A brief review of the history of the rules will serve to demonstrate the truth of this statement.

There have been two divisions of the rules within the last thirty years.

In the Forty-sixth Congress (1880) the rules were revised under the direction of the Committee on Rules, consisting of Speaker Randall and Messrs. Stephens, Blackburn, Garfield, and Frye. The changes then made consisted mainly in dropping a number of rules that, by reason of changed conditions had become obsolete, in consolidating a number of others and changing their arrangement, and in the introduction of a very few new rules. The Committee in its report, which was unanimous, said:

> The objective point with the committee was to secure accuracy in business, economy of time, order, uniformity, and impartiality, and to prepare, if possible, a simple, concise, and nonpartisan code of rules, which would neither surrender the right of a majority to control and dispose of the business for which it is held responsible, nor, on the other hand, invade and restrict the powers of a minority to check temporarily, if not permanently, the action of a majority believed to be improper or unconstitutional, and to attain, if possible, the great underlying principle of all the rules and forms by which the business of a legislative assembly is governed, whether constitutional, legal, or parliamentary in their origin, viz., "to subserve the will of the assembly rather than to restrain it, to facilitate and not to obstruct the expression of its deliberate sense."

The rules then adopted remained in force until the Fifty-first Congress (1890), when they were revised by the Committee on Rules, consisting of Speaker Thomas B. Reed, Messrs. McKinley, Cannon, Carlisle, and Randall. By this revision, out of the total number of forty-seven rules, twenty-nine were allowed to remain unchanged, and in the remaining eighteen such changes as were made were only formal, except in four fundamental particulars. These related to (1) dilatory motions, (2) the counting of a quorum, (3) the number which should constitute a quorum in Committee of the Whole, and (4) the order of business. This last revision was found necessary in order to carry out the announced objects sought to be attained by the revision of 1880, viz., "Economy of time, order, and the right of a majority to control and dispose of the business for which it is held responsible."

Prior to this last revision, under then existing rules, the practice known as filibustering had grown to such an extent as to waste much valuable time and to threaten the power of the majority to deal with the business of the country. By the use of the privileged motions "to adjourn to a day certain," and "to take a recess," and the practice on the part of Members of remaining silent and refusing to vote, thus breaking a quorum, it was in the power of the minority at any time effectually to obstruct the passage of any legislation. A motion to adjourn to a day certain was subject to two amendments, on each of which, as well as on the original motion, the yeas and nays could be ordered. The same was true as to the motion to take a recess; these motions could be repeated without limit, and thus days could be consumed in useless calls of the roll. In point of fact, in the Fiftieth Congress on one occasion the House remained in continuous session eight days and nights, during which time there were over one hundred roll calls on the iterated and reiterated motions to adjourn and to take a recess and their amendments. On this occasion the reading clerks became so exhausted that they could no longer act, and certain Members, possessed of large voices and strenuous lungs, took their places. If this was not child's play it would be difficult to define it. Then, again, when a measure to which the minority objected was likely to pass, the yeas and nays would be ordered.

The objecting minority Members, sitting in their seats, would fail to respond when their names were called, and when the count was made it would appear that there was no quorum present to do business, and thus the measure would fail. It seems now strange to realize that many eminent men acting as Speakers of the House maintained that for this manifest evil no remedy existed. It remained for the Speaker of the Fifty-first Congress, Thomas B. Reed, the greatest parliamentary leader in the history of English-speaking people, to make an end of this manifest absurdity. He declared that physical presence and constructive absence was impossible; that the quorum called for by the Constitution was a present and not a voting quorum; and so, on a certain historic occasion, he added to the names of those voting the names of those present and not voting and announced the result accordingly. He has no greater glory than that the principle he announced and put into practice has not only been indorsed by the Supreme Court of the United States, but also by his partisan foes when they came into power in the House, and by the practical results which recent years of wise legislation unobstructed by foolish tactics have put on the statute book. Under present rules the motion to adjourn to a day certain and the motion to take a recess are not privileged, and, furthermore, the Speaker is not allowed to entertain any dilatory motion. If a quorum has been ascertained by actual count to be present, a measure voted on passes or fails in accordance with the recorded vote, whether all Members have voted or not.

In the Committee of the Whole 100 now constitutes a quorum instead of a majority of the whole House. This is in the interest of the expedition of business.

Bills are now introduced by filing and not by presentation in the open House, and thus much time is saved. Business once entered upon is continued until concluded instead of, as under prior rules, being limited to a certain time for its consideration and then not having been concluded being sent to the graveyard of the calendar of unfinished business.

In the last Congress (Fifty-ninth) there were 386 Members (in this Congress there are 391), and there were introduced a total of bills and resolutions numbering 27,114. It goes without saying that not all of these bills could be considered, nor could all of these Members have a hearing. Theoretically, every Member of the House is the equal of every other Member; every constituency is entitled to equal recognition with every other constituency, but practically there can not be 391 Speakers; there can not be 391 chairmen of committees, nor equal recognition for debate given to 391 Members. The real purpose, then, to be accomplished by the rules is the selection from the mass of bills introduced those proper to be considered. There is no limitation on the right of a Member to introduce bills; as many as he likes and of whatever character he pleases. Every bill introduced goes to an appropriate committee for consideration, and whether or not it gets upon a House Calendar for action depends upon its being reported by the committee. It may never be reported, and, of course, if not reported can never be considered in the House. In the last Congress, of the 27,114 bills and resolutions introduced, there were 7,823 reported; the others remained in the pigeonholes of the various committees. Of the bills reported, 7,423 were considered, and passed. Bills when reported go upon certain calendars of the House, according to the character of the bills.

1. Revenue and appropriation bills. These are few in number, not to exceed, perhaps, 20. They come from the Committee on Ways and Means, whose office it is to provide revenue for the Government, and from the Committee on Appropriations, and from the several committees having to do with the maintenance of the Government in its various arms, such as the Naval Committee, the Military Committee, and others. These bills when reported go to a calendar known as the Union Calendar, but they are highly privileged, as they ought to be, for without their passage the Government wheels would stop. They can be called for consideration at any time. They take precedence of all other bills, and the Speaker has no alternative but to recognize the Member calling them up. These bills are considered not in the House, but in Committee of the Whole; the Speaker leaves the chair and another Member takes his place.

2. Another class of bills are such as relate to some public purpose, but carry no appropriation, such, for instance, as bridge bills and the

like. To a large extent bills from the important committees on the Judiciary and on Interstate and Foreign Commerce are of this class. These bills go on the House Calendar and are entitled to consideration in the morning hour. There being no privileged bills for consideration, the morning hour is the regular order. The Speaker must call the committees in their alphabetical order, and then the chairman of the committee which has the call is entitled to recognition by the Speaker, as of right. The House then proceeds to the consideration of such bill reported by the committee in question and then on the House Calendar as the chairman calls up, and continues its consideration until a vote is had, subject only to a possible interruption at the end of sixty minutes, to which I will refer hereafter. But even if interrupted, its consideration thereafter, when business of that character is in order, until it is finally disposed of.

3. In addition to public bills such as I have enumerated, some carrying an appropriation and others not, there is another class of bills, the most numerous of all — private bills providing for the relief of private individuals or corporations. These have a Calendar of their own called the Private Calendar and are in order on every Friday of each week. They are, generally speaking, bills from the Committee on Claims, from the Committee on War Claims, and from the Committee on Pensions. As to these bills the Speaker has no independent right of recognition. When addressed by the chairman of the appropriate committee on a Friday he must recognize him, and unless the House declines to consider these bills the Speaker must leave the chair and nominate a Member to preside in his place. In the last Congress there were reported 6,834 private bills; 6,624 were passed, leaving 210 undisposed of.

There is another class of bills that, like private bills, have a day of their own under the rules, viz., District of Columbia bills. As is well known, there is no right of suffrage in the District of Columbia, and the Senate and House act as its select and common councils. District of Columbia bills are in order on two Mondays of every month. As to these bills, again the Speaker has no alternative but to recognize the chairman of the District Committee when, on his allotted day, he calls up his business.

4. A fourth class of bills provide for various matters of public concern and are such as involve a charge upon the Treasury. These go to the Union Calendar, and when considered must be considered in Committee of the Whole. At the end of the morning hour (sixty minutes) a motion may be made to go into the Committee of Whole for the consideration of bills on the Union Calendar or for the consideration of some particular bill thereon. This motion the Speaker is bound to entertain.

Then, a large part of the business of the House is done wholly outside of the rules, by unanimous consent. Some gentleman, for instance, arises in the House and, being recognized by the Speaker, asks "unanimous consent for the present consideration of the following bill." Unless objection is made the bill is considered and voted on. It is in connection with this practice and because of it that autocratic power is without any reason ascribed to the Speaker. But the rules have nothing at all to do with this. The applicant for recognition asks that all rules be set aside. To this any Member of the House may object. Why should complaint be made if the Speaker exercises his right of objection by refusing to recognize an applicant for recognition in any particular case? Because he is Speaker he is no less a Member of the House; no less a Representative of his Congressional district. If he were on the floor he could interpose an objection to any request for unanimous consent. Should he be less able to interpose that objection because he is in the chair? Certainly not. That the Speaker's power in this regard is only, in the last analysis, that of a Member may easily be illustrated. During the latter part of the Fifty-fourth Congress, when Mr. Reed was Speaker, there was a Member from Nebraska named Kem who announced that he would object to any consideration of bills by unanimous consent. After the announcement, on the first day, the Speaker's room was crowded, as usual, with applicants for recognition. Mr. Reed promised to do the best he could, but recalled to his applicants Kem's threat to object. Still members persisted, one of them was recognized, and Kem objected. The next day the throng at the Speaker's room was not so great, but still of large proportions. Members had faith that Kem would not persist. Again Mr. Reed promised to do his best; again a recognition was had, and again Kem objected. On the third day the Speaker's room was deserted, while an anxious throng surrounded the desk of Mr. Kem, and from that time on, Kem being persistent, the Speaker had peace; Mr. Kem was the autocrat, and the business of the House proceeded under the regular order.

There is no doubt that a great many measures of questionable character are passed by unanimous consent. Members can not keep the run of all bills reported and are loath to object, both because ignorant of the merits of the particular measure proposed and because they may have measures of their own to be considered and they fear a reciprocity of objection. In a majority of cases the only real intelligent objection made to measures proposed for unanimous consent is that made by the Speaker, who has had opportunity to examine, as was his duty, the bill. On two Mondays in every month and during the last six days of a session a motion is in order to suspend the rules and pass bills, which requires for its adoption a two-thirds vote of a quorum. The object of this rule, of course, is to expedite business by getting rid of bills to which two-thirds of the House are agreed. But the demands for recognition to move to suspend the rules are so far in excess of any possible power of grant upon the Speaker's part that he is confronted by the embarrassing necessity of making a choice. There is no doubt that he performs his unpleasant duty with due regard to his obligation to the public service.

It is manifest that even under the methods provided by the rules for the consideration of all classes of business there must necessarily be measures of great public importance that, by reason of their late report from a committee or for some reason or another, can not be reached in the regular order of business. These are provided for by special orders reported by the Committee on Rules, which consists of the Speaker, two Members from the majority, and two from the minority. Like the rules themselves, the Committee on Rules is made the subject of much unjust criticism. Autocratic power is ascribed to it. But it must be recognized first that the existence of such a body is a necessity, and second that the only power it exercises is the power of the House. The Committee on Rules does not dictate, it simply suggests. Its report is of no consequence until it has been adopted by a majority. The fact that the committee's reports are uniformly adopted, so far from being any evidence of undue authority or power on the part of the committee, is evidence of the discretion of the committee in recognizing and making possible what the House wants to do. The real temper of the House upon any question at any given time, it may be assumed, is better known by the Committee on Rules than by any one else. The committee, so far from being the master, is the servant of the House. Of the 7,423 bills considered last year, only twenty-four were brought forward by the Committee on Rules.

All of these were of large national importance, and consideration of them was in accordance with the well-known desire of a majority of the House, as for instance, among others the following: The statehood bill, the immigration bill, Philippine tariff bill, pure food bill, railroad rate bill, bills relating to Isthmian Canal, etc.

While it is true that the authority of the Speaker as to recognition is very much limited, it would be useless to deny that he exercises a great power upon the business of the House. But this is not due to the rules in the first instance, but to the personality of the Speaker himself. Much of his power lies back of his office. It is because of his character, his experience, his service, his position as a party leader that he is Speaker. He comes to his high office because he is *primus inter pares*. A leader on the floor, he does not cease to be a leader when he becomes Speaker. One who was himself a distinguished Speaker of the House of Representatives, James G. Blaine, in that most eloquent eulogy pronounced upon his chief, President Garfield, said:

There is no test of a man's ability in any department of public life more severe than service in the House of Representatives; there is no place where so little deference is paid to reputation previously acquired or to eminence won outside ; no place where so little consideration is shown for the feelings or failures of beginners. What a man gains in the House he gains by sheer force of his own character, and, if he loses and falls back, he must expect no mercy, and will receive no sympathy. It is a field in which the survival of the strongest is the recognized rule, and where no pretense can survive and no glamour can mislead. The real man is discovered, his worth is impartially weighed, his rank is irrevocably decided.

Undoubtedly the rules contribute to the Speaker's power in so far as they place in his hands the appointment of committees. He can, by a judicious selection of committee membership, to a limited extent, shape legislation in advance to accord with his views. But, after all, his power in this respect is limited by a number of considerations. In the appointments to committees he must recognize the claims of localities, the qualifications and length of service of his appointees, and various other things. Above all things, he is interested in the success of his administration, in the standing of his party, and in his own reputation for fairness. What he does he does in the open, where all men can see. And, besides, how else could committees be selected in a House of so large a membership as the present House of Representatives? Caucus selection would mean selection by combinations representing localities or special interests; would turn over the power of the House to the States having large delegations. Caucus selection has been tried in the past, and abandoned as impracticable. Committees can best be selected by an authority that can with certainty be located and made to bear the burden of responsibility.

I know of nothing more interesting in the history of Congress than those passages which relate to the expedients to which the majority has been compelled to resort to obtain control as against obstructive tactics upon the part of the minority.

Early in our history unlimited debate was resorted to to prevent legislative action, and the result was the adoption of the previous question in the House. According to Mr. Calhoun it was adopted —

in consequence of the abuse of the right of debate by Mr. Gardenier, of New York, remarkable for his capacity for making long speeches. He could keep the floor for days.

But Mr. Gardenier was only a type, and the adoption of the previous question marks the first step in our Congressional history taken by the majority toward securing its right to rule. The next step was the adoption of the hour rule, pursuant to which a Member of the House is confined to the use of one hour in debate.

It must be confessed that in a House constituted of so large a membership as the House of Representatives unlimited debate would be impossible, having any due regard to the dispatch of the public business. There is little if any complaint about the hour rule. Anyone familiar with the record of the last few Congresses will concede that notwithstanding the existence of the hour rule there has been practically no limitation on the opportunities for debate. All parties desiring to be heard have been furnished an opportunity, and when greater latitude as to time has been asked it has readily been granted by unanimous consent. The House will always listen to the Member who really has something to say.

With each decennial apportionment the House of Representatives increases in numbers. As the numbers increase in the very nature of things the importance of the individual Member decreases and the influence of a few increases. What the remedy for this is I do not undertake to predict, or what new or modified rules may in the future become necessary. But under present conditions the rules of the House of Representatives are as efficient as present wisdom and past experience have been able to devise "to subserve the will of the assembly rather than to restrain it, to facilitate and not to obstruct the expression of its deliberate sense."

CRITICISM OF THE RULES, APRIL 5, 1906

[The sentiment of individual members upon the rules is brought out in the following extracts. There will be abundant illustrations also from other discussions, which will be given later on, especially in the matter of special rules and finance legislation.]

MR. MOON. I have no objection to drastic rules in a body of this size. It is unwieldy, and we need the power of the rule even to force legislation, but we do need rules that will operate justly and equally upon every Member and every party in this House. It is unwise for us, in view of the needs of this Government, to tie the Representatives of the people upon this floor. The present rules of the House of Representatives, in my judgment, are dangerous to the welfare of the people; and yet, take them altogether, leaving a few rules out of consideration, it is perhaps as good a code as we could obtain for a body of this size.

The power, though, which the Speaker has, or exercises if he chooses, under the construction of the rule, to turn from a Member and decline to recognize him for the purpose for which he rises, after once recognizing, is a most dangerous power in any parliamentary body. That power which you have given him, and which he exercises as your servant, is a power that ought never to be invoked against the interests of the people in the consideration of legislation. It denies equal opportunities to the membership of the House. It degrades the Representative.

Another rule to which I have referred is this: You prevent upon the consideration of an appropriation bill new legislation. Don't you think it would be wise to modify that rule to the extent that legislation which is germane to a particular subject of consideration may be presented? That is a wise rule to prevent riders being placed on an appropriation bill, riders foreign to the subject of consideration; but right here, right under this bill, at this hour if that rule were modified this House could consider the question of railway mail-pay; it could consider the question of changing the rate of second-class matter; it could consider the question of a usurpation of power under the statute in the Post-Office Department. But you are powerless under the rule which shackles you by your own will to do so. What further remedy have you? Can you appeal to the committee for consideration of these questions by separate bills? You have found those things vain and futile. If you clothe the Speaker with the power to name the committee instead of letting the House of Representatives select its own committeemen as the Senate does, you place it within his power to so organize the committees of this House as to forever defeat legislation coming before the committee, and then you put it beyond your power in this House by the rule to which I have referred of resuming the sovereign power to which you are entitled yourself. You have yielded away your power, you can not help yourselves. The result of this, Mr. Chairman, is that when gentlemen on the floor of this House find that it is impossible to be heard in the interest of their constituents, they yield. When a question arises in this body upon which they ought to have independent judgment ——

Mr. SIMS. Mr. Chairman, I thoroughly agree with what the gentleman has been saying about this rule of not being permitted to legislate on an appropriation bill; but it is not a fact that it does not prevent that new legislation, provided that in the Senate they put on the same amendment that we rejected here in the House. It comes back then, and under the rules, and it is not out of order to consider that which has been once solemnly ruled out of order.

Mr. MOON of Tennessee. Of course, we agree on that question. It can legislate, while this House can not, under the rule.

Mr. SIMS. But the Senate forces us to do it.

Mr. MOON of Tennessee. The Senate, of course, forces us to do it. The Senate forces us to do nearly all we do. The Republican majority is not to blame alone for this.

Mr. SIMS. Mr. Chairman, I think the gentleman is right about that.

Mr. MOON of Tennessee. The Republican majority in this House has surrendered beyond all question freely and voluntarily all of the reserved rights of a Representative, save one or two, to the Speaker of the House. Now, if anybody has to exercise that power on the Republican side, I would as soon have the present Speaker do it as anybody in the world. It is not a question of the Speaker individually. I believe everybody in this House is personally fond of him. It is a question of the abrogation of the power of the Representatives so as to prevent legislation that is wholesome and just.

I have now demonstrated to the House, I trust, legislation that is needed upon this bill. I defy anyone to get one particle of it. You can not put it on here. You are tied by your rules; you can not put it through your committee, for the Speaker has tied your committee. What are you to do? Gentlemen, there are reserved rights, but only one or two to the House of Representatives.

If without the spirit of revenge or anger, if in obedience to the high dictates of duty, if in recognition of those representative rights which you all possess, you will say to the House of Representatives, "Be bound by the chains you have forged; no business shall be done in this House save by and in accordance technically with every rule that this House has adopted for the transaction of business," and you do that for a few weeks, then this majority and the Speaker will find themselves utterly powerless to move one inch in legislation. They will break the chains themselves, and they will tell the Speaker that he is no longer a master, but a servant of the House of Representatives. How was it in the days that are past? Was this a body in which the will and decree of a political coterie was registered? This was the great forum in which the battles of the people were fought. Here every great battle for American liberty and American citizenship has been fought out in behalf of the people, and to-day, like craven cowards, you have surrendered every right you have given to the Speaker of the House of Representatives and the Committee on Rules, and without the slightest deliberation you pass for consideration to the other end of the Capitol every bill nearly that is before you.

Without naming any particular bill, but to show the evil effect of that and of ill-considered legislation, a bill is to-day pending, upon which this House has acted, affecting a great Territory proposed to be made a State, greater than the State of Missouri, where this House actually failed to extend, so far as some necessary provisions were concerned, the benefit of the law proposed to be enacted to a part of the Territory — unintentionally, of course. No consideration in committee, no consideration anywhere, until the Senate of the United States pointed out, to the shame of the House of Representatives, the patent defect. You gentlemen can not go back to the country and accuse the Republican party of all the wrongs that the people suffer at the hands cf this once great but now degenerate body. The Democracy of the House of Representatives must exercise the reserved power of refusing and forbidding anything to be done, save in obedience to the law that the House has made for its government, and then the people will see where the chains are and who forged them, and they will put an end, I trust, to the wrongs and injustices that exist here.

Mr. SIMS. We witnessed the spectacle a few days ago of two Representatives on this floor, one a member of the Republican party and one a member of the Democratic party, who undertook to have one bill passed according to the general rules of this House, and the Committee on Rules got together and decided that the general rules were the worst thing possible to apply to that appropriation bill; and they brought in a special rule, repealing the general rules and making in order everything that had gone out on points of order as well as all that remained.

* * * * * * * *

Mr. SIMS. What are you going to do about it? Let us get down to something practical.

Mr. MOON of Tennessee. I was just suggesting to you a practical solution of it. Suppose when a gentleman gets on the floor of the House of Representatives and asks unanimous consent and the Speaker recognized the gentleman for unanimous consent; suppose you have no objection to the bill, but have objection to the exercise of that power emanating from one source alone, a power that practically controls the operations of the House, you have the reserved right as a Representative to say, "I object." That places the gentleman who made the motion in his seat. How is he going to get his bill up?

He can not do it except upon call of committees on the day when it is reached, and the chances are only one in a hundred he can reach it then. He can not go to the Union Calendar and take a bill off that Calendar. There are three-fourths of the important bills of the House upon that Calendar, and that Calendar, by virtue of the power of the Speaker, has not been called for general consideration in ten long years in the House of Representatives. You can consider on it those things he favors only without unanimous consent or a special rule, and he controls recognition and is chairman of the Committee on Rules.

Mr. SIMS. Then what is to hinder the Committee on Rules from selecting out these very bills to which objection has been made and bringing in a special rule that they shall be considered without any reference to unanimous consent?

Mr. MOON of Tennessee. Well, what hinders the House of Representatives from exercising its power to overturn the Committee on Rules?

Mr. SIMS. Well, I thought the gentleman answered a while ago that we had lost about all self-respect and courage and everything else.

Mr. MOON of Tennessee. Oh, I think not; I did not mean to say and did not say that, Mr. Chairman. I meant to say that we had lost the power of resistance.

Mr. RICHARDSON of Alabama. Mr. Chairman ——

The CHAIRMAN. Does the gentleman from Tennessee yield to the gentleman from Alabama?

Mr. MOON of Tennessee. I yield to the gentleman from Alabama.

Mr. RICHARDSON of Alabama. I heard you say something in your remarks relative to the degeneracy of the Democracy on this side of the House. I ask the gentleman the question — inasmuch as you called us degenerate — if when we were in power and Mr. Crisp, of Georgia, was Speaker the same rules were not substantially adopted then as are adopted now?

Mr. Moon of Tennessee. Yes; and.they were just as infamous then as they are now. [Applause on the Democratic side.]

Mr. Towne. Mr. Chairman, I desire to subscribe very cordially to some of the remarks — indeed, practically to all of them — of the distinguished gentleman from Tennessee who has just resumed his seat, addressed to the subject of the rules of this House; but I wish to enter one important qualification in respect to the criticisms that are passed ' upon the Speaker. The Speaker is, in my judgment, almost as much sinned against as sinning. The fact that under both Republican and Democratic régimes very largely the same complaint has been made in respect to the exercise of quasi-autocratic power by the Chair is itself a recognition to a considerable degree that the necessity for exercising that kind of power inheres in the duties of the office itself as it has evolved in our system.

Now, sir, I am not prepared at this moment to enter upon a careful discussion of certain matters that I wish merely to indicate for the sober consideration, in this connection, of the men who, as I hope, are to participate in the framing of the rules for the Sixtieth Congress. [Applause.] I mean the Democrats of this body. [Renewed applause.]

The Speakership of this House, sir, in its origin was not a political office. It is interesting to contrast it with the history of the speakership of the English House of Commons, whence we borrow very largely the model upon which this House is constructed. In the House of Commons the speaker is a mere moderator, who presides over a parliamentary body for the purpose of enforcing ordinary parliamentary rules. The office has no political significance. That fact is illustrated by the recent re-election of Mr. Lowther, the Conservative speaker, by the new enormous Liberal majority in the House of Commons.

If a speaker is a competent parliamentarian, a fair man, and a man of ability, no majority in the English Parliament cares to which party he belongs. But originally the English speaker was a political officer. His name signifies it. He spoke for the Commons with the King, and to a considerable degree was able to direct the deliberations of the House and to select the subjects upon which it should deliberate. In process of time there developed the English ministry, the responsible element in the control of the legislative in the British system. The ministry determines all the initiative in legislation, marks out the programme for the Commons, determines what propositions of legislation shall come before that body; and the opposition — I may interpolate at this point — has always the right to propose and discuss amendments. That function is ever the great factor in that general system of government to which the English Commons and this body belong, a system that the great commentator Bagehot has called a government by discussion; and if at any time this House shall ever have its ancient dignity and power restored and shall again appeal to the imagination and respect of the people of America, it will be when it shall have vindicated for itself the right to discuss all public measures proposed here. [Loud applause.] But in America we have never evolved anything that answers to the British cabinet or ministerial system. There must, however, in every majority temporarily controlling the deliberations of this House, be somewhere an initiative, the power of determining the policy according to which the majority shall choose to proceed, and how it shall exercise that power. It is interesting to note how this function has become an asset of our Speakership, an evolution in that office having occurred directly opposite from that which marked the English speakership. Speaker Muhlenberg, the first Speaker of the House of Representatives, nearly one hundred and twenty years ago, was a mere presiding officer, but in the course of time the officer who commenced as a mere moderator has developed into the most powerful political functionary in our Government.

I do not propose at this moment, and without preparation, to undertake a discussion of the philosophy implied in the fact I have cited. I shall merely suggest whether in this proposed and desirable reform of the rules of the House we are not face to face with more than a mere question of convenience, a deep question of government indeed, complicated with the evolution of our system itself. But there are some things that those who propose to reform these rules can entertain little difference about. One of them was suggested very ably by the gentleman from Tennessee in answer to a question. We can change the rules of the House. We can if we will. We will not if we submit ourselves to the dictation of a few men on grounds of alleged party interest and refuse to stand in favor of the inherent legislative rights of the House. The majority party can, if it will, make a few simple changes in the rules that will go a great way to restore the ancient capacities and prestige of the House.

For instance, now, if a man on the floor of this House desires to challenge the attention of the Chair he must arise in his place and address the Speaker; and, as I think the language of the rule is — although I have not seen it lately — "upon being recognized, he shall proceed in order." If he is not recognized he can not proceed, and we witness this anomalous and insulting thing — although the Speaker is not in a personal sense to blame for it, let me say, it is inherent in the rules — that a man representing a great American constituency, with something to speak about and to think about and to propose to this great body on his individual and political responsibility, arises in his place here and the Speaker says to him, "For what purpose does the gentleman rise?" And if the purpose does not suit the Speaker the Member has not, to any effectual purpose, arisen at all, but has to take his seat.

Now, sir, when two or more men are contemporaneously challenging the attention of the Chair, it is a mere necessity that he shall choose which one to recognize. No rule can ever obviate that; but it has happened time and again — it happened in my own case in the Fifty-fourth Congress — that but one Member is asking recognition from the Chair, and that he can not get the floor. Now, I undertake to say that any Representative of a great constituency of the American people upon this floor has a right, or ought to have the right, to ask the attention of the Chair and the House to anything he wishes to bring to the attention of this assembly when nobody else is claiming the floor at the same time. [Applause.]

REPRESENTATIVE CUSHMAN ON THE RULES[1]

MR. CUSHMAN. I for one expect to live to see the day in this House, not when the Speaker shall tell the individual members of this House what he is going to permit them to bring up, but when those individual members constituting a majority will inform the Speaker what they are going to bring up for themselves.

THE CALENDAR OF THE HOUSE

I for one expect to live to see the day in this Hall, when this House has leisure in the interim between the passage of the great appropriation bills that this House will go into the Committee of the Whole House on the state of the Union for the consideration of bills on the Union Calendar. I expect to live to see the day when the Union Calendar will be called oftener than once in a lifetime.

Does anybody say that it is lack of time that prevents this? I have seen this body adjourn three and four days at a time when the Union Calendar was freighted with the hopes of voiceless millions. No, sir; it does not lie in the mouth of this body or any member of it to say that it is lack of time. It is lack of inclination and not lack of time that ails this body — or at least those who dominate it.

It does not require any longer time to pass the same bill when we are in the Committee of the Whole House on the state of the Union than it does to pass it under unanimous consent. The only difference is the first is entirely within the power of the members themselves, while the unanimous consent route is entirely controlled by the Speaker. But, sir, I have seen the Speaker's room black with members, like flies around a honeycomb, each one wondering if he was going to be able to persuade the Speaker to recognize him. I will tell you, sir, all we have to do to regulate this matter is not to put in so much time trying to get the Speaker to recognize us, but to rise up in our dignity and our might and recognize ourselves. [Applause.]

When we go into the Committee of the Whole for the consideration

[1] *Congr. Record*, Apr. 17, 1902.

of bills on the Union Calendar, every man with a bill on that Calendar has, or ought to have, an equal chance to get his bill considered.

But under the other system — the unanimous-consent route — unfair and inequitable, the Speaker of this House stands up and passes out recognitions for "unanimous consents" like so many sugar-coated doughnuts. He recognizes those he desires to recognize, and he does not recognize those whom he does not wish to recognize.

What is the Union Calendar of this House and what bills go upon that Calendar? Every bill containing an appropriation of money or creating an office goes upon that Calendar. It is difficult to conceive of any important bill which would not include in its provisions one or the other of those features.

That being true, the most important bills that are introduced in this House go upon the Union Calendar. I would like to stand up in one crowd the 70,000,000 in this Republic and have each one make a guess as to how often there is a call of the Union Calendar in the House of Representatives. It is never called. Only once in the last seven years has this House gone into the Committee of the Whole House on the state of the Union for the consideration of bills on the Union Calendar. Why do we have a Calendar in this House? Did any man ever hear in his lifetime before of a Calendar that is never called? Under the present system of running this House we have no more need of a Calendar than a man with both arms cut off above the elbows needs a pair of fur-trimmed mittens. [Laughter.]

A friend of mine some time ago said to me, "Cushman, what makes you so thin?" I will tell you what makes me so thin. I have behind me an honest but infuriated constituency. A half a million worthy, honest, patriotic people who are demanding, and rightfully demanding, that I secure certain needed legislation for them. That is the pressure on me from the rear. Then in this House whenever I try to secure the consideration of matters of legislation in which my people are interested I run up against the stone wall that surrounds the Speaker of this House and the Committee on Rules. That is what constitutes the pressure in front. And I tell you frankly that between the pressure that has been brought to bear on me from the rear and the pressure I have encountered in front that I have become thinner than a cancelled postage stamp. That is what is the matter with me. [Laughter.]

THE RIGHTS OF A LEGISLATOR

Under the rules of this House as they are administered, the rights of the individual legislator in this body are simply limited to his right to vote "yes" and "no" on the various propositions that are brought before this House.

I say to you that one of the rights inherent in and appertaining to the individual membership of every deliberative legislative body is not only the right to vote on the questions that are brought up, but the broader and higher right to have his voice heard and his vote recorded in determining what questions shall be brought up for consideration. And any man who denies that, denies the existence of every principle that lies at the base of a republican form of Government.

What do we amount to as individual units in this House — this House that was once the great House of Representatives, the popular forum of a patriotic people? What is it now? It is an annex to the committee room of the Committee on Rules. Here is where we meet and go through the stupid formality of ratifying the legislation that is determined upon by the Speaker and his Committee on Rules. To me one of the amazing things that occur in this House is to have some man arise and select for his subject "Government without the consent of the governed," for the Speaker invariably strains his eyes and cracks his voice trying to discern and draw pictures of an alleged condition of that kind in a region 7,000 miles away. Talk about government without the consent of the governed. If my brief legislative experience counts for anything, that system has reached its greatest perfection and found its most perfect flower right here in this Hall.

REPRESENTATIVE COCKRAN ON THE HOUSE PROCEDURE[1]

MR. COCKRAN. Anyone who has followed the course of this general debate must have become impressed with two radically distinct and conflicting emotions; admiration for the high capacity shown by the speakers and regret that under the rules which govern us the speeches themselves were directed not to some question pending before the House, but delivered into the empty air. By this, Mr. Chairman, I would not be understood as saying that they were irrelevant to matters deeply affecting the public welfare and vividly before the public mind. With hardly an exception they all turned upon questions of vital and pressing political importance, yet hardly one touched a subject with which the House will be suffered to deal. If years from now some student should undertake to study the *Record* which chronicles our proceedings, he would be driven to the conclusion that while nearly every one of those speeches taken by itself was of such excellence that it might have been addressed to a council of sages, yet the whole debate taken together suggests the incoherence, discordance, and dissonance of a lunatic asylum rather than the debate of a highly intelligent, deliberative body. [Laughter.]

[1] *Congr. Record*, reported Apr. 20, 1906.

Mr. Chairman, my object in taking the floor now is to bring before the House the rules which have caused this profligate waste of such excellent material, in the hope that through discussion of them means may be found by which these abundant talents, these great potentialities of efficient service, will be utilized for the public benefit — not dissipated to the public discredit.

Mr. Chairman, the recent history of this House shows conclusively that there is not in all this world a body capable of higher legislative service or animated by loftier civic virtue. And yet, sir, it is a melancholy spectacle that this body, which, when controlled by the judgment, the intelligence, and the patriotism of its membership, has succeeded in producing the most important and triumphant legislative results, when hampered, fettered, and restricted by absurd rules, often sinks to an almost ludicrous incapacity, of which this very debate is a striking illustration. That I do not exaggerate is, in my judgment, conclusively proved by the triumphant success of the House this session in framing and passing a railroad rate bill, when it was free to control its own Members, and its utter failure to pass an effective measure last session when it was bound and gagged under restrictions imposed by the Committee on Rules.

Last year when this House was called upon to deal with the intricate, perplexing, and almost wholly unexplored field of railroad rate legislation it was placed under a rule which restricted its power to adopting the measure recommended by the majority of the Committee on Interstate Commerce, or else adopting the measure recommended by the minority. No power was left in a Member to offer an amendment, or in the House to consider it. As amendment is the only object and purpose of discussion, where a body is practically unanimous on the principle of a bill, as the House was on that railroad measure, the passage of such a rule simply meant that we threw over upon the Senate the important duty of originating amendments, which all conceded to be necessary. That was not only an abdication of our functions and a renunciation of our duty, but it was a confession of incapacity. For my part, sir, I declined to be a party to such an abasement of this House, membership in which I consider a distinguished honor, and so when the measure was on its passage I refused to vote, asking simply to be recorded "present."

That measure met the fate which the method of its passage invited. It fell stillborn on the threshold of the other Chamber. It was never even considered by the Senate. It was thrown in the wastebasket, its proper destination. There it remained, useless for every purpose, except as a monument to the folly, the incapacity — aye, sir, I will say the disloyalty — with which we renounced our functions, turned our backs upon our obligations, fled from our obvious duty.

Now, Mr. Chairman, contrast with that dreary record of incapacity, of folly, and of failure, the triumphant progress of the bill dealing with the same subject which passed the House this year. When it came before us, the House was left free to deal with the measure as it pleased. Full power to offer amendments was left in the hands of every Member. The limit of debate was fixed by a unanimous vote. Every amendment offered was considered and action taken freely upon it. The result was a measure which I venture to say will stand for a long time as a monument to the patriotism in which it was conceived, the wisdom in which it was framed, and the resolution with which it was passed. [Loud applause.]

I say this, sir, notwithstanding the fact (and largely because of the fact) that since this measure passed this House it has been the subject of vigorous animadversions and very bitter criticism. I take it that these criticisms are in the highest degree a compliment to its merits. The wrongdoers with whom it was intended to deal testify by the vehemence and fury with which they assail it how deeply they realize its efficiency. But, sir, the abuse of miscreants whose crimes it is intended to prevent weighs little in the minds of honest men against the approval of the people whose rights it is drawn to protect. And this it enjoys beyond all question. Conceive for a moment the change in public attitude toward this measure since closing debate. Recall the objections that were advanced to it in this House with so much vehemence this year and last year, and then you have but to examine from day to day the adverse comments in newspapers, the speeches delivered against it, the interviews with railway officials and railway attorneys who condemn it, to measure the distance between the grounds occupied by its opponents before discussion in the House began and since its close. Then you will be able to realize the distance that public opinion has traveled under the light and guidance of our proceedings in this body.

When this measure was pending here, the point dividing its supporters and opponents was the question whether we had any constitutional or moral right to pass it. Some of its opponents said it violated the letter and others the spirit of the Constitution, but they were all unanimous in describing it as a long step toward socialism. Well, these objections have all been quieted. Not one of them has been audible since the close of debate here. If one is heard occasionally it is in a voice so feeble and so rare that it merely serves to attest the overwhelming preponderance of public opinion. Gentlemen who were then most vehement in opposing it now claim to be its most ardent supporters. One after another popularly supposed to be bitterly hostile to it objects strenuously now to being counted among its opponents. But while he wants to be recognized among its supporters, he protests that he wishes to perfect it.

Mr. Chairman, no one among the supporters of the bill objects to any suggestion for its improvement. But I believe its friends should be vigilant, and I am sure they will be vigilant, to see that under cover of attempts to perfect the measure its enemies will not be permitted to emasculate it.   We must see that it is not destroyed by mutilation disguised as amendments, now that efforts to destroy it by open opposition are no longer considered safe.

Mr. Chairman, it is quite true that although the grounds of criticism which were advanced in this House have been abandoned, new ones have been evolved, which, though less weighty, enjoy the advantage of not having been subjected to the test of our scrutiny.   Of these the most formidable now directed against this bill is that we have omitted to provide for a judicial review of all orders made by the Interstate Commerce Commission.   For that reason this House has been denounced as incapable, negligent, and indifferent.   Now that I have the floor I do not know how I can better improve the time at my disposal than by employing some of it in refuting this criticism, and sending it to join all its predecessors.   I do not think, sir, that will be a very difficult task; I think the very slightest examination of this last objection will show that among criticisms it deserves to be classed as survival of the loosest. [Laughter.]

First, Mr. Chairman, let me say a word as to its source.   This objection is not advanced openly by the interests chiefly affected by the bill. It proceeds ostensibly from a rather new product of our constitutional evolution — the constitutional lawyer — the great constitutional lawyer, who chooses a legislative body, rather than a judicial tribunal, for the display of his qualities.

It is well to observe that the constitutional lawyer of a legislative body is always a "great" constitutional lawyer.

Now, I confess that I regard this legislative constitutional lawyer with something of the awe which attaches to everything beyond our comprehension.   [Laughter.]   I do not know that I am able to describe him. I think I know him when I see him, for he has certain unmistakable characteristics.   But to describe you must understand, and I admit he is far beyond the power of my intellectuals.   Ordinarily our conception of law is a uniform rule of conduct made binding upon all members of a community, or at least on the large majority of them, by the sovereign authority, whatever it may be; and the function of the lawyer, we plain mortals believe, is to ascertain this rule, to define and expound it, and thus promote unanimous obedience to it.   But while the essential function of the ordinary lawyer is to promote uniformity of the law, the activities of the great constitutional lawyer in a legislative body produce radically different results.   Whenever we find him active in either branch of Congress we find just as many different constitutions as there are great constitutional lawyers to expound the organic law.

In this particular case the constitutional lawyers all declare that this bill is constitutionally infirm somehow or other, but no two of them agree in pointing out the precise seat of infirmity. The constitutional lawyer is always vehement in warning us that before we undertake any measure we must be sure of its constitutionality; that he alone is competent to advise us; that next to the duty of accepting him as infallible comes that of regarding all other constitutional lawyers as unsound, if not worse; that we must be wary even of trusting their quotations lest instead of giving us the judgment of a court they mislead us into accepting as its decision the language by which a minority seeks to show that the authority of the majority depended entirely upon the number of judges who constituted it, not upon the weight of reasons which justified it.

Mr. Chairman, if we must wait until the great constitutional lawyers agree upon any subject, it is plain that we would never take a step in any direction.

We would stand paralyzed at the threshold of every legislative enterprise, amazed and bewildered — puzzled to distinguish amid the din of their vociferation how much of it is advice to us and how much of it denunciation of each other. I defy any man to define Congress itself according to the constitutional lawyers after he has read three of their speeches. [Laughter.] Some of them say that we have all power, others that we have no power. Some that we can establish our authority over the courts, that we can not only confer jurisdiction on them or withhold it, as we please, but even after we have granted t that we can control its exercise — at least so far as to determine what persons or classes may have the benefit of it; that we can give it to the courts, as it were, with a string, so that a writ may be left within reach of our favorites and pulled far beyond even the view of any person or corporation whom we dislike or distrust. Others, again, tell us that we are not even an independent or coördinate department of government, but, so to speak, an antechamber to some other department; that our power consists in merely proposing laws, which, by the permission of another body, may acquire the force of statutes.

Now, Mr. Chairman, to me — an ordinary citizen, an humble Member of this House — a constitutional lawyer is an imposing personage before a court whose authoritative interpretations of the Constitution he aids by his arguments. For that very reason, sir, it seems to me that a legislative body is not the proper theater for disputatious attorneyship, but essentially one for constructive statesmanship. I can not believe that the function of Congress is a mystery difficult to comprehend or the duty of its Members a puzzle too perplexing for the ordinary mind to solve, as these gentlemen would persuade us.

It seems to me that the duty of Congress is to examine closely the condition of the country and keep itself constantly informed of everything affecting the common welfare. Wherever a wrong is found to exist with which the nation can deal more effectively than a State, it is the business of Congress to suggest a remedy. If the courts hold that the legislation we consider essential is beyond our power to enact, our duty to suggest a remedy is none the less binding, except that instead of proceeding by the enactment of a law we should proceed by proposing a constitutional amendment. Our duty to propose an amendment to the Constitution when advisable is just as binding as our duty to change the law when that is within our power and we believe it is essential to the welfare of the citizens. [Applause.] If, therefore, we find that a wrong exists anywhere which the National Government in our judgment has the power to redress, and some great constitutional lawyer should undertake to raise objections with that wonderful ingenuity which enables us always to distinguish him, not by numerous decisions of courts upholding his contentions, but by the wonder and awe of his legislative associates at the multiplicity of his quotations, the strangeness of his phrases, the majesty of his mien, and the mystery of his meaning [laughter and applause], it is not for us to waste time in abstract and fanciful speculations about the course which the courts may pursue toward the remedial measures we may enact. Face to face with a wrong which we believe a State can not cure, it is our duty to find a remedy some way or other. Our first step must be in the direction of legislation. The only way we can ascertain definitely whether a law which we believe will prove effective is constitutional or unconstitutional is not by abandoning ourselves to a maelstrom of speculations about what the court may hold or has held on subjects more or less kindred, but to legislate, and thus take the judgment of the court on that specific proposal. We can tell whether it is constitutional or unconstitutional when the court pronounces upon it and not before. Even if the court declares it unconstitutional its decision will not reduce us to helplessness. When it drives us from establishing a remedy by legislation it will by that very act direct us to propose a remedy by constitutional amendment. Having framed a suitable amendment and proposed it to the legislatures of the States, our duty will have been accomplished. The final step toward full redress will then be with the bodies most directly representative of the people affected by the wrong.

*   *   *   *   *   *   *   *

THE COMMITTEE SYSTEM [1]

[The following extracts are taken from an extended debate on the distribution among the House committees of the various parts of the President's annual message. This question was made the occasion of discussions covering the entire field of national policy. The particular debate here reproduced took place immediately after the resolution for the distribution had been reported to the House by Mr. Payne, chairman of the Committee on Ways and Means.

[1] *Congr. Record*, Dec. 13–15, 1905.

The controversy turned especially on the question whether bills dealing with insurance should be referred to the latter committee.]

MR. HEPBURN. Mr. Chairman, I have no objection to the resolution as it was introduced at the time of its reference. I do object to the amendment made in the fourth line, by inserting the words "and insurance." The effect of that is to carry all matters of legislation concerning the control of insurance to the Committee on Ways and Means; and the reason assigned for that is that in the opinion of the Chairman the only manner in which Congress can have jurisdiction over that subject is through the exercise of the taxing power.

Mr. Chairman, even if that were true, that would not indicate, necessarily, the direction which this class of business should take in assignment to committees. It is true that all matters of taxation, where taxation — the raising of revenue — is the object to be attained, should be considered by the Committee on Ways and Means; but where taxation is resorted to solely for the purpose of securing jurisdiction, solely for the purpose of the exercise of a power, I submit that it is not the rule of this House to send matters of that kind to that Committee — notably the legislation with reference to oleomargarine. A tax nominal was resorted to only to give power to the Congress, or justify it in the exercise of power. Yet you will remember that that matter was considered and reported by the Committee on Agriculture. They had jurisdiction of it, recognizing the fact that the assumption upon the part of the Committee on Ways and Means was a mere fiction. The object was not to secure revenue. The object was to secure the right to exercise a power. Therefore the taxing power was resorted to, or taxation was made the pretext. There are a number of instances that might be given where this rule has been observed and where jurisdiction of the Committee on Ways and Means has been denied, notwithstanding the fact that a nominal tax was provided for in the legislation sought.

Mr. Chairman, I am willing to concede that there is more than one decision of the Supreme Court in which it has been held, in a casual way, that insurance was not commerce; but I want to call attention to the fact that that was not the major proposition considered by the Supreme Court, that but little attention was paid to that question in the argument, that that was simply one of the incidents in the case; and it is the opinion of a great many men learned in the law that when the proposition is fairly made, when the attention of the Supreme Court is called to the fact of the immense interest there is in insurance, interwoven inextricably with trade, when it is remembered that the annihilation of insurance would well-nigh annihilate commerce, that thousands and tens of thousands of commercial enterprises would never for a moment be considered or undertaken but for the auxiliary of insurance; when it is shown how interwoven insurance is with all commercial transactions, with the millions of money invested in trade and commerce, that another view of that subject may be taken. And I want to call attention to the fact that I have in my possession a bill prepared by the secretary of the National Bar Association, and, as I understand, a bill that met with their approval, from which it is clear that, in their opinion — in the opinion of the National Bar Association of the United States — the regulation of insurance companies is a power given to Congress under the commerce clause of the Constitution. The language of these gentlemen, as used in the bill, declares that the writing of policies and other business of that character is commerce, and therefore it is a power conferred by the commerce clause of the Constitution.

This is a matter of importance. I want to call attention to the fact that, so far as there is any precedent upon the part of the House, you will discover from that precedent that the Committee on Interstate and Foreign Commerce had jurisdiction over this subject. The only legislation that we have upon that subject emanated from that committee. That committee reported the bill creating the Department of Commerce and Labor, by which there is created a Bureau of Corporations, and in express terms, with the other conferments of power, is the one including insurance. So that, so far as precedent goes, I think the gentleman is wrong in his assumption that the committee he has referred to and over which he presides (the Committee on Ways and Means) is the sole committee that may take jurisdiction of this subject.

I reserve my time, but I will yield to any gentleman who desires me to do so.

*   *   *   *   *   *   *   *

Mr. LACEY. If the Committee on Interstate Commerce should conclude that the only remedy in this matter is by taxation, I presume they would scarcely report a bill upon that question for fear of trespassing upon the jurisdiction of the Ways and Means Committee. That is a question we will worry about when we get to it; but here is the President's message that only points out one way through commerce, and that would go to the Committee on Interstate Commerce, not the Committee on Ways and Means. There is not a single suggestion anywhere in the message that there is any thought in the mind of the Executive that the question can be handled through the taxing power. Possibly it could be legislated upon in that way, but the message does not consider anything of that kind or suggest anything of the kind to the Congress, and therefore it seems to me clear we ought not to adopt this amendment, but to leave revenue measures to go to the Committee on Ways and Means, and matters connected with commerce in the message go to the Committee on Interstate Commerce.

The CHAIRMAN. Before the Chair recognizes the gentleman from Illinois, does the gentleman from Iowa desire to reserve the balance of his time?

Mr. HEPBURN. I desire to reserve the balance of my time, and if I can be recognized I would desire to yield five minutes to the gentleman from Minnesota [Mr. Stevens].

Mr. STEVENS of Minnesota. This subject is an important one, but the proposition to be immediately settled is not novel. It seems to me that similar subjects which should be precedents and a basis for our action here have been settled by the House in previous Congresses with the assent of the Committee on Ways and Means, and especially of its distinguished chairman. Now, he did relate somewhat the history of the oleomargarine legislation, but he omitted especially the significant course of legislation in the Fifty-sixth and Fifty-seventh Congresses, which is of the greatest interest and bearing now. The history of that legislation in those two particular Congresses is that which is appropriate to the present settlement of this proposition. There were several bills introduced in the Fifty-sixth Congress to regulate and control the sale of oleomargarine by means of the taxing power. I have here the index to *Congressional Record* of the first session of the Fifty-sixth Congress. From it there appears to have been six bills introduced in the House, three of which were referred to the Committee on Ways and Means.

The *Record* shows that the Committee on Ways and Means took no action with the bills referred to them. The *Record* also shows that the Committee on Agriculture did take action on one of the bills — H. R. 3717 — referred to it, and that the House received the report without objection by anybody as to jurisdiction, but no bill passed. The *Record* of the Fifty-seventh Congress shows that there were eight bills introduced in the first session of the Fifty-seventh Congress. Seven of them were referred to the Committee on Agriculture — and one, containing other provisions, was referred to the Committee on Ways and Means — H. R. 6534, by Mr. Underwood, of Alabama, which by its terms amended the revenue act of October 1, 1890. The especially noticeable fact which the House should know is this: There were two of the bills introduced in the Fifty-sixth Congress providing for the control and regulation of the subject of oleomargarine by means of the taxing power, one introduced by my colleague from Minnesota [Mr. Tawney] and one by my friend from Wisconsin [Mr. Davidson], which were referred to the Committee on Ways and Means in the Fifty-sixth Congress. In the Fifty-seventh Congress those almost identical bills, introduced by those same gentlemen, were referred to the Committee on Agriculture by the officials of the House without any objection from the chairman of the Committee on Ways and Means or from the Committee on Ways and Means itself. And the bill which was considered in the Fifty-seventh Congress, the bill which actually passed, was a bill introduced by Mr. Henry, of Connecticut — H. R. 9206 — which was referred to the Committee on Agriculture, reported by that Committee to the House and considered on the floor from that reference, and no objection was made by the Committee on

Ways and Means or by anyone else to the jurisdiction of the Committee on Agriculture, although the taxing power of the Government was invoked by the measure. So that the history of that legislation which bears the closest analogy to this proposition before this committee shows, although it contained provisions for the taxing powers, which were even the basis for its action and existence, yet the Committee on Ways and Means, although at first it assumed or received jurisdiction of the bills, afterwards yielded the control of them, for the very good reason that the main subject of those bills and the main purpose of that legislation was not the exercise of the taxing power, but the power to regulate and control a certain subject-matter which should be considered by another committee. Now, the House has considered and settled just this sort of matter. The Committee on Ways and Means has already considered them and yielded jurisdiction on a similar subject when the same question was involved, and that seems to me ——

Mr. LITTLEFIELD. May I ask the gentleman from Minnesota a question?

Mr. STEVENS of Minnesota. Certainly.

Mr. LITTLEFIELD. I have listened with a great deal of interest to the analysis of what was or was not legislation. Now what I would like to inquire is why these bills that went before the Committee on Agriculture and which are so parallel to this proposition did not go before the Interstate and Foreign Commerce Committee, the committee that now wants to get possession of this subject?

Mr. STEVENS of Minnesota. That is just the point I wanted to make. The House evidently considered — and the Committee on Ways and Means evidently considered, and it should be considered now — that the reference of any bill as to any subject should be to the committee which has general charge of the subject-matter which is the general main purpose of the bill. If the general purpose of the bill, if the general scope of the legislation, if the primary object for its enactment, is to raise revenue, even if it taxes insurance companies and insurance policies, or whatever it may do, and because of that regulate them in certain ways — if the main purpose of that legislation is to raise revenue, then it unquestionably should go to the Committee on Ways and Means. But if the main purpose of the legislation is to benefit the general or any particular agricultural interests of the country — is to vitally affect the agricultural interests of the country — and its incidental purpose is to use the taxing power, this House has decided that bill should go to the committee which had general charge of the agricultural interests of the country.

Now, if the main purpose of this bill be to regulate commerce, is to regulate the business which is incidental to or may be an integral part of commerce, regulate the general object which concerns commerce, it should go to the committee which has general charge of the subject of commerce, even though one of its incidental features concerns the subject of taxation, just exactly as did the question of control of oleomargarine in the Fifty-seventh Congress go to the committee which had charge of the interests which were most and vitally affected.

That has been the rule in the past. It seems to me to be a safe and salutary rule now and in the future, one that ought to be adopted in this House on all sorts of subjects. That kind of a rule is always safe and fair to all interests and all committees; and under that rule this subject should go to the Committee on Interstate and Foreign Commerce.

Mr. LITTLEFIELD. Now let me suggest to the gentleman, if he pleases.

Mr. STEVENS of Minnesota. Certainly.

Mr. LITTLEFIELD. That very reason you have given why this bill should go to the Committee on Interstate and Foreign Commerce applies with equal force to the oleomargarine proposition, as to which we could not legislate at all except under the interstate-commerce clause of the Constitution. Now, why did not your Committee on Interstate and Foreign Commerce at that time assert the jurisdiction that they are now undertaking to assert, when there were just exactly the same reasons for it? You had one bill referred to the Committee on Interstate and Foreign Commerce, and that committee quietly let that bill die in the committee.

The CHAIRMAN. The time of the gentleman from Minnesota has expired. The gentleman from Iowa has eight minutes remaining.

Mr. LITTLEFIELD. I ask unanimous consent that the gentleman from Minnesota may have five minutes more.

The CHAIRMAN. Unanimous consent is asked that the gentleman from Minnesota have five minutes in his own right. Is there objection? [After a pause.] The Chair hears none.

Mr. LITTLEFIELD. It seems to me that the very reason you have given why this bill should go to the Interstate Commerce Committee, and all the reason you have given why it should go to that committee, is that it is interstate commerce; all the reason why you say the oleomargarine proposition went to the Committee on Agriculture was because it related to agriculture. Now, this proposition relates not to interstate commerce, but to insurance. There was a Committee on Agriculture, and the oleomargarine proposition was one that related to agriculture, and it went to the Committee on Agriculture, and the only provision under which that committee could get jurisdiction of legislation of that kind was that it was interstate commerce, and that is exactly the same jurisdiction over that subject that you have over this. Why did you not assert that jurisdiction then?

Mr. STEVENS of Minnesota. I do not think the gentleman from Maine quite apprehends the point I make. It seems to me that the true rule should be that the main purpose of the bill should be primarily considered in its reference. The object which is mainly and primarily sought to be accomplished should determine the reference of the bill. Now, in the oleomargarine bill the main purpose of the bill was to assist the agricultural interests of the country. It was subsidiary and an incident that it related to the question of interstate commerce. The main purpose of that legislation was to assist the agricultural interests; but for that it would not have been passed or enacted. This House did exactly right in considering the main purpose and object of that legislation in making the reference to the committee which had charge of the principal subject-matter of agriculture. Now, in this case, insurance is incidental at least to commerce; it is part, an integral part, of a business which is concerned with the subject of commerce; if it exists at all, it must be as a part of the great business interests of the country and of the great commercial interests of the country, and that subject-matter goes, by our rules, to the Committee on Interstate and Foreign Commerce.

*   *   *   *   *   *   *   *

Mr. PAYNE. Mr. Chairman, to return to the subject of this resolution and the amendment offered to it referring this message, so far as it relates to matters of insurance, to the Committee on Ways and Means, I wish to discuss that question briefly.

There can be no doubt but that all bills raising a tax go to the Committee on Ways and Means, no matter what may be their nature. They go there under the rule.

The gentleman from Iowa [Mr. Hepburn] yesterday, in speaking of the matter, announced a rather novel and strange doctrine. He said:

Therefore the taxing power was resorted to. The taxation was made the pretext —

And from reading the context it would seem from the tenor of his remarks that in various laws passed by Congress taxation was made the pretext to give Congress the jurisdiction of the subject-matter. Now, of course, it is patent to every lawyer in the House that if the House should enact a law and put into the law itself the statement that the taxation was simply a pretext to get jurisdiction over the matter the Supreme Court would promptly declare the law unconstitutional; and where any of these laws which the gentleman characterizes in this manner have gone to the Supreme Court on their constitutionality the Supreme Court has examined the law, and when it found that the law imposed a tax they have promptly said that under the Constitution Congress had jurisdiction, but if the tax was a mere pretense Congress would have no jurisdiction. No committee would have any jurisdiction. Congress has no jurisdiction over the subject of insurance unless it can get it under the taxing power of the Government, as I shall proceed to show later on in numerous decisions of the Supreme Court of the United States where that subject was involved in the decision of the case.

Mr. SMITH of Iowa. Mr. Chairman, may I put a question to the gentleman?

Mr. Payne. I would rather the gentleman would not interrupt me now. If he will wait until I finish, then he can put his question.

Mr. Smith of Iowa. Very well.

Mr. Payne. The gentleman from Iowa [Mr. Hepburn] yesterday cited what he said was a precedent for this action, and that was the bill imposing a tax on oleomargarine. I have quite a vivid recollection of what occurred at that time, because it occurred during my early service in Congress, and I was curious to see how the House would get at a subject when it was bent on doing so, rule or no rule.

The bill came here first in 1882. That was before I broke into Congress, and it was referred to the Committee on Ways and Means under the rules. It was a bill to tax oleomargarine. There was a suspicion in the House, as well as in the country, that the object of that law was to tax oleomargarine out of existence. Nevertheless, the bill went to the Committee on Ways and Means. Why.? Because it raised revenue; because by its terms it imposed a tax. No one doubted then but that that was the proper reference.

In 1886 the same bill was introduced in the House and the same bill was referred to the Committee on Ways and Means. I think it was referred there in the first instance properly under the rules of the House. Mr. Hatch, of Missouri, chairman of the Committee on Agriculture, had very pronounced views on the subject of the suppression of oleomargarine. I do not remember whether the bill was introduced by him or not, but he had a suspicion that the bill would go to sleep in the Committee on Ways and Means. They had not reported it. It was rumored that that committee was opposed to the bill and opposed to the proposed legislation, and in order to get the bill out of the Committee on Ways and Means and get it into more friendly atmosphere Mr. Hatch made the motion in the House to discharge the Committee on Ways and Means from the further consideration of that bill and to refer it to the Committee on Agriculture, of which he was chairman.

After some debate, from which it appeared that the House was overwhelmingly for the bill, a very large majority representing their farmer constitutents here on the floor of the House having gotten the idea that this law, if enacted, was going to greatly improve the condition of agriculture, and especially the dairy farming in the United States, anxious as they were to have an immediate action upon this bill and get it before a committee that would report it to the House, by a vote of 67 to 40, as I am informed, the bill was taken from the Committee on Ways and Means and referred to the Committee on Argiculture, and the bill was reported and afterwards became a law. That is the origin of the oleomargarine law.

Since that time in various Congresses, since my friend from Iowa has become chairman of the great Committee on Interstate and Foreign Commerce, various bills of like character — a bill taxing filled cheese, the bill taxing impure flour, and bills of that nature — have been introduced in the House and referred invariably to the Committee on Ways and Means and reported by that committee, and have become a part of the law of the country from such reference and reports.

No one ever doubted that the proper place for these bills was with the Committee on Ways and Means. I do not know whether the gentleman from Iowa claims that his committee has jurisdiction over the subject of insurance or not, but it seems to me that if any legislation is proposed on this subject the Committee on Interstate and Foreign Commerce has no more pretense to a right of jurisdiction than has the Committee on Expenditures in the Interior Department.

TACTICS OF THE OPPOSITION. ACCOUNT OF THE OPPOSITION MOVEMENT

[The parliamentary tactics employed by the leader of the minority in the first session of the 60th Congress, 1908, are of great interest. They were avowedly planned not for the purpose of obstructing legislation, but enforcing action of the House upon certain measures. The method of obstruction employed by the minority leader was to make use on every possible occasion of the constitutional right to have the yeas and nays taken on a motion. The first extract is an account of the whole proceeding, from the point of view of the opposition. The attitude of the majority leaders toward the movement is brought out in the debate itself.]

BY REPRESENTATIVE HENRY T. RAINEY [1]

MR. RAINEY said:

Mr. Speaker: Under the general leave to print I desire to submit the following brief review of the attempt by the Hon. John Sharp Williams, of Mississippi, the Democratic leader in the House of Representatives, to compel the enactment of the legislation demanded by the country at the present time. In his effort to compel the enactment of certain needed legislation Mr. Williams received the united and active support of the Democratic minority in the House from the moment the movement commenced until the adjournment of Congress.

At the opening of the Sixtieth Congress the following legislation was universally demanded:

1. An employers' liability bill.
2. A bill providing for publicity of campaign contributions.
3. A bill placing wood pulp and print paper on the free list.
4. An anti-injunction bill.

The first session of the Sixtieth Congress commenced at noon, December 2, 1907, and from that time until January 7, when Congress reconvened, after the holiday recess the House was in actual session just

---

[1] *Congr. Record*, June 5, 1908.

fourteen hours and five minutes. During that time the House adjourned for two weeks on account of the holiday recess. Up to the 24th day of March the House was in session ninety days. The average daily length of each session was three hours and sixteen minutes. From the beginning of the session until the 24th day of March only three bills of public importance had been passed, to wit:

An act providing for an immigration station in Philadelphia, and appropriating $250,000 therefor;

The urgent deficiency appropriation bill; and

The bill to increase the efficiency of the personnel of the Life-Saving Service.

Up to that time only one joint resolution had been passed, to wit, a resolution inviting other countries to send representatives to the International Congress of Tuberculosis.

The above bills and the above joint resolution represent the sum total of the activities of the Sixtieth Congress for the first four months of the session which closes to-day.

There is not much a minority can do to compel legislation on the part of the majority. A minority, however, has certain rights under the Constitution which can not be taken away. Among these rights is a right to demand roll calls, and this right the minority have asserted from the 24th day of March until to-day.

On the 24th day of March, 1908, Mr. Williams, the minority leader, on behalf of the Democratic minority, demanded the enactment of certain legislation. [His speech on that occasion is given on p. 271.]

The first roll call demanded by Mr. Williams in pursuance of his announced purpose occurred on March 30, just two months prior to the adjournment date, and the period of the activity of the Sixtieth Congress commenced also on that date. During the remainder of the Session following the inauguration of the aggressive campaign of the Democrats, under the leadership of Mr. Williams, for needed legislation between the 30th day of March and the 30th day of May the House passed thirty-one important public bills and four important public joint resolutions. During that period of time the Committee on Rules exerted its strength against the aggressive policy of the minority leader and, among other rules, it reported out the following, all of which were passed by a strict party vote:

(P. 4462.) Mr. Payne, from the Committee on Rules, reported out an order for the consideration of H. R. 233 for the distribution of the President's message; and

(P. 4467.) Moves closure of debate.

(P. 4495.) Mr. Dalzell, from the Committee on Rules, brought in a rule the effect of which was to revoke the previous unanimous consent of the House for eight hours of debate on the District appropriation bill, allowing two hours only.

(P. 4513.) A sweeping rule was brought in by Mr. Dalzell, which provided that all Senate amendments to general appropriation bills should be agreed or disagreed to en bloc. The rule also provided that a motion for a recess should be a privileged motion. It also provided for closing debate by motion in the House before going into the Committee of the Whole — the motion not to be subject to debate or amendment. In his speech reporting this rule Mr. Dalzell admitted that the rule was brought in for the purpose of counteracting Mr. Williams's tactics. [See p. 273.]

(P. 4675.) A rule was brought in declaring recesses in advance from day to day for the current week. It also provided for the closing of debate on the naval appropriation bill.

(P. 4684.) A rule was reported providing that whenever a general appropriation Bill is reported favorably from the committee on the bill it shall be in order to apply to it in the House a motion to suspend the rules under the conditions prescribed in Rule XXVIII, except a vote shall be by a majority instead of two-thirds.

The above are some of the arbitrary rules brought in to counteract the effect of the tactics of the minority leader. More time was consumed in discussing and in voting on the above rules than would have been required to have discussed and to have passed bills on all the matters referred to by Mr. Williams on the 24th day of March.

On the 26th day of March the President sent to Congress a special message advising, among other things, in substance, the legislation demanded by the minority leader. The Democrats, under the leadership of Mr. Williams, compelled the adoption of an employers' liability bill, which was approved April 22, 1908, and is known as "Public bill No. 100."

The other three demands of the minority leader have not been complied with by the Republicans.

PUBLICITY OF CAMPAIGN CONTRIBUTIONS

The Republican majority, in pretended compliance with the Democratic demands for publicity of campaign contributions, compelled the passage by a strict party vote in the House of Representatives on the 12th day of May, 1908, of the following bill:

An act (H. R. 20112) providing for publicity of contributions made for the purpose of influencing elections at which Representatives in Congress are elected, prohibiting fraud in registrations and elections, and providing data for the apportionment of Representatives among the States.

The above measure is a combination of the McCall publicity bill, the Federal election bill, and an effort to take the preliminary steps toward reducing Southern representation in the House of Representatives. It was passed through the House against a protest of the Democrats, and with the knowledge that it could not possibly under any consideration pass the Senate. The country was demanding an act providing for publicity of campaign contributions. The investigations of the life-insurance companies in New York, recently finished, disclosed the necessity of legislation of this character. The tremendous corrupting influences of contributions by the Standard Oil Company, the steel trust, the life-insurance companies, and other great corporations of the Republican campaign funds from 1896 to date discloses the immediate necessity for publicity. This legislation was universally demanded. The bill met its fate in the Senate, as predicted in the House, on the 28th day of May — two days ago. It was impossible to get it through the Senate with the objectionable provisions attached.

I quote from a part of the debate in the Senate on that day on the subject. (*Congressional Record*, p. 7505, first session Sixtieth Congress):

Mr. CULBERSON. There is another important matter, Mr. President, which the Senator, I trust, will pardon me for calling his attention to at this time, measures which are pending with reference to the publicity of campaign contributions. I ask the Senator if we may expect any legislation on that subject at this session?

Mr. ALDRICH. I am also without authority to speak for anybody but myself. There is a measure pending in the Committee on Privileges and Elections which comes here from the House of Representatives, and I can only say, as far as I am personally concerned, if the Senator desires a vote on that measure this afternoon or any hour to-day or to-morrow, without further debate, after the pending conference report is disposed of, I certainly shall make no objection to that request.

Mr. CULBERSON. Does the Senator refer to what is known as "the McCall publicity bill?"

Mr. ALDRICH. I refer to the bill which came here on that subject from the House of Representatives, and which is now pending in the Committee on Privileges and Elections.

Mr. CULBERSON. But my inquiry was with reference to a publicity bill pure and simple, unmixed with other political matters.

Mr. ALDRICH. The publicity bill that is before the Senate is associated with other provisions in regard to changes in election laws. The Senate cannot disassociate those two items. It the Senator desires legislation upon the subject, of course it must be legislation with the concurrence of the House of Representatives, and those two things cannot be separated. Of course, if we should agree to take a vote upon the subject and fix a time and the Senate should disagree to that provision, then the matter would be in conference. But I am quite willing, speaking for myself, to fix a time immediately after the disposition of the pending conference report for a vote upon the House proposition without further amendment.

Mr. CULBERSON. The Senator, then, I assume, so far as he is concerned — and of course we know the extent to which he speaks — is unable to give us any assurance that a publicity bill pure and simple, unmixed with the bill, I will state frankly, concerning representation, will be acted upon at this session and be passed.

Mr. ALDRICH. There is no possible way in which the Senate can bring the matter to a test vote except by taking up the House bill, so far as I can see. If we are to have effective legislation upon the subject, it must be, as I said before, by concurrence of the two Houses; and I shall join with pleasure the Senators upon the other side, if they desire to have a time fixed for a vote upon that proposition, in acceding to their request.

Mr. BACON. With the permission of the Senator from Texas, I desire to make a suggestion to the Senator from Rhode Island in that connection. There are some things in which parties and Senators are at variance. Of course we recognize that there are some things in which there is controversy, some things in which there is a diversity of opinion and of wish. There are other things in which there is, on the part of Senators of both political parties, a profession of unanimity of purpose and of desire.

Now, both parties represented in this Chamber, and those outside of this Chamber who are recognized as the leaders of the parties in the country at large, avow that they are at one upon one subject, that they are in perfect unison and accord on the subject of the requirement of publicity in connection with campaign funds and contributions.

Mr. ALDRICH. Will the Senator from Georgia state to whom he refers? I would be glad to have the Senator state definitely to whom he refers as the leaders of the two parties.

Mr. BACON. I can only speak of what appeared in the press. I am not speaking otherwise than what has been given out in an authoritative manner. There are some who in the public press assume to be leaders and express themselves in that way. But I am not speaking of that except simply by way of a side matter. I am speaking about what concerns us in this Chamber, to wit, the profession on the part of Senators on each side of the Chamber that we are in favor of the passage of a law which shall make public the contributions for campaign purposes prior to an election. I suppose there is no Senator here who will rise in his place and say he does not favor that.

Now, that being a matter in which we are professedly in absolute accord, the suggestion I wish to make to the Senator is that if in truth we are in accord, if it is true that in good faith that profession is made, then the matter which is thus without controversy can be easily disposed of without debate and without reference to committees or anything else. We can pass the measure in five minutes if it is limited to the publicity feature, whereas the Senator well knows that to attach to it a matter which is in controversy and about which there is not a concord of sentiment it must necessarily at this time defeat the one about which there is no diversity of opinion.

That being the case, I suppose of course it has occurred to the Senator — but I thought I would take the liberty of suggesting it — that the plain, simple way, we desire really to carry out our professions relative to requiring publicity of campaign contributions, is to limit our consideration and our action to that matter about which there is professedly no diversity of opinion.

I said I supposed there was no Senator in this Chamber who would rise in his place and say that he did not favor the publicity bill. Then I would ask every Senator to ask himself the question whether it is acting in good faith to attach to that measure relative to publicity another measure which does produce controversy and about which we are disagreed and the inevitable consequence of which must be to defeat that which they profess a desire to accomplish.

It it be true that our profession is sincere on both sides, if it be true that each of us, without exception, favors the enactment of a law which shall require publicity as to contributions for campaign funds, why is it that we cannot make good that profession by an act which it is easy for us to accomplish by simply saying that we will pass a bill which shall relate to that and to nothing else?

Mr. CULBERSON. Mr. President, I am obliged to the Senator from Georgia for the suggestion which he has made and to which no reply so far has been made by the Senator from Rhode Island, to whom I yield if he desires to make a reply now. If he does not see proper to reply further, I assume — and if my assumption is not well founded, I hope that I may be corrected — that there is no possibility of passing an anti-injunction bill at this session of Congress, nor is there any probability or any possibility of passing a bill providing for the publication of campaign contributions, pure and simple.

WOOD PULP AND PRINT PAPER

No attempt was made to pass this legislation so universally demanded by the newspapers of the country. A committee was appointed to investigate the matter. The method usually adopted for the postponing of legislation is by the appointment of committees. The committee met and heard the complaints of the publishers. They are still meeting. The investigation is not over.

THE ANTI-INJUNCTION BILL

No attempt was made to pass this legislation. The majority leader [Mr. Payne], however, introduced the following bill:

A bill (H. R. 21359) relating to injunctions.

Be it enacted, etc., That hereafter no preliminary injunction or restraining order shall be granted by any judge or court without notice to the party sought to be enjoined or restrained, unless it shall appear to the satisfaction of the court or judge to whom application for such injunction or restraining order is made that the immediate issue of such injunction or restraining order is necessary to prevent irreparable damage.

SEC. 2. That any such injunction or restraining order granted shall contain a rule on the opposite party to show cause within five days why such injunction or restraining order shall not be continued.

The above bill may therefore be considered to be the Republican measure relating to injunctions. I submit that if enacted into law it would not afford the slightest relief.

The Democratic minority in the House has done all it could to compel the enactment of the legislation so universally demanded on these questions. We are willing to go to the country on the record we have made. The charge that the Democratic party as represented in Congress will not follow a leader has been answered on all of the above questions. The party was united always and presented a solid front to the enemy.

The only measure passed by the Republicans in response to the universal demands of the people was an employers' liability bill of doubtful constitutionality. If its constitutionality had been clear it probably would not have been by the majority permitted to pass.

REPRESENTATIVE J. S. WILLIAMS ANNOUNCES HIS POLICY [1]

[The following extracts embody illustrations of the progress of the attempt of Mr. Williams to force certain action by the House. On March 24, he announced his policy. Thereafter there was much debating combined with the dilatory tactics. Special rules were brought in on April 4, April 20, and other days for the purpose of shackling the opposition; and on May 13, Mr. Williams compared his methods with those of earlier filibusters. The incidental illustration which this action affords in the matter of rules and practice in the House is very important.]

MR. WILLIAMS. Now, Mr. Chairman, I believe that the country, and I believe that the Members of the House upon the Republican side of the aisle will agree with me that, acting as minority leader, thus far this session I have given the majority perfectly "smooth sailing." I have not wanted to be regarded as factious; I have not wanted the country to think that the minority on this side was trying to assume responsibility for legislation. I knew that responsibility rested with the majority, and I did not want to appear to coerce the majority — and very little coercing can the minority do — until that majority had made absolute demonstration before the country of the fact that it does not intend to do anything at this session of Congress. [Applause on the Democratic side.] And that, too, notwithstanding the fact that your President has issued a programme that he calls upon you to execute, and notwithstanding the fact that the distinguished gentleman from Iowa [Mr. Hepburn] announced early in the session that unless you did execute that programme somebody was going to "get run over" and "get hurt."

I have waited like a Democratic lamb ready for the slaughter, waiting for the Republican party to do something. I have finally come to the conclusion that the Republican party in this House has forgotten how to do anything; it has become the party of negation, of passivity, and, as

[1] *Congr. Record*, Mch. 24, 1908.

far as I can see, has no idea of doing anything. [Applause on Democratic side.] It is plain now that without some method of parliamentary coercion you are going to be deaf to every demand of the country. The minority can not exercise much power, but it has some power, and I want to make the announcement now, that from this moment on to the balance of this session this is not going to be a lie-easy, wait-on-the-enemy campaign [applause on the Democratic side], and that the little parliamentary power the minority has under the rules is going to be exercised. The minority has a right to refuse unanimous consent to legislation. It has the right to call for the yeas and nays upon every affirmative matter of legislation. I now make the announcement that no requests for unanimous consent from that side of the aisle, unless it be to adjourn or to take a recess — in which two cases I believe it is not from a parliamentary standpoint necessary to have unanimous consent — will not be granted during the balance of this session until the majority shows that it is alive to the demands of the country sufficiently to report for consideration in this House, or to give me satisfactory assurance that they will report for consideration, the following bills:

First, an employers' liability bill. [Applause on the Democratic side.] You have been wasting too much time over it. You have been permitting your Judiciary Committee to have hearing upon hearing, and you have been using that bill merely as a buffer in order to prevent hearing upon other essential legislation before that committee, which legislation you hope to evade.

Second, I shall refuse unanimous consent until you report to this House for its consideration some publicity of campaign contributions bill [applause on the Democratic side], whether it be the bill offered by the gentleman from Missouri [Mr. Rucker] or some other bill. I care not whose name is attached to it, Republican or Democrat.

Third, I shall refuse unanimous consent for any request upon that side of the Chamber until the Ways and Means Committee of this House, in response to the overwhelming demand of the entire newspaper and magazine fraternity of this country, Republican as well as Democrat, shall bring to the consideration of this House a bill for free wood pulp and free print paper. [Applause on the Democratic side.]

Fourth, I shall make the same declination until the Clayton bill, now pending before the Judiciary Committee, or some other bill embodying like provisions, shall have been reported out of that committee for the consideration of this House. What the Clayton bill does is this: It prevents mere ex parte and temporary injunctions, where only one side has been heard from, acting as a supersedeas of a law passed by a sovereign State.

I do not deny the right, upon final hearing of the injunction when it is made permanent, to set aside a State law, if in the opinion of a Federal court it violates the Constitution of the United States, but I do deny the right, upon a mere ex parte hearing by means of a temporary injunction without hearing the State's side at all, of a subordinate court of the United States to sit in judgment on the constitutionality of the legislation of a sovereign State. [Applause on the Democratic side.] I am reinforced in that opinion by the fact that under the original judicial act the courts had no such power, and for years and years afterwards had no such power, and could not issue an injunction until they had heard both sides, with reasonable notice to both sides. Mr. Chairman, in order that there may be no misunderstanding about that, and how far I am going, I desire to read this Clayton bill, though I do not insist upon this particular bill. Bring in a bill in the name of the chairman of the committee; bring in a bill in the name of a Republican, claim the credit for it, go before the country and get the credit for it — you have a right to do it; that I admit, and I would be glad to see you do it, for I am never better satisfied than at the unusual spectacle of the Republican party serving the country. [Laughter and applause on the Democratic side.]

Thomas Jefferson said we ought to preserve the rights of the States as the best security for individual liberty and local self-government. He also stated that we ought to guard with equal care the delegated powers of the Federal Government as our only safeguard for national independence and national peace and progress. I would not take from the Federal Government one of the powers that have been delegated to it. I would not for a moment join in an attack upon the courts of the United States for declaring a State law or a Federal law unconstitutional when in their honest opinion they deem it to be so, but I do say that it is as little as any man who loves his State and believes in local self-government can demand to ask that no mere subordinate Federal court should exercise this newly derived power to set aside an act of a State upon a mere ex parte hearing from the attorney and the witnesses of a railroad corporation or of anybody else, much less to forbid a State to be heard in its own defense. [Applause on the Democratic side.] Now, Mr. Chairman, if after some time I do not notice signs of amendment on that side of the Chamber and a disposition to do something — to quit this policy of passivity and mere negation and "standpatism" — if I do not note some disposition to awake to the idea that you are representatives of the American people and ought to be doing something in their interests, then I shall use about the only other power that the minority has, and that is to call for a yea-and-nay vote upon every affirmative proposition, however insignificant, presented to this House for passage. [Applause on the Democratic side.]

REPORT OF A SPECIAL RULE, APRIL 4, 1908

Mr. Dalzell. Mr. Speaker, I submit the following privileged report from the Committee on Rules.

18

The SPEAKER. The gentleman from Pennsylvania submits a report from the Committee on Rules, which the Clerk will report.

The Clerk read as follows:

Resolved, That immediately upon the adoption of this rule, and at any time thereafter during the remainder of this session, it shall be in order to take from the Speaker's table any general appropriation bill returned with Senate amendments, and such amendments having been read, the question shall be at once taken without debate or intervening motion of the following question: "Will the House disagree to said amendments en bloc and ask a conference with the Senate?" And if this motion shall be decided in the affirmative, the Speaker shall at once appoint the conferees, without the intervention of any motion. If the House shall decide said motion in the negative, the effect of said vote shall be to agree to the said amendments.

And further, for the remainder of this session the motion to take a recess shall be a privileged motion, taking precedence of the motion to adjourn, and shall be decided without debate or amendment.

And further, during the remainder of this session, it shall be in order to close debate by motion in the House before going into Committee of the Whole, which motion shall not be subject to either amendment or debate.

[Applause on the Republican side.]

Mr. SULZER. Mr. Speaker, would it not be well to add to that, "That hereafter the Democrats shall have nothing more to say?" [Laughter.]

Mr. DALZELL. Mr. Speaker, the purpose of this rule, like the purpose of the rule that was introduced yesterday, is to expedite the public business.

Mr. WILLIAMS. Mr. Speaker ——

The SPEAKER. Does the gentleman from Pennsylvania yield to the gentleman from Mississippi?

Mr. DALZELL. Yes.

Mr. WILLIAMS. I wish to ask the gentleman a question. I wish to ask, before we proceed, whether the minority members of the Committee on Rules will be accorded the usual twenty minutes?

Mr. DALZELL. They will not.

Mr. WILLIAMS. They will not! I just wanted the House and the country to know that fact before we start this debate.

Mr. DALZELL. As I say, the purpose of the rule is to expedite the public business and release the House from the grasp of this idiotic filibuster inaugurated by the gentleman from Mississippi [applause on the Republican side]; to prevent the waste of public time at the public expense [laughter on the Democratic side and applause on the Republican side]; to enable the majority to consider and enact into law the great supply bills upon which the existence of the Government depends. [Laughter on the Democratic side and applause on the Republican side.]

Mr. Speaker, let me explain at some length, perhaps, this rule.

Mr. SULZER. It needs explanation.

Mr. DALZELL. I do not think I could make an explanation that would reach the gentleman from New York. [Laughter on the Republican side.]

Mr. SULZER. Not on anything like this.

Mr. DALZELL. When the House is acting in the usual orderly and decent way in the conduct of its business, when a general appropriation bill with Senate amendments comes over to the House it is taken from the Speaker's table by unanimous consent, and the Senate amendments are concurred in or disagreed to. This is the ordinary courteous way of doing business between the two Houses. That is the orderly method whereby the minds of the two Houses are brought together and law is enacted. But if unanimous consent be not granted, if the minority of the House be indulging in useless obstruction of public business in a disgraceful filibuster, then the bill must in the natural course go to the Committee on Appropriations. When it comes back from the Committee on Appropriations a motion to go into Committee of the Whole for the consideration of its report is subject to the statesmanlike demand of the yeas and nays on the motion. Nay, more. There may be possibly three demands for the yeas and nays on the motion to go into Committee of the Whole, on the previous question, and possibly on another motion. After the bill has been treated in the Committee of the Whole and the usual statesmanlike call for tellers and other dilatory proceedings have been indulged in, it comes back into the House and it may be subject to hundreds of calls of the roll if there be so many Senate amendments, and the call of the roll on the adoption of the previous question, a call of the roll on the adoption of the report of the Committee of the Whole, and so it will be observed that it is in the power of the minority in the exercise of an abused constitutional right to obstruct the business of the House, waste the people's time and the people's money, and all for no purpose save delay. [Applause on the Republican side.]

Another provision of this rule is that from this time forward a motion to take a recess shall be a privileged motion and take precedence of the motion to adjourn, and not be subject either to amendment or debate. In this way it will be in the power of the majority to cut off many of these useless roll calls. A further provision is that it shall be in order to close debate by motion in the House before going into Committee of the Whole, which, I think, outside of this rule, would be a sensible rule at all times.

Now, Mr. Speaker, the gentleman from Mississippi [Mr. Williams] says that he is not indulging in any filibuster. Does he believe that he can fool the people of this country by any such statement as that?

Does he believe that the people in this country can be persuaded that any principle is involved in a demand for the yeas and nays on the approval of the *Journal* and then voting for the approval of the *Journal?* Can any man conceive of a more asinine performance than that? [Applause on the Republican side.] Does he believe that he can fool the people of this country; that there is any principle involved in a demand for the yeas and nays on a motion to go into Committee of the Whole to consider the passing of the great supply bills on which the existence of the Government depends? Does he believe that he can persuade the people of this country that there is any principle involved in a call for the yeas and nays on a motion to adjourn at half past nine in the evening?

The gentleman from New York is complained of because he spoke of this performance as puerile. Nay, it is childish and a disgrace to grown men of full stature. [Applause on the Republican side.] What a sweet little story we heard yesterday about old black Lucy and little Johnny at Grand Junction running away from a Chinese gong! I could not help thinking of what a wave of pride would have passed over that old black Lucy's face could she have foreseen little Johnny rising to the heights of a sublime statesmanship in demanding the yeas and nays on a motion to adjourn in the House of Representatives. [Laughter on the Republican side.]   ·

After playing all day, little Johnny is unwilling to take his dolls and dishes and go home without the exhibition of this last piece of statesmanship in calling for the yeas and nays on a motion to adjourn.

Mr. Speaker, I now move the previous question.

Mr. SULZER. Mr. Speaker, will the gentleman yield to me for two minutes?

Mr. DALZELL. No; I will not yield to the gentleman for two seconds. [Prolonged laughter and applause on the Republican side.]

Mr. SULZER. That is because the gentleman does not dare to do it.

The SPEAKER. The question is on ordering the previous question.

DISCUSSION ON THE BRIDGE BILL, MAY 13, 1908

MR. TOWNSEND. Mr. Speaker, this is what is known as the "omnibus bridge bill." It is a bill which contains all of the bridge bills which have been sent to the Committee on Interstate and Foreign Commerce and which have received a favorable report from that committee and have been indorsed by the Secretary of War. All are to be constructed under the provisions of the law known as the "general bridge law of 1906." I do not understand that there is any objection to the bill, and therefore, believing as I do that everybody understands it, I will reserve the balance of my time.

Mr. ADAMSON. Mr. Speaker, the bill was put in this shape in order to insure consideration of all projects for bridges which were pending before the Committee on Interstate and Foreign Commerce. Exigencies in the House are such, at this time, that it was necessary to resort to this device in order that Members might secure all their projects. Therefore we took a bridge bill which came from the Senate and attached to it by amendment every single meritorious bridge proposition that was pending before the committee, thus forming this omnibus bill. It is a good bill in its present shape, and it is a necessary to pass it in this way in order to secure all these bridges. I request gentlemen on this side not to regard its origin on the other side as a badge of suspicion, but to accept it as being all right, and, notwithstanding the circumstances, to vote for the bill. [Applause.] I have no request, Mr. Speaker, for further time ——

Mr. WILLIAMS. I will take a minute or two.

Mr. ADAMSON. Mr. Speaker, I yield to the gentleman from Mississippi such time as he wishes to use.

Mr. WILLIAMS. Mr. Speaker, if I had been wanting a mathematical demonstration of the fact that I had been engaged in saving the public time and expediting the public business, this bill would have furnished me with it. It contains twenty-three bridges. Ordinarily these twenty-three bridges would have come up each as a separate bill; something like ten minutes would have transpired in asking unanimous consent and in inquiries as to whether the bill conformed with the provisions of the general law, as to whether it was unanimously reported by the committee, and in the gentleman offering it explaining why that particular bridge was requisite. If ten minutes had not been required, five would have been required on each. Twenty-three times ten is two hundred and thirty minutes. Twenty-three times five is a hundred and fifteen minutes.

Now, we are going to get twenty-three bridge bills through in forty minutes of debate, if all the time upon that side is consumed — and I take it for granted that it will not be — and if all the time on this side be consumed — and I take it for granted that it will not be — plus thirty-five minutes of time necessary to call the roll, making a total of seventy-five minutes, a saving, Mr. Speaker, of forty minutes of the people's time on one calculation and a hundred and fifty minutes of the people's time on another calculation. [Laughter.] Now, Mr. Speaker, I hope I will hear no more from the leader of the majority about our wasting the public time when we are expediting it in this remarkably expeditious manner. Not only that, but we have accomplished the same purpose in connection with pensions. We used to stand here and pass one little pension bill at a time, and now under this new régime you put them all in one, and we pass them after forty minutes' debate and thirty-five minutes of roll call. There never has been anything that hurried up public business equal to the mustard-plaster policy that has been applied to the Republican body politic by the Democratic party during this Congress.

Mr. GILLETT. Will the gentleman from Mississippi permit a question?

Mr. WILLIAMS. If the gentleman wants to ask a question germane to the bill which I am discussing, I will be glad to answer.

Mr. GILLETT. It is germane to your argument.

Mr. WILLIAMS. Of course the argument is germane to the bill.

Mr. GILLETT. I want to ask the gentleman if he thinks this is a good way to legislate, to combine a great number of bills, so that if one vicious bill is there, you have got to vote down all the good bills in order to defeat that?

Mr. WILLIAMS. Mr. Speaker, I have been admonished by the leader of the Republican party on this floor and by the Speaker's rules deputy from Pennsylvania that the Democratic Representatives are not Members of the House except nominally, and that the Republican party is "responsible for all omissions and commissions." If this be a bad method of legislation, as the gentleman from Massachusetts would infer, then by the confession of the majority leader this is a Republican bad way of doing business. I am not at all responsible for it. The galled jade can wince, my withers are unwrung. Now, this morning, Mr. Speaker, the gentleman from New York [Mr. Payne] referred to my calling the roll upon motions to take a recess and upon motions to adjourn, and said the framers of the Constitution never had an idea that a man like that would be here!

When I first came to Washington as a Representative it was as a Member of the Fifty-third Congress, and the great Thomas B. Reed was minority leader at that time. He organized a real filibuster, not a movement like this. This movement is for the purpose of coercing the majority into legislating. But he organized a real filibuster — that is, to prevent the majority from doing anything, even routine business. And what do you reckon was the reason that he gave to the country for his filibuster? It was that he was going to force the Democratic majority to manacle the Republican minority, in order that he might be justified in history for having manacled the Democratic minority when he was Speaker! And day after day the roll was called upon the adoption of the *Journal*, upon every motion that was or could be made; unanimous consent was refused upon everything; the point of no quorum was made on every occasion. I just happened this morning to be reminiscing a bit, and, with the help of the gentleman from New York [Mr. Fitzgerald], I came on the proceedings of July 8, 1892, in the *Congressional Record*, page 5920, a yet earlier period than I have just referred to, and at that time the distinguished gentleman from New York [Mr. Payne] was not the Republican leader, but he was a distinguished man in the councils of the party and was doing their agreed work.

Upon that occasion a bill for the government of Utah was brought up, providing for the manner of electing delegates, and all that. When the bill was finally passed it was passed with only one vote in opposition. There sprang to his feet upon that occasion, when the motion was made by the gentleman from Tennessee [Mr. Washington] to suspend the rules and pass the bill, the gentleman from New York [Mr. Payne], and I find recorded:

Mr. PAYNE. I move that the House do now adjourn.

The SPEAKER. The gentleman from Tennessee had been recognized to make a motion to suspend the rules and pass the bill that he has indicated.

Mr. PAYNE. I supposed that the gentleman had made the motion and it was pending.

Showing that he was not only frequent, but premature. Then the bill was read. Then the gentleman from New York [Mr. Payne] said:

Mr. Speaker, I make the motion that the House do now adjourn.

Who has heard me move "that the House do now adjourn?" Who has heard me make the point of no quorum? At that time Mr. Payne and other Republicans made it all the time, and the Republican leader announced that the "Democrats must keep a quorum here" themselves, as the Republicans were not going to help them do so.

We go down in this pleasant history and find after the gentleman had made his motion to adjourn, and that motion had been defeated, the gentleman from New York [Mr. Payne] said:

I ask for a division.

The House divided, and there were — ayes 31, noes 134.

Mark the paucity of ayes! The gentleman said that he did not understand that the forefathers had "anticipated" me or anybody that would come to the House and call for the yeas and nays, and move divisions and tellers, except when they really did want them and had a large crowd of people behind them ready to enforce legislation or negation of legislation. But *revenons à nos moutons*. After that announcement was made, of 31 to 134, the gentleman from New York [Mr. Payne], in his desire to accelerate the public business, arose and said:

I ask for tellers.

Tellers were refused, only 31 voting in favor thereof.

Mark once more the noble thirty-one only! But the gentleman from New York, who apparently also was not "anticipated by the forefathers," upon a proposition where he could not even get tellers, much less the yeas and nays (and who has heard of my failing to get the yeas and nays when I asked for them this year?), the gentleman from New York, in those historic days, rose and said:

I ask for tellers.

They were refused — not a sufficient number.

Then he said:

I demand the yeas and nays.

Great Hercules! Think of it! The yeas and nays! The question was ordered on the yeas and nays and they were refused — not a sufficient number.

Then the gentleman from New York [Mr. Payne] arose — a much more replete and complete parliamentarian than I — and I find recorded:

Mr. PAYNE.   I demand tellers on ordering the yeas and nays.

Who has heard me demand tellers on ordering the yeas and nays? and tellers were ordered on the question of ordering the yeas and nays, because there was a fair Speaker in the chair.   And then:

The House divided, and the tellers reported — ayes 34, noes 158.

Then the gentleman from New York, in his great desire to accelerate and expedite public business and to prove that the forefathers had foreseen him as an expediter and accelerator, said:

I demand a second on the motion to suspend the rules.

Mr. Washington said:

I ask unanimous consent that a second may be considered as ordered.

And then objection was made.

Then the Speaker appointed tellers, the gentleman from New York being one of the tellers.   Then the gentleman from New York said:

I ask that the gentleman from Iowa [Mr. Perkins] be substituted.

[Laughter.]

Why, he was so tired "expediting public business" that he had to get somebody else substituted for him to count as a teller.   Who ever heard of my being tired of expediting public business to the point of physical exhaustion?

Mr. ADAMSON.   I would like to know if that interesting record discloses anything that was ever said about dilatory?

Mr. WILLIAMS.   It does not disclose that anything was *said* about "dilatory."   But, Mr. Speaker, it is an old maxim that actions speak louder than words.   Then I found that when matter was finally voted upon ——

Mr. AMES.   Will the gentleman allow me?

Mr. WILLIAMS.   I want to finish this branch of this very interesting story.   I find there was one vote cast in the negative, and I presume, out of charity, it was the vote of the gentleman from New York. [Laughter and applause.]   Now, I yield to the gentleman from Massachusetts.

Mr. AMES.   Is there not a material difference between the position of the gentleman from New York at that time and the position of the gentleman from Mississippi at this time?

Mr. WILLIAMS. There was; thank God for the difference! I will tell you what the difference was.

Mr. AMES. Will you let me finish my question? Is there anything in the *Record* you allude to there which indicates that the gentleman from New York claimed that he was expediting public business?

Mr. WILLIAMS. Oh, now, Mr. Speaker, why it was not necessary for him to claim it then; he has claimed it, as his constant and chronic habit, only this morning; and it is the modern instance and not the ancient saw that has aroused my discursiveness. All this contention now is to show that nobody should ever do these things except when he wants to defeat a particular bill.

The gentleman says there is a difference. Yes; there is a difference. I am endeavoring and trying to rivet the attention of the country on the fact that I want to make the Republican majority pass legislation that not only we, but the majority of the American people and their own President — accidentally right — wants. [Laughter and loud applause on the Democratic side.] What was he engaged in? What was the great Thomas B. Reed engaged in during the Fifty-second and Fifty-third Congresses, followed by his lieutenants, the gentleman from New York [Mr. Payne] and the gentleman from Pennsylvania [Mr. Dalzell]? Oh, a puny effort, a spiteful effort, with a senseless purpose — to make the majority manacle the minority, when he himself was in the minority. [Applause on the Democratic side.] And he succeeded to a very large extent.

He had, as Speaker, applied the so-called "Reed rules," throttling debate, and since that moment this House has never been a deliberative assembly. He announced to the Democrats, when they came into power, substantially this: "In order to prove to you that much of your criticism of me for throttling debate and preventing deliberation and manacling a minority are unjust, I am going to prove to the country that you can not do business without manacling us, and I am going to refuse all unanimous consents; I am going to call the roll whenever I can find occasion; I am going to make the point of no quorum every time I can; I am going to move to adjourn whenever the rules will allow it; I am going to move to take a recess whenever the rules will allow," and so forth, ad infinitum, on the adoption of the *Journal*, and so forth, and he did it all, until they were forced in a Democratic House to adopt in part, in part only the gag rule for the origination of which [laughter and loud applause on the Republican side] the Republican party still applauds itself, strange to say. [Laughter and applause on the Democratic side.]

Why, Mr. Speaker, into what contempt has the American House of Representatives sunk! The Constitution speaks of three independent, coördinate, separate branches, and then refers to the executive, the judiciary, and the legislative. Do you know what the three separate, independent, and coördinate branches are now? The executive, the judiciary, and the Senate of the United States. [Applause on the Democratic side.] What do you amount to over there, either one of you Republicans, individually? [Laughter.]

Mr. GREENE. What do you amount to?

Mr. WILLIAMS. What do I amount to? I confess I amount to nothing, politically and personally, but then, I am a member of the minority party; but what do you individually amount to, any one of you, in the matter of legislation? [Applause on the Democratic side.]

Why, you have got to the point of actually being afraid to sign a respectful request to your own Speaker to recognize somebody to ask consideration of legislation that you yourselves are in favor of.   Deny it if you dare, and I will prove it on you. You dare not indite a note to him of the most respectful and polite character without having previously obtained his consent. [Applause on the Democratic side.] You have got to the point where you introduce bills to do things; you make speeches in favor of doing them, and you dare not address a billet doux to the Speaker asking him for a chance to vote on them. You dare not lovingly write:

DEAR MR. SPEAKER: I most respectfully and humbly and considerately request that you will permit consideration by the House of H. R. —, introduced by me.

You are going to the country that way, too, are you not? Why, Mr. Speaker, somebody stepped across the aisle this morning and said I had made a humorous speech. I have not made any humorous speech. My speeches have all had a serious purpose. The only humorous thing about these little lectures that I have been delivering is the perplexed gravity with which they are received by the gentleman from New York [Mr. Payne]. [Laughter.] The only man who has been physician enough to successfully diagnose your case is the gentleman from Washington [Mr. Cushman], when he said that we were giving you "mustard-seed politics." We are putting a blister upon you every day that brings a boil unless you assert your individual independence as Representatives sufficiently at least to have the courage to make a request of your own Speaker without previously getting his consent to make the request; then have the modesty and sense of eternal fitness to resign as Members of the House. [Applause on the Democratic side.]

The gentleman from Washington has diagnosed it right. It is mustard-plaster politics, and it is not bringing any blisters over here. The blisters are over there. You say it is puerile; you say it is silly; you say that there is no sense in it; you say it is childish; you say it is vaudeville. Well, then, why do you not laugh. What makes you so infernally serious about it? [Laughter on the Democratic side.] And why do you not do something? You are going to the country after a while and tell them that I "would not let you pass important and popular measures," when I am standing here every day pleading and praying with you that you will legislate. Why, I would pray literally to the Higher Power, that you might do something, except for my recollection of the fact that the Bible says that "the prayer of the righteous man availeth much," and I am afraid that my prayer would not, because I can not class myself that way. But just a few of you that introduced free wood-pulp bills — just a few of you that introduced campaign contribution publicity bills, get up a few little notes and send them in to the Speaker; our petition he already has. Dare you add yours? [Applause on the Democratic side.]

The SPEAKER pro tempore. The time for the gentleman from Mississippi has expired.

Mr. TOWNSEND. Mr. Speaker, I have been entertained on various occasions by the endeavors of the gentleman from Mississippi to apologize for the filibustering course that he has pursued up to date. He never neglects any opportunity of trying to explain himself, and I do not blame him, because I understand some of the trials that he has been undergoing, brought about by the dissatisfaction on his own side, at the senseless policy which he has pursued in this filibuster. [Applause on the Republican side.]

He ought to have gone further in his mathematics to-day, when he was demonstrating how much time he had saved to the House by bringing about a condition which he himself has condemned so many times on the floor, viz., the passage of legislation without giving anyone an opportunity to express himself on the measure. He ought to have gone further and shown that he has saved this House from the Democratic party, as led by the gentleman from Mississippi, from twenty-three roll calls on this bill, which would have aggregated something like eight hundred and five minutes, or eleven hours and a half. He would have imposed upon the House for eleven and one-half hours on such calls could he have had his way and the Republican Rules Committee had not presented the rule for the purpose of allowing us to do business.

Mr. WILLIAMS. Do you not think that before they got through with those roll calls they would have brought in some of this legislation that you and I want, and then I should have stopped?

Mr. TOWNSEND. It is also amusing to me, Mr. Speaker, to notice the audacity (I think perhaps that is the proper word) which the gentleman displays on every occasion when he states what he and his party are proposing to bring to the attention of the majority, certain measures of legislation, nearly all of which, all the sane parts of which, had been presented here from Republican sources, and that part of it which has been reached would have been reached in the orderly procedure of the business of the House.

Now, Mr. Speaker, there have been times when I have become impatient at the action of the House in not doing things which to me seemed necessary.

Yet I have learned since I have been a member of this House that all legislation should be given careful and most considerate attention. I now would like to have certain measures brought up. I am not charging anyone with bad faith because I can not have my way about everything. But I submit, Mr. Speaker, that when the record of this session of the Sixtieth Congress shall have been completed, the Republican party can go before the country with the statement of things done which will redound to the credit of the majority party that has had control of this Sixtieth Congress. [Applause on the Republican side.]

I wish to say further, Mr. Speaker, that this House and the country is not going to be deceived by the statements of gentlemen who are at this time advocating legislation which, if they were in the majority, they would not dare to present. [Applause on the Republican side.] The country should be thankful sometimes for failure of Congress to pass certain proposed bills. It is an easy thing for gentlemen to find fault; it is an easy thing for gentlemen not charged with responsibility to criticise; it is quite a different thing to take charge of positive legislation and carry it to completion.

Mr. SHERLEY. Will the gentleman yield?

Mr. TOWNSEND. I do not wish to yield, because I do not wish to carry on this controversy any further.

Mr. SHERLEY. Will the gentleman enumerate the legislation urged by us and which we would not stand for?

Mr. TOWNSEND. I will take this time to say that you will have an opportunity, as I understand it, to-morrow afternoon to present certain amendments to the currency bill, to present your notions of what you want enacted into law, and I want to see you do it. Instead of advocating your opposition and saying, "We oppose the Republican bill," present a positive scheme that you are willing to stand for and go before the country upon.

Mr. WILLIAMS. Will the gentleman permit an interruption?

Mr. TOWNSEND. I do not want to be interrupted, for I do not want to enter into a controversy that I did not introduce in the House. This discussion was injected not by any desire of mine.

I had not expected to say a word, but I would suggest to the gentleman from Mississippi and to the House that there are certain methods of reform, certain methods for expediting business which would expedite and which could be adopted. One of them is the policy of discussing the questions before the House, instead of giving gentlemen an opportunity to exploit themselves before the country on every possible occasion. [Applause on the Republican side.]

Mr. WILLIAMS. How are we going to discuss a question if you will not let it come before the House?

Mr. TOWNSEND. This bill is before the House, and I apologize for occupying any of the attention of the House in discussing any matter not germane to it. This is a bill which, I take it, everybody is going to vote for, and yet, under the filibuster inaugurated by the gentleman from Mississippi and persisted in by him, we will have to take thirty-five minutes to pass it, and I call for a vote.

REMARKS OF REPRESENTATIVE CLARK [1]

[The power of the organization in the House in controlling legislative action is illustrated in a humorous way in the following discussion, by Mr. Champ Clark of Missouri. This extract will also serve as an example of Congressional humor. It may be noted in passing that in the matter of wit the House is not always very exacting, but is as ready to be amused as an audience at a theatre.]

*　　*　　*　　*　　*　　*　　*　　*

MR. CLARK of Missouri. Let me ask the gentleman a question now, while he is on his feet. Turn about is fair play.

Mr. GROSVENOR. That is right.

Mr. CLARK of Missouri. Are we going to have any river and harbor bill at this session?

Mr. GROSVENOR. If we need one.

Mr. CLARK of Missouri. The gentleman knows that we need it. Don't try to get out of it in that way. [Laughter.]

Mr. GROSVENOR. My recollection is that under a Democratic Congress, during which I had the honor to be on the Committee on Rivers and Harbors, at the end of the second session we passed a moderate river and harbor bill, and a Democratic President vetoed it. Now, last year, at the end of the Fifty-eighth Congress, we passed a large river and harbor bill. Under our new system of contracting we shall not need a new river and harbor bill except for new or comparatively new projects, so that the sundry civil bill will carry the amount of appropriation for the rivers and harbors far in advance of any that the Democrats have ever passed.

Mr. CLARK of Missouri. Now, gentlemen, I want you to bear witness to that testimony. That statement is made ex cathedra. The gentleman well speaks as "one having authority."

Mr. GROSVENOR. But not as a scribe.

Mr. CLARK of Missouri. He belongs to the great triumvirate in this House that runs things, composed of the Speaker and the gentleman from Pennsylvania [Mr. Dalzell] and the gentleman from Ohio. He is one of the "Three Czars," and you men who want anything done for the rivers and harbors in your districts hearken unto his voice, for ac-

[1] *Congr. Record*, Jan. 8, 1906.

cording to his statement just made there is not going to be anything done except on work that has already been started.

Mr. GROSVENOR. I hope the gentleman will not misrepresent the organization of the House. The river and harbor bill is a privileged bill, and does not require the action of the Committee on Rules. I hope the gentleman will remember that in all the future of his life.

Mr. CLARK of Missouri. Yes.

Mr. GROSVENOR. I hope the gentleman will remember that all the future of his life.

Mr. CLARK of Missouri. I will; and I will tell you what else I will remember — that whenever they get up a bill of any importance and get it through the House without the consent of the Committee on Rules I will be willing to exclaim with one of old: "Now, Lord, lettest now Thy servant depart in peace." [Great laughter and applause.] I do not want you kindergarten Congressmen here, especially, to labor under any misapprehension as to what is going to happen to you, because the gentleman from Ohio has told you. If there is any work going on in your district that has to be continued to keep it from going to ruin you will get a little money; but if there is any new work, no matter how important or pressing, you are not going to get a cent for it, because they have not got the money to give. This blessed Dingley bill, the fount of every blessing, has produced a deficiency in the revenues to the amount of sixty or seventy millions of dollars. Now, I will ask the gentleman from Ohio ——

Mr. PAYNE. Now, the gentleman wants to be fair.

Mr. CLARK of Missouri. Certainly.

Mr. PAYNE. Which bill do you refer to?

Mr. CLARK of Missouri. The Dingley bill. If you had a good tariff bill you would have had enough money to carry on these improvements.

Mr. PAYNE. Such a one as the Wilson bill?

Mr. CLARK of Missouri. A revenue-producing bill, such as I would draw if I had the power to do so.

Mr. PAYNE. The Wilson bill, under which we were running behind every year.

Mr. CLARK of Missouri. If the Supreme Court had not held the income-tax provision unconstitutional we would have got plenty of revenue from the Wilson bill.

Mr. PAYNE. I want to say to the gentleman that the income-tax provision would not have produced money enough to make a grease spot under the Wilson bill.

Mr. CLARK of Missouri. The only reason why it would not was stated by Mr. Cockran, of New York, who said that it would have made the wealthy men of New York get into the habit of committing perjury to keep the taxes from being collected on their incomes.

Mr. PAYNE. The gentleman is quoting from a distinguished Demoerat upon that. To return to what I was just saying, as to there not being any deficit this year because there will be no river and harbor bill. It would not make any difference whether there was a river and harbor bill this year or not. All that money would not come out of the Treasury until the end of the fiscal year. In the last session we provided liberally for rivers and harbors, and that money is now being paid out of the money in the Treasury.

Mr. CLARK of Missouri. Now, let me ask you whether there is going to be any public-building bill reported this year? Now, answer that — yes or no.

Mr. PAYNE. I am not a member of that committee.

Mr. CLARK of Missouri. But you are the floor leader in this House.

Mr. PAYNE. If any such bill was brought in here as was brought in during the last Congress I should oppose it with the utmost vigor I have.

Mr. CLARK of Missouri. Gentlemen, I am sorry to see the chairman of the Committee on Ways and Means resort to dodging in this debate. [Laughter.]

Mr. PAYNE. What does the gentleman mean?

Mr. CLARK of Missouri. What I mean is that you you do not tell us frankly whether we are going to have a public-building bill or not.

Mr. PAYNE. I do not know.

Mr. CLARK of Missouri. Why don't you know? [Laughter.]

Mr. PAYNE. Because, like the gentleman from Missouri, I have not been consulted on that subject.

Mr. CLARK of Missouri. Why do you not consult the Speaker and those gentlemen on the Committee on Rules?

Mr. PAYNE. So far as I am concerned, I am not interested in public buildings.

Mr. CLARK of Missouri. Oh, yes; that's it; you have got yours. [Great laughter.]

Mr. PAYNE. The gentleman is right about that. I commenced in a Democratic Congress many years ago.

Mr. CLARK of Missouri. You have been here a long time. When these kindergarten statesmen have sat here as long as you have they will get some too.

Mr. PAYNE. On that I had little experience, and if I were commencing with the "kindergarten class" I would not introduce a bill for a public building in my district.

Mr. CLARK of Missouri. What does the gentleman from Ohio say about a public-building bill? I want to get at the facts. [Laughter.]

Mr. GROSVENOR. On that question I am a single Member of the House of Representatives.

Mr. CLARK of Missouri. Yes, you are; and much more. You are one of the governing trio — one of the ruling elders.

Mr. GROSVENOR. I shall pass upon a public-building bill exactly as I pass upon other questions that come before this House.

Mr. CLARK of Missouri. I will ask you a leading question: Do you know whether it is the intention of the managers of this Congress that there shall not be any river and harbor bill, except as you have described, and there shall be no public-building bill at this session, in order to make buckle and tongue meet?

Mr. GROSVENOR. I do not understand either branch of that question in the affirmative.

Mr. CLARK of Missouri. All right.

Mr. GROSVENOR. I have a suspicion on the river and harbor question, because of an interview given out by the chairman of the committee. As to the public-building question I have no knowledge, no information, and no belief.

Mr. CLARK of Missouri. I want to state to you that unless you gentlemen who want public buildings in your districts and improvements of your rivers and harbors do not break away from and overthrow this Republican machine in the House, which dominates in all things, you are not going to get any at this session of Congress. You can write that on the tablets of your memory now. This is an argumentum ad hominem. I have seen that game played two or three times since I have been here.

CONGRESS AGAIN DEBATING, 1902

[The following articles from the *New York Evening Post* bring out certain important points with respect to the action of Congress. 1. The character of Congressional debate. 2. The importance of permanence of service in Congress, and, 3. Illustrations of slipshod methods in legislation. There is added to these a brief description of the practice obtaining in the House by which members obtain leave to print speeches which have not actually been delivered.]

AN unusual interest has been manifest in the proceedings of either house of Congress for the past few days. One sure sign of this is the increased space which the newspapers have given to Washington dispatches. Congressmen sometimes complain that the press does not report their debates as it formerly did. The fault is in themselves. Let them make their debates interesting, and the newspapers, which always search for interesting reading as they do for hidden treasure, will jump at the chance of printing them. Consider the columns gladly given up to the Cuban debate in the House, and to the arguments on the Chinese Exclusion Bill in the Senate. They show how press reports increase directly as the square of public interest in the doings of Congress.

What has been the secret of this revived attention to Congressional oratory? It is not far to seek. In the first place, these animated discussions of public policy have been free from the deadening influence of a foregone decision on strict party lines. There has been an open give-and-take of argument, and votes have been changed by it. We have not seen a party leader, beaten in his logical contentions, rise and taunt the master of the better reasons with the fact that the heavier battalions were against him, and say, "Well, talk as you will, you are bound to lose when the roll call comes." Now it is the very breath of life for public debate to have this possibility of persuasion in it. Merely to apply "a fine brute majority" is the way not simply to crush your opponents, but to destroy the interest and real significance of debating at all. When men can feel compelled to say, as the honest English Squire did to the able Parliamentary orator of the other party, "You have changed my opinion by your speech, but no man can change my vote," then we need no longer inquire why Congressional debates have decayed, or why public interest in them has declined.

It is obvious that the discussion of the Chinese Exclusion Bill actually brought about a vote in the Senate very different from what would have been cast but for the searching analysis of the measure. Undebated, it would have gone through triumphantly. But it could not stand exposure. Its improprieties and indecencies, its illegalities and absurdities, its lack of business sense and of humanity alike, were so driven in upon the general conviction that it was beaten off the field. The New England conscience rose in revolt, every Senator from that section voting against it except Mr. Lodge. He preferred to side with Tillman and the other advocates of barbarous methods in dealing with the Chinese; but the reason and conscience of New England — indeed, we may say of the Republican party — were against the bill as it passed the House. One could wish for no more complete demonstration of the value of free debate by legislators whose minds are open, and whose votes are at liberty to follow their judgment.

In the House the case has been different, but there, too, we have been given a vivid illustration of the cause of public interest in Congressional proceedings. It is not simply that the subject under discussion is large and important. So was the Philippine Tariff Bill, but it went through amid universal indifference. The reason was that then we had the certainty of a party majority at the end, while debate was limited, and a rigid rule shut out the possibility of so much as offering an amendment. That is the sure way to kill a debate. Of course, men in the Opposition will present their views for the sake of a "record," and in order to put the party in power "in a hole"; but argument for such purposes only is obviously a dead-and-alive affair, and can never have the directness, the fire, the power and point of a speech which may change votes and really affect the course of legislation. Note the great contrast offered by the progress of the Cuban Bill through the House. It was attended by the stir and interest of an uncertain result. Party lines were broken up. Amendments could be and were offered. Tactical positions were eagerly manœuvred for.   Far-reaching, indirect results might follow in national politics.   Hence the kindling and continuous interest with which the debate was followed by press and public; hence the new appeal to the debating power of the members themselves, with the discovery, in some cases, of an unexpected talent; and hence the restoration to the House of a measure of that national attention which used to be fixed upon it as the theatre of great debate.

The example ought not to be lost on those leaders of the House who have the shaping of its methods in their hands.   Let them abolish some of their hard-and-fast rules for stifling debate, or else making it perfunctory.   Let them take the sense of the House freely on all great subjects, instead of so hedging it about that the conquered cause is too often the one really pleasing to the majority, if it could find free expression, as well as to Cato.   Let them open the true parliamentary career for talent by showing the aspiring orator that it is within his power to produce conviction and lead to action.   In a word, let them make Congressional debate what debate ought to be everywhere — a means of bringing out the better reason and the wiser policy — and we shall hear much less of the decadence of Congress, or the growing indifference of the people to what goes on in the Capitol at Washington.

INFLUENCE IN CONGRESS, 1906

WASHINGTON, June 5. — New York's representation in Congress in recent years is something that citizens of the State have not found much pride in talking about.   To all intents and purposes it is wholly unrepresented in the Senate.   This is a matter of common notoriety, and requires no comment.   Its thirty-seven representatives in the House form the largest delegation from any one of the States.   Pennsylvania ranks next with thirty-two; Illinois has twenty-five, Texas sixteen, and Massachusetts fourteen.   Though first numerically, the New York delegation is not first in importance.   How many citizens of New York could name the whole delegation, or even the representatives from New York city?

Representative Perkins of the Rochester district had something to say the other day about the State's past representation in Congress, which has attracted some attention.   He spoke with special reference to the tenure of office of members, and made the point that the men who were sent here after civil service reform principles were established in the Federal Government had retained their offices longer than the representatives of other days, who depended on the spoils system to keep them here.   Mr. Perkins found from an examination of the records that New York State, from the time of its organization down to 1860, was represented by about 600 members of Congress.   Of these, 400, or about two-thirds of the entire number, served only one term in Congress.

One hundred and fifty were able to stay here for two terms. Of the whole 600 that came during the period from 1789 to 1860, only 50 were allowed to remain in Congress more than two terms, and there was only one out of the 600 during the period of seventy years who was elected by his constituents for ten terms in Congress. Mr. Perkins had to confess that he had forgotten the name of that man whose career is so unique in the early history of New York.

Those were the days when members of Congress controlled Federal patronage and eked out their days of political life by the free disposal of jobs to their followers. Mr. Perkins asked this pertinent question: "What does it show when 400 members of Congress, although possessed of this political patronage, were cut off at the end of their first term of Congress? Does it show that political patronage is, as is supposed by some, a means to lengthen political life, or does it show that it is a means of hastening political death?"

From 1860 to 1880 the New York experience was almost precisely similar, but since that time there has been a great change in the length of service on the New York members, and of the members from other States. At the present time only about one-sixth of our delegation are first-term men, and nearly three-fourths have served more than two terms, where formerly two-thirds of the delegation were first-term men. Of the present membership of the whole House, more than one-half have served more than two terms. Whether this change is entirely due to the partial abolishment of the spoils system, or whether electors in the various States have waked up to the fact that ordinarily the longer a man stays here the more important he becomes, and the more power he secures in the House, is not definitely established. Whatever the cause, a distinct tendency on the part of the people to give their representatives in Congress longer tenure of office is noticeable. Mr. Perkins offers this explanation of the change:

"It seems to me that the reasons are perfectly apparent. Our predecessors had unlimited patronage. Where they appointed one man they necessarily disappointed ten men. These men at once formed a coherent body, who said, 'If we can get out the man who is in, the man who is out will get us in.' There was, when a new man came up for nomination to defeat the sitting member, a coherent body of workers who were actuated by the hope that, if they could get their man in, there was a $1,200 job down in Washington waiting for them. Well, there is no use in promising those jobs now, because even the boys in the wards know there are no such jobs to give, and it results that, instead of the constant presence of this united group of men working to get out the sitting member in hopes of furthering their personal interests, a member is left undisturbed unless he has given dissatisfaction to the community as a whole. This is the explanation, it seems to me. It must be the chief and almost the only explanation of the notable fact of the gradually increasing tenure

of office in the House of Representatives during the last twenty years."

Of the present thirty-seven New York members these are chairmen of committees: Payne, Ways and Means; Wadsworth, Agriculture; Southwick, Education; Driscoll, Elections No. 3; Ketcham, Expenditures in the State Department; Sherman, Indian Affairs. Or course, these chairmen are necessarily limited to the twenty-six Republican members of the delegation. Three of these are important committees — Agriculture, Indian Affairs, and Ways and Means.

Mr. Perkins himself is the third man on the Committee on Foreign Affairs, and the ranking member next to the chairman of the Committee on Printing. Mr. Vreeland is the sixth in rank in the Naval Affairs Committee, and is also a member of the Committee on Labor. He is a "big-navy" man and may be chairman of that committee some day. Littauer, of "gloves and gaunts" fame, is a member of the important Appropriations Committee, and has charge on the floor of the House of the legislative, executive, and judicial appropriation measures. None of the New York city men is strongly placed on committees. The city representatives are new men, and, of course, had to give way to men of longer service, and Democratic members of committees are not doing much business under the present organization of the House.

It would be difficult to imagine a person of less consequence than a new member of the House of Representatives in his first term. They are practically negligible quantities, and must do as they are told, or be of little service to their constituents. Mr. Lamar of Florida and Mr. Murphy of Missouri are two shining examples of the fate that befalls the disobedient. Early in the session Mr. Lamar had a row with John Sharp Williams, the minority leader, because he was not placed on the Committee on Interstate Commerce. He kicked over the traces and publicly denounced Mr. Williams on the floor of the House. Since that time, despite his efforts, he has been only a figurehead. Murphy of Missouri is one of the new representatives who came in on the Roosevelt landslide. He beat his Democratic opponent by only thirty-six votes. That narrow squeak, it would seem, should have made him cautious, but he has bucked against the speaker several times at this session. Whether the Republican Congress campaign committee will find it advisable and wise to pay much attention to his very close district in the autumn, falls under the head of debatable questions.

Iowa and Maine are two States that long ago discovered that they would get more than their share of what good things were coming by electing good men and keeping them here. These two States in recent years have exercised a great influence on legislation merely through the length of tenure of their representatives. There are no two more important men in the Senate than Hale of Maine and Allison of Iowa. Representative Hull of Iowa is chairman of the great Committee on Military

Affairs in the House. Hepburn is chairman of the Committee on Inter-state and Foreign Commerce, which this session, at least, has been the most important committee of the House. Lacey of the same State is chairman of the Committee on Public Lands.

Mr. Ketcham of New York has had seventeen terms in the House, not continuous. Speaker Cannon has had sixteen terms, skipping only the Fifty-second Congress. Representative Bingham of Pennsylvania has served fourteen continuous terms, and Mr. Hitt of Illinois has had thirteen continuous terms. Mr. Payne is the next oldest man in point of service. He has had eleven terms, not continuous, however, but skipping the Fiftieth Congress.

SLIPSHOD LEGISLATION, 1903

WASHINGTON, April 5. — "The decadence of the art of legislation" is the term which is applied to the tendency in the last few decades of Congressional history by a public officer who has recently had occasion to make an exhaustive and critical examination of the Federal statutes. The earlier laws, in his opinion, such as those regulating navigation, the internal revenue laws, and the administrative features of the customs laws, are, for the most part, models of construction. They are precise in their wording, comprehensive and exact in providing for all possible contingencies, and so clear and perspicuous as to leave little difficulty in their construction and application.

These were passed, it is cynically suggested, at a time when the surprising notion obtained that the business of the legislative department of the Government was to legislate. The last thirty years have shown a great change in the quality of legislation, not in its purport, but in its workmanship. The statute books have been disfigured by slovenly, ambiguous, and nugatory provisions to an extent that surprises every one who comes to study the matter.

A year or two ago a publishing house issued a compilation of the United States statutes, and in the prospectus summed up the difficulties of the undertaking in these words: "In preparing this compilation the editors have found a number of amusing proofs that the complexity of bills passed was too much even for members of Congress itself to unravel. They have come upon amendments to laws that have been repealed, amendments that overlook previous amendments, new laws that re-enacted existing and forgotten laws, etc."

But even this falls short of an adequate statement of the conditions that exist. For example a law found in 32 Statutes at Large, 786, begins as follows:

An act to amend an act approved March 2, 1895, relating to public printing. *Be it enacted, etc.* That the first and tenth paragraphs of the Printing of January 12, 1895, following the paragraph which reads: "The public printer shall furnish the *Congressional Record* as follows, and shall furnish no others gratuitously in addition thereto," be amended, etc.

It will be noted that the act mentioned in the title is not the one amended by the text, and reference to the statute book shows that these two have no relation whatever to each other. Moreover, the act of January 12, 1895, was not divided into numbered paragraphs at all, so that part of the description furnishes no guide as to where the amendment is intended to be inserted, and is simply misleading. By reading through the twenty-four pages of the law the weary seeker finds in section 73 the language quoted, and thus is able to locate the passage to which the amendment refers.

Another instance might be cited where Congress solemnly repealed certain words in an act designated when no such words, or any of like purport, could be found anywhere in the act.

But the most prolific source of confusion is the mischievous and growing practice, so often attempted during the past weeks, of inserting general legislation in appropriation bills. Some curious results have been brought about by the inhibition in House rule 21: "Nor shall any provision changing existing law be in order in any general appropriation bill or in any amendment thereto." While this is on its face an absolute prohibition, yet in practice it means that any provision can be inserted in an appropriation bill, as long as no member objects. Thus new legislation can be put in by unanimous consent. Since each member's pet measure, if offered in the form of a rider, must run the gantlet of his 386 colleagues, any one of whom could give it a death stroke by rising in his seat and uttering eleven words, he makes it as inconspicuous as possible in phraseology. The House is very frequently willing to let a bit of legislation go through without objection when it does not show on its face that it is a change in the existing law, but a clause would not stand a moment's chance if it said in so many words, "Section 41,144 of the Revised Statutes is hereby amended to read as follows."

Thus comes about an evasion. The provision desired is drawn as if it had no relation to any previous act, and so passed. There are then two provisions, more or less conflicting, on the same subject-matter, and the officers charged with their execution are left to guess how far the later supersedes the earlier. The confusion is carried into almost every department of the Government.

As to a remedy for the evil, the critic already quoted is of the opinion that Congress, in order to consider adequately all measures of needed legislation and mature them with respect to their phraseology, should remain in session for at least nine months in every year. He further believes that the state of affairs which his researches disclose furnishes one of the best possible arguments against Congressional interference in executive matters. Without pointing such a moral as might be drawn from the postal scandal, it is safe to say that if legislators confined their duties to legislating their work would be better done.

While the number of slovenly enactments actually in the statutes is startling enough, those which are headed off in the House and Senate committees are almost past counting. The individual members, who introduce the greater part of their bills at some one's request, and with little scrutiny, do not feel the responsibility of looking up the antecedents of each such piece of legislation. Any one who has examined the mass of reported bills at a session must have noticed the great number of instances in which a committee has recast a bill entirely without changing in any way its purport. For instance, a member is asked by some body of his constituents to put through a bill authorizing the erection of a bridge across a stream in his district. They suppose, and he supposes, that no one ever planned such a bridge before. The bill, therefore, is introduced on the supposition that the project is new, and contains the usual clause authorizing the secretary of war to determine whether the bridge will interfere with navigation. The committee, however, looks up the law, and discovers — what the bill's sponsor should have ascertained before introducing — that a bridge at the same point on the same river was provided for years ago, and all that is necessary is some slight amendment of the former law, or an extension of time. The committee reports the bill with the comprehensive amendment, "strike out all after the enacting clause, and insert the following."

Often enough, the committee or its clerk, has to perform the functions of a teacher of rhetoric, cutting out slipshod English and ambiguities.

The clerks of important committees in the House and Senate are veterans, some of them having served under a half-dozen different chairmen of both political parties, and these men are experts in the technique of legislation. But the clerk of a less important committee comes to that position merely as the private secretary of the chairman, has divided duties, is less experienced, and takes less pride in his work.

The real fundamental difficulty, perhaps, is that a congressman may have the most sound and statesmanlike views as to what he wants to accomplish, and still be careless and neglectful on such points as those described. Some good and wise laws have been tacked to appropriation bills, or have been enacted in apparent ignorance of the existing laws on the same subject. This very fact furnishes an added argument for care for the form as well as the subject-matter of legislation.

GENERAL LEAVE TO PRINT [1]

MR. PAYNE. Mr. Speaker, I move to suspend the rules and agree to the following order, which I send to the desk and ask to have read.

The Clerk read as follows:

Ordered, That general leave to print be granted Members from the adoption of this order until five days after the adjournment of the present session of Congress.

The SPEAKER. Is a second demanded?

Mr. WILLIAMS. I demand a second.

The SPEAKER. Under the rule, a second is ordered. The gentleman from New York is entitled to twenty minutes and the gentleman from Mississippi to twenty minutes.

Mr. PAYNE. Mr. Speaker, I reserve my time.

Mr. WILLIAMS. Mr. Speaker, in my opinion, at all times it is a bad policy to encumber the *Record* with speeches undelivered upon the floor, especially when the speeches do not go out with any notice to the people that they were not delivered here. They are, without that notice, a sort of deception of the people of the United States. If there had been no sharp partisan clash between the two parties this year I would still have objected, as I did successively in the Fifty-eighth Congress, to a resolution of this description. I believe that what purports to have been said upon this floor ought to be said upon this floor, in the presence of one's colleagues, with an opportunity for reply. I believe that especially the habit of printing after Congress has adjourned and printing whatsoever one may evolve out of one's inner consciousness, without any opportunity of reply at all, especially upon the eve of an election, printing anything or everything, is peculiarly an advantage for an unscrupulous man as it is peculiarly unfair to the honest man, because the letter will publish only what he knows or believes to be exactly true. This is a reward, therefore, to men who are unscrupulous, who are dishonest of statement, who are careless and reckless of what they are willing to say. Mr. Speaker, I understand, of course, why this is offered by the leader of the majority at this particular time.

The majority party has pretty nearly gone into commission. It has organized commissions to consider nearly everything. It has abdicated its legislative functions. It has delegated to commissions of one sort or another many, and it is going to delegate to more commissions a great many more, public questions of every description. It has spent unparalleled sums of money belonging to the people, a great deal of it wastefully. It requires very much explanation. It would be cheaper and

---

[1] *Congr. Record,* May 26, 1908.

better for it to be made by a few selected men to whom there would be no opportunity of reply, whose remarks in the *Record* will not be seen by any Democrat, will be printed after adjournment, so that a reply can not be made in such a way as that the reply could be, like the observations themselves, franked to the country. The Republican party, as I said a moment ago, has appointed so many commissions that it had better appoint just one more. In Great Britain when a king goes crazy — and I am not saying that the Republican party is a king, only that it is here in Congress crazy — the great seal is put into commission for some time. After you get through with the currency commission and all the other commissions you have appointed, too numerous for me to remember at this moment, it would be very well for you to appoint one more commission and call it a commission upon Republican defense, and Republican defense through the *Record* after the House has adjourned, with no opportunity to reply to it. [Applause on the Democratic side.]

You have had your day in court just as much as we have had. There have been more of you than there have been of us. You are at least of equal ability with us — or you claim to be, and we will discourteously deny it. The only disadvantage that you have had is that you have had a bad, weak cause, or many bad, weak causes. You have been doing nothing, and you are going now to try to defend the policy of doing nothing. You have proudly, even vauntingly, asserted that you were "responsible for commissions and omissions of legislation." You will have some degree of explanation to make concerning your "commissions," and you will have a great deal of explanation to make concerning your "omissions." Of course you will undertake to say that one reason why you have not done a great many things the country demands and things which your President has demanded and things which Democracy has joined in demanding, was because the Democracy by demanding them, so far as it had the parliamentary power to demand and cry out aloud for them, had "prevented you" from doing them.

Mr. Speaker, it seems to me that in ordinary fairness, in ordinary honesty, if there were no sharp party clash, this sort of resolution ought not to pass this House. I say that one reason why the House of Representatives has sunk so low is this: "Its *Congressional Record* has become so bulky that nobody reads it. The people of the United States get their information of what occurs from the press, and the press tries to be accurate, but it necessarily can not do it. The press, of course, can not be full in its reports.

The reason why the *Congressional Record* is so bulky that nobody can keep up with it is because what goes into it is not what is said upon this floor. In an ordinary Congress 50 per cent of what goes into the *Congressional Record* are things never said upon the floor — put in there under leave to print upon particular bills, under general leave to print, and under orders such as this. I say that this resolution, if carried, is especially unfair and deceitful, not to one another as Representatives alone, but to the American people. To introduce a resolution to allow men to shove into the *Congressional Record* what they please for five days after Congress has adjourned, without any opportunity for anybody to read it and reply to it with equal frankable privilege is disingenuous, if not worse, and I hope that this resolution will not pass. [Applause on Democratic side.]

Mr. Speaker, I reserve the balance of my time.

Mr. PAYNE. Mr. Speaker, I have but a few words to say. It has been the custom of the House always toward the close of the session to grant by unanimous consent general leave to print for a period of from five to ten days. That has been almost a universal custom, and the gentleman while he has been here has assented to it by not making objection. It is more imperative that this resolution pass at this session of Congress because of the three or four weeks of time wasted — it is not necessary to say any longer how or by whom — in the House during the past two months. If that time could have been utilized in general intelligent debate, perhaps there would have been no necessity for this resolution at this time, but it was used otherwise.

VIII

FINANCIAL LEGISLATION

JAMES A. GARFIELD ON REVENUE BILLS [1]

[Under the constitution, the House of Representatives has the exclusive power of introducing bills to raise revenue. Controversies have arisen with the Senate concerning the power of the latter body to propose amendments which would materially alter the character of the original measure. This matter has already been taken up in Mr. McCall's article, on page 135. The following extract from a speech by James A. Garfield, in April, 1872, is important in this connection.]

At the second session of the Forty-second Congress the question of originating revenue bills came up in a new form. This is shown by the following resolution, adopted by the House, April 2, 1872, on the motion of Mr. Dawes, of Massachusetts:

Resolved, That the substitution by the Senate, under the form of an amendment, for the bill of the House, entitled "An Act to repeal existing Duties on Tea and Coffee," of a bill entitled "An Act to decrease existing Taxes," containing a general revision, reduction, and repeal of laws of imposing impost duties and internal taxes, is in conflict with the true intent and purpose of that clause of the Constitution which requires that "all bills for raising revenue shall originate in the House of Representatives"; and that therefore said substitute for the House bill do lie upon the table.

Mr. Garfield made a brief speech on the respective rights of the two houses, but only his remarks on the new question are given.

Mr. Speaker, — The case now before us is new and difficult. I think the same point has never before come into controversy. It raises the question how far the Senate may go in asserting their right to "propose or concur with amendments, as on other bills."

We must not construe our rights so as to destroy theirs, and we must take care they do not so construe their rights as to destroy ours. If their right to amendment is unlimited, then our right amounts to nothing whatever. It is the merest mockery to assert any right. What, then, is

---

[1] See Works of James A. Garfield, I, 698.

the reasonable limit to this right of amendment? It is clear to my mind that the Senate's power to amend is limited to the subject-matter of the bill. That limit is natural, is definite, and can be clearly shown. If there had been no precedent in the case, I should say that a House bill relating solely to revenue on salt could not be amended by adding to it clauses raising revenue on textile fabrics, but that all the amendments of the Senate should relate to the duty on salt. To admit that the Senate can take a House bill consisting of two lines, relating specifically and solely to a single article, and can graft upon that bill in the name of an amendment a whole system of tariff and internal taxation, is to say that they may exploit all the meaning out of the clause of the Constitution which we are considering, and may rob the House of the last vestige of its rights under that clause. I am sure that this House, remembering the precedents which have been set from the First Congress until now will not permit this right to be invaded on such a technicality.

Now I will not say, for I believe it cannot be held, that the mere length of an amendment shall be any proof of invasion of the privileges of the House. True, we sent to the Senate a bill of three or four lines, and they have sent back a bill of twenty printed pages. I do not deny their right to send back a bill of a thousand pages as an amendment to our two lines; but I do insist that their thousand pages must be on the subject-matter of our bill. It is not the number of lines, nor is it — I now respond to my friend from Maine,[1] who asked me a question — nor is it the amount of revenue raised or reduced, of which we have a right to complain. We may pass a bill to raise $1,000,000 from tea or coffee; the Senate may move so to amend it as to raise $100,000,000 from tea and coffee, if such a thing was possible; or they may so amend it as to make it but one dollar from tea and coffee; or they may reject the bill altogether.

Mr. PETERS. May not the Senate add other articles?

If we refer to the practice of the two houses, doubtless the Senate has usually, without any question having been raised by the House, added other articles. And I do not say that this would be trenching on our privileges on a general revenue bill. But the bill on which these amendments were made was in no sense a general revenue bill. It was an act relating exclusively to a single article. There was nothing, either on the title or in the bill itself to indicate that it was intended as a general revenue bill. Furthermore, it was well known that the proper committee of the House were preparing a general bill, in which the whole subject was to be opened for consideration. Considering all the circumstances of the case, and particularly the fact that on the single clause of our bill relating to but one article of taxation, the Senate has ingrafted a general

---

[1] Mr. Peters.

bill, embracing not only the tariff generally, but our whole system of internal taxation, it is clear that the ground we now take is not questionable ground, and it becomes the undoubted duty of the House to stand on its rights, and refuse to consider this bill.

Mr. PETERS. Then allow me to ask the gentleman if the rule is a fixed one, or one in the discretion of the House.

I will say this: it is a fixed rule. If the House has ever slept on its rights it ought not to be now concluded from asserting them because of its past neglect; and if there ever was a time in the history of the government when this House should reclaim and assert its rights, it is now and here, when on the naked lay figure of a two-line bill, the Senate proposes to impose the entire revenue system of the government. If the bill from the Senate now on your table, Mr. Speaker, be recognized by us, we shall have surrendered absolutely, not only the letter, but the spirit of the rule hitherto adopted, and with it our exclusive privilege under the Constitution.

If it be said that this resolution, which the House is asked to adopt, is an unusual one, I answer that the circumstances under which it is proposed are equally unusual. It is well known that the Senate, even in the recess, have been deliberately at work preparing the tariff bill; and they have only been waiting the slight opportunity afforded by the two lines which the House sent them, to initiate and take control of our tariff legislation. It is this course of procedure which the House is called upon to resist.

ANNUAL STATEMENT OF APPROPRIATIONS[1]

[The general character of fiscal legislation, the difficulties confronting the Committee on Appropriations, and the size of the annual appropriations, will be apparent from the annual review of appropriations and expenditures given by Mr. J. A. Tawney, the chairman of the Committee on Appropriations. The reader will note that the Committee on Appropriations has jurisdiction over none of the special appropriation bills, such as that for agriculture, the army, the navy, the post office, etc. The control of these appropriations was distributed among the committees dealing with the subject-matter of these interests in the eighties. This step has greatly complicated fiscal legislation and has made it impossible to have a unified budget.]

MR. TAWNEY said:
Mr. Speaker: The annual expenditures of our Government exceed those of any other government in the world. The work of analyzing the estimates for them, of inquiring into their necessity, together with the

---

[1] *Congr. Record*, May 30, 1908.

needful inquiry into the methods of the Departments in administering and in expending previous appropriations, is rapidly becoming the most important duty and the most prodigious task to be performed in connection with the legislative department of the Government, a task whose magnitude is not appreciated, nor is the labor necessary in its performance understood. It requires constant application from the beginning until the close of the session and the most careful discrimination to prevent needless appropriations for the Federal Government or unauthorized appropriations for the exercise of governmental functions belonging to the States or for the doing of that which belongs exclusively to private interests.

So far as this work has devolved at this session upon the committees of this House having appropriating jurisdiction, I know it has been performed conscientiously and faithfully. Speaking for the Committee on Appropriations, I can say that it has been performed with no other thought or purpose than to supply the actual needs of the public service within the prescribed functions of the Federal Government, without reference to the personal desires of those from whom the increased estimated expenditures or the recommendations for increased appropriations emanated. I would not be worthy of the position I occupy on the Committee on Appropriations if I did not acknowledge the gratitude I owe to its members for their loyal support and the efficient and intelligent service they have rendered in the committee's endeavor to prevent needless or extravagant appropriations or the authorization of new services outside of the legitimate functions of the Federal Government.

Mr. Speaker, with the passage of this bill all the great supply bills of the Government for the fiscal year 1909 will have been passed, and the session will practically end. It is a custom as well as a duty we owe to the people to state, at the close of each session, the amounts appropriated and the estimated revenues for the fiscal year for which the appropriations have been made. In doing so the people are afforded an opportunity to know and compare our appropriations with those of previous sessions, and to determine whether or not they have been wisely or unwisely made; whether or not they are extravagant in amount, or are no larger than are necessary to meet the needs of the public service.

The responsibility of the House of Representatives in respect to the appropriation of money from the Federal Treasury is a direct responsibility we owe to the people. It is a non-partisan responsibility. No political party, when in control of the Government, can have any other policy in respect to appropriations than that of appropriating no more and no less than is necessary for the exercise of the constitutional functions of the Government. To us, as the direct representatives of the people, the Constitution intrusts the power and the duty of originating the bills that authorize the distribution of the public revenue.

THE DEMOCRATIC FILIBUSTER

It is a matter of sincere regret that, to accomplish a political purpose or to gain some partisan advantage in the coming Presidential campaign, the minority in this House deemed itself justified in disregarding its responsibility in this respect by pursuing the policy it has followed for almost two months, under the leadership of the distinguished gentleman from Mississippi [Mr. Williams], a policy which made it necessary for the majority, in order to transact any public business, to adopt rules of procedure under which nonpartisan questions in relation to the appropriation of public moneys could not be considered with that freedom of discussion and action that otherwise would have enabled this House to have prevented many of the increases that were finally agreed to. As the result of these increases, the aggregate of the appropriations made at this session is larger by many millions than it otherwise would be.

The constitutional right of one-fifth of the membership of the House to have a yea-and-nay vote on any measure, invoked by the minority and applied to every important and unimportant step in legislation in order to make effective their prolonged and unprecedented filibuster, instituted two months ago and persisted in until these very last hours of the session, compelled us of the majority to resort to the drastic rule under which we have operated in order to enact before the close of the fiscal year the requisite supply bills to maintain the life of the Government. Without the rule and policy thus forced upon us the appropriation bills, containing enormous increases by Senate amendments, particularly for the Army and Navy, would have received from the membership of this body deliberate and, I believe, different and more effective consideration. We could devise a rule that would compel the minority to permit a vote and conclusion on these absolutely necessary measures for support of the Government, but we could not deprive them of their power, in the exercise of a constitutional prerogative, to so consume the time of the House as to effectually preclude discussion and deliberate consideration of many of the appropriation bills.

UNUSUAL DEMANDS FOR APPROPRIATIONS

While the action of the minority in this House is not responsible for the increased estimates and the demands for increased appropriations, the policy which the minority has pursued is responsible to a greater extent than any other cause for the lack of complete success which has attended the efforts of those who resisted these demands for increased appropriations.

The extent of these demands and the sources from which they came should also be stated, in justice to this House. A review of these demands as they appear in official documents presented to Congress will show that the estimates for the established public service and for previously authorized public works for the next fiscal year were more than $156,000,000 in excess of appropriations made for the same purposes during the last session of the Fifty-ninth Congress. These demands or increased estimated expenditures, many of us believe, did not rest in fact upon the necessities of the public service. They were supported mainly by official recommendations to Congress backed by the approval of the press of the country, and they consisted largely of increased compensation to those in the civil and military branches of the public service.

In addition to the demands for increased appropriations for the established public service came the demand for the authorization and establishment of many new services and new activities upon the part of the Federal Government. Many of these were wholly without the constitutional functions of the Federal Government. Demands of this character are rapidly increasing. They are the result of, and are supported by, a general tendency throughout the country to increase the power of the Federal Government where the exercise of that increased power would relieve the States and private interests of the expense incident thereto. These demands come from all of the States, but more particularly from the States south of Mason and Dixon's line. The many bureaus and offices of the Executive Departments here at the seat of Government are always eager to take on new services and the exercise of new powers whenever there arises among the States or the people of any section of the country a demand that they should do so. Demands of this character were greater at this session of Congress than ever before, and they may be expected to increase in the future unless the executive and legislative branches of the Government unite in resisting propositions for the exercise of these extra constitutional powers and the consequent encroachment upon the revenues of the Federal Government.

Efforts for Economy Received Scant Support

Because of the nature of the demands and the sources from which these demands emanated, prominent Members of both Houses of Congress, and especially on both sides of this Chamber, whose voice and influence otherwise would have been most potential in checking these increased appropriations, sat here silent or aided those who sought their fulfillment. I am not criticising anyone. I am only stating for the record an indisputable fact. I do not deny that some of the increases made were just, but I do say that, in view of the present and prospective condition of our revenues, these increases in pay and increased expenditures on account of newly authorized Federal services could well have been postponed, and that, too, without detriment to the public service.

In our endeavor to check and keep down these increased expenditures and increased appropriations, we were throughout this session without support either from the public, from the press, from the minority, or from the Executive Departments of the Government. The increased appropriations of more than $43,000,000 on account of the Army and Navy, or for preparation for war to the end that we may have peace, were not, in the judgment of many, necessary, and yet this increase was not as great as the amount demanded. The demand for these enormous increases in war expenditures did not originate with the representatives of the people. It originated elsewhere, and was supported largely by a misdirected public sentiment, to such an extent that a majority of this House and a majority in the other branch of Congress, including Representatives of both political parties, supported them because they did not dare oppose them, while those who did oppose them were restricted in their efforts by the meaningless filibuster by the minority.

ANALYSIS OF APPROPRIATIONS

The history of the appropriation bills for the session, which I will print, shows in detail and in aggregates the estimates of appropriations submitted to the Congress; the bills, as reported by the House committees, as passed by the House, as reported by the Senate committees, as passed by the Senate, and, finally, as they became laws after the differences between the two Houses were reconciled in conferences; and also for purposes of comparison the appropriations made for 1908 are shown.

The estimates submitted to Congress by the executive as a basis for the appropriations made, including regular annual expenses, deficiencies, miscellaneous, and permanent charges, amounted to $1,079,449,288.96, or an excess over the total of all appropriations as finally approved by Congress during this session of $70,644,394.39, and $158,651,145.16 excess over all appropriations made at the last session of Congress.

The twelve regular annual appropriation bills for 1909, as passed by the House, appropriated only $743,907,820.97. The last sum is a reduction under the regular estimates submitted to Congress at the beginning of the session of $98,847,172.87.

Adding to the latter sum the additional estimates submitted to Congress since the session began, and carried in the table under estimates as miscellaneous at $25,500,000, a total reduction by the House is shown in estimates for the ordinary operating expenses of the Government of $124,347,172.87.

The Senate passed the twelve regular annual appropriation bills by increasing them over what they carried as passed by the House to the amount of $73,453,553.76.

The twelve regular annual appropriation bills as finally enacted appropriate —

Less than the estimates, including additional or miscellaneous estimates, $73,640,368.04;

More than as passed by the House, $50,706,804.83;

Less than as passed by the Senate, $22,746,748.93; and

More than the regular appropriation acts for the current fiscal year $36,850,701.53.

The grand total of all appropriations made at this session, including the regular annual bills, deficiencies, miscellaneous, and permanents, exceed those of last session by $88,006,750.77.

A comparison of each of the general appropriation bills and other general titles of appropriations with those of the last session of Congress is shown in the following table:

DIFFERENCES IN THE APPROPRIATION MEASURES OF THIS SESSION, COM-
PARED WITH THOSE OF THE LAST SESSION OF CONGRESS

Title of Bill	Increase	Reduction
Agriculture	$2,224,816.00	. . . .
Army	16,747,664.86	. . . .
Diplomatic and consular	485,130.19	. . . .
District of Columbia	. . . .	$322,929.78
Fortifications	2,419,134.00	. . . .
Indian	. . . .	871,728.28
Legislative	707,487.20	. . . .
Military Academy	. . . .	1,084,068.55
Navy	23,703,977.97	. . . .
Pension	16,910,000.00	. . . .
Post-office	10,871,199.00	. . . .
River and harbor (none this session) .	. . . .	37,108,083.00
Sundry civil	2,168,101.92	. . . .
Deficiencies	44,586,974.74	. . . .
Miscellaneous	2,261,099.38	. . . .
Permanents	4,307,975.12	. . . .
Total	127,393,560.38	39,386,809.61
	39,386,809.61	. . . .
Net increase	88,006,750.77	. . . .

DEFICIENCIES IN APPROPRIATIONS NOT LARGE

The total appropriations made apparently on account of deficiencies at this session, amounting to $56,995,973.65, exceed the amount of the last· session by $44,586,974.74. This unusual sum is due not to any violation of the antideficiency legislation so recently enacted, or to ill-advised or inadequate appropriations made last session, but is more than accounted for by the sum of $12,466,750 for public buildings authorized at this session, and by two other sums, one of $10,000,000 for the payment of pensions required on account of the law passed at this session to increase the pensions of widows of soldiers, and another of $12,178,900 to continue the work on the Panama Canal. At the last session of Congress all the money was appropriated that was asked for or that could, under the expectations then entertained, be expended during the current fiscal year in the construction of the canal; but the rapid progress under the splendid organization at work on the Isthmus made it necessary to supply as a deficiency in the current appropriations the sum given in order to avoid a suspension of the work.

Deducting the three sums named, together with $11,791,342 for the Army and Navy expenditures, to which the prohibitive deficiency legislation does not apply, and the sum left for deficiencies, only $10,558,981.65 is gratifyingly small, and much less than the ordinary deficiencies for any of the recent years.

RELATION OF EXPENDITURES TO WEALTH

At the request of the Committee on Appropriations the Director of the Census has recently prepared and furnished, for their information, tables showing the actual expenditures of the Federal Government from 1791 to 1907, by fiscal years, and by four-year periods corresponding to the several Administrations.

In connection with these statistics Director North has furnished an analysis so valuable and informing to all who are interested in the problem of governmental expenditures that I shall ask its insertion in the *Record* as a part of my remarks.

The most significant fact to be derived from an inspection of the relationship of expenditures for the maintenance of government to the aggregate wealth of the nation is the uniformity for a long series of years of the proportion shown. This uniformity, as indicated in the tables and analysis, exists not only in the expenditures for the Federal Government, but also in the tax levies for State, municipal, and local government. Practically no variation whatever appears in the proportion of expenditure for the Federal Government per $1,000 of national wealth, but such increase as appears is indicated in the tax levies made for government other than Federal. The figures presented suggest a tendency to increase expenditures for State or local government more rapidly than for the Federal Government.

The truth of this apparent tendency is confirmed by the fact that the census report of 1890, the first to present the aggregate payment for all expenditures of all classes, as distinguished from mere tax levies, for States, counties, cities, and minor civil divisions, including schools, amounted to $569,252,634, or $9.30 per $1,000 of national wealth. In 1902, however, the year in which the next census inquiry upon this subject was made, the aggregate payment for expenditures of this class had nearly doubled, amounting to $1,156,447,085, or $12.80 per $1,000 of national wealth.

In general, therefore, it appears to be an established fact that while the expenditures for the maintenance of the National Government have steadily increased during the whole period of national existence, and latterly much more than I believe they should, they have maintained an almost uniform proportion, except during the period of the civil war, in comparison with each $1,000 of national wealth; but that the expenditures made for the maintenance of State and local governments of all kinds have shown a decided tendency to increase in proportion to each $1,000 of national wealth, thus reflecting the general tendency of the age and of the nation, as wealth increases, to make more liberal expenditures for the maintenance of various classes of government and governmental institutions.

The actual per capita expenditure for the maintenance of the Federal Government during the first period, from 1791 to 1796, as shown by the Census Office, was $1.34. It would be natural to contrast this figure with the per capita of annual expenditure for the last fiscal year, amounting to $8.91; but it will be evident upon reflection that there is no comparison possible between the mere per capitas themselves without consideration of the resources of the nation at the two periods mentioned. Except in time of war or in periods of great depression, there is of necessity in every nation a rough relation between the expenditures for the maintenance of government and the ability of the nation to furnish such resources. Unfortunately, there exists no information concerning the aggregate wealth of the United States at the beginning of the nineteenth century. The earliest data upon the subject was collected at the Seventh Census in 1850.

This Congress Deserves Praise

Mr. Speaker, in conclusion I want to commend this Congress as it is concluding the labors of its first session, and pay tribute to the courage it has manifested in its acts of commission as well as those of omission. Whatever the unthinking or the superficial critic may now say, the impartial and nonpartisan historian will hereafter record and truthfully state that, in the affirmative work performed and in contending against and successfully resisting unconstitutional demands upon the powers and the treasury of the Federal Government, the work of no previous session is comparable with the work of the first session of the Sixtieth Congress. [Great applause on the Republican side.]

The history of the appropriation bills of this session and the analysis of public expenditures made by the Census Office to which I have referred follow, pp. 310–311.

REVIEW OF APPROPRIATIONS ON BEHALF OF THE MINORITY [1]

[It is customary that after the chairman of the committee on appropriations has made his statement, he is followed by the principal member of the minority on that committee with a criticism of the fiscal policy of the majority.]

Mr. FITZGERALD said:

Mr. Speaker: Speaking for the Democratic members of the Committee on Appropriations and at their direction, I desire to present the following review of our appropriations and of the country's financial condition:

It is a prodigious task to examine the Departmental estimates. The gentleman from Minnesota [Mr. Tawney] has not overstated the difficulties of those upon whom the burden is placed. The country would have been benefited had the recommendations of the committees charged with the preparation of the supply bills been more generally heeded by the House. The importunities of those outside are sufficiently difficult to resist, without having the membership of the House take sides against its committees on questions of expenditure.

The gentleman from Minnesota [Mr. Tawney] enunciated a new doctrine. It will be a surprise to the country to hear his explanations of the enormous appropriations of this Congress. He attributes the wastefulness, the recklessness, and the extravagance of his own party, in complete control of the Government, to the fact that the Democratic minority of the House has exercised its constitutional right to call the roll upon every question submitted to the House. The purpose of the minority was to center the attention of the country on the work of Congress, and that purpose has been successfully accomplished.

Mr. Speaker, I recall when the naval appropriation came back from conference it was not due to the vigilance of the majority, but to the vigilance of the minority that it was discovered that the conferees on that bill, in violation of all rules of parliamentary law, had inserted a provision carrying a large sum of money. It was not the action of the minority that prevented that report being rejected, but it was the partisan action of a Republican Speaker who permitted the conference report to

[1] *Congr. Record*, May 30, 1908.

HISTORY OF APPROPRIATION BILLS, FIRST SESSION OF THE SIXTIETH CON-
AND APPROPRIATIONS FOR

[Prepared by the clerks to the Committees on Appropri-

Title.	Estimates, 1909.	Reported to the House.
Agriculture	$10,666,351.00	$11,431,346.00
Army	89,755,833.75	85,007,566.56
Diplomatic and consular	3,960,320.91	3,508,963.91
District of Columbia	13,798,126.35	9,561,449.35
Fortification	38,443,945.36	8,210,611.00
Indian	8,219,272.87	8,020,597.87
Legislative, etc.	35,040,066.13	32,336,573.00
Military Academy	977,087.87	825,837.87
Navy	125,791,349.80	103,967,518.43
Pension	151,043,000.00	150,869,000.00
Post-Office	230,441,016.00	220,765,392.00
River and harbor	. . . . .	. . . . .
Sundry civil	134,618,623.80	105,715,369.48
Total	842,754,993.84	740,220,225.47
Urgent deficiency, 1908 and prior years		24,074,450.26
Additional urgent deficiency, 1908 and prior years	57,000,000.00	2,025,500.00
Deficiency, 1908 and prior years		17,342,572.89
Total	899,754,993.84	783,662,748.62
Miscellaneous	25,500,000.00	. . . . .
Total, regular annual appropriations	925,254,993.84	. . . . .
Permanant annual appropriations	154,194,295.12	. . . . .
Grand total, regular and permanent annual appropriations	1,079,449,288.96	. . . . .

Amount of estimated revenues for fiscal year 1909 . . . .
Amount of estimated postal revenues for fiscal year 1909 . . . .
Total of estimated revenues for fiscal year 1909 . . . .

[1] This amount includes $17,806,645 to carry out contracts authorized
of the Isthmian

GRESS; ESTIMATES AND APPROPRIATIONS FOR THE FISCAL YEAR 1908–9, THE FISCAL YEAR 1907–8.

ations of the Senate and House of Representatives.]

Passed the House.	Reported to the Senate.	Passed the Senate.	Law, 1908–9.	Law, 1907–8.
$11,508,806.00	$11,642,146.00	$12,152,406.00	$11,672,106.00	$9,447,290.00
84,207,566.56	98,820,409.12	98,840,409.12	95,382,247.61	78,634,582.75
3,508,963.91	3,967,805.91	3,597,230.91	3,577,463.91	3,092,333.72
9,560,499.35	11,494,887.35	11,575,513.85	10,117,668.85	10,440,598.63
8,210,611.00	11,510,187.01	12,116,187.01	9,317,145.00	6,898,011.00
8,179,097.87	9,904,920.93	10,532,826.87	9,253,347.87	10,125,076.15
32,302,913.00	32,945,631.00	32,965,631.00	32,833,821.00	32,126,333.80
825,837.87	914,967.37	914,867.37	845,634.87	1,929,703.42
105,405,768.43	112,984,799.88	123,115,659.88	122,662,485.47	98,958,507.50
150,869,000.00	163,053,000.00	163,053,000.00	163,053,000.00	146,143,000.00
222,355,892.00	229,027,367.00	229,706,367.00	222,962,392.00	212,091,193.00
. . . . .	. . . . .	. . . . .	. . . .	37,108,083.00
106,972,864.98	118,032,263.22	118,791,275.72	112,937,313.22[1]	110,769,211.30
743,907,820.97	804,298,384.79	817,361,374.73	794,614,625.80	757,763,924.27
23,725,188.25	24,083,267.12	24,083,500.48	24,050,125.48	
2,110,500.00	2,163,000.00	2,163,000.00	2,163,000.00	} 12,408,998.91
17,344,322.89	18,374,811.43	18,385,316.88	30,782,848.17	
787,087,832.11	848,919,463.34	861,993,192.09	851,610,599.45	770,172,923.18
. . . . .	. . . . .	. . . . .	3,000,000.00	738,900.62
. . . . .	. . . . .	. . . . .	854,610,599.45	770,911,823.80
. . . . .	. . . . .	. . . . .	154,194,295.12	149,886,320.00
. . . . .	. . . . .	. . . . .	1,008,804,894.57	920,798,143.80

. . . . $658,000,000.00
. . . . 220,123,011.30
. . . . 878,123,011.30

by law for river and harbor improvements and 29,187,00 for construction
Canal for 1909.

History of Appropriation Bills, Firs

[Prepared by t

	Tho
Agriculture	
Army	
Diplomatic and consul	
District of Columbia	
Fortification	
Indian	
Legislative, etc. . .	
Military Academy .	
Navy	
Pension	
Post-Office	
River and harbor .	
Sundry civil	
Total . . .	
Urgent deficiency, 1908 and prior years .	
Additional urgent deficiency, 1908 and prior years	
Deficiency, 1908 and prior years	
Total	
Miscellaneous	
Total, regular annual appropriations	
Permanent annual appropriations . .	
Grand total, regular and permanent annual appropriations	

Amount of estimated revenues for fiscal year 1909	
Amount of estimated total revenues for fiscal year	
Total of estimated revenues for fiscal year 1909	

[1] This amount includes $17,806,645 t

ng has apparently
demoralized and
ority.
te the enormous

ountry's finances
itrasted with ex-
t at Republican
y's future. Ex-
:perity were still
imbling into the

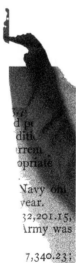

d p(
dith
rrem
opriate

Navy on
year.
32,201.15,
Army was

7,340.23;

for the
7.40.
is coun-

come up under a motion to suspend the rules instead of being brought up as the conference report on this bill is in the regular and orderly manner that enabled the Republican conferees, in violation of the rules, to insert and retain in the bill an item that was never considered in either House of Congress. The record vote upon the adoption of that report will show that more Democrats voted to reject the report, because of the improper action, as well as the unjustifiable extravagance of that bill, than did Republican Members of this House. I challenge the chairman of the Committee on Appropriations now, and I shall yield to him to answer, to name a single item of large appropriation where the *Record* does not show more Democrats recorded against it than there are Republicans recorded against it. [A pause.]

The gentleman does not care to answer. I make the assertion that in every instance when his committee was overridden, or when appropriations were improperly enlarged, more Republicans voted the reckless appropriation than did the Democrats, and more Republicans in proportion to their numbers in this House than Democrats. With a majority of fifty-seven Members in this House it is a pitiable spectacle for the chairman of the great Committee on Appropriations to have to plead that the majority of fifty-seven was unable to prevent the minority from looting the Treasury. Despite, Mr. Speaker, what I consider an extraordinary attempt of the gentleman from Minnesota to place the sins of his party upon his political opponents, and despite the extraordinary character of his statement at this time, we of the minority desire to pay a highly deserved tribute to the industry, the fearlessness, the patriotism and the high purpose which have characterized the labors of the chairman of the Committee on Appropriations [Mr. Tawney]. It has been a source of keen gratification to have worked with him, knowing that his only ambition has been honestly to serve the country and to conserve the public interests. He deserved more loyal support from his party associates. Had he received that aid and coöperation from his own party which should have been freely given, all honest men would now have great cause to rejoice.

The Congress is now about to adjourn. This session has been the most profligate in our history. Extravagance has run riot; the Treasury has been depleted; the public money has been shamefully squandered.

On January 13 of this year I stated that "preparations have been made to squander the public treasure with a lavishness heretofore unknown." The record of this session is in complete harmony with that declaration. No other nation in the civilized world could be so reckless with its treasure and escape disaster.

The responsibility rests with the Republican party. It can not evade the issue. Every energy seems to have been concentrated upon the task of emptying the Treasury and of making imperative the issuance of bonds by the next Administration in order to defray the ordinary expenditures of the Government. The dreaded handwriting has apparently been seen upon the wall, and the Republican party is demoralized and shaken; it can not shift responsibility to a helpless minority.

The appropriations for the next fiscal year aggregate the enormous sum of $1,008,804,894.57.

To those who have given only slight attention to the country's finances the statement will undoubtedly be startling; when contrasted with expenditures for other periods in our history amazement at Republican recklessness quickly gives way to alarm for the country's future. Expenditures have been authorized as if the wave of prosperity were still rolling high instead of having broken, as is has, and tumbling into the trough of a severe industrial depression.

Under Cleveland the per capita appropriations for the Army for four years were $1.35; for the Navy, $1.54; for fortifications, 20 cents; the average per capita for the four years for such service, $3.90.

Under Roosevelt, in his second Administration, the per capita appropriations for the Army for the four-year period are $3.66, more than two and one-half times the amount under Cleveland; for the Navy, $4.91, more than three times the amount under Cleveland; for fortifications, 32 cents, more than 50 per cent increase over Cleveland, and the average per capita cost for the three services under Roosevelt is $8.90, two and one-fourth times as great as under Cleveland.

The appropriations for the Army for the next fiscal year are $16,747,664.86 more than for the present fiscal year. It has already been pointed out by the gentleman from Virginia [Mr. Hay] that $3,000,000 additional will be required next year to meet the demands of the service, so that in reality the Army, without the addition of a single man, will cost at least $19,747,664.86 more next year than during this year.

The appropriations for the Navy for next year are $23,703,977.97 more than for the present year. So that in a time of profound peace our military establishments will cost, including the $2,419,134 additional for fortifications, $45,870,776.83 more next year than for the current year. This increase in one year is practically the total amount appropriated in 1894 to maintain the Army and Navy, to wit, $46,329,701.16.

In other words the entire expenditure for the Army and Navy only fourteen years ago is equalled now by the increase in a single year.

In 1907 the expenditures for the British army were $121,232,201.15, and an army at least two and one half times as large as our Army was maintained.

In 1907 the expenditures for the French army were $138,707,340.23; for the German army, $176,842,187.20.

For the British navy the expenditures were $149,364,556.75; for the French navy, $62,732,182.88; for the German navy, $63,165,747.40.

These nations have repeatedly been pictured to the people of this country as staggering under the burdens of militarism. It has been our boast that this free land has not been so afflicted, yet our expenditures for the two military services for the next year will be practically the same as those made by the great military nations of Europe.

The gross receipts of the United States for 1907 were $846,725,329.62; of Great Britain, $704,737,686.26; of Germany, $617,941,200.80; of France, $715,883,610.08.

Evidently the receipts of these four governments, are very much alike, and the expenditures for maintenance of military establishments not widely different.

In a report prepared by the Census Bureau for the Committee on Appropriations this statement is made:

In the fiscal year ending June 30, 1907, the per capita expenditures of the United States National Government were 6.65 times as great as was the average of such expenditures during the six years of Washington's administration for which complete reports are available. National expenditures have increased in one hundred and eleven years that much faster than the population. This increase is attracting the attention of statesmen, newspaper writers, and students of public affairs.

It may be that the increasing expenditures of the Federal Government are attracting the attention of the persons mentioned in this excerpt. Evidently, however, it has completely escaped the attention of every responsible official of the administration of Theodore Roosevelt. [Applause on the Democratic side.] Surely these significant facts have not permeated the recesses of the White House nor found even a temporary lodgment in the active brain of the President. No other conclusion can satisfactorily be reached; for upon no other theory is it conceivable that the Administration would have submitted estimates, as has been repeatedly pointed out during the session, at least $128,000,000 in excess of the revenues estimated for the coming fiscal year. Since these estimates were submitted to Congress the country has been afflicted with a panic. The business and industrial depression is growing rather than lessening. Yet in the plethora of messages to the Congress from the Chief Executive there has not been a single warning to safeguard the interests of the people by resolutely repelling all attempts to raid the Treasury. Indeed, when the history of this session is impartially and truthfully written, as it will be some day, the wielder of the " big stick " will be pictured in heroic size at the head of those who, openly encouraged or secretly abetted by him, have successfully rifled the people's strong box. [Applause on the Democratic side.]

How are these extraordinary authorizations to be met? If the Treasury were overflowing and money unnecessarily taken from the people through various forms of taxation were being withheld from the channels of trade, it might be sufficient excuse for some to make lavish appropriations. Or if the party in power adopted the policy of the tyrants of old and expended enormous sums upon public works to keep the unemployed from awakening to the truth of the country's position, such reasons might be urged in defense of these appropriations.

But of the total of $1,008,804,894.57 appropriated at this session not a single dollar is to be spent on new projects for the improvement of water routes and harbors and but $30,000,000 is for newly authorized public buildings.

From the daily statement of the Treasury Department for May 23, 1908, it appears that the excess of expenditures over receipts for the fiscal year to and including that day was $61,421,301.82.

     *   *   *   *.   *   *   *   *

The gentleman from Minnesota [Mr. Tawney] does not prophesy idly when he warns his associates, as he has on several occasions during the past few months, that within the next fiscal year it will be necessary to issue either certificates of indebtedness or bonds to obtain the money to pay the current expenses of the Government.

It would appear as if the Republicans were preparing to repeat their conduct in the closing months of the Harrison Administration [applause on the Democratic side] of preparing the plates, as was done by Secretary Foster, for the printing of bonds for use by a Democratic Administration because of Republican folly. [Applause on the Democratic side.]

Mr. Speaker, in striking contrast with the management of the nation's finances by the Republican party is the situation in Great Britain to-day. On the 7th of this month the budget was presented to the House of Commons by the premier, Mr. Asquith, acting for the chancellor of the exchequer. A perusal of his speech would be of incalculable benefit to every Member of this House. Whatever opinions may be entertained of the British system of government, the conduct of its finances can not do other than elicit admiration.

Mr. Asquith pointed out that in presenting the budget a year previously he had estimated the revenues for the fiscal year, ending March 31, 1908, at about $765,000,000 and provided for the expenditure of $762,510,000. The revenue had actually been $782,690,000, $17,000,000 in excess of his estimate, and the actual expenditures $759,060,000, about $3,000,000 less than provided. As a result at the end of the year there was a surplus of receipts over expenditures of $20,000,000 and the public debt had been reduced $85,000,000. Highly impressive when contrasted with the labors of the Republican party, which produces a deficit this year of $78,000,000, and then in the face of falling revenues is asked by the executive officials to appropriate at least $128,000,000 more than the estimated revenues and actually appropriates $223,000,000 more than the reasonably anticipated revenues, and then the gentleman from Minnesota [Mr. Tawney] puts the blame on a Democratic filibuster at this time! [Applause and laughter on the Democratic side.]

The estimated revenues of the British Government for the next fiscal year, as pointed out by Mr. Asquith, are $788,850,000; the expenditures provided aggregate $764,345,000, a surplus of about $25,000,000. With this surplus revenue it is proposed to remove certain annoying stamp taxes, to initiate a system of old-age pensions, to reduce the tax on sugar 1 farthing a pound, with a consequent loss of revenue of $17,000,000, so as to afford some relief to the masses from the burdens of taxation, and still have a surplus of receipts over expenditures available for unforeseen contingencies.

With estimated revenues practically identical with our probable revenues — Great Britain, $788,850,000; United States, $785,000,000 — Great Britain will support an army three and one-half times as large as our Army, and a navy, estimating by the number of men, about three times as large as our Navy; will initiate a system of old-age pensions, will apply about $75,000,000 to the reduction of its debt, will reduce substantially the tax upon sugar, a universally used foodstuff, and still have a surplus of receipts available for contingencies, while the United States proposes to expend $223,000,000 in excess of its probable revenues, with military establishments only one-third as large as Great Britain, and without relieving the people from a single dollar of taxation.

It is little to be wondered that the British premier exultantly declared that —

When people talk about the demands of democracy, I may be allowed to say that there is not a more credible chapter in the annals of democratic finances than that which records the fact that during three years, with a passionate desire for diminution of expenditure and for the mitigation of popular burdens, there has been the application of the enormous sum of between thirteen and fifteen millions (sterling) a year out of taxation to redeem the principal of our national debt.

Mr. Speaker, while I have not as much admiration for the British Government as for our own, I can not withhold my admiration for the manner in which their finances are conducted, particularly when contrasted with the Republican party's Administration of this Government.

Within the last few days there seems to have been an awakening on the Republican side of the House. Feeble protests have been made against the extent of appropriations and some complaint against the Senate for presuming to add to the appropriation bills as passed by the House.

Mr. Speaker, with the exception of the gentleman from Minnesota [Mr. Tawney], there has not been a single Republican in this House with sufficient influence to be considered an important factor in the deliberations of this body who has, prior to this week, raised his voice in protest against the unjustifiable extravagance of the House and of Congress. [Applause on the Democratic side.]

DIVIDED AUTHORITY AND APPROPRIATIONS

[The following extract from a speech by Mr. Livingston on July 2, 1906, brings out the opinions of leading men upon the policy of distributing the appropriation bills among a number of committees.]

MR. LIVINGSTON. I wish to bring to the attention of Congress the fact that the division of appropriations among several committees was a serious mistake. Mr. Randall, in the Forty-ninth Congress, on a report on this subject, said:

The best interests of the people require that the subject of appropriations should mainly be committed to the charge of one committee — not that one set of men is abler or more honest than another set, but because experience has shown it is the safest course to pursue. Such body of men can make careful scrutiny into every detail by itself, and, in connection with others, and taking a survey of the whole field of receipts and expenditures, it will be responsible to the House to see to it that the latter shall be reduced to an economical basis, and kept within the limits of the public revenue.

If, in place of the responsibility and certainty of keeping appropriations within economical limits, we are to inaugurate a system of making appropriations by many committees, without regard each to the other or the amount of money involved, increased expenditures will ensue, and the party in power and responsible for the control of legislation in this House will be held to strict account by the people.

If you undertake to divide all the appropriations and have many committees where there ought to be but one, you will enter upon a path or extravagance you can not foresee the length of or the depth of, until we will find the Treasury of the country bankrupt.

Mr. Garfield, of Ohio, said:

It is a fact within the experience of every Member who has been here long, that the Committee on Appropriations always finds itself confronted with a demand from each of the committees having a special subject in charge for larger appropriations than the Committee on Appropriations think should be made. There never was a time, within my knowledge since I have been here, when the Committee on Military Affairs did not resist the tendency of the Committee on Appropriations to cut down the appropriations for the Army. The Committee on Naval Affairs has always been found resisting the reduction of the naval appropriation bill. For this reason, I say that if each of these several committees had charge of getting up the appropriation bills on these several subjects, the amount of the bills would be very large; they would outgrow the grasp of the House, and there would be no unity in the appropriations of public money.

I do say, sir, without the slightest question in my own mind of the truth of the statement, that the scattering of these appropriations as suggested by gentlemen here will be absolutely breaking down all economy and good order and good management of our finances. It cannot be otherwise.

Senator Beck said:

The Agricultural Committee will frame the law and vote all the money they can, and no man not on that committee will know anything about it. So of the Post-Office Committee, so of the Naval Committee, so of the Military Committee, so of the District of Columbia Committee. They become autocrats, not only in the framing of the law, but in the appropriation of the people's money to carry it out; and outside of that committee room no man can get the information to enable him to contradict what they say if they are wrong; and they are selected because they are special friends of the Department they are appointed to represent; for each Secretary ought to have men he can trust, before whom he can present the wants of his Department here.

*   *   *   *   *   *   *   *

Senator Sherman said:

Sir, I would not do anything at all to weaken the restraint or power of the Committee on Appropriations. I believe that it is necessary, as my friend from Vermont says, to bring all the items of expenditures for the nation under the eye and control of one committee, so that they may limit the amount of expenditures.

*   *   *   *   *   *   *   *

Senator Hale said:

I know from my own experience that the tendency of the mind of a member of either of the other committees calling for appropriations each year— the Military or Naval Committee (I will speak of the latter because I have had service upon that committee) — is to gain all the power in appropriating money possible, and connected with that is the unerring result of desiring to have the power to appropriate more money. There has never been any exception to that. I think few Senators will dispute the statement that if all the business of the Committee on Appropriations was taken from it and given to the several committees we should then be confronted with a general scramble upon the part of each committee for more money.

Mr. Cannon said:

That committee having the exclusive power to propose legislation, and also to report the appropriations for the service, would be an autocratic committee without any check upon it with any other committee of the House. Now, I undertake to say when you give a committee of that kind that kind of power— you may put my friend from Maine [Mr. Reed] upon it, or you may put my friend from New York [Mr. Hiscock] upon it, or the gentleman from West Virginia [Mr. Gibson], or the gentleman from Pennsylvania [Mr. Randall]— they might make fair appropriations this session, and possibly next session, but, as the years roll around, so sure as the sun rises, that committee having exclusive jurisdiction of legislation and appropriations for that subject would abuse its jurisdiction and magnify its department.

Why, Mr. Speaker, when you come to select the committees which are to have charge of the business of the War Department, or the Navy Department, or the Post Office Department, I take it, sir, that it will be your duty to select able men that have a knowledge of these different Departments; and not only that, but men who are friendly, if you please, to the Navy of this country, to the Army of this country, and to the Post Office Department. You ought not, sir, to pick out enemies, and I do not believe you would do so. So when you have placed the power in the hands of the friends of these various Departments, and given them this exclusive jurisdiction of legislation and of appropriations, you have at once this abuse ready to come into this House and from Congress to Congress to run riot, blossoming and bearing the fruit of bad legislation and inordinate appropriations.

How truly did this our present Speaker predict the conditions of to-day. These committees that have power to legislate and appropriate

APPROPRIATIONS FOR FISCAL YEARS 1898 AND 1907

Title	Appropriations made for fiscal year 1898, the first full fiscal year under Mr. McKinley's Administration	Appropriations made for fiscal year 1907, under Mr. Roosevelt's Administration
Agricultural	$3,182,902.00	$9,932,940.00
Army	23,129,344.30	71,817,165.08
Diplomatic and consular	1,695,308.76	3,091,094.17
District of Columbia	6,186,991.06	10,138,692.16
Fortifications	9,517,141.00	5,053,993.00
Indian	7,674,120.89	9,260,399.98
Legislative, etc.	21,690,766.90	29,741,019.30
Military Academy	479,572.83	1,664,707.67
Navy	33,003,234.19	102,071,650.27
Pensions	141,263,880.00	140,245,500.00
Post-office	95,665,338.75	191,695,998.75
River and Harbor (including amounts in sundry civil, deficiency, and special acts)	20,832,412.91	....
Sundry civil	34,490,370.47	98,274,574.32
Deficiencies	9,096,417.34	39,119,246.62
Total	407,907,801.40	712,106,981.32
Miscellaneous	749,057.90	28,000,000.00
Total regular annual appropriations	408,656,859.30	740,106,981.32
Permanent annual appropriations (estimates)	120,078,220.00	140,076,320.00
Grand total	528,735,079.30	880,183,301.32

are merely the representatives of specific Departments, and as foretold by Mr. Cannon are "bearing fruit of bad legislation." If this pernicious practice can not be changed, our appropriations will continue to "run riot." Mr. Cannon at that time suggested that all conferees between the House and Senate upon money bills should be selected from the appropriations committees of the House and Senate, with power to cut out unnecessary appropriations and scale down extravagant ones. Congress and the country need not look for retrenchment in expenses or appropriations under the present methods. Each of these committees with power to legislate and appropriate will continue to strive for the advantage to their particular Departments in the disbursement of the Government's revenue.

DEBATE ON AN APPROPRIATION BILL

[Under the rules of the House the general appropriation bills are not allowed to contain any new legislation, but only appropriations for services already provided for by former laws. In 1906, this rule was put in operation against various appropriation bills in order to keep them within proper limits. It has been the practice of the House to allow much legislation of this kind to go through without objection by unanimous consent, but, of course, the objection of even a single member is sufficient under the rules to throw out an appropriation for which there is no legal warrant. In this manner it was easy for the members on the Committee on Appropriations to exercise a certain control over the bills brought in by other committees, through their right of objection as individual members. But when on March 23, 1906, the Committee brought in one of its own bills, the Legislative and Judicial Appropriation Bill, certain of the members of the House took it upon themselves to enforce the rules against the Committee on Appropriations itself. Item after item was objected to and under the rules of the House a great many sections were stricken out. The attitude of the members and the committee is brought out in the following extract from the debate of March 23, which also illustrates the opinions held by some members upon the rules of the House.]

MR. PRINCE. I will not oppose any measure which has for its purpose the betterment of the service of the United States in any of its branches; but under the rules of this House this is no way to legislate. No man in this House can tell how these rolls may be padded. There is no means of getting at it. We may be criticised by some for doing what we are doing, but we want to know how these men are placed on the rolls; we want to know by what authority of law they are placed there, and some of us have stood here under the rules making objection; and in every instance practically where we have made objection under the rules, Chairman after Chairman occupying the position that you now occupy, Mr. Chairman, has held in accordance with the rules of the House. Why criticise us for doing our duty?

I am not here criticising gentlemen of the committee, but I am only asking them to live under the rules that they want us to live under. The rules of this House are invoked time and again, and when the time comes it is a rare instance for me to oppose the rules. More than ten years have I been in this House, and at no time when a rule has been brought in along the lines of party policy have I ever refused to stand by it. I have stood for the rules of this House and stand by the rules to-day, and I am insisting upon the rule; and the gentleman very properly says that these provisions are subject to the rule, and he makes no objection to the point of order. Then what is his answer for bringing them in here when he knows that they are contrary to the rules of this House?

Mr. TAWNEY. Mr. Chairman, I wish to make an observation in reply to the gentleman from Illinois [Mr. Prince], who attempts to justify his course and the course of his colleague from Georgia [Mr. Hardwick] in their opposition to certain provisions in this bill upon the ground that under the rules of the House the House can not consider a provision in an appropriation bill providing for the salaries of the clerks that are engaged in carrying on the public service. Now, if you will follow to its logical conclusion the position of the gentleman from Illinois, this House for the next five years would have no time to do anything else than to take up in the several Departments the necessity for legislation, for the purpose of increasing one clerk in one bureau and a number of clerks in another bureau, and in another division, and it would absolutely make the House of Representatives ridiculous.

The course which the Committee on Appropriations has followed in this bill has been the practice ever since I have been a Member of this House, which has been fourteen years. When the departmental officers submit their estimates to Congress they submit an estimate not only for the clerical force they then have on the rolls, but if the growth of the service in their respective Departments has been such as to necessitate an increase in that force that increase is included in the estimate, and the demand for it is investigated by whom? Investigated by the committee that reports the appropriation for carrying on that service, and if, in the judgment of that committee, the additional clerical force is necessary, the committee invariably reports in its legislative, executive, and judicial appropriation bill the necessary increase in positions and the necessary increase in salaries.

There is no other way to provide for the increasing demands of the Departments except by introducing bills for the increase of specific salaries and then have these bills go to the respective legislative committees; these committees consider the necessity, and then bring in a bill providing for an increase, say, of one clerk in the Post Office Department and perhaps one or two clerks in the Civil Service Commission, or an increase in the salaries or an increase in the number of chief clerks, etc.

I say the enforcement of this rule as interpreted makes the House absolutely ridiculous. I am not finding any fault with the rulings of the Chair, but when these gentlemen make their points of order and explanations are made for the necessity for the changes in current law or the reasonableness of the increase in salaries that have been reported, even though these changes result in an aggregate decrease in the expenditure of the public money, they nevertheless are not satisfied.

It is not to enforce the rules of the House, it is not to protect the House against any violation of its rules, that this policy has been inaugurated by these gentlemen; that is not their motive. If it were they would accept the statements made here on the floor as to the necessity for these changes in the interest of better administration and in the interest of economy.

Mr. Chairman, we may as well face this situation now as any time. If this rule is to be enforced, then more than one-half of the provisions of this bill will have to go out. More than one-half of the provisions of a legislative bill that has been reported to this House for the last ten years could not have been considered. We have certain provisions in this bill where clerks were employed under a lump-sum appropriation, a practice that has been criticised by this House, and the Committee on Appropriations has been the particular object of that criticism for not bringing in specific appropriations defining these places and salaries to be allowed to each one of them.

As the result of the investigation made by the Committee on Appropriations, in three or four instances were found lump-sum appropriations, in almost every instance we find that where the head of a Department is employing clerks under a lump-sum appropriation the salaries are a great deal higher than when the salaries are provided for specifically in appropriation bills. As the result of the changes we have reported to the House in three bureaus a reduction, a saving to the Government, of $12,511 is accomplished. But under the policy of the gentleman from Illinois [Mr. Prince] and his colleague from Georgia [Mr. Hardwick], if their policy of making points of order is pursued by them, it is absolutely impossible for this House to effect any reform or any reduction in the salary or any improvement in the public administration by reclassification or otherwise, for the reason that to do so would be obnoxious to the rule. Similar provisions have heretofore been reported from the Committee on Appropriations in this same bill, but they remained in the bill notwithstanding they were obnoxious to the rules. They remained in the bill because in the interest of good administration and in the interest of economy there was no man on this floor who objected to the enactment of provisions of that kind. Now, no matter how great the economy may be, no matter how beneficial these reclassifications may be in the administration of public affairs, these two Members say they can not be considered. They even refuse to allow this House to consider any one of these proposed changes. If they were acting in good faith they would at least permit the House to consider propositions of that kind when they are informed that as a result of this legislation we are saving the people's money and improving the public administration of our public affairs.

Now, if these provisions did not suit the House, or any Member of the House, that Member has a perfect right, under the rules of the House, to amend, if he desires to do so. If the salaries which have been reported here are in excess or greater than what they think they ought to be, they have the right to offer an amendment if they see fit to do so. I speak of this, Mr. Chairman, merely for the purpose of emphasizing the fact that if we are to go on here day after day under the technical policy of these gentlemen I want the country to know who is responsible for it and why they are pursuing the course that they are. I do not want them to give it out to the country that they are actuated by motives of economy when they refuse to allow this House to consider a proposition which results, if enacted into law, in saving money to the public or improving the public service. Now, they have a perfect right — any Member has a right, if he sees fit to exercise it — to make points of order against these provisions, but this House ought to remember and the country ought to know that a point of order deprives the House of an opportunity to consider whether or not the provisions are wise or unwise — whether or not they would result beneficially to the Government. And when, contrary to the uniform practice of this House of considering provisions of this kind by unanimous consent, the country will know that these men set themselves up as censors, not in the interest of good administration or in the interest of economy — when the country knows that they are depriving the House of an opportunity of considering provisions in the interest of economy — I imagine that their course will not meet with that popular approval which it is evident they hope or anticipate it will· by their claiming that they are doing this for that purpose. Why, just a few minutes ago, as a result of their policy, they have made it necessary to increase the public expenditures. They have by their policy made it impossible for us to improve the efficiency of one of the branches of the Government. Now, Mr. Chairman, I submit, in all candor, that if this policy is to be followed out we may as well proceed with the reading of this bill, have everything stricken out, whether it reduces or does not reduce public expenditure, and then rewrite the bill in the language of the current legislative bill and let it go to the other branch of Congress, where these proposed reforms and changes may be considered. I will not say that there is any purpose or intention on the part of the Committee on Appropriations to do this, because it is not necessary. Those things can be corrected under the parliamentary procedure of the House, and they will be, but it will involve simply going over this bill again. It will simply involve the time necessary for reconsidering every one of these provisions which, by the policy of these gentlemen, the House is

now deprived of the opportunity of considering. The House is competent to determine whether these changes should be made or not. The plan
proposed by the gentleman from Illinois [Mr. Prince] is absolutely impractical. If these changes are not right, or if these provisions should
not be enacted into law, if we should not cut down the forces in the Executive Departments as we have done in this bill, if we should not change
around and reclassify as we propose in this bill, it is a matter that the
House can by a majority vote determine. But the attitude and the policy
of these gentlemen is to deprive the House of the opportunity of accomplishing anything of this kind.

Mr. PRINCE. Mr. Chairman, I ask unanimous consent to answer in a
brief time the speech of the gentleman from Minnesota, the chairman
of the Committee on Appropriations.

The CHAIRMAN. The Chair is ready to rule on the point and will do
so, and then submit the gentleman's request. The Chair sustains the
point of order. The gentleman from Illinois asks unanimous consent to
proceed for five minutes. Is there objection. [After a pause.] The
Chair hears none.

Mr. PRINCE. Mr. Chairman and gentlemen of the House, the chairman of the Committee on Appropriations, the gentleman from Minnesota [Mr. Tawney], says that if we persist in asking for the rules of the
House to be observed, we are obstructionists; that we are not acting in
the interests of economy; that this bill and many of its provisions will
fail, and, in fact, half of the bill, as he stated before, would go out on a
point of order. Now, Mr. Chairman, in the first place, speaking for
myself only, I have not made a point of order against any reduction of
expenses in this bill.

Mr. TAWNEY. I beg the gentleman's pardon, he did.

Mr. PRINCE. Wherein, sir?

Mr. TAWNEY. In respect to the Civil Service Commission.

Mr. PRINCE. You have brought in a bill which, you say, reduces it,
have you not?

Mr. TAWNEY. Yes, sir; $2,590.

Mr. PRINCE. Very well. In the first instance, let us see what it
means. On page 34 I have asked two chiefs of divisions, at $2,000 each,
be stricken out. That cannot be an addition. I have asked twenty-two
clerks be reduced to six clerks. That cannot be an addition. I have not
changed any provision of the law. Can that be an addition? That is
subtracting, not an addition. On page 35 I have asked that seven clerks
be reduced to six. Is that an addition?

Mr. LITTAUER. But you know the force as you have emasculated it
cannot remain so, that it has to be put back one way or another, else the
work of this bureau be given up.

Mr. PRINCE. Is it possible that one clerk at $1,000 can disarrange
the entire bureau?

Mr. LITTAUER. Your statement covered more than one clerk.

Mr. PRINCE. Can it be possible that two examiners who heretofore have never existed can disarrange the entire bureau?

Mr. LITTAUER. The work that these examiners are designed to perform has been going on, and they are now in this service.

Mr. PRINCE. In the old bill there were none of them there, and this Commission has existed ever since when? Will the gentleman from Ohio tell me when the first civil-service bill was passed?

Mr. GROSVENOR. It was passed in 1883.

Mr. PRINCE. And it is the only one that has been passed, has never been modified or amended?

Mr. GROSVENOR. Never.

Mr. PRINCE. So the machinery is there as it is and in running order and now I say and deny I have reduced it. Very well, what else?

Mr. LITTAUER. How many clerks do you reduce in that paragraph?

Mr. PRINCE. I mean I have not increased it; I have reduced it.

Mr. LITTAUER. Nine clerks in one paragraph.

Mr. PRINCE. Six clerks in one paragraph. Can that be an addition?

Mr. LITTAUER. No; but you render it incompetent to do the work.

Mr. PRINCE. I will answer any question you put to me.

Mr. LITTAUER. We might be able to get along without the whole force, but we cannot get along without a well-ordered force.

Mr. PRINCE. You gentlemen representing the Committee on Appropriations have declined to restore the old law. I have offered an amendment on the floor of this House to restore the old law, and you decline to do it. You stand here and cripple the service, not I.

Mr. TAWNEY. Will the gentleman yield?

Mr. PRINCE. I will.

Mr. TAWNEY. As a result of your point of order you have been recognized for further time.

Mr. PRINCE. The main contention, as I gather, is this: The gentlemen in charge of the bill charge that we are invoking the rule when we ought not to invoke the rule. What are the rules for? If it should appear to the country that here is a great body of 386 Members who have rules that they cannot do business under, it may be suggested in the country that the rules ought to be modified in a way so that the expressions of the American people through their representatives can have a voice upon the floor of this House. [Applause.]

And I trust and hope that, aside from the discussion of this bill, it will rivet the attention of the country upon the rules of this House. Tell us what they can do, and what they cannot do. And in the coming Congress, which, in my judgment, will be overwhelmingly Republican, we will adjust the rules in a way that things will be carried on and policies carried out in accordance with the wishes of the people; and as one of their representatives I am perfectly willing to stand before my people, as I expect to this fall, and give an account of what I am doing here on the floor of the House to-day. I have no question what the result will be. Now, if you want to bring in a proposition here which will make these various propositions in order, bring it in and let us vote on it. [Applause.]

Mr. UNDERWOOD. Mr. Chairman, I move to strike out the last word. I listened a while ago to a speech by the chairman of the Committee on Appropriations in reference to the rules of the House. I served at one time on the Appropriation Committee, and I certainly have a kindly feeling for the committee, and I am sure in violating the rules of the House the general Appropriation Committee of this House have often passed meritorious, economic, and good legislation.

I do not think there is any doubt about the fact that the law that was written on the statute book in the last session of Congress which prohibited Department officers from creating deficiencies was a good law, an economic remedy; but notwithstanding that it is a fact that this committee has written good law on the statute book in violation of the rules of this House, I do not think it lies within the mouth of the great Committee on Appropriations, or any other committee, to come into the House of Representatives and attempt to justify themselves in the violation of the rules of the House. We all violate the rules of the House every now and then, and ask unanimous consent to do so, but when we do it it ought to be understood that we do it with the unanimous consent of every Member of this House.

Mr. Chairman, the object of the rules of this House is not simply to prevent the House of Representatives from being an unorganized mob of men. The object of the rules of this House more than anything else is to protect the rights of every individual man upon the floor of the House, and more than all, Mr. Chairman, the object of our having a set of rules in this House is to protect the rights of the minority of this House. It is to see that the minority here has justice, and to regulate the majority so that they shall not trample on the rights of the minority and the rights of the individual Members of this House.

I therefore say that no man has the right to complain that an objection is being made to what he is doing if his course of action is beyond and outside of the rules of the House. Now, the gentleman said that we could not legislate. A great deal of legislation that goes on appropriation bills belongs to other committees in this House. If the Appropriation Committee of this House did not legislate in appropriation bills that legislation would be enacted after coming from other committees in the House; and if it came from other committees it often would receive a more careful consideration, and a better consideration, than when it comes in here to be enacted on an appropriation bill.

I do not think there is any rule in this House that is wiser, that is better, that is safer for the good government of this House, than Rule XXI, which prohibits the enactment of new legislation on appropriation bills, and I think the Members of the House will recognize that fact when they realize that if you put new legislation on an appropriation bill and bring it into this House you go into the Committee of the Whole, you have no chance to call the roll, you have no chance to put the membership of this House on a record vote on that direct question. If you allow this to be done, to enact new legislation on a general appropriation bill, you can put law through this House without complying with the constitutional requirement that one-fifth of the membership of this House shall be entitled to have a record vote, because you can only have the record vote on the adoption of the bill itself.

The CHAIRMAN. For what purpose does the gentleman rise?

Mr. SMITH of Iowa. For the purpose of moving to strike out the last word.

The CHAIRMAN. The gentleman from Iowa moves to strike out the last word.

Mr. SMITH of Iowa. Mr. Chairman, during the consideration of this bill there has apparently arisen something of bitterness as between Members of the House sitting in the committee which, it seems to me, we might well avoid, if possible. The growth of appropriations for the support of the Federal Government has been so great that under the most favorable circumstances it is almost impossible for the House to consider properly the separate items of expenditure. Hampered as we are by the difficulties incident to the appropriation of money for the public service, we ought, at least so far as possible, to approach the consideration of these questions free from excitement and free from anger. I do not mean by this remark to criticise at all the gentlemen who have seen fit to raise points of order during the consideration of this bill. I was myself engaged in a greater or less degree in presenting points of order during the consideration of the Army bill. Some of my colleagues upon the Appropriations Committee were also engaged in that, and I am not here to criticise in others those things I practice myself. Of course, there has sometimes arisen the question as to whether the points of order made against this bill are in memory of the points of order made against the Army bill.

Mr. SHACKLEFORD. Mr. Chairman, a point of order.

The CHAIRMAN. The gentleman will state the point of order.

Mr. SHACKLEFORD. The gentleman is not speaking to anything before the House.

Mr. SMITH of Iowa. I am speaking to an amendment under the invariable practice of the House which I had a right to propose. The question has arisen in my mind whether the fate that overtook the bill to abolish the grade of Lieutenant-General in the Army may have had anything to do with arousing the feeling that is displayed now upon the floor of this House, but whatever may have been the provocation upon our part and whatever may have been the direct cause that induced our distinguished friends to raise these points of order, I am not seeking to criticise them nor in any sense to rebuke them. I assume no right or authority to rebuke them, but it does seem to me that misapprehension exists here as to the purposes of the rules of the House. The rules of the House are not like the criminal laws of the land. The criminal laws of the land should be enforced or repealed, but the rules of the House contemplate their being set aside by numerous methods. We set apart special days on which to suspend the rules and for the time being set them aside. We pass more measures here by unanimous consent, perhaps, than by all other methods combined and not in accordance with the rules — the bills not being entitled to consideration under the rules.

Mr. PRINCE. May I ask the gentleman a question?

Mr. SMITH of Iowa. Oh, most certainly.

Mr. PRINCE. You say we pass many bills by unanimous consent.

Mr. SMITH of Iowa. I do.

Mr. PRINCE. Is it not the invariable rule of the Speaker of the House, when, for instance, the gentleman from Iowa rises and asks unanimous consent for the present consideration of a bill, that the bill is sent to the Clerk's desk and read, and the Speaker asks if there is objection, and pauses for an objection?

Mr. SMITH of Iowa. The gentleman is certainly correct as to the practice of the House.

Mr. PRINCE. And unanimous consent can be objected to if we desire to do so.

Mr. SMITH of Iowa. I am simply seeking to point out, Mr. Chairman, that while we have rules that we are entitled to insist upon, they are not, under the practice of the House, insisted upon in season and out of season as though they were statutes, but that most of the legislation of the House is done either by motion to suspend the rules or by unanimous consent, and bills are taken up which could not come up under the rules, save by unanimous consent. So that most of our legislation is legislation enacted not in obedience to the rules laid down, but by either unanimous or through two-thirds approval by a departure from the ordinary rules. So it has been the practice from the early time to make such changes on appropriation bills as are made upon the bill now before the Committee of the Whole House on the state of the Union. That does not deny to anyone the right to raise a point of order or object, and what I am seeking to get at is this: That the rules are made that they may be insisted upon by any Member, in the exercise of his best judgment, for the advancement of good legislation, but that the objection ought not to be raised unless the proposed matter is objectionable.

The CHAIRMAN. The time of the gentleman has expired.

Mr. SMITH of Iowa. I ask unanimous consent to proceed for ten minutes.

The CHAIRMAN. Is there objection? [After a pause.] The Chair hears none.

Mr. SMITH of Iowa. I want to say this to those who have objected: That it is their strict legal right; but if a meritorious measure is brought in here to reduce expenditures, that it is not a wise time, in my judgment, that they should seek to control the judgment of others by insisting upon a rigid enforcement of the rules. These rules are not enforced as to the greater number of bills that pass the House. Here is a proposition to reduce public expenditures. It is a laudable enterprise; a commendable effort; and yet these rules that strike down alike meritorious propositions and those lacking in merit are cited for the purpose of preventing the reduction of public expenditures. No criticism will be heard from me upon my distinguished friend from Illinois. Between us there have always existed most pleasant personal relations, and I trust they will always so continue. But I ask the question here: Passing over, free from anger and free from offense, whatever may have been given by any man in the past, should these rules be resorted to for the purpose of preventing a reduction in public expenditures? If we are to come here to discharge our duty dispassionately to the whole country, we should insist upon the rules when their violation would be detrimental to the public service, and waive these rules whenever we can thereby promote the public welfare. So I hope that whether the offense originally emanated from one side or the other in this matter, that the rules will be enforced whenever asserted, as they will be by the Chair; but that no Member will feel that it is his duty to raise a point of order against any portion of any bill when the enactment of that provision would be beneficial to the public welfare.

Mr. SHERLEY. Will the gentleman allow me to ask him a question?

Mr. SMITH of Iowa. Certainly.

Mr. SHERLEY. I will ask the gentleman if he does not think the rule that he is speaking in favor of, that should actuate Members not on the committee, ought to also actuate the Members on the committee?

Mr. SMITH of Iowa. I do.

Mr. SHERLEY. Does not the gentleman think they ought to consider amendments offered in good faith by Members not on their committee with regard to whether the amendment is for a good purpose or not, and not simply make the point of order, irrespective of the merits of the proposition?

Mr. SMITH of Iowa. I will answer that question with great pleasure. The committee, at least the subcommittee, has given a most patient and careful investigation to the items of this bill. It could have given no consideration to an amendment here proposed from the floor. An amendment, therefore, proposed by the committee after full consideration should not, in my judgment, be put upon an equality with a proposition made on the floor that had never been submitted to the committee.

Mr. SHERLEY. There is something in that; but does not the gentleman realize that the practice of the committees having in charge these various appropriation bills has been to make the point of order universally, without regard to the matter, whether wise or unwise; and is not the gentleman now in a rather peculiar position when he appeals to the House to accept the wisdom of the committee, that never has accepted the wisdom of the Members of the House?

Mr. SMITH of Iowa. I can not agree that it has been the practice universally to raise the point of order, but the general practice has arisen because the great body of amendments offered from the floor has not been considered by the committee; and it is a matter of common knowledge that wise and orderly legislation ordinarily can not be prepared here upon the floor of the House, but ought to be prepared in the committee room.

Mr. FITZGERALD. The rules of the House were adopted in a manner that prevented any Member of the House attempting to effectuate a change. As soon as the House was organized a motion was made that the rules be adopted which were in force in a previous Congress, the previous question was demanded and ordered, and no Member of the House practically had any voice whatever in the make-up of the rules under which the House operates.

So that when some Member of the House now insists on exercising the rights that are conferred upon him under those rules, it comes with poor grace from those who have shackled the House with the rules to complain of their enforcement.

It may be — and I have no doubt it is the fact — that some of the points of order that have been interjected during the course of this bill have prevented reforms and economies, but the House must realize that in giving gentlemen the power to prevent the consideration of legislation the House itself is responsible for that action and not the gentlemen who undertake to exercise their rights.

Even, Mr. Chairman, though a member of the committee reporting the bill should rise to interpose a point of order, gentlemen are inclined to criticise him seriously for that action. I am not at all in sympathy with that prevalent feeling in this House, that committees are so impeccable, that they are so virtuous, that they are so wise, that when they have determined by a majority vote that certain things should be reported to the House it is high treason for any Member to exercise his right under the rules to prevent, if he desires, the consideration of those matters in violation of the rule. [Applause.]

I am not going to criticise my own committee. I believe that the committee has done its full duty in calling the attention of the House to abuses that exist, and I am indifferent to what happens to any provision in this bill. I will vote for each provision or against it, as my judgment dictates that I should. I am perfectly willing that every other Member of this House shall exercise freely all the rights that he has under the rules in the consideration of this bill, and let each Member do as the committee is compelled to do, assume the responsibility for his own action. When that is done, Mr. Chairman, if it prevents reforms being made on this bill, it may result in vitalizing some of the dead committees of the House. It may result in effecting a reform by accomplishing it through the proper machinery of the House, and there may no longer be the spectacle of seventeen or eighteen committees organized for the purpose of working, but existing merely to give places of refuge to the gentlemen fortunate enough to be appointed as chairmen of these committees.

So I would say to my colleagues on the committee, in the best of good nature, whatever be the course followed by these gentlemen or any other gentlemen, and whatever may be the fate of any provision in the bill, that we rest content in the knowledge that we have performed our duty, and satisfied that everybody else is endeavoring to perform his according to his best judgment and according to his rights.

Mr. SMITH of Arizona. Mr. Chairman, it seems to me that they have gotten into a difficulty here that could be very easily and peacefully and properly settled. Why does not this committee rise and report to the House their inability to handle an appropriation bill, refer it to the Committee on Territories of this House, get a rule passed by the Speaker and pass this bill, and don't let anybody read it? [Laughter.] What is the use of talking about it and wasting time in this way? Two millions of people can be disposed of in twenty minutes' debate, and here you are quibbling over what a clerk gets in some Department. I am ashamed to see my friends forgetting how to attend to public business. [Laughter.] They have got no business to consider this bill, anyway. It has come to a point in the consideration of public business in this House that consideration of a bill is folly. Why, you can not even send it over to the Senate in a shape to suit you. This skeleton is going over there, and the gentlemen who have been trying so hard to maintain the dignity of this body will be crawling on their stomachs to the Senate to get these items put back in the bill. Abuse it with the lips and serve it with your hearts every minute when you want something done. [Applause.] That is what will become of this bill.

Mr. PAYNE. Mr. Chairman, I am reluctant to take any of the time of the committee, because I think this bill would have made much more progress if there had been less debate upon the method of procedure of some of the gentlemen in the House. Now, the House is amply able to take care of itself, even without the aid of the Delegate from Arizona [Mr. Smith], and to pass such legislation as the majority of the House shall deem best to have passed and to defeat such legislation as the majority shall deem best to defeat. Of course, it is in the province of any

Member of the House in Committee of the Whole to raise a point of order, and if the point of order is well taken, the chairman will promptly rule. These rules are in the interest of economy, so far as they relate to appropriation bills, in order that the Committee on Appropriations or anyone else shall not come in here and create new offices unless it is considered by the appropriate committee, the committee having that legislation in charge. They are purposely framed so that any Member can defeat any such attempt on the part of the Committee on Appropriations by raising the point of order, and it does not disturb me in the least to see two gentlemen sitting here and raising points of order. It has generally been the custom of the House, Mr. Chairman, in such cases, for a gentleman to reserve the point of order on a provision in the bill which he thought was out of order and which he could not see the merit of until the item was explained, and if it was explained satisfactorily to him, to waive the point of order and let it go in the bill; but gentlemen have the right to insist upon the point of order. Now, I hope they will insist to their hearts' content, and I hope that when similar points of order are raised upon these items which must go out, that the matter will be left speedily to the Chair to rule upon and to rule whether they are in order or not, and with less debate upon each proposition we can get through with the consideration of this bill in the Committee of the Whole, each Member finding out what he thinks ought to be in and what he thinks ought to be out. Afterwards the House can very easily pass the bill, and pass such a bill as the majority of the House is in favor of, and no two Members or any number of Members less than a majority of the House can prevent it; we can do it with fair consideration, and we can send a bill over to the Senate which does not need to be deliberated upon by making a speech, when three or four Members are present, of three or four hours in length; we can have here when necessary the five-minute debate, when the Members can be brought into contact with all the reasons for or against a single item in the bill, and we can proceed in an orderly manner.

Gentlemen declaim against the rules of the House and they want a sort of town meeting, where every one of 386 Members, clamoring for recognition of the Speaker, shall each receive recognition at the same time to make his motion or to make his speech. They want pandemonium. The rules of the House, Mr. Speaker, are not the result of any one man's work. They are the result of the experience of many more years than most of us have ever seen either in the House or out of it. They are the result of the best thought of the best men who have adorned the halls of Congress in the past on both sides of the House. They were made for the protection of the minority as well as for the advantage of the majority in having its will preferably in this House. And no such exhibition as has been made here to-day and no such declarations as we have just heard from the gentleman from Arizona will change the rules of the House. The rules of the House will remain after we have left it and they will remain substantially as they are to-day, and the House will transact its business under these rules in an orderly and proper manner. I want to say that gentlemen who are opposing this bill will finally see the bill pass in the shape that the majority of the House desire it passed and it will go over to the Senate and they will perform their functions upon it by way of amendment.

SPECIAL RULE ON THE LEGISLATIVE, EXECUTIVE, AND JUDICIAL APPROPRIATION BILL [1]

[In order to save the Legislative, Executive, and Judicial Appropriation Bill from ruin, the committee appealed to the Committee on Rules which came to the rescue on March 28, by reporting a resolution which marks a great advance in the power of centralized leadership in the House. The special rule, as will be seen, virtually cut off any further right on the part of members to enter objections against the bill under consideration. This action illustrates perfectly how absolutely the procedure of the House is controlled by the Committee on Rules. This special rule and the discussions thereon are of the highest importance to an understanding of our Congressional procedure.]

MR. DALZELL. Mr. Speaker, I submit the following privileged report from the Committee on Rules.

The SPEAKER. The gentleman from Pennsylvania submits a report from the Committee on Rules, which the Clerk will read.

The Clerk read as follows:

The Committee on rules, to whom was referred the resolution of the House No. 383, have had the same under consideration and respectfully report in lieu thereof the following:

Resolved, That hereafter, in consideration of the bill (H. R. 16472) making appropriations for the legislative, executive, and judicial expenses of the Government, and for other purposes, in Committee of the Whole House on the state of the Union, it shall be in order to consider, without intervention of a point of order, any section of the bill as reported, except section 8; and upon motion authorized by the Committee on Appropriations it shall be in order to insert in any part of the bill any provision reported as part of the bill and heretofore ruled out on a point of order.

Mr. DALZELL. Mr. Speaker, on that I ask the previous question.

Mr. SULZER. Mr. Speaker, I should like to have some explanation in regard to this rule. It seems to be a very extraordinary departure from the general rules of the House.

Mr. DALZELL. I do not wish to discuss the rule until after the previous question is ordered, because any debate before the ordering of the previous question would cut off all debate thereafter.

[1] *Congr. Record*, March 28, 1906.

The SPEAKER. The gentleman from Pennsylvania moves the previous question upon agreeing to the resolution.

The question being taken, on a division (demanded by Mr. Dalzell) there were — ayes 120, noes 71.

Accordingly the previous question was ordered.

The SPEAKER. The gentleman from Pennsylvania is entitled to twenty minutes, and the gentleman from Mississippi [Mr Williams] to twenty minutes.

Mr. DALZELL. Mr. Speaker, I shall occupy but a very brief time in explanation of the rule.

The House is familiar with the fact that in the consideration of the legislative appropriation bill in Committee of the Whole a great many paragraphs have been stricken out by reason of an appeal to the rule of the House which prevents legislation on appropriation bills. The trouble has been mainly with respect to the number of employees provided for in the bill and with respect to the salaries of employees. The point of order has been made that employees not provided for by existing law are included in the bill and that salaries not provided for by existing law are included in the bill; and it is fair to say that it seems to me that in all cases the point of order has been well taken.

The difficulty with which the House is confronted arises out of the fact that the law fixing the number of employees and the salaries of employees in the various Departments is in most cases an old law, in some cases as old as thirty years, and, of course, during the passage of those thirty years the service of the Government has largely increased, the necessity for new employees has arisen, and the necessity for changes of salary has arisen. Those changes ought to have been made by general law. The fault lies not wholly with the Committee on Appropriations, but largely with the various committees of the House, who ought to have secured the passage of general laws which would authorize the Committee on Appropriations to insert these provisions in the appropriation bill. A custom, however, has grown up during all these years not to make points of order upon items in the appropriation bill which were recognized by the House as appropriate under the circumstances, and the custom therefore has justified the Committee on Appropriations from year to year in putting into the appropriation bill these increases of salary and these increases of appropriation. As I say, the fault lies with the committees of the House, who ought to have provided general legislation. In illustration of that proposition, let me call your attention to what appears on two pages of the *Record*. An appropriation in this bill for the employees at New Orleans went out on a point of order because it infringed a provision of existing law on the subject. That provision was over thirty years old; nevertheless, during all these thirty years since its enactment, without any additional legislation, appropriations corresponding to this have been made by the sufferance of the House.

Now, on the opposite page of the *Record*, you will find a like appropriation for employees at New York, but that did not go out on a point of order, because there appears on the statute book this provision:

The assistant treasurer at New York may appoint from time to time, by and with the consent and approbation of the Secretary of the Treasury, such other clerks, messengers, and watchmen, in addition to those employed by him, as the exigencies of the business may require.

In other words, we ought to have, to avoid the confusion into which we have fallen in this case, such general legislation upon the statute books. It is apparent, however, that the House can not now stop, the business of the country can not be held up, because of the lack of this general legislation. The Government needs must be met, and therefore the only way in which the present needs of the Government can be met is by the adoption of this rule.

The rule provides that these items which have already gone out on points of order may be inserted at the will of the House. In other words, it submits to the House the right to say whether or not upon the merits the items shall go into the bill. The rule also provides that, as to the items not yet reached, they shall be passed upon on their merits irrespective of the technical rule; all except section 8, which relates to superannuated clerks, so called. Your committee felt that that was a piece of legislation that was entitled to be considered by the House as a separate proposition, and therefore that is excepted from the operation of the rule.

Mr. CURTIS. Under the rule that section would be subject to a point of order?

Mr. DALZELL. Yes.

Mr. CURTIS. I think that provision unfair to the clerks who have devoted many years to the service, many of whom were Union soliders, and it should be stricken from the bill.

Mr. JONES of Washington. The rule does not make anything in order that may be offered to be inserted by a Member?

Mr. DALZELL. No; it does not make anything in order except what was reported by the Appropriation Committee and an amendment to it which would be germane.

Mr. JONES of Washington. Does n't the gentleman think that the Members of the House ought to be allowed to offer amendments to be considered on their merits?

Mr. DALZELL. They will have that privilege.

Mr. JONES of Washington. If subject to a point of order, they would go out.

Mr. DALZELL. They would go out anyway.

Mr. MANN. Under this rule the amendment which the Committee on Appropriations offers — that is, to increase the salaries — is in order.

Mr. DALZELL. If it is in the bill.

Mr. MANN. Whether it is in the bill or not, if the committee reports it, it is in order.

Mr. DALZELL. Only as reported in the bill.

Mr. MANN. In that case, then, the amendments offered by any Member of the House to increase that amount would necessarily be in order.

Mr. DALZELL. But subject to a legitimate point of order, of course.

Mr. MANN. If the proposition offered by the Committee on Appropriations is in order, an amendment to that proposition is also in order.

Mr. DALZELL. I should say so.

Mr. NORRIS. I would like to ask the gentleman from Pennsylvania if the Committee on Appropriations puts in the bill an appropriation for a salary, for instance, greater than that allowed by existing law, it would not be subject to a point of order; but if a Member on the floor of the House offers an amendment that increases the salary in the bill greater than that allowed by existing law, that would be subject to a point of order?

Mr. DALZELL. Not if the amendment was to a paragraph in the bill that under the rule was not subject to a point of order.

Mr. NORRIS. So that the gentleman may understand my proposition suppose it makes an appropriation for a salary that is in exact accordance with existing law, and a Member on the floor of the House offers an amendment to increase it beyond that limit, would that be in order?

Mr. DALZELL. I should think not; I should think it would be subject to a point of order. If the committee's proposition was in accordance with the law, and the amendment not in accordance with the law, I should think it would be subject to a point of order.

Mr. NORRIS. In other words, the committee can propose amendments that go beyond existing law, but Members of the House can not. This privilege exists only in favor of the committee. In other words, it is a rule that does not work both ways.

Mr. DALZELL. Not at all. It is a rule that allows the bill as reported by the Committee on Appropriations to be considered without being subject to points of order, except as to section 8. That is all it is.

Mr. WM. ALDEN SMITH. It is to be considered on its merits.

Mr. DALZELL. In other words, it submits to the House the bill as reported by the Committee on Appropriations on its merits. The committee may vote on each proposition without respect to points of order upon the merits of the proposition.

Mr. BROOKS of Colorado. Mr. Speaker, to be more specific on the question asked by the gentleman from Nebraska [Mr. Norris], then if the committee has reported an item which is entirely legal, or an amendment, and the House by amendment attempts to change that in any way, that proposition is open to a point of order.

Mr. DALZELL. Not unless it is against the law.

Mr. Brooks of Colorado. In any way, so that it transgresses the rules.

Mr. Dalzell. For instance, if there is an amount named in the bill. that is subject to amendment.

Mr. Brooks of Colorado. One further question. Then if the committee has reported an item which if objected to would go out on a point of order, that item may be further amended also in the direction that would have been, without the rule, open to a point of order.

Mr. Dalzell. I think so; yes.

Mr. Fitzgerald. Mr. Speaker, will the gentleman yield to a question?

Mr. Dalzell. Yes.

Mr. Fitzgerald. Did the Committee on Rules proceed upon the theory that the Committee on Appropriations was unanimously in favor of having considered in this way all of the legislative provisions excepting section 8?

Mr. Dalzell. I do not understand the gentleman's question.

Mr. Fitzgerald. Did the Committee on Rules proceed upon the assumption that the Committee on Appropriations was unanimous in desiring to have all of the legislative provisions considered in this way excepting section 8?

Mr. Dalzell. Why, we did not think anything about what the Committee on Appropriations wanted especially.

Mr. Fitzgerald. I think the gentleman did, because his rule provides that all the things reported in the bill by the Committee on Appropriations shall be considered regardless of the rules, excepting section 8. Now, there are several other distinctively legislative provisions in the bill not excepted by the rule, but to which there was objection in the committee, about which notice was given that points of order would be interposed and which this rule takes out of the operation of the rules of the House. I would ask the gentleman to explain why the Committee on Rules singled out one legislative provision and not other legislative provisions equally offensive?

Mr. Dalzell. Because we thought that that one legislative provision was so radical in its character, so much more radical than any of the others, that it ought to have separate consideration in the ordinary way.

Mr. Speaker, I reserve the balance of my time. How much more time have I?

Mr. Bartlett. Mr. Speaker, I would like to ask the gentleman a question.

The Speaker. The gentleman has seven minutes remaining.

Mr. Dalzell. Then, Mr. Speaker, I reserve the balance of my time. I can not yield any more.

Mr. Williams. Mr. Speaker, the object of this rule is to make points of order which are in order under the rules of the House out of order under this rule. It is an apt illustration and object lesson, indeed, of the defectiveness of the rules of the House. I shall not consume the time of the committee by arguing that question. Others want to be heard, and I shall yield to them. I now yield five minutes to the gentleman from Illinois [Mr. Prince].

Mr. BARTLETT. Mr. Speaker, may I ask the gentleman from Mississippi a question before he sits down?

Mr. WILLIAMS. Mr. Speaker, I do not want to consume any time if I can help it. I desire to yield to others.

The SPEAKER. The gentleman from Illinois is recognized for five minutes.

Mr. PRINCE. Mr. Speaker, the whole trouble that the House is now in is due to paragraph 2 of Rule XXI of the House of Representatives, which is as follows:

No appropriation shall be reported in any general appropriation bill, or be in order as an amendment thereto, for any expenditure not previously authorized by law, unless in continuation of appropriations for such public works and objects as are already in progress; nor shall any provision changing existing law be in order in any general appropriation bill or in any amendment thereto.

The honorable gentleman from Pennsylvania [Mr. Dalzell], who has just taken his seat, says the points of order have been well taken. So much for the obstructionists. The points of order have been well taken. Now, what does the chairman of the committee say? On page 4281 of the *Congressional Record* of March 23, 1906, Mr. Tawney says:

If this rule is to be enforced, then more than one-half of the provisions of this bill will have to go out.

Properly taken! More than one-half of it is to go out! What is the rule? "No appropriation shall be reported" — confessedly in order are these supposed obstructionists. "The points of order are well taken," says the gentleman from Pennsylvania. The chairman of the committee says that half of it will go out. Why did he knowingly, willfully, deliberately, and flagrantly violate the rules of this House to bring in a bill of which he himself says one-half would go out on points of order if they were made? Now, then, let us turn to the effect of the rule. Here is a rule that applies to one Committee on Appropriations. How many appropriation bills are there, gentlemen of the House?

Look at your Calendar of date March 26, 1906, and you find the following: Urgent deficiency; pensions; fortifications; Army; Indian; legislative, executive, and judicial; post-office; agricultural; diplomatic and consular; District of Columbia; general deficiency; Military Academy; naval; public buildings; rivers and harbors, and sundry civil appropriation bills — sixteen appropriation bills in this House.

If this provision is good for one committee, why is it not good for every committee that passes appropriation bills in this House? [Applause.] Will you tell me? I say now, and wait for answer, if the Committee on Rules will make this special a general rule that will apply to every appropriation committee of this House I will vote for the rule now. Will you do it? What answer have you to make to these other committees that you single out one as against ten others?

What is your reply for doing it when you confessedly admit your bill is out of order, when you confessedly admit every point of order that has been made against the bill is in order and under the rules of this House? Now, who have passed upon the objections? Two honorable Members of this House, none higher in the estimation of this body than those two, sitting day in and day out in the chair as Chairman of the Committee of the Whole House on the state of the Union. The honorable gentleman from Pennsylvania [Mr. Olmsted] held time after time that practically every one of those points of order are in order, and the provisions had to go out. They changed horses for a few minutes, and the distinguished Member from New York [Mr. Payne] took the chair, and he held likewise upon these very same provisions. Where is the obstruction? Now, gentlemen of the House, let me say this to you, that we are all here as Members. You have heard me ask the Committee on Rules if they will make this rule a general rule to apply to your committees on which you are serving and the committees on which I am serving. They have not said they would do it. What will you say to your constituents? Will you vote for a special rule which allows the increases of salaries, changes existing law, and enacts new and original legislation? What will you say to the committees of which you are members, over which have presided for more than a hundred years some of the most distinguished men who have sat in this body ——

The SPEAKER. The time of the gentleman has expired.

Mr. PRINCE. I ask leave to extend my remarks if I so desire.

The SPEAKER. The gentleman from Illinois asks unanimous consent to extend his remarks in the *Record*. Is there objection? [After a pause.] The Chair hears none.

Mr. WILLIAMS. Mr. Chairman, I now yield five minutes to the gentleman from Missouri [Mr. De Armond].

Mr. DE ARMOND. Mr. Speaker, I am one of those who are not opposed to suitable legislation upon an appropriation bill. I am opposed, however, to this way of getting at that legislation. It would be very easy, as matters now stand, to have every item in this appropriation bill considered by the committee and by the House. Of course, when the point of order is made it is the duty of the presiding officer to rule upon that point of order, under the rules. A point of order against new legislation on a bill like this is a good point, and under the rules, the presiding officer has to sustain it. Now, when the point of order is sustained, if there be real occasion for the legislation proposed, what is the reason that the chairman of the subcommittee on appropriations, or the chairman of the Committee on Appropriations, or any other gentleman favoring the proposed legislation, should not frankly admit that the proposition is obnoxious to the rules, but that, owing to its merits, owing to the necessity for legislation at the time and of the kind proposed, the rule as to that item ought to be set aside and the particular matter proposed ought to be enacted into law? Upon that proposition, with a majority of those present sustaining it, the item would remain in or go into the bill. Now, that is a very much safer and a very much better way of proceeding than by a wholesale rule, an omnibus rule. While undoubtedly there are good provisions offered in this bill which are not in accord with existing law, it probably is not saying too much to say that there are also bad provisions offered, also not in accordance with existing law. In the case of a good provision, a necessary provision, upon appeal to the House it is reasonable to believe that the House would sustain the appeal, and would enact the good provision — would put it into the bill or retain it in the bill.

Every provision offered in the way of new law, everything obnoxious to the rules of the House, is protected and covered by this rule; everything suggested by the Committee on Appropriations and incorporated in the bill, including those items that were opposed and knocked out — all are legitimized. Provisions already eliminated are to be brought forward, and no point of order shall be tolerated against any of them or against anything in the bill except section 8, when, no matter how meritorious a proposition offered from the floor may be, the rules may be invoked against it; and if it be a change of existing law, or a proposed change of existing law, it must be denied consideration.

This rule is neither in the interest of good legislation, nor is it fair. Allow the rules to stand, if you will; you made them, made them without consideration, without giving opportunity for any particular consideration. When you see proper to set aside one of them, or any order of this House with reference to any particular piece of legislation, appeal direct to the judgment of the House, and if the judgment of the House sustains you the rules will be waived for the time being, and the meritorious piece of legislation will be incorporated in the bill; and let that apply not only to the Committee on Appropriations — that one committee to be singled out for favor over all other committees — but let it apply to all the other committees, and let it apply also to the entire membership of the House. Whenever a proposition is offered from anywhere and ruled out as new legislation, if the proponent of it, or anybody else, sees proper to ask the judgment of the House upon this proposition, and if the majority see proper to incorporate it, let the rules be then and there set aside as to that matter, and let it be incorporated. There is neither necessity for nor propriety in this rule; it is dangerous in its tendency, and will be bad in its effect. [Loud applause on the Democratic side.]

Mr. WILLIAMS. I will ask the gentleman from Pennsylvania to consume some of his time.

Mr. DALZELL. I propose to close on this side.

The SPEAKER. The gentleman from Pennsylvania has seven minutes and the gentleman from Mississippi ten minutes.

Mr. WILLIAMS. I yield five minutes to the gentleman from Georgia [Mr. Hardwick].

Mr. HARDWICK. Mr. Speaker, it is perfectly apparent that one of two things is true. Either the bill is wrong or the rule is wrong. If the rule is wrong, this bill ought to pass, and the rule ought to be repealed; and if the rule is wrong, then the rule ought to be repealed, so that any bill can pass.

I do not think, Mr. Speaker, that there has ever been in the legislative history of the country such a measure proposed as that contained in this rule. I want to make the statement here in my place that never before in the history of the American Congress has such a proposition been made to any House of Representatives as that contained in this rule. There are two or three precedents in which the Committee on Rules have taken some one single proposition and passed a rule to make a matter in order when a point of order would lie against it and had been urged against it. In the second session of the Fifty-second Congress such a provision was made by the Committee on Rules on one single proposition, namely, the creation of a commission to investigate the various Executive Departments of the Government. In the last session of the Fifty-eighth Congress we had another rule from the committee, authorizing the committee to consider an increase in the salary of the rural carriers, and we had the same proposition at the second session of the Fifty-seventh Congress on a bill providing for the levying of a personal tax in the District of Columbia. Each one of these propositions was segregated and distinct, and the House of Representatives understood what it was voting for. Now, in this proposition, by this omnibus rule, we are offered what? To make everything in order, involving forty-seven separate paragraphs, involving a general increase of appropriations; thirty-eight separate paragraphs, involving different amounts of increase of salary; in other words, in my humble judgment — and I have investigated it to some extent — you are proposing by this rule to legalize about seven hundred things that would not be legal if this rule did not pass.

No member of the Committee on Rules and no Member of this House who votes for this rule will know what on earth he is voting for. Now, if we are going to let the Committee on Appropriations have certain special rights to pass any legislation as riders on appropriation bills. — new legislation — let us have the same rights for everybody. Why should we not? I want to call the attention of the House to the fact that during the progress of the consideration of the pending bill, the gentleman from Mississippi [Mr. Humphreys] arose and asked that the House be allowed to vote on a simple proposition, viz., that the internal-revenue offices of the Government should be required to furnish certified copies of their records to any coördinate court, State or Federal, to be used as evidence, as to what licenses had been taken out for the sale of liquor. That proposition had been recommended by the unanimous vote of just as strong a committee as the Appropriations Committee, to wit, the Ways and Means Committee; and yet the gentleman from New York [Mr. Littauer], in charge of this bill, made the point of order against that and insisted upon it. Now, I say this is not fair. There are good reasons why riders putting new legislation to appropriation bills ought not to be allowed. Under the rules of the House 100 Members constitute a quorum in Committee of the Whole, and fifty-one Members may, if this sort of thing be kept up, enact all sorts of legislation. Indeed, I have seen thirty-six members of the Committee of the Whole decide a question, less even than a quorum of the committee. But even if the rules are invoked, fifty-one Members — less than one-seventh of the membership of the House — can decide a question in committee. There are good reasons back of Rule XXI and it ought to be enforced. I understand the Senate has no such rule, and it may be that when these propositions are meritorious they will be restored in the Senate. With that I am not concerned; but I say that our general rule is a good one and it ought to be enforced, and that it ought not to be varied simply because certain gentlemen want to pass legislation to suit themselves, or because a certain committee wants to do about seven hundred things that the law will not allow them to do, in their own way. [Applause.]

Mr. WILLIAMS. Mr. Speaker, I now yield three minutes to the gentleman from New York [Mr. Driscoll].

Mr. DRISCOLL. Mr. Speaker, this is a very extraordinary method of attempting to pass a very ordinary bill. A measure similar to this, making appropriations for the legislative, executive, and judicial expenses of the Government, is passed every year without any unusual friction and without appealing to the Committee on Rules for assistance. This bill was debated during several days, and when the reading was commenced under the five-minute rule the Committee on Appropriations found itself in trouble. Subdivision 2 of Rule XXI of the Rules of the House of Representatives is as follows:

No appropriation shall be reported in any general appropriation bill, or be in order as an amendment thereto, for any expenditure not previously authorized by law, unless in continuation of appropriations for such public works and objects as are already in progress; nor shall any provision changing existing law be in order in any general appropriation bill or in any amendment thereto.

A few Members of this House on both sides of the Chamber examined the bill with considerable care and they found that this rule of the House was violated in almost every section; that many appropriations of small and large amounts were reported in the bill which were not previously authorized by law, and that there were in it several provisions changing existing law. These were all obnoxious to the rule and liable to be stricken out on points of order. The gentlemen who examined the statutes and this bill commenced to raise these points of order against increases of salaries and clerks and other provisions increasing expenditure, and also against the new provisions changing existing law. In my judgment, those gentlemen who have given much time and attention to this matter and have sat here day after day insisting that the rule be observed have been rendering a signal service, not only to the other Members of this House, but to the country. For their courage or temerity, if we may so describe it, they are entitled to great credit, because there is altogether too much of "you tickle me and I'll tickle you" in this appropriation business. That is why the expenditures increase from year to year, and it is practically impossible to keep them down. Not every Member, especially if there is in the appropriation bill some benefit for his district or constituents, wishes to object to any other appropriation, no matter how extravagant or unreasonable. Therefore these gentlemen are entitled to the thanks of the country for their courageous and unselfish action in behalf of the Treasury.

After a few objections of this character were made the distinguished chairman of the Appropriations Committee, in an able and vigorous speech, undertook to criticise and censure those gentlemen for objecting, and attempted to arouse public sentiment in the House against them. In this he failed, for they continued to raise points of order, which were sustained by the Chair. The gentleman from New York, who has charge of this bill, undertook to lash one of the objectors — the gentleman from Illinois [Mr. Prince] — into silence by twitting him about a little crumb of patronage in the form of a janitorship. This did not avail, and later on another member of the Appropriations Committee took the floor, raised the white flag of truce, and, in a most conciliatory address, sued for peace; and that failed to accomplish the object desired. Now, these gentlemen throw up their hands and surrender at discretion, and acknowledge that they can not pass an ordinary appropriations bill under the ordinary rule which has obtained for many years, and have applied to the all-powerful Committee on Rules for a special rule or resolution giving them extraordinary powers and privileges. Why? Is it claimed that the Chairman of the Committee of the Whole House who presides during the consideration of this bill is unfair or partial? He has had before him the book of rules, and has ably and honestly applied them to each point of order raised; and a gentleman stands at his elbow who writes and revises the book, and who the Speaker said could give any man on the floor of the House cards and spades and beat him in parliamentary law. Now, what is the trouble? The gentlemen in charge of this bill do not assert that they have not received fair treatment in the consideration and application of the rule, and admit that a very large part of this appropriation bill will have to be stricken out if the rule be insisted on. The conclusion is forced on every Member of this House that the rule is a very bad one, or the bill is a very bad one. If the rule is insufficient and antiquated, let it be amended or repealed. If the rule is a good one, let it be applied. If the bill is an extravagant one, let it be trimmed down to come within the limitations of the law.

That is the best way to determine whether it is a good or bad measure. And the best way to determine whether a rule or law is good or bad is by its enforcement. Let the law be applied. Let the rule be enforced. Let the balance of this bill be read, and let the gentlemen who are raising points of order continue to do so and hew to the line and let the chips fall where they may. When it is concluded the country at large will be informed how much of this bill is in violation of law, how much of it represents extravagance, and how much of it is padded, and the Members of this body will be enlightened as to the wisdom of maintaining the rule.

In ordinary proceedings in this House this rule is invoked more perhaps than any other, and we have from time to time been told that for the proper discharge of business and for the sake of economy and wise legislation, it is necessary and should be maintained in its full force and vigor. If any Member of the House suggested to the Appropriations Committee that the number of clerks in a bureau be increased or the salary of any employee be advanced, and it did not suit them, he was told very politely that it was unauthorized by existing law and would be stricken out on a point of order, and he subsided gracefully in deference to the rule. These gentlemen, who have disposed of so many applications by invoking the rule, should be the last to seek relief from the force of its application. They should be willing to take their own medicine.

There are perhaps fifteen other committees of this House who bring in appropriation bills and are expected to have them enacted into law. Why should this rule be suspended as to this committee and this appropriation bill and enforced as to all the others? If a good rule, why should it not be enforced as to all? If a bad rule, why should it not be suspended as to all?

There are 386 Members of this House, and only 17 of them are on the Appropriations Committee. Under this special resolution or rule sought to be adopted here no further points of order can be raised. No objections can be made no matter how many appropriations there are in it which are unauthorized by existing law. Thus the Appropriations Committee will be permitted to submit to the consideration of the House all amendments they have inserted in the bill which will increase salaries and employees, while if any other Member offers an amendment for the same purpose, it will be ruled out on a point of order. If you insist on suspending this rule in its application to the Appropriations Committee, why not suspend it in its application to all the Members and let each of them have the same privilege of offering amendments whether within the provisions of existing law or not? Why should not each Member have the privilege and opportunity of offering an amendment and having it considered on the merits without being ruled out on a point of order, which privilege and opportunity will be accorded the Appropriations Committee under this proposed resolution? The ordinary Member of the House is sufficiently hampered and circumscribed already. Many of you have been complaining and wincing under the application of the rules in force. If you adopt this resolution, you will surrender one of the prerogatives vouchsafed you. You will tie yourselves hand and foot and deliver yourselves bound and gagged into the power of the Appropriations Committee. So far as practical results go, you may as well go home and send so many wooden Indians in your places. [Applause.]

This proposed legislation should not be adopted. We should stand by the rule in force, which seems to have served its purpose pretty well in the past and avoided much unnecessary extravagance. This seems to be a "stand-pat" Congress. Only yesterday the distinguished gentleman from New York, chairman of the Committee on Ways and Means, in a very able and eloquent address, notified the Members of this House and the whole country that there will be no revision of the tariff schedules; that this House will stand pat. For the sake of consistency, for the sake of economy in the public service, and for the protection of our own rights and dignity as individual Members of this body let us "stand pat" on the existing rule and reject this resolution.

The SPEAKER. The time of the gentleman has expired.

Mr. WILLIAMS. I yield the two remaining minutes to the gentleman from New York [Mr. Fitzgerald].

Mr. FITZGERALD. Mr. Speaker, while I have no sympathy with the action of the gentlemen who have been taking matters out of the legislative bill without regard to their merits, yet I do not favor this rule. It is more sweeping in its character than I have been able to find in a search of the precedents. It makes it possible to keep in this bill indefensible increases of salary for favorites of some men in this House, while those who are without influence are ignored entirely. The committee, indeed, might be said to have been tyrannical in reporting this bill, because, in defiance of the rules, points of order submitted in committee were ignored, although the rules of the House are binding there, and matters that should not be in the bill are in it and are going to be continued in it under this rule. There are other legislative provisions equally indefensible, equally offensive, equally as important for separate consideration as section 8; and yet the Committee on Rules, without knowing what is in the bill, includes the good with the bad and compels the House to consider on this bill provisions with which few of the Members are familiar.

If this rule was framed so that these matters of importance — the matters that had real merit — would be considered in this way, I would gladly support this rule, but unless this rule is so framed that other committees with appropriating powers are permitted to report legislation and have it considered, the exception should not be made in this case.

This rule — Rule XXI, under which the points of order have been made — is of great importance and value, having originated in 1837, or else it is absolutely worthless. If it is worthless, it should be modified to meet the changed conditions. In my judgment, the action of these two gentlemen, of which complaint is made, while it has done great harm in some instances, yet they have effected considerable good in the position they have taken during the past few days. It would be an extraordinary thing to permit the Committee on Appropriations, of which I happen to be a member, to say that increases of salaries for certain persons should be considered in order on the legislative bill while increases for other men who have no friends could not be considered. [Applause.]

Mr. DALZELL. Mr. Speaker, I now yield the balance of my time to the gentleman from Ohio [Mr. Grosvenor].

Mr. GROSVENOR. Mr. Speaker, the rule of the House which has been so often invoked by the gentleman from Georgia [Mr. Hardwick] and the gentleman from Illinois [Mr. Prince] is an old and time-honored rule of the House. It was not made by a Republican House; it originated in a Democratic House. I found it in active operation when I came here twenty years ago, and it has been pretty effectually enforced ever since. On the present occasion I wish first to state, so that the Members of the House will not be misled, that the proposed rule operates upon provisions subject to a point of order made against them in the pending bill in this way: In the first place, it leaves exactly where we find it all that part of the bill which relates to aged or superannuated clerks that has gone out of the bill, and it is not proposed to put it back into the bill by the operation of this rule.

Mr. KEIFER. That provision has not yet gone out.

Mr. GROSVENOR. It has gone out under the rules as effectually as if it had never been put in. The various rulings of the Chair have that effect. Now, what next? The next operation is to make it in order that the other provisions of the bill, to which exceptions have been taken and which have been sustained by the Chairman, will still be in order, but subject to the action of the House upon each one of these provisions separately. So that a majority of the Committee of the Whole House can either adopt one of these provisions, or amend one of these provisions, or reject it altogether. It simply affords the House the full opportunity to pass upon every one of these objectionable provisions.

Mr. Speaker, the Committee on Appropriations, after very careful study, apparently — and I think I may safely say so — have brought here a provision that looks to me, and, I think, looks to gentlemen even on the other side, as a proposition of great improvement, as it will completely reorganize certain of the clerical forces of the various Departments here. It is true it comes here without the sanction of the rule of the House. The gentleman from Illinois [Mr. Prince] seems to take it for granted that to bring a bill into the House with a paragraph or section in it obnoxious to the rule of the House is a sort of parliamentary crime, a crime for which the Committee on Appropriations ought to be indicted. Why, I have never known of an appropriation bill of any considerable length that did not have some provision in it that was held by the Chairman to be obnoxious to the rule that has been invoked here against provisions of the pending bill.

·Mr. Speaker, here is what we have got to meet: We must abandon our proposition of reform and improvement and send a bill to the Senate that would be disgraceful to the House of Representatives — a bill that does not and would not provide for any considerable completeness in the appropriations — or else, having ascertained what ought to be done, we temporarily set aside this rule for the purpose of doing exactly what the House of Representatives will decide ought to be done. It is not a revolutionary proposition; it is a proposition looking to the action of the House itself, an action which they may just as well take in this form as to take it in some other form. How can you get this proposition before the House anywhere else during this session of Congress than in an appropriation bill and in this appropriation bill?

There is a large number of appropriations for salaries of clerks employed in the various bureaus of the Government that have gone out of the bill under the ruling of the Chair, which was a proper ruling and had to be made. Now, shall we stumble about here and act unwisely and inconsiderately, or shall we take up these amendments one by one and act wisely and judiciously and in keeping with a rule of the House that is higher than a written rule in the books? Gentlemen seem to think that this action in the House is in some way or other revolutionary. It is just as exactly and as completely in order and just as proper as it would be to create a new rule. Gentlemen say, "Send the rule back to the Committee on Rules and let them make a new rule." That is no more in consonance with good judgment and wise legislation than will be the correction of the difficulty by this action, this temporary action, upon this particular appropriation bill. Mr. Speaker, this is the shortest and best way to give to the House a fair opportunity to be heard upon every one of these propositions and to act intelligently and wisely. Therefore I think that gentlemen who have delayed this bill all these days ought not now to appeal to the House to destroy the bill and compel it to go back to the Committee on Appropriations to have a new investigation and a new bill. [Applause.] [1]

MR. TAWNEY ON URGENT DEFICIENCIES [2]

Mr. Tawney. Prior to the Fifty-eighth Congress deficiencies in appropriations made for the public service had become so common and had increased to such an extent that that Congress deemed it essential to enact legislation to prevent such deficiencies. Theretofore many of the Executive Departments proceeded on the theory that they, and not Congress, should fix the standard of public expenditure, and if the amount appropriated for the service under their jurisdiction was not in their judgment adequate, they proceeded to expend the appropriation upon the basis of their estimates and then at the next session of Congress would submit deficiency estimates which, if not allowed, would necessitate the suspension of the service.

It was this practice which prompted a distinguished Cabinet officer during this session to state before the Committee on Appropriations that this policy was the policy of coercive appropriations and should be stopped. In view of these increasing deficiency estimates the chairman of the Committee on Appropriations, the Hon. James A. Hemenway, now serving in the United States Senate, reported in one of the general appropriation bills at the last session of the Fifty-eighth Congress a provision requiring the heads of the Departments at the beginning of each fiscal year to apportion appropriations, by monthly allotment, or otherwise, so as to prevent a deficiency, and that such apportionment when made could not be waived except by the head of the

[1] Commentary of the *New York Evening Post* upon this legislative incident:

All students of legislation have agreed in denouncing the Congressional practice of passing general legislation as part of the appropriation bills. This year, at the hands of a group of embattled members, the House of Representatives got, as the phrase is, "just what was coming to it." Out of a difficulty of its own creation it extricates itself by an action which, however "practical," is without justification in logic, law or precedent. In the face of the absolutely definite rule against expenditures not authorized by existing law, the Appropriations Committee has followed its own sweet will so far that the Legislative, Executive, and Judicial bill has been "riddled " by perfectly valid points of order, and can be saved only by a special rule to the effect that it shall be passed whether legal or illegal. The point of order in Congress has long been regarded simply as a club. The speaker does not enforce the rule against new legislation or provisions not germane unless somebody brings the case to his attention. Thus many of the most necessary bills, as in the present instance, come upon the floor in a shockingly vulnerable state. As for the extraordinary expedient adopted to save the measure, we hope the incident will merely be a salutary warning to the House, and not the beginning of a line of precedent that will still further tighten the grip of the Speaker and the Rules Committee upon the organization.

[2] *Congr. Record*, reported July 2, 1906.

Department. The waiver was required to be in writing, stating the reasons therefor.

At the beginning of this session, when the deficiency estimates were presented, it was discovered that this act was defective in that it did not restrict the waiver of the apportionment beyond the giving of a reason. This enabled the head of the Department to waive the apportionment for any reason, and proceed to expend the appropriation regardless of whether such expenditure would create a deficiency or not. In some instances it was stated as a reason for waiving the apportionment that Congress had failed to appropriate the amount estimated by the Department to be necessary for a specific service, and the amount appropriated for the entire year having been practically all expended at the end of the third quarter, Congress was obliged to appropriate for the remaining quarter or suspend the service.

To correct this, and to prevent the Departments from determining how much should be expended for the public service regardless of the amount appropriated, the first appropriation bill reported at this session of Congress amended this so-called anti-deficiency law by expressly providing that the apportionment, when made, shall not be waived except upon the happening of some emergency or unusual circumstance which could not be reasonably anticipated at the time of making the apportionment. While the law as it was enacted by the Fifty-eighth Congress had a very salutary effect in preventing deficiencies, as it enabled this Congress to reject many deficiencies that otherwise might have been appropriated for, nevertheless it is believed that this law as amended at this session will practically wipe out all deficiencies in annual appropriations that must be apportioned, except in case of an emergency or other unusual circumstance which could not be anticipated either by the Department or by Congress.

The penalties which are imposed by this law on account of the failure to comply with it are such that it is believed that those who are charged with the responsibility of expending appropriations will so administer the service under their jurisdiction as to keep their expenditures within the amounts appropriated for the entire year.

There have been reported in other appropriation bills many legislative provisions, many of which have been enacted into law, restrictive in their character and imposing limitations upon departmental officers that will tend to improve administrative methods and effect economy in the public expenditures.

One provision reported in the legislative, executive and judicial appropriation bill is worthy of special mention. It is the provision enacted to put a stop to the practice of the several Executive Departments of the Government competing with each other for clerical services. It will have the effect also of preventing the demoralization which now happens as a result of clerks, as soon as they are appointed in one Department, seeking positions in another Department where the compensation is greater than that in the Department in which they are employed. This provision prohibits the transfer of any clerk from one Department to another until he has served in the Department from which he desires to be transferred at least three years.

Another, and still more important provision, as viewed by the Committee on Appropriations, is the one which is now a law as a part of the Sundry Civil appropriation Act, requiring the heads of each Department in the future to report to the Secretary of the Treasury, within thirty days after the close of every fiscal year, a statement of all money received by them during the previous fiscal year for or on account of the public service or in any other manner in the discharge of their official duties, other than as salaries or compensation, which was not paid into the general Treasury of the United States, together with a detailed account of all payments, if any made from such funds during said year.

It was ascertained by the Committee on Appropriations in the course of its investigations that in some fiscal years many millions of dollars, representing proceeds of public property or money derived from some source no account of the public service was being handled by Department officials without any account of the same being taken as a part of the receipts or expenditures of the Government. The fact that no dishonesty or irregularity has occurred because of this unbusiness-like method in the public service did not argue, in the opinion of the committee, that this effective precaution should not be taken against the possibility of breach of trust encouraged, or at least not guarded against, by the law.

While the expenditures of our Government are constantly increasing, and while the appropriations made therefor by Congress are in the aggregate very large, yet when we take into consideration the marvelous growth of the country, the extent to which the people demand that the Federal Government shall perform services that should be paid by the States, none but the unthinking or misguided who do not stop to consider the care with which the estimates for appropriations for the public service are scrutinized by the several committees having jurisdiction of appropriation bills can find any reason to criticise appropriations made during this session of Congress.

During the seven months of this session the Committee on Appropriations has spent practically all of the time in endeavoring to ascertain what appropriations can be eliminated without detriment to the public service, and what changes in administration should be made to reduce expenditures. The hearings on the several appropriation bills reported from the general Committee on Appropriations during this session cover nearly 4,000 printed pages, and comprise three large volumes. These hearings have been more extensive during this session than in any previous Congress — all for the purpose of avoiding unnecessary or extravagant appropriations.

REPRESENTATIVE LITTAUER ON APPROPRIATIONS [1]

MR. LITTAUER. Mr. Chairman, the legislative, executive, and judicial appropriation bill as presented to the House makes provision for the annual salaries of 14,406 public officials. It carries appropriation in all of $29,134,181. The annual Book of Estimates as submitted to Congress called for appropriation in connection with this bill of $447,000 increase over the bill of last year. The bill we present to you is $1,135,572 less than the estimates, or, in other words, $688,000 less than is carried in the bill for the current year.

The Departments have asked for an increase of force of one hundred and seventy-one. The bill carries two hundred and thirty-two less than was submitted to us, or a decrease of force of sixty-one.

Mr. Chairman, it requires much more than a cursory examination of a bill of this character, regulating the salaries of the entire governmental service, to appreciate the hundreds of details it contains. In fact, your committee after weeks of labor on the bill has been unable to consider each one of its many details. We must necessarily be guided in large measure by the detail of former appropriation bills and consideration of the various submissions of the Book of Estimates — submissions for increase of force, increase of compensation, and for new projects. We have, however, in late years had frequent occasion to refer to many facts to demonstrate that the annual estimates were often prepared with less care and scrutiny than they deserved. The estimates come to us through the heads of Departments, the Secretaries of the President's Cabinet, whose many duties, established by law and by custom, take up so much of their time that it seems impossible for them to enter into details which they submit to us. The result is that in general practice they are compelled to rely upon statements, estimates, and submissions of their bureau chiefs, as we have to depend upon theirs.

The result of this custom is that in matters of submission of estimates the bureau chief is in reality supreme and soon grows into the habit of thinking he ought to be supreme. So that, if, in the course of events, the Secretary sees fit to eliminate any of his estimates, to cut them down or to cut them out in part, or if the judgment of Congress, as declared in its appropriations, takes a like course, the gentlemen at the head of these bureaus seem to have taken it upon themselves to study out means and methods of drawing from the general appropriations — the indeterminate appropriations — for their departments and bureaus such sums as in their own good judgment are necessary to carry out the purposes of their bureaus as they believe they ought to be carried out. Their impulse, as is generally stated, is that they seek to carry on the necessary work of their bureaus as they believe it ought to be carried on. The

[1] *Congr. Record*, March 13, 1906.

system has resulted in placing the opinion of the bureau chief over that of his superior officer; it negatives the action of Congress, and leads, as we have frequently demonstrated in this bill, to a diversion of public funds and extravagant expenditure, thwarting the purpose of Congress, paying higher salaries, bringing about abuses in promotion, and applying funds intended for one purpose to the accomplishment of others.

Your Committee on Appropriations has sought in this bill to limit every diversion of public funds from the exact purpose for which they were appropriated, and if gentlemen will examine the report accompanying the bill, they will find that we have placed many limitations on the expenditure of appropriations. For instance, in the State Department we have placed a limitation on the use of the emergency fund given to the President for the emergencies in the diplomatic service, used for clerk hire in the Department in Washington. In the War Department we have limited the use of general appropriations for the detail of civil officers and clerks to bureaus in the Department from other branches of the service in the District of Columbia.

In the Navy Department we found contingent expenses in the bureaus were drawn not only from the contingent fund of the Department, but from the general appropriations for the bureaus and for the increase of the Navy. We intend to put a stop to that practice. In the Treasury Department we found an appropriation for the restoration of old rolls and vouchers. All the old ones seem to have been restored. The fund was used to supplement the clerks in the various bureaus of the Department, and we have omitted that appropriation. And then we took it upon ourselves to wipe out every lump-sum appropriation that we could get at. We found that certain forces had been provided for year after year, as, for instance, in the Bureau of Engraving and Printing, forces that were devoted to the executive work of that office; we took them over and specifically provided for them. In the Office of the Supervising Architect there was a like condition. Gentlemen all know that about 5 per cent is drawn from the appropriation made for new buildings and applied to work of design and engineering for draftsmen and clerks here in the Supervising Architect's Office. We took over as much of that force as seemed to us to be permanent. We have covered into this bill specifically every force that we could get at, carried by lump-sum appropriation. There were a few in regard to which we felt that it was not yet the proper time to appropriate specifically, and notably the administrative force of the Government Printing Office, concerning the work of which we held elaborate hearings, but found that the Public Printer, recently appointed to that office, had not yet such comprehensive idea of the work and had not yet begun the elimination of the force that was necessary to properly conduct the office, and hence was not able to advise us in reference to specific salaries for the necessary force.

It is becoming gradually more and more difficult for us to ferret out what is going on in the Departments. Our hearings lasted for weeks, extending over 700 pages in the pamphlet before you. The fact is constantly before us that we should have at our service some sort of aid which would examine into the expenditure after the appropriation has been made, so as to get at the facts in the bureaus of what is actually taking place there in order to control with fullest intelligence appropriations for the future. The machinery provided by Congress for the examination of accounts and expenditures, of economy, justness, correctness of expenditures, of conformity with appropriation law, of retrenchment, abolishment of useless offices, of the reduction and increased pay of officers is evidently not in working order; at any rate, some gear is out of place which needs looking after by the engineers in charge. Without some aid from those who have made examinations of the actual conduct of expenditures in the bureaus your Committee on Appropriations probes away, in the ascertaining of these facts, largely in the dark. We follow up leads which come to us through rumors or through our own experience and casual observation. Our efforts in forming such an appropriation bill as this toward getting at necessary facts can amount to nothing but a scratch on the surface, astounding though such revelations scratched up actually are. The diversion of appropriations, setting aside the will of Congress, despite such limitations as we place upon expenditure to prevent the diversion of funds intended for one purpose to the accomplishment of another, will go on unless we can provide active and live means for greater scrutiny and vigilance over the operation of the Departments. Actual violations of the law can not be charged, but the intention of Congress is constantly thwarted by unauthorized use of its appropriations, diverted through the study of various appropriation bills to find the technical right for the diversion of funds.

Now, Mr. Chairman, the consideration of a bill of this character naturally leads us to an examination of the conditions we find in the public service, and we have this year been greatly impressed by many serious consequences — matters that have grown worse in the course of time in connection with the appointment, the methods of promotion, and the tenure of office.

Mr. Chairman, I want first to call the attention of the committee to what to-day seems to be an absolute necessity — a reclassification of the Government service for the purpose of establishing the principle that like work should receive like pay. To-day we find forces of men receiving salaries at $900, at $1,000, at $1,200, and even at $1,800 a year performing exactly the same work. This is most demoralizing to the force and works detriment. It is as unjust as it is unfair. Unjust to the man who performs the same work as his neighbor and at a lower salary, and unfair in the distribution of the public funds. We find by our system of promotion that a clerk working at one time at a thousand dollars will perform just the same work when thereafter, in the course of years, he has been promoted to $1,200 or $1,400, or to a compensation of $1,800 per year. Such a system of promotion is manifestly wrong. I do not see how we can reform these matters in our appropriation bill. I feel that there ought to be appointed a commission of the two Houses of Congress to consider this subject of inequality of pay and the subject of the methods of promotion, and the causes why in one Department a larger force is required to accomplish the same result as a much smaller force in another Department.

It seems to me that we ought to have a commission to consider these problems with power to report their recommendations with every privilege. If we do not take some action, the inequality of compensation will continue to grow from year to year until its growth will be a serious detriment to the proper conduct of our Departments.

Mr. Chairman, the Government offers a very attractive field of occupation in its service. Our salaries, especially those in the ordinary clerical force, are not only generously liberal, but even extravagantly high in comparison with what is paid throughout the country. I make bold to say that if the conduct of our service could be the same as that which obtains in the great manufacturing and trading concerns of the country, in the railroads, such as the New York Central or the Pennsylvania Railroad companies, that the service of the Government could be conducted by three-fourths of the force now employed and at practically little more than half its cost. Our salaries are higher, our hours of work are less, our leaves of absence with pay are longer, our holidays are more frequent, and the relative productive gait at which our clerks work is decidedly lower, with the result that the wide-open doors of our public service, barred only by an examination for competency, are always crammed jam full with numerous applicants. Once inside the doors, safely within the public service, those not blessed with more than the usual ambition or independence remain until death makes a vacancy in their positions. Under the operation of civil-service regulations, with its wide-open door at the entrance, there is no other outlet, except by resignation, than a door wide enough to let a coffin through. [Applause.]

Now, Mr. Chairman, our conditions are daily growing worse, until the time has come when we must devote our best endeavors to correct this state of affairs. With the right of continuous tenure in office must go the demand that the clerk remain competent. When through any infirmity, mental or physical, he is no longer competent to deliver an equivalent for his salary, he must make room for those able to do so. Our Government is no charitable institution.

Mr. GROSVENOR. Mr. Chairman, I should like to ask the gentleman a question.

Mr. LITTAUER. Certainly.

Mr. GROSVENOR. I should like to inquire of the gentleman in charge of this bill, and whose statement is very interesting, if there is no power anywhere to get rid of an incompetent clerk?

Mr. LITTAUER. There is. The law makes amp.e provision for getting rid of an incompetent clerk to-day; but I was just about to comment on the fact that the law is never carried out.

Mr. GROSVENOR. Can you make a law that will be lived up to?

Mr. LITTAUER. I believe we can make provision that would eliminate incompetent and incapacitated employees.

Mr. GROSVENOR. Would it not be a good idea to eliminate some of the people who refuse to obey the law?

Mr. LITTAUER. It would be, and they are the heads of bureaus and heads of Departments, who seem to be overcome with sympathy.

Mr. CHARLES B. LANDIS. And are some of them in the same class?

Mr. LITTAUER. And many of them are in the same class. But, Mr. Chairman, as I was saying, this Government is not a charitable institution. Our Departments must not be turned into homes for the aged and infirm. We must demand that our clerks continue competent, and we must find means of getting rid of those who prove that they are not competent. For years this House has included a provision in this very bill declaring that no appropriation carried in the bill should be applicable to the payment of the salary of an incapacitated clerk; but when our bill reaches another body we find insistence there that this incapacity must be "permanent" incapacity, or it must be incapacity "other than temporary." Then the administration of the law falls into the hands of the heads of the Departments and the heads of the bureaus, and these gentlemen declare that they are not gifted with divine foresight, that they can not tell whether the incapacity of the day, in the case of any clerk, will not be cured at a future day. They say they can not tell whether the clerk stricken with paralysis may not at some future day be drawn out of his trouble. Consequently the law is nothing but a dead letter.

It was never the intention of Congress that tenure in the civil service should be for life, but only during efficiency, and yet the action of these heads of Departments and heads of bureaus, permitting their sympathies to carry them away, has evidently thwarted the intention of Congress. While appointment to office is no longer the spoil of the victorious partisan, retention in office has become the spoil of the incapacitated clerk.

REPRESENTATIVE GILLETT ON THE INFLUENCES IN LEGISLATION TOWARDS EXTRAVAGANCE [1]

"What the Appropriations Committee has to consider in making up any bill is not how small it ought to be, but how small we can make it,

[1] *New York Evening Post*, May 29, 1905.

and still have it go through the House," said Representative Frederick H. Gillett, a member of that committee, in discussing to-day the influences which were operative in national legislation toward extravagance. The recently retired chairman of that committee, Mr. Hemenway, has lately expressed his opinion that we needed no tariff revision and no increase of internal revenue; that what we really needed was the elimination of needless expenditures. Mr. Gillett thus shows how difficult that task would be. He has had some experience in the troubles of an economist, for he has been pilloried and lampooned in the Washington newspapers for extending the working day in the departments from four to half-past, in accordance with the law. Speaking of the needs of economy, Mr. Gillett said:

"The great difficulty is to find the spot where Congress will agree to economize. Most of the members say they are for economy, and I believe they are sincere, but when it comes to applying their principles to any particular case, there is apt to be some special reason against it, and so, while favoring economy in the abstract, they oppose it in practice. The most common instance is, of course, where money is to be spent in a man's district, for a public building, or for river or harbor improvements. Some districts seem to gauge their representative's ability and usefulness by his success in extracting money from the Treasury to be spent at home. When constituents set up such a standard, it is hard for a member not to be influenced by it.

"Gradually the men who want different things compare their needs, combine and agree to help one another, tacitly or avowedly, and thus a majority may be rounded up, which is quite insensible to argument, because each one is earnest for his own appropriation, and knows that the only way to get it is to support the other claims, regardless of their merits. This is, of course, the time-honored system of log-rolling, but I fear that as the country has grown larger, its interests more diverse, and its sections more separate and mutually unknown, the tendency develops for a member to feel that he can not grasp and master the needs of the whole, and that therefore he will be content to look out for his district and himself. There was a striking instance not long ago when an influential State delegation were intent on securing a large appropriation, and, apparently fearing argument would not win it, set about gaining votes by promising to support other schemes, and their independence and judgment were mortgaged throughout that Congress by the trades they made.

"Every member will denounce such methods in theory, and admit that they are destructive of good legislation, but many honorable men will stoop to them under the belief that it is the only way to achieve some most deserving end, and to maintain their popularity at home.

"The Appropriations Committee in making up the large bills is subjected to great pressure from members of the House — never for economy, but always for larger expenditure in each man's district. Naturally the committee has a pride in carrying its bills through the House without substantial amendments, and consequently, in formulating the bills, must take into account not only the merits, but the popularity of each proposition, and it will be discouraging to friends of economy to know that the committee never has any fears that the House will reduce any expenditure — the danger always is of increases. There is no selfish interest enlisted on the side of economy, while every member has pressure from home for increased expenditure, and naturally the Government suffers. Experience on the Appropriations Committee, when one sees how defenseless the Treasury is against the constant assaults upon it, is bound to make a man an economist unless he reaches that hopeless stage where he concludes that resistance is vain, and that he might as well join the scramble, take what he can, and wait for the deluge. Unless public opinion is aroused to the dangers of this constant attack upon the Treasury, by endorsing the members who oppose it, constantly increasing deficits must be expected."

CAPITALIZING EXTRAVAGANCE, 1901 [1]

MOST of the Congressional alarm and lamenting over swollen public expenditures is beside the mark. Senators with hands all adrip with extravagance of their own reproach others for wanting to do what they themselves have already done. That is neither edifying nor convincing. Nor does it advance the cause of economy, which, like charity, begins at home. As little are we profited by charges and proof that the minority party is just as extravagant, just as eager to fasten its own little local jobs upon the Treasury, as the party in control of the Government. The pot may be perfectly justified in calling the kettle black; but it is the pot which is responsible, and which will be smashed if an overtaxed people ever takes to looking about for an object of vengeance. Republicans may taunt and expose Democrats to their hearts' content; but if there is inexcusable extravagance, and if anybody is to be held to stern account for it, the Republican party will be the sole sufferer, as it is really the sole offender. Under party government no other result is possible or desirable.

One reason why the party responsible for the Government is less able, if not less willing, than it used to be to keep down appropriations, has often been pointed out in these columns. Our system does not lend itself to rigid financial control. Unlike all other governments in the world, the American has no man, or committee of men, to make up a yearly budget, to determine income and fix outgoes. Our method is a

[1] Editorial in the *New York Evening Post*, 1901.

happy-go-lucky plan of allowing one set of men to make laws for revenue, another to frame bills for expenditures. That we have not gone to smash under such chaotic management is due partly to our traditional good fortune, partly to our expanding wealth — which has operated in the same way that robust health enables a man to order his life recklessly, for a time — and partly to the fact that we have had a rough system of financial control. But this has been badly broken down.

At the close of the civil war the Committee on Ways and Means had charge of all the appropriation bills as well as the revenue bills. That was something like a budget-framing body. Then came the creation of the Committee on Appropriations, to take sole charge of outgo as the Ways and Means Committee did of income. What this meant in the days when Samuel J. Randall was Chairman of the Appropriations Committee, everybody whose memory goes back to 1874–76 will recall. But, under malign influences, the House has been induced, from time to time, to scatter the annual appropriation bills among thirteen or fourteen different committees, each intent on log-rolling its own measure up to the top notch, and with no firm and centralized control existing longer anywhere. Responsibility has thus been dissipated, and so have the funds. Chairman Cannon may still protest that it is his main business not to make appropriations, but to prevent their being made, and Senator Allison may warn and protest; but effective control has largely escaped from them, and their complaints are unheeded. Some day Congress will see this hugger-mugger system driving us straight to national bankruptcy, and will be compelled to set up a responsible government in financial matters — something that we are now alone among the nations in not having.

One serious aspect of national extravagance is commonly overlooked. People do not see how one spendthrift Congress makes the next one almost inevitably as prodigal. The reason is that the extravagant legislation fixes a permanent charge on the Treasury. No step backward, is the rule. There was loud outcry against a "billion-dollar Congress"; but its successor was able to save little or nothing. Now we are rapidly approaching a billion-dollar session, and no dam for the rising flood is in sight. Each succeeding Congress inherits a legacy of extravagance from its predecessor. Its own hands are partly tied by anterior legislation committing the Government to continuing appropriations for this and that scheme, this and that enlargement of the public service and creation of new offices. It is this which makes retrenchment so difficult, if not practically impossible. To abolish places, to consolidate offices, to cut down regular expenses — why, this is almost treason, from the party point of view. It is flat villainy in the minds of men whose sinecures are threatened. So that extravagance always tends to perpetuate itself. The lavish appropriations of one Congress become a kind of annual interest charge which must be paid upon a capitalized extravagance.

A common fallacy in all this business is the urging of an analogy from private life. Congress will economize, it is said, when it has to, just as a man will when his income is cut in two. We are now in the presence of an overflowing Treasury; there will be a surplus after all the bills are paid; the country is prosperous; no one complains of taxes — so what are you afraid of? When the lean years come, the appropriations will be lean. A man gives up his carriage and his box at the opera in hard times, and Congress will do the same. Ah, but Congress's coach-. man will simply refuse to be discharged. The federated coachmen all over the country — *i. e.*, the officeholders — will prove stronger than Congress. They will tell it that it has brought them into the world, and now it must fill their mouths. What, will Congress be worse than an infidel, and not provide for its own? It is not merely in war expenses that Congress has been lavish. Every appropriation bill has been increased, new offices created, new entering wedges driven, a permanent charge on the Treasury laid in many a swollen item. The point is that flush times are setting a pace which will have to be kept up in the lean times. If economy is disregarded now, it will be declared impossible then. It is easy enough to let the jinn of extravagance *out* of the bottle, but to get him back in again — that is the labor. Thus we see that the evil which an extravagant Congress does lives after it; and the good, if good there be, is interred with its bones.

PRESIDENT CLEVELAND'S VETO MESSAGE ON THE RIVER AND HARBOR BILL, 1896

To the House of Representatives:

I return herewith without approval House bill, No. 7977, entitled "An act making appropriations for the construction, repair, and preservation of certain public works on rivers and harbors, and for other purposes."

There are 417 items of appropriation contained in this bill, and every part of the country is represented in the distribution of its favors.

It directly appropriates or provides for the immediate expenditure of nearly $14,900,000 for river and harbor work. This sum is in addition to appropriations contained in another bill for similar purposes amounting to a little more than $3,000,000, which have already been favorably considered at the present session of Congress.

The result is that the contemplated immediate expenditures for the objects mentioned amount to about $17,000,000.

A more startling feature of this bill is its authorization of contracts for river and harbor work amounting to more than $62,000,000. Though the payments on these contracts are in most cases so distributed that they are to be met by future appropriations, more than $3,000,000 on their account are included in the direct appropriations above mentioned. Of the remainder nearly $20,000,000 will fall due during the fiscal year ending June 30th, 1898, and amounts somewhat less in the years immediately succeeding. A few contracts of a like character authorized under previous statutes are still outstanding, and to meet payments on these more than $4,000,000 must be appropriated in the immediate future.

If, therefore, this bill becomes a law, the obligations which will be imposed on the Government, together with the appropriations made for immediate expenditure on account of rivers and harbors, will amount to about $80,000,000. Nor is this all. The bill directs numerous surveys and examinations which contemplate new work and further contracts and which portend largely increased expenditures and obligations.

There is no ground to hope that in the face of persistent and growing demands the aggregate of appropriations for the smaller schemes, not covered by contracts, will be reduced or even remain stationary. For the fiscal year ending June 30th, 1898, such appropriations, together with the installments on contracts which will fall due in that year, can hardly be less than $30,000,000; and it may reasonably be apprehended that the prevalent tendency toward increased expenditures of this sort and the concealment which postponed payments afford for extravagance will increase the burdens chargeable to this account in succeeding years.

In view of the obligation imposed upon me by the Constitution, it seems to me quite clear that I only discharge a duty toward our people when I interpose my disapproval of the legislation proposed.

Many of the objects for which it appropriates public money are not related to the public welfare, and many of them are palpably for the benefit of limited localities or in aid of individual interests.

On the face of the bill it appears that not a few of these alleged improvements have been so improvidently planned and prosecuted that after an unwise expenditure of millions of dollars new experiments for their accomplishment have been entered upon.

While those intrusted with the management of public funds in the interest of all the people can hardly justify questionable expenditures for public work by pleading the opinions of engineers or others as to the practicability of such work, it appears that some of the projects for which appropriations are proposed in this bill have been entered upon without the approval or against the objections of the examining engineers.

I learn from official sources that there are appropriations contained in the bill to pay for work which private parties have actually agreed with the Government to do in consideration of their occupancy of public property.

Whatever items of doubtful propriety may have escaped observation or may have been tolerated in previous Executive approvals of similar bills, I am convinced that the bill now under consideration opens the way to insidious and increasing abuses and is in itself so extravagant as to be especially unsuited to these times of depressed business and resulting disappointment in Government revenue. This consideration is emphasized by the prospect that the public Treasury will be confronted with other appropriations made at the present session of Congress amounting to more than $500,000,000.

Individual economy and careful expenditure are sterling virtues which lead to thrift and comfort. Economy and the exaction of clear justification for the appropriation of public moneys by the servants of the people are not only virtues but solemn obligations.

To the extent that the appropriations contained in this bill are instigated by private interests and promote local or individual projects their allowance can not fail to stimulate a vicious paternalism and encourage a sentiment among our people, already too prevalent, that their attachment to our Government may rest upon the hope and expectation of direct and especial favors and that the extent to which they are realized may furnish an estimate of the value of governmental care.

I believe no greater danger confronts us as a nation than the unhappy decadence among our people of genuine and trustworthy love and affection for our Government as the embodiment of the highest and best aspirations of humanity, and not as the giver of gifts, and because its mission is the enforcement of exact justice and equality, and not the allowance of unfair favoritism.

I hope I may be permitted to suggest, at a time when the issue of Government bonds to maintain the credit and financial standing of the country is a subject of criticism, that the contracts provided for in this bill would create obligations of the United States amounting to $62,000,000 no less binding than its bonds for that sum.

GROVER CLEVELAND.

IX

THE DEPARTMENTS

[The compass of this collection does not permit the giving of a complete account of Departmental Work in all its branches. It has been the purpose of the author to include selections which would illustrate in a particularly interesting manner the functions of government. Not all the Departments are dealt with nor all important functions in the Departments described. In some cases only a certain bureau, *e. g.*, the Bureau of Corporations, has been selected for description. For a complete account of the organization and work of the Departments, the student is referred to Fairlie's "National Administration of the United States," Gauss, "Government of the United States," and also to a very excellent series of articles on the work of Government which appeared in *Scribner's Magazine*, volumes 33–35, from which a few selections have been included in this collection. The work of the Departments of State, War, and Navy, is dealt with in other portions of this collection, *e. g.*, the Senate debate on foreign affairs.]

THE TREASURY [1]

By Frank A. Vanderlip [2]

Astonishment at the extent and diversity of interests embraced in the Treasury Department must have been one of the first sensations of most Secretaries of the Treasury after taking up the duties of the office. Even if the Secretary had been active in public life, and possessed passing familiarity with the great Department, he would scarcely have clearly comprehended its scope, but if he were a man coming from an active business career, without opportunity for intimate acquaintance with the treasury, the first few weeks of his official life, it is likely, were marked by daily discoveries of new and entirely unanticipated functions.

The bureaus which are bound together in the Treasury Department are, by all odds, the most diverse, and at the first casual glance it would seem the most unrelated that are to be found under the jurisdiction of

[1] Extracts from an article in *Scribner's Magazine*, April, 1903. Reproduced by permission. Copyright 1903.
[2] Formerly Assistant Secretary of the Treasury.

any of the cabinet officers. The public thinks of the Treasury Department as the fiscal division of the Government's executive system. It is a fact, however, that for a good many years probably not less than two-thirds of the time of the Finance Minister has been devoted to problems bearing little or no relation to the strictly fiscal business of the Government. The organization of a Department of Commerce, drawing, as it will, its principal bureaus from the Treasury Department, will bring needed relief to a cabinet officer who has quite enough to occupy his attention in the administration of affairs closely related to the Government's financial business.

The responsibility for raising the revenues and for their disbursement, now that the totals have come to aggregate more than one thousand million dollars, would seem to be quite enough to lay upon the shoulders of any man, particularly if he must take up those duties without thorough familiarity with their details, as does each new Secretary. But in addition to that duty, there is the further responsibility for the solution of the problems of an intricate and diverse currency system. The Secretary, too, occupies indirectly, through the Comptroller of the Currency, a supervisory relation to the whole national banking organization of the country. He is the indirect custodian of $800,000,000 of gold and silver coin, stored in the Treasury vaults, against gold and silver certificates in circulation representing that coin, and, through his subordinate, the Treasurer of the United States, he shares the responsibility for the care of more than two hundred million dollars, representing the cash balance which the Government carries. All the Mints and Assay Officers are, through the Director of the Mint, under his control. He directs the operations of a great factory employing 3,000 operatives in the printing of money and Government securities, and he must there meet the same problems of organized labor that other great employers have to meet. He is responsible for the collection of commercial statistics, and is fortunate in finding a bureau for that purpose which has a record for the best statistical work done by any of the great Governments. He is at the head of the greatest auditing offices in the world, where every dollar of income and every item of expenditure is checked over with minute exactness, so that at the end of the year it is safe for him to say the whole billion dollars, the total on both sides of the ledger, has been collected and disbursed with absolute fidelity and legality and without error.

All these functions are naturally related to the management of the fiscal affairs of the Government, but there are many other bureaus that do not apparently bear such close relation. The Secretary will discover that there are almost as many vessels which would fly his official flag should he come on board as there are ships of war to fire salutes to the Secretary of the Navy. He has large fleets engaged in light-house and coast-survey work, while the revenue cutter service, in which are many swift and modern vessels, does police duty at every port. He is the final authority in all official judgments relating to the more than five hundred thousand immigrants who land on our shores annually, and he is the responsible executive for carrying out the immigration laws and the Chinese Exclusion Act. He is the official head of the Bureau of Public Health and Marine Hospital Service, which guards our ports from contagious diseases, maintains quarantine service and stations, and a great system of hospitals for disabled seamen. The Government's Secret Service Bureau reports directly to him, and he watches day by day the unfolding of detective stories more interesting than the dime novels of his boyhood days, and there accumulate in his files packages of reports, tied with red tape, more thrilling than the choicest examples of yellow-covered literature. Not only is the Secret Service Bureau devoted to the detection of counterfeiting, but its services are called into play in connection with any secret service work which the other Departments may wish to have done. The Bureau of Standards, to which all questions of weights and measures may be finally referred, is under his direction. No steamship may sail in American waters, nor leave an American port, the boiler of which does not bear the stamp of official inspection by one of his subordinates. He is the responsible head of a Life Saving Service, with 272 stations and a cordon of men patrolling 10,000 miles of coast; of a Light-house system, marking the course of mariners with a chain of lights from Maine away around to Alaska; of a Coast Survey, which has for its business not only the charting of navigable waters, but the scientific investigation of the earth's curvature; of the Architect's Office, which has already constructed and has the care of 400 public buildings, most of them architecturally bad, and which is at the moment engaged in planning and building 149 others, many of which, happily, are showing great architectural improvement.

All these duties are in addition to the fundamental one of collecting the public revenues, a work requiring the maintenance of a corps of 6,300 officials at 168 ports of entry, and of a body of internal revenue employees, whose eyes are literally upon every foot of the country's territory.

By no means the least of the manifold duties of this official are those which are connected with the administration of the Civil Service, for his complete corps numbers 26,000 subordinates. There must be endless appointments, promotions, and changes, and in regard to them all the Secretary of the Treasury is the final authority.

The mere enumeration of such a list of responsibilities carries with it the conviction that the Treasury of the United States must be a wonderfully well organized machine, else it would be impossible for any man to step into the responsibilities of its direction without the change being seriously felt by the entire Treasury organization and the whole country. The Treasury Department *is* a wonderfully well organized commercial machine. Taking it all in all, I believe there is no organization in the commercial life of this country, look where you will, that is its superior; in many respects one will not find its equal.

We are apt to have none too good an idea of our Government administration, and sometimes, with scant knowledge of facts and conditions, condemn the executive branches of the Government. Naturally the Treasury has come in for its full share of criticism, for it touches every citizen in the tender spot of his pocket-book. For my own part, however, every day of greater familiarity with the organization was a day of growing admiration for it and of increasing pride that the multitude of affairs entrusted to the head of this Department are administered so intelligently, so promptly, and above all with such absolute integrity and entire devotion to the Government's interests.

Not only does the Treasury Department handle, in the ordinary income and expenditures, cash transactions aggregating more than a billion dollars annually, but it is responsible for the custodianship and the renewal of currency, the printing of paper money, the coinage of specie and the handling of public securities, and the figures on both sides of the ledger representing the total of all these transactions reach the incomprehensible aggregate of three and a half billions.

Such great sums are handled year after year with absolute integrity, with books that balance to a penny, with cash drawers that are never short, with a trust not betrayed. Whatever opinion home-coming European travellers may have of Treasury methods, after more or less successful attempts to avoid custom regulations, they must, on the whole, give respect to an organization which accepts a responsibility for annual financial transactions aggregating $3,500,000,000, and has discharged that responsibility year after year, under one political administration after another, through the vicissitudes of cabinet changes, and presents a clean record having on it no important blot of a betrayal of a trust.

A new Secretary of the Treasury approaching the responsibilities and duties of the great position with an appreciation of their importance must, in years past, have been greatly surprised to find how little time apparently he could devote to the consideration of great national questions, and how much he must give to the small routine details of the administration of the civil service. The 26,000 employees under the direction of the Secretary of the Treasury make the Treasury Department only second to the Post-Office in point of numbers. When the civil service blanket was only partly drawn over these places, the time which the head of the Department was forced to give to the discussion of appointments, matters in most part of minor consequence so far as the efficiency of administration was concerned, was something that must have discouraged more than one Secretary. While such appointments may have been of minor consequence in the actual administration of the Department, they were of great importance if regard was to be had for maintaining cordial relations with the legislative branch of the Government.

Washington wishes to see evidence of democracy about the Departments. Neither Senator nor Congressman is satisfied to cool his heels in an ante-room for any length of time, nor are political leaders who come to the Capitol on a mission likely to be pleased if the Secretary's engagements are such that an appointment can not be made without notice or delay. So it came about that a business day in the Secretary's office was, in times past, almost wholly given up, during the periods in which Congress was in session, to the reception of visitors, and most of these visitors came to discuss matters of small consequence to the administration of the Department. The Secretary of this great Department must give heed to innumerable trifles such as would never reach the head of even a comparatively small business organization. Requests come from people of importance, and they must be taken up with the care which the position of such persons demands rather than with any thought of their importance in relation to the administration of departmental affairs.

There is vast improvement in the Treasury Department in this respect compared with former conditions. The Secretary now has power to make but few appointments outside the classified service, and by recent executive order he may not consider outside recommendations in regard to promotions in the classified service.

Early in the administration of Secretary Gage it was recognized by the Secretary that, if he was to give consideration to the unusual number of important public questions which were pressing, he must be relieved of much of the detail of the administration of the civil service; so he delegated to a committee, consisting of an Assistant Secretary, the Chief Clerk and the Appointment Clerk, consideration of all questions of civil-service administration effecting the employees in Washington. This plan continues in force. Political considerations have always been absolutely excluded from the deliberations of this Committee. I can speak for that positively, and I mean to say that such a statement is literally true. The Committee has considered many thousands of promotions and changes in the classified service, and there has been no more discussion of politics than would be found in the consideration of promotions in a great banking or insurance institution. The recommendations of heads of bureaus, the length and character of service, the regularity of attendance, and the results of examinations which are made to cover both academic and practical qualifications, are the factors taken into consideration. So far is political influence eliminated, indeed so far as promotions governed strictly by merit may be considered the goal in an ideal civil-service administration, I believe the conduct of the civil service in the Treasury Department is to-day practically all that could be asked.

* * * * * * * *

A notable difference between the position of the Secretary of the Treasury and that of the head of a great business organization is the time which the Secretary must devote to the discussion of public questions with newspaper representatives. No small part of his success will depend upon his adaptability to that new condition, for the view which most of the people of the country will form of his administration will naturally be much colored by the attitude of the newspaper correspondents through whom the public is informed regarding official matters.

Newspaper conditions in Washington are unlike those in other cities. There are innumerable representatives of papers, covering the whole range of the country, each one of whom serves a constituency of great importance. As a body, the newspaper correspondents of Washington are incomparably superior to the average newspaper representatives in other cities. Many of them have been intelligent observers of public affairs for a generation, and have been the confidants and advisers of many Cabinet officers. There is hardly an important newspaper man in Washington who is not at times the trusted custodian of state secrets, and the relation of these men to public affairs is entirely different from the relation of the average reporter in other cities to the business questions of local interest. It is important that the Secretary of the Treasury recognize this, for the Treasury Department is one of the chief sources of news at the Capital, and that he should learn to meet fairly and frankly the newspaper correspondents. This requires much time, much tact, and a discrimination in determining those who can be fully trusted and kept confidentially informed of the progress of affairs, and those who must be talked to with guarded politeness.

The sacrifice of time is by no means without its recompense. Many a Cabinet officer has received quite as good counsel from conservative and experienced newspaper correspondents as he could get from members of Senate or House. This confidential relation with newspaper representatives is unique, and unless a Secretary of the Treasury has been trained in the official atmosphere of Washington, it is likely to take him some time to recognize it and adjust himself to the condition.

In a most important particular the Treasury Department differs from the Finance Ministries of other countries. Elsewhere the Finance Minister occupies an authoritative relation to legislation affecting income and expenditure. With us, the Government has always gone on with the most happy-go-lucky lack of coördination between legislation affecting income and legislation affecting expenditure. The Finance Ministers of other countries draw up a budget, which forms the basis of Parliamentary legislation in financial matters. They make careful estimate of probable Government income and of the demands for the executive administration, and Parliament, as an almost *pro forma* matter, passes legislation affecting taxation which will conform to the proposals in the budget and limits appropriations within lines which the budget may prescribe.

With us, however, the Secretary of the Treasury is little more than an agent who, without comment, transmits to Congress from the heads of the various Departments their estimates regarding appropriations. Congress, in turn, does not pay close heed to these estimates, frequently declining to make appropriations asked for and not infrequently making appropriations which the executive head of the Department has declared are not needed.

With us there is little flexibility on the income side of the great public ledger. The Secretary of the Treasury may make general recommendations regarding the necessities for greater income or the opportunity for decreasing taxation, but Congress does not look to the head of the Treasury Department with much solicitude for advice regarding tax legislation or suggestions concerning conservative limits of appropriations. The sources of our Government income are so intimately bound up with the economic theory of protection that we are likely to formulate our tax laws with little or no regard to the amount of income they will produce, and to make appropriations on as liberal a scale as the income will permit, and the Finance Minister has little if any responsibility either for a cash balance or a Treasury deficit.

Congress is not disposed, either, to give very much heed to Departmental recommendations regarding expenditures.

For many years, for example, every Secretary of the Treasury, in each of his annual messages to Congress, recommended that no appropriation be made for maintaining certain customs districts which have become commercially obsolete and which are maintained apparently for no other purpose than to give the Senator or Congressman most concerned an opportunity to recommend a Presidential appointment. There are 12 customs districts, which are officered at an expense of $15,578.14, where the total income from customs in a single year was only $275.26, and the cost of collection, therefore, reaches $56.59, for each dollar collected. In spite of repeated recommendations that we accept the changed conditions which have made these old-time customs districts quite deserted by commerce, Congress insists year after year that they shall be maintained, that officers shall be appointed, and the expenses of salaries and office administration appropriated.

A saving of $200,000, a year could easily be made without any sacrifice of efficiency in the customs service, but Congress hesitates to give up the privilege of naming the appointees who are to receive in salaries this $200,000 of useless expenditure.

Sometimes this apparent spirit of perverseness goes farther and actively puts obstacles in the way of administration. An illustration of that is found in recent efforts to introduce improved methods into the Bureau of Engraving and Printing. The Government printing of currency is done upon the same form of old-fashioned hand-press that was used when the first greenback and the first national bank-note were turned out. The process is slow and expensive. The growth of the country created a demand upon the Bureau which it was almost impossible to keep pace with, and so it was decided to put in power presses to print the backs of notes. An expenditure of $25,000 was made, with results so economical that a saving of the whole cost of the machines was effected in a few months. Tests were made by mixing hand-printed and machine-printed bills and submitting them, unmarked, to numbers of expert money counters; and invariably the machine-printed bills would be selected as the best examples of plate printing.

Labor organizations were opposed to this introduction of power presses, however, and when Congress convened brought active pressure to bear at the Capital, with the result that riders were tacked upon the appropriation bills prohibiting the expenditure of any appropriation for the maintenance of power presses; and this was done without any communication with the Secretary of the Treasury on the part of either Senate or House committee, without any opportunity for presenting the Treasury's side of the matter, and without any effort to secure information as a basis for intelligent legislation except such as was presented by labor leaders who were not even in the employ of the Government.

The Ways and Means Committee and the Appropriation Committees of Congress take upon themselves the responsibility for adjusting the relation between income and expenditure. A great tariff bill may be framed with little more than nominal reference to the Treasury Department, and legislation formulated which may enormously affect one side or the other of the Treasury accounts without the voice of the Secretary being heard or his advice asked for. Income is provided and expenditures are appropriated, without Congress being advised by the head of the Treasury as to the balance between the two sides of the budget.

A phase of Treasury affairs emphasized in the public mind is the relation of the Treasury to the money market. At certain seasons much is to be heard about the cries of Wall Street for Treasury help, and of the relief measures which the Secretary of the Treasury may bring to bear upon an unsatisfactory banking position. An ideal fiscal situation for the Government, President Harrison once said, would be one in which the income each day just equalled the expenditures. In such a situation there would be no problem regarding the relation of the Treasury to the money market. So long as we must work with our present Sub-treasury system, however, founded as it was in ignorance and suspicion of proper banking functions, we must periodically face a situation in which the operations of the Treasury are of great import in the general financial situation. Laws which have been allowed to stand unchanged since Jackson's hatred of the banks was crystallized into statute, prevent the deposits of the receipts from customs anywhere but in the actual budget and lists appropriations within lines which the budget may prescribe.

With us, however, the Secretary of the Treasury is little more than an agent who, without comment, transmits to Congress from the heads of the various Departments their estimates regarding appropriations. Congress, in turn, does not pay close heed to these estimates, frequently declining to make appropriations asked for and not infrequently making appropriations which the executive head of the Department has declared are not needed.

With us there is little flexibility on the income side of the great p ledger. The Secretary of the Treasury may make general recomm tions regarding the necessities for greater income or the opportu decreasing taxation, but Congress does not look to the head Treasury Department with much solicitude for advice regar legislation or suggestions concerning conservative limits of a tions. The sources of our Government income are so intimat up with the economic theory of protection that we are likel late our tax laws with little or no regard to the amount of i will produce, and to make appropriations on as liberal income will permit, and the Finance Minister has littl sibility either for a cash balance or a Treasury deficit.

Congress is not disposed, either, to give very much mental recommendations regarding expenditures.

For many years, for example, every Secretary of each of his annual messages to Congress, recommend priation be made for maintaining certain customs di become commercially obsolete and which are maintai no other purpose than to give the Senator or Congr cerned an opportunity to recommend a Presidential ap are 12 customs districts, which are officered at an exp where the total income from customs in a single yea and the cost of collection, therefore, reaches $56.59, lected. In spite of repeated recommendations that we conditions which have made these old-time customs serted by commerce, Congress insists year after year maintained, that officers shall be appointed, and the ex and office administration appropriated.

A saving of $00,000, a year could easily be made wit of efficiency in the customs service, but Congress hesita privilege of naming the appointees who are to receive $200,000 of useless expenditure.

Sometimes this apparent spirit of perverseness goes fart puts obstacles in the way of administration. An illustr found in recent efforts to introduce improved methods i of Engraving and Printing. The Government printing

done upon the same form of old-fashioned hand-p... that
when the first greenback and the first national ba...
out. The process is slow and expensive. The gr... of
created a demand upon the Bureau which it was a... impossible to
keep pace with, and so it was decided to put in pow...s to
the backs of notes. An expenditure of $25,000 was m... with
so economical that a saving of the whole cost of the m... was
in a few months. Tests were made by mixing hand pr...ed and
printed bills and submitting them, unmarked, to m... of
money counters; and invariably the machine-print... b... ...
selected as the best examples of plate printing.

Labor organizations were opposed to this introduction of power p...
however, and when Congress convened brought activ... pressure to...
at the Capital, with the result that riders were tacked upon the a...
priation bills prohibiting the expenditure of any appr...iation for
maintenance of power presses; and this was done with...t any commu...
cation with the Secretary of the Treasury on the part... either Senate...
House committee, without any opportunity for presenting the Treasury
side of the matter, and with...t any effort to secure information a...
basis for intelligent legisl...ion except such as was p...ented by lab...
leaders who were not eve... in the employ of the Government.

The Ways and Means Committee and the Appropriation Committee...
of Congress take up...... the responsibility ... adjusting th...
relation between income ... expenditure. A great ...iff bill may be
framed with little m...e ... ...inal reference to th... Treasury Depart...
ment, and legislation ... ... which may enorm... affect one side
or the other of the T...... without the v... of the Secretary
being heard or his a...... Income is pr...ed and expenditures are appropri...... Congress being adv... by the head of
the Treasury as to ... ... be... the ... sides of the budget.

A phase of Treas...... m...erialized in the p...ic mind is the
relation of the Treas...... money market. At cert... seasons much
is to be heard ab... the ... of W... Street for Tre...ry help, and of
the relief measures w... ... ...retary of the Treasury may b...g to
bear upon an unsa...... ... ... f...al situation
for the Govern...... Harrison once said, ...ld be one in
which the income ... ... the expenditures. In such a
situation there w...... regarding the ...s of the Treasury
to the money m...... ... work ...her present Sub-
treasury syste...... ... ...nerals and suspicion
of proper ba...... ... ...riod... In a situation in
which the oper...... ... ... are of great ...t ... the general
financial situ...... ... ... and unchanged
since Jackson's ....
the deposits .... the actual

vaults of the Treasury or Sub-treasury. The country is in such a position as a great business firm would be whose receipts at times enormously exceeded its expenditures, if it should decide to lock up its daily income in safety deposit vaults, turning all credits into cash and locking up the actual currency just at a time when there might be a most active demand in the ordinary channels of trade for the currency which would thus be abstracted.

Of course, it is impossible to have such an ideal situation as President Harrison suggested; so long as the laws relating to the Sub-treasury system stand unchanged it is useless to talk about taking the Government out of the banking business. The operations of the Treasury inevitably draw it into the situation, and it becomes one of the great problems of the Secretary to keep, as nearly as may be, an unchanging total of currency in the Treasury vaults and neither withdraw from the circulating medium in active use great quantities of currency when income is excessive nor suddenly add to the currency in circulation when the Government has great payments to make in excess of its daily income. The problems of that character were unusually frequent and difficult during Secretary Gage's administration. The successful settlement of the Pacific Railroad indebtedness brought a payment of $58,000,000 to the Treasury in December, 1897, just at a period of most active commercial demand and when the withdrawal of so much currency would have been disastrous to reviving business. A few months later came the sudden expenditures resulting from the $50,000,000 appropriation made by Congress at the beginning of the Spanish War, and soon after that were poured into the Treasury the proceeds of $200,000,000 of Spanish War bonds. Twice during the administration issues of Government bonds matured, and payment of many millions had to be made on that account. This period was the most remarkable since the Civil War for violent fluctuations in the Treasury's balance, and it is one of the best evidences of genius in the administration of the Department at that time that the stock of money actually in the Treasury vaults, in spite of this period of irregular income and expenditure, was always kept at comparatively the same level, and Treasury operations were not permitted seriously to affect the currency of the country.

It is such problems as that which a Secretary of the Treasury must always find recurring, so long as our present Sub-treasury system is maintained and the best evidence of ability on the part of a Secretary is that these sudden influxes of funds or exceptional expenditures are handled so that the public has no reason to recognize the intimate relation which must exist under present conditions between the Treasury and the banking situation.

With a currency system which has largely been the growth of exigency rather than of forethought, there is always a desire for legislation which will bring the country's currency into line with the best economic ideas.

Both the country and Congress have come to look to the head of the Treasury Department as a natural source for suggestions regarding needed currency and banking legislation, and one of his most important duties is the preparation of that portion of his annual report to Congress, which contains recommendations of such character. That has been true particularly during those recent years in which fundamental currency discussion has been so prominent in political affairs, and during which there has been formulated legislation which is an important part of the ground-work of our financial system. It requires a wide range of ability to pass easily from the innumerable practical problems of executive administration which the Treasury presents, to the writing of State papers given to theoretical and economic discussion of some of the subtleties of finance and currency. The annual reports of the heads of the Treasury Department for many years, however, show that we have been fortunate in having men of such breadth of ability that they could do this and do it well.

Not only must the Secretary successfully grasp theoretical problems in finance and be capable of building up in his message to Congress sound recommendations for financial legislation, but he has to face a much more trying ordeal when he is invited to appear before either the Senate Finance Committee or the House Committee on Banking and Currency — a thing which is usual whenever important financial legislation is under consideration. It is a comparatively easy matter, with ample time and good counsel, to evolve satisfactory recommendation for legislation, but it is far more difficult to advocate those recommendations in an inquiry by ingenious and hostile members of a Congressional Committee. Anyone who has studied the proceedings of Senate or House Committees when prominent business men have been brought before them to express their views upon financial legislation must have been struck by the lamentable showing which some of the most prominent financiers may make under a fire of questions from keen-witted and experienced members of this Committee. Men who are rulers in practical finance are frequently unable to hold their own in anything like creditable shape in a discussion of fundamental financial measures which it may be proposed to enact into law.

English Cabinet Members must appear in Parliament to answer interpellations, but notice of the question is given the day before and a member of the Cabinet has ample time to confer and to study his answer, and he may even decline for state reasons to make any answer, if he sees fit. Our own Finance Minister is put in a much more difficult position, however, when he appears before a Congressional Committee. He knows only the general line that the inquiry will take. If he is called before the Banking and Currency Committee, he faces seventeen members, of whom a large minority are politically hostile and who are thoroughly trained in the art of asking difficult questions. His answers become a part of the published records, and he is placed in a position where, if he is to make a satisfactory showing, he must reply off-hand to any question that is propounded by any member of the Committee. To go through such an ordeal with satisfaction needs thorough understanding of the subject and readiness of comprehension and retort.

The most important bureau in the Treasury Department is the one charged with the duty of collecting the customs. Not only must this bureau, in order that there shall be no smuggling, keep a watchful eye upon 15,000 miles of coast, a Northern frontier more than three thousand miles long, and a Southern boundary stretching the full breadth of Mexico, but it is charged with the administration of the most intricate tariff schedule, requiring not only fidelity and integrity where vast sums are concerned, but great expert knowledge in regard to commodities and the keenest intelligence in the application of that knowledge. The great work of this bureau is, of course, in the collection of the customs levied on regularly imported merchandise, and that work goes on with little criticism and without much friction. Another phase, the collection of duties on articles brought home by returning travelers, is comparatively insignificant in point of income, but to a large number of citizens it is the one point of contact which they have with the Department, and it not infrequently leaves them ready to condemn and upbraid. One of the difficulties in this part of the administration lies in the palpable fact that it is not easy to obtain a corps of inspectors, when Congress limits their salaries to four dollars a day, who will serve long hours at trying duties, always maintain their equanimity, and be courteous in the face of much provocation to be otherwise, and always retain their integrity and repel efforts to corrupt them made by people occupying positions of high standing and respect in the community. Under President McKinley's administration it was determined to make the enforcement of the law, as it applied to returning travellers, much more rigid than had been the case, and the stricter enforcement which has since been in vogue has led to more criticism of the Treasury, probably, than has any other phase of its affairs.

In the minds of most people a customs law seems to be quite unlike other laws. It is a statute which it is more or less of a credit to evade, and methods of false witness and bribery may be brought to bear without troubling the traveller's conscience. It is this peculiarity of human nature that makes the task extremely difficult. There is much complaint about the Treasury treating returning travelers as if their word was not to be trusted, and submitting their baggage to search after sworn declaration has been made. Brief experience, from the inside, with this part of the Treasury administration will convince one how necessary such an attitude is. As an illustration of that statement, the case might be cited of fifteen prominent citizens of New York City who went abroad two or three years ago, and, on their return, all submitted sworn statements in regard to the contents of their trunks. Twelve declared they had no dutiable articles, and the remaining three paid an aggregate of $538. The next year the same fifteen citizens made their annual European pilgrimage and, on their return, were met by the stricter administration of the same law. In addition to their sworn declaration their baggage was carefully examined, with a result that they paid over $34,000 of duty. Is it small wonder that, after endless experiences, of which the foregoing is but an average illustration, a strictness of inspection should be put in force which is galling to men who have both honor and good memories and make out correct schedules of their purchases when they give their sworn declaration to a customs inspector?

In the administration of the customs there have undoubtedly been men who were not true to their oath of office and have accepted bribes. A considerable number of inspectors have at one time or another been summarily dealt with for such offense. In the handling of the vast sums of money which are a part of the Treasury's operations, there have, in very rare cases, been instances of petty pilfering. Taken by and large, however, the Treasury Department is a splendid great commercial machine, administered with an integrity reaching all the way from the head of the Department through the whole army of its thousands of subordinates, an integrity of which the country may well be proud. Everywhere in the administration the interests of the Government are paramount to all else.

THE TREASURY AND THE MONEY MARKET

[The vast sums of money paid to the United States government in the form of taxes, fees, and postal charges (considerably over $1,000,000,000 per year), bring the administration of the treasury into close connection with the banking industries and the money market of the United States. The manner in which the treasury has from time to time interfered in order to give relief to the money market is illustrated by the following brief article from the *New York Evening Post*, March 8, 1907.]

WHEN it became known that George B. Cortelyou was to become Secretary of the Treasury on March 4, many persons went to him and asked what his policy or policies would be, and whether he intended to "come to the aid of the market" when Wall Street, through speculative excesses, needed money. Mr. Cortelyou told all these inquirers that he had formulated no cut and dried programme; that he was going to take up the problems of his new office as they confronted him. Nearly every one who talked with the incoming secretary, however, came away with the impression that he would not be so ready to heed the cries for help from the New York financial district as Mr. Shaw had been.

In his last annual report, Secretary Shaw reviewed his financial policy

with respect to the Treasury's relations with the money market. He set
forth with detail and explanations his reasons for extending aid in 1902,
1903, 1904, 1905, and 1906. What follows is Secretary Shaw's own
account of the reasons which influenced him, and which have been so
widely discussed and criticised. It is set forth again at this time to
refresh the memory of those who may be interested, and may be used
as a basis of comparison with whatever line of action Secretary Cortelyou may determine to pursue.

Conditions in 1902

During the summer of 1902 surplus bank reserves throughout the
country ran relatively very low. "Preparatory for the crisis certain to
ensue," the Secretary of the Treasury caused to be printed as much un-
ordered national-bank circulation as the Bureau of Engraving and Printing could turn out, in addition to the ordinary demands upon it, and in
September of that year offered to accept satisfactory security other than
Government bonds for deposits of public money then held by the banks,
for which this additional circulation had been printed, on condition that
the released bonds should be immediately made the basis for circulation.

He also anticipated the payment of November interest due on outstanding obligations of the Government, and offered to purchase for the
sinking fund any United States 4 per cent bonds of the loan of 1925 that
might be offered at 137¾ and interest to date of purchase. He also
increased deposits in national banks in a considerable sum. In these
several ways be restored to the channels of trade somewhat over
$57,000,000 and stimulated national bank circulation to the extent of
$18,000,000. He also issued an announcement that he would not exer-
cise the discretion given him by statute to liquidate banks which fail to
maintain their reserve should they fail to maintain the same against
deposits of Government money.

These operations were not begun, however, "until a condition existed
which in the opinion of many leading bankers of New York city justified
the issuance of Clearing House certificates, and when a resort thereto
was being seriously considered." Two of these methods (the acceptance of other than Government bonds as security for deposits, and the
announcement that the discretion with which the Secretary of the Treasury is clothed by statute would not be exercised against banks failing to
maintain reserve against Government deposits) received their full meed
of criticism at the time, "but no lawyer ever doubted their legality and
no business man now questions their necessity.

"Financiers generally now recognize, and some of the best known
have publicly announced, that but for what was then done a panic would
have ensued rivalling in severity any in our history, and which would

possibly have continued until industrial conditions were disastrously affected."

AID GIVEN IN 1903

The law authorizes the Secretary of the Treasury to deposit in national banks only internal revenue and miscellaneous receipts. Having found it impracticable to relieve a monetary stringency with current internal revenue receipts, amounting only to about $500,000 per day, Secretary Shaw early in 1903 ordered their segregation and the accumulation of a separate and distinct fund composed entirely of internal revenue and miscellaneous receipts, so as to be prepared in case of an emergency to grant prompt relief by large deposits. This practice has been continued.

During the fall of 1903 there was restored to the channels of trade an aggregate of $27,000,000. This was accomplished by purchasing outstanding Government bonds for the sinking fund amounting to $13,000,000 and by direct deposits in national banks aggregating $14,000,000. National bank circulation was also stimulated to some extent.

CANAL PAYMENT IN 1904

In the spring of 1904, by direct appropriation of Congress, $10,000,000 was paid to the Government of Panama, and $40,000,000 to the Panama Canal Company for the right of way on which to construct the canal across the Isthmus. Preparatory to making these payments pro-rata transfers were made of Government deposits from all depository banks outside to those within the city of New York, and the amount thus transferred distributed pro rata among depositories in that city.

The payment of $40,000,000 to the Panama Canal Company on May 9, 1904, was accomplished by the appointment of J. P. Morgan & Co. special disbursing agents for the Treasury Department, and a pay warrant for $40,000,000 was then issued to Clearing House. Morgan & Co. at once deposited an equal amount through the same channel in the banks, from which the money was drawn with which to pay the warrant.

As the transaction worked out, only a few thousand dollars actually changed hands, money rates were not affected in the slightest degree, and not a dollar of gold was shipped from this country. The transfer to France was skilfully effected by Morgan & Co. through the purchase from time to time of foreign exchange. Neither was there any expense to the Government, the disbursing agents volunteering to represent the Government gratis, and look to the French Canal Company for their pay. The Republic of Panama invested most of the purchase price of her cession in the United States, and thus shipments of money to that country were avoided. No purchases for the sinking fund were made during the year.

OPERATIONS IN 1905

"For reasons which cannot be fully explained," revenues fell off during the calendar year 1904 and the early months of 1905, which, coupled with the extraordinary expenditures, caused a deficit for the fiscal year ending June 30, 1905, of $23,000,000. To make good this deficit and to meet these expenditures, $50,000,000 was withdrawn from depositary banks. "These withdrawals, however, were insufficient to inspire conservatism," and during the summer the surplus reserve of the associated banks of New York City fell below $7,000,000, while the rate on call money, fluctuated from below 1 to 3½ per cent, averaging for the season, perhaps, about 2 per cent. The anticipated stringency was deferred, however, possibly in part by extensive refundings of Government bonds into consols of 1930, which, in conjunction with withdrawals of deposits, lowered the price of consols to a point where banks found the maintenance of circulation profitable, and an increase of $25,000,000 resulted. "The crisis inevitable came, though some months belated."

RELIEF MEASURES IN 1906

In February of 1906, $10,000,000 was deposited in national bank depositaries in seven of the principal cities, and satisfactory security other than Government bonds accepted, but with the distinct understanding that it would be recalled in July of that year. "This relief was not sufficient, however. Banks, everywhere, West as well as East, found themselves in the spring with surplus reserve exhausted. The foreign exchange market responded sympathetically in a very marked decline in sterling exchange sufficient to have insured the importation of gold if the banks had been in position to buy the exchange with which to secure it."

Secretary Shaw then offered to make deposits, satisfactorily secured, equal in amount to any actual engagements of gold for importation, the same to be promptly returned when the gold actually arrived. In this way approximately $50,000,000 (more than six carloads) in gold, largely in bars, was brought from abroad. Most of this came from Europe, but part from Australia and South Africa.

"This was accomplished without expense to the Government, and without profit to the importing banks, but with great benefit to the business interests of the country. The various banks which imported this gold lost in the transactions several thousand dollars, as established by their books; the price of exchange promptly advanced so that merchants and exporters of grain and cotton having exchange to sell were benefited in excess of $150,000, and interest rates dropped sufficiently to effect a saving to borrowers in New York city alone of more than $2,000,000."

This means of relieving financial stringencies, which has been once since repeated, attracted far more attention throughout Europe than in the United States, though it has been widely commented upon in both places. "It has at least demonstrated that the United States is in a position to more effectually influence international financial conditions than is any other country, and justifies great caution lest, while protecting our own interests, we cause distress elsewhere, which will soon be reflected here."

THE UNITED STATES DEPARTMENT OF JUSTICE [1]

By Professor John A. Fairlie

The Department of Justice has been developed from the English office of Attorney-General, with important features added in the course of American experience. As early as the reign of Edward I, almost contemporaneous with the appearance of a special legal profession in England, we find Crown Attorneys (*Attornati Regis*) employed for guarding the royal privileges in the courts. By the time of Edward IV the official title of Attorney-General appears for the first time. A little later, as the distinction between barristers and solicitors became established, the Crown lawyers are distinguished as the King's Attorney and the King's Solicitor.

These law officers acted as the legal advisers of the King and his ministers, and also conducted public prosecutions in important criminal cases. But there was not developed, and has not yet developed in England any system of local public prosecutors. Nor has the English Attorney-General become one of the leading political officials with a seat in the cabinet, since political and administrative functions, which have become attached to the office in this country, are there performed by the Lord Chancellor and other officials.

Most of the colonies had Attorneys-General; and these officers were continued under the State governments. In the national government the office of Attorney-General was provided for in the Judiciary Act of 1789. For a good many years the work of the office did not require the entire time of the Attorney-General and he was permitted, if not expected, to continue in private practice. The salary was only $1,500 a year, less than that of the other cabinet secretaries; and not until 1814 was he required to reside in Washington. From the first the Attorney-General was a member of the President's cabinet; but his office was not formally recognized as an executive department until in 1870 the Department of Justice was established.

The functions of the Attorney-General and the Department of Justice

[1] *Michigan Law Review*, 1906.

may be considered in four main divisions: (1) as legal adviser to the President and the executive departments; (2) as attorney for the United States before the courts, either as prosecutor or defendant; (3) administrative supervision over officers of United States courts and over United States penal and reformatory institutions; and (4) as adviser to the President in the exercise of his pardoning power.

It is the duty of the Attorney-General to give his advice and opinion upon questions of law when required by the President or by the heads of departments on any matter concerning their departments. Questions not involving the construction of the Constitution of the United States may be referred to subordinates; and their opinions when approved by the Attorney-General have the same force and effect as the opinions of the Attorney-General himself. Officers in the Department of Justice must give opinions and render legal services to the President or officers of other departments.

In the discharge of these duties the action of the Attorney-General is quasi-judicial. "His opinions officially define the law in a multitude of cases, where his decision is in practice final and conclusive — not only as respects the action of public officers in administrative matters, who are thus relieved from the responsibility which would otherwise attach to their acts, — but also in question of private right, inasmuch as parties, having concerns with the government, possess in general no means of bringing a controverted matter before the courts of law, and can obtain a purely legal decision of the controversy, as distinguished from an administrative one, only by reference to the Attorney-General. Accordingly, the opinions of successive Attorneys-General . . . have come to constitute a body of legal precedents and exposition, having authority the same in kind, if not the same in degree, with decisions of the courts of justice." "The Supreme Court will not entertain an appeal from his decision, nor revise his judgment in any case where the law authorized him to exercise his discretion or judgment."

But the Attorney-General is under no obligation to render an award, or determine a question of fact in cases referred to him; nor does an appeal to him lie from another department by any party assuming to be aggrieved by its action, and seeking to have it reviewed; nor is he to give advice to heads of departments on matters which do not concern their departments, and in which the United States have no interest; nor is he authorized to give official opinions not falling within the scope of his duties, so as to connect the government with individual controversies, in which it has no concern; nor is he in general to give official opinions to subordinate officers of the government; nor in cases not actually presented for action by an executive department. He will not answer abstract or hypothetical questions of law; nor purely judicial questions in controversy before the courts; nor construe department regulations. He may, like the heads of other departments, be required to furnish information to Congress; but he does not furnish legal opinions to Congress, or its committees.

More specifically, it is the duty of the Attorney-General and his assistants to examine all titles to land purchased by the United States for the purpose of erecting public buildings; and no money can be expended for land until the title has been approved.

As chief advocate for the government, the Attorney-General has supervision over all actions at law or suits in equity to which the United States is a party or in which the United States has an interest. Suits begun by the government are brought before a District, Circuit or Supreme Court of the United States under the provisions of the statutes regulating the jurisdiction of these courts. Criminal cases include only crimes in violation of the statutes of the national government. The largest number of prosecutions are for violation of the internal revenue laws; a considerable number are for violation of postal laws, custom laws and pension laws; while a great variety of other statutes are involved in other cases. Civil suits are brought most largely in connection with customs and internal revenue administration; but all of the departments are involved in some cases. Besides cases in which the United States is itself a party, it has been held that in a suit between States where the United States has an interest, the Attorney-General may appear and introduce evidence and argument without making the United States a party for or against whom judgment may be rendered.

Following the rule of English law, suits against the United States government are not allowed as a matter of right.[1] But provision has been made for trying some kinds of claims against the government by the creation of a Court of Claims and a Court of Private Land Claims;[2] while claims for small amounts may be brought before the District and Circuit Courts of the United States, and claims under treaty stipulations are investigated by special commissions. In all these cases the officers of the Department of Justice act as attorneys for the defense on the part of the government.

According to the statutes the Attorney-General is to conduct and argue cases before the Supreme Court and the Court of Claims, except where other provision is made for particular cases. In part, cases in the Court of Claims are now placed in the hands of one of the Assistant Attorneys-General; and even before the Supreme Court many cases are conducted without the personal appearance of the Attorney-General. In the subordinate courts the Attorney-General very seldom appears in person.

In the countries of continental Europe the Minister of Justice appoints, or at least selects, the judges; and exercises through his department a

---

[1] Not even the Attorney-General can waive the exemption of the United States from judicial process or submit United States property to the jurisdiction of the court in a suit brought against its officers. *Stanley* v. *Schwalby*, 162 U. S., 255.

[2] The Court of Private Land Claims was abolished June 30, 1904.

large administrative control over the judiciary. Even in England, the Lord Chancellor selects most of the judges and has disciplinary powers over the judges in the lower courts, as well as some minor supervision over the higher courts. Compared to the practice of foreign countries the powers of the Attorney-General over the judicial administration are very limited. He has no power of appointing judges; and while he may be consulted by the President in reference to a judicial appointment, there is no established custom of asking his advice, still less of accepting his recommendations. And the position of the judiciary as an independent branch of the government, coördinate with the legislative and the executive, prevents any control over their judicial acts. Nevertheless the Attorney-General has some powers of administrative supervision over the executive officers of the courts, similar to those of a European Minister of Justice, which serve to make his position of more importance in the national administration than that of the Attorneys-General in the States.

Local government attorneys were unknown both in England and the American colonies. . Criminal prosecutions were ordinarily begun by private individuals; while the specially important criminal cases and civil cases requiring a government attorney were attended to by the Attorney-General and his immediate staff. But the Judiciary Act of 1789, organizing the United States courts, provided that in each district there should be an attorney of the United States appointed to conduct government business in the courts. At first these district attorneys were paid by fees, and probably gave only a part of their time to government matters. But with the development of public prosecutions in criminal cases, they have become permanent salaried officials; while a corresponding class of officials has also been developed in the States.

District attorneys are now appointed, by the President and Senate, for each of the eighty-six judicial districts of the United States. Their terms are four years, and their salaries vary from $2,000 to $6,000. In most districts there are one or more assistant attorneys and clerks.

It is the duty of each district attorney to prosecute, in his district, all delinquents for crimes and offenses cognizable under the authority of the United States, and all civil actions in which the United States are concerned. In certain cases he must act as attorney in suits where officers of the United States are parties; unless otherwise instructed by the Secretary of the Treasury, he must appear in behalf of the defendants in all suits against collectors, or other revenue officers in connection with their official duties; and he must conduct suits and proceedings under the national banking law which involve United States officers.

From this statement it will be seen that the duties of the district attorney are analogous to the court functions of the Attorney-General. The district attorneys in fact stand in much the same relation to the District and Circuit Courts as does the Attorney-General to the Supreme Court. They are, as has been noted, under the general superintendence of the

Attorney-General; but it has been held that this does not authorize him to control the actions of the district attorneys by general regulations.

One of the most important branches of the work of district attorneys is their control over criminal prosecutions. Limited as they are to crimes against the authority of the United States, this function is of less importance than that of the prosecuting attorneys in the States; but within their own field they have the same influence. It depends to a large extent on their action to secure an indictment, and to carry on the prosecution so as to secure conviction. But in case of neglect of duty, the supervision of the Attorney-General is more likely to secure the removal of the delinquent official than in the States.

United States Marshals were also a new creation of the Judiciary Act of 1789; but their functions correspond to those of the old English office of sheriff. Marshals are appointed by the President and Senate for each judicial district of the United States for a term of four years. Each marshal has a number of deputies to assist in the duties of the office.

It is the duty of each marshal to attend the District and Circuit Courts of the United States when sitting in his district; and to execute throughout the district all lawful precepts directed to him and issued under the authority of the United States. The marshals and their deputies have in each State the same powers in executing the laws of the United States as the sheriffs in such State have in executing its laws. They make arrests and carry out the judgments of the courts, seizing and selling property under civil judgments, and transferring convicted prisoners to the place of confinement. They stand in the same relation to the peace of the United States as a sheriff to the peace of the State. Under the Act of 1789 it was considered that they had implied power to summon the military forces of the United States as a *posse comitatus;* but the Act of 1878 prohibited the use of the army in this way except when expressly authorized by the Constitution or Acts of Congress.

THE POST OFFICE: ITS FACTS AND ITS POSSIBILITIES [1]

By R. R. BOWKER

UNCLE SAM meets his folks face to face at the post office. It is the post which brings each citizen, who may have no other relations with his government in mind, into daily touch with the United States. The United States Post Office Department is the largest business system and does the largest single business in the world. In the year ending June 30, 1904, it transmitted through 71,131 post offices approximately 9,500,000,000 pieces of postal matter, an average of 115 to each

[1] From the *Review of Reviews*, 1904. Reproduced in part, by permission.

man, woman, and child in the country, received from all sources $143,582,624, and paid out $152,362,116, leaving a deficit of $8,779,492 to be paid from taxes.

United States Postal Figures

Under the first Postmaster General, the 75 post offices of 1789 served an average of 52,400 persons each. Under his forty successors, there has been an increase of post offices from 1,025 in 1800–01, serving an average of 5,000 persons each, to a maximum of 76,945 in 1900–01, or a post office for less than each thousand of population. The increase in rural free-delivery routes, making unnecessary many fourth-class offices, has reduced the number to 71,131 in 1904. These are connected by 31,513 mail routes, 469,818 miles in length, with annual travel in 1904 of 505,585,526 miles. Of these 421 were electric car routes, covering 4,945 miles. A hundred years ago, the yearly postal receipts were about half a million dollars, out of which as high as $100,000 profit was returned to the Government. In 1900, the receipts passed the hundred-million point, but showed a deficit exceeding $5,000,000. The largest deficit, in 1897, exceeded $11,000,000, but it is estimated that the deficit for 1905 will exceed $14,000,000.

When, in 1845, our American Post Office made a half-hearted adoption of Rowland Hill's reform, letter postage became 5 cents per half-ounce under and 10 cents over 300 miles; in 1851, the rate was made 3 cents under and 6 cents over 3,000 miles; in 1863, the rate became 3 cents for all distances, and in 1883, 2 cents; finally, the weight unit at the 2-cent rate was increased to one ounce. The 1-cent postal card came into use in 1872.

Classification of Mail Matter

Under the present classification, written communications, including all matter of the nature of individual correspondence, even though printed and all matter closed against inspection, constitute the *first class*, at the rate of 2 cents for each ounce or fraction thereof, up to the limit of four pounds, or 1 cent for postal cards or private mailing cards (officially known as "post-cards"). "Drop-letters" at rural post offices, not involving free delivery, may be posted at 1 cent each. The domestic rates extend to Canada, Mexico, Cuba, possessions of the United States abroad, the "Panama Canal Zone" and the United States Postal Agency at Shanghai, China. Periodicals "entered at the post office as *second-class* matter" can be prepaid by publishers or news-agents in bulk, at the rate of 1 cent per pound. The *third class* includes, at the rate of 1 cent for each two ounces or fraction thereof, or 8 cents per pound, to a limit of four pounds, except in the case of a single book, books, papers, and other printed matter, including "point" for the blind, and proof-sheets and manuscript copy therewith; but periodicals of the second class may be sent individually at 1 cent for four ounces, or 4 cents per pound. Books printed for the blind may be sent between public libraries or public institutions and blind people, free of postage. The *fourth class* includes merchandise at the rate of 1 cent for each ounce or fraction thereof, or 16 cents per pound, to a limit of four pounds, except that seeds, plants, etc., may be sent for 1 cent for each two ounces or fraction thereof. The difficulty and needless cost of discriminating between third and fourth class matter, and the prohibitory rate for the latter, have induced the department to recommend the inclusion of both these in a new third class, at the rate of 1 cent for each two ounces or fraction thereof, or 8 cents per pound, a wise proposal, which is now pending before Congress. Third and fourth class matter must be prepaid by stamps, except that under a recent law 2,000 or more identical pieces may be prepaid in money without stamping.

NEWSPAPER POSTAGE

With the purpose of encouraging the printing of newspapers for the education of the people, it was early provided that newspapers should be sent free of postage within thirty miles, and later, within the county of publication, except at letter-carrier offices. In 1879, a "bulk rate" of 2 cent per pound was enacted for periodicals "entered at the post office as second-class matter," permitting publishers to prepay periodicals in bulk without affixing individual stamps requiring individual cancellation, a saving both to the publisher and to the post office. This second class was defined by law to cover "newspapers and other periodical publications, regularly issued, at stated intervals, and as frequently as four times per year, bearing a date of issue and numbered consecutively, issued from a known place of publication, without substantial binding, and originated and published for the dissemination of information of a public character, or devoted to literature, the sciences, arts, or some special industry, and having a legitimate list of subscribers," — exclusive of "publications designed primarily for advertising purposes, or for free circulation, or for circulation at nominal rates."

Foreign periodicals were included, and later, publications of institutions of learning, etc. In 1886, this bulk rate was reduced, perhaps as a sop to papers of political power, to 1 cent per pound, a rate below average cost, which reduction further stimulated the Post Office Department to hedge about this second-class rate with restrictive regulations. These restrictions were aimed especially against cheap libraries or books issued serially, which the Supreme Court has recently decided may not be classed as periodicals; the "return privilege" accorded to news agents; extravagant numbers of "sample copies"; periodicals from institutions of learning which are really private affairs; and advertising sheets with circulations forced by nominal rates or premiums, such as are published in great numbers at Augusta, Me. The aggregate amount of periodicals mailed free or at pound rates in 1904 was 610,149,073 pounds, or over 305,000 tons.

Unfortunately, in the endeavor to prevent abuses, "such regulations as the Postmaster General may direct" have developed and degenerated into an elaborate and perplexing system of restrictions, now so complex and detailed as to occupy 24 pages of the Postal Rules and Regulations of 1902, arbitrarily applied and resulting in a petty interference with the periodical press comparable only with Russian censorship. This bureaucratic spirit has come to such a pass that well-known periodicals have been "held up" in the post office for days because a page of illustration or advertisement was slightly shorter or narrower than other pages, and the legitimate business of the country has been subject to incessant annoyances. When President Roosevelt's attention was called to these absurdities, with an apology that such trivialities should be brought before the President of the United States, he expressed with characteristic vigor his regret "that such trivialities should exist to be brought before the President." But even the hands of a President may be tied by red tape, and the appeal found lodgment, as usual, in the pigeon-holes of the very official appealed from, the statutory provision that "the Postmaster General shall have the determination of appeals from the action of the several Assistant Postmasters General" being practically a dead letter. The Third Assistant Postmaster General, though pursuing this policy of restriction, says, sensibly, in his recent report that "it would undoubtedly facilitate the work of the department and subserve the interests of the publishing business if the conditions of admissibility were made to depend upon considerations of a more material and less ideal character, and class and class distinguished only by physical tests."

Rate Complexities

The law itself provides a sevenfold confusion of rates for periodical publications of the second class: first, free to actual subscribers within the county of publication, except through letter-carrier offices; second, at 1 cent a pound to all offices, letter-carrier or otherwise, except the office of publication if that be a letter-carrier office; third, the same rate for weekly publications even at the letter-carrier office of publication; fourth, at 1 cent per copy for "newspapers," except weeklies, for delivery by the letter-carrier office of publication; fifth, at 1 cent per copy for other periodicals within two ounces in weight for delivery by the letter-carrier office of publication; sixth, at 2 cents a copy for the same exceeding two ounces in weight, — all these six rates applying to publisher or news agent only; a seventh rate of 1 cent for each four ounces or fraction thereof being payable under all these circumstances by the public for "second-class" periodicals, though for other printed matter the rate is 8 cents per pound.

The contradictory result is that weeklies printed in New York will be delivered in New York, San Francisco, or elsewhere for a cent a pound; that any other periodical published in New York will be delivered in San Francisco or anywhere except New York for 1 cent a pound, but in New York, if a "newspaper," must pay 1 cent for a copy of any weight, or if not a weekly or a "newspaper," 1 cent a copy under two ounces, or 2 cents a copy thereover. These complexities, which propably are not paralleled in any postal system in the world, are the direct result of haphazard and piecemeal legislation. "This multiform classification rate," says the Third Assistant Postmaster General, "is a relic of the days when the postal business was in a more or less primitive state. In this day of business methods, in government service the lack of business simplicity and uniformity is keenly felt." As free county circulation is now of diminishing importance, a simple uniform system might include all regular periodicals formally registered in the second class at the rate of 1 cent per pound to all regular subscribers, and 2 cents per pound for all other copies; or at the rate of 1 cent per pound except for delivery by carrier, which should be at 2 cents per pound.

THE PARCELS POST

A "parcels post" has been a chief lack of our postal system. In Great Britain, a parcel up to three feet in length may be sent for threepence, or 6 cents, for one pound or less, and a penny, or 2 cents, for each additional pound, making thirteen pence, or 26 cents, for the maximum weight of 11 pounds. The presence in the Senate of the United States, as Senators from New York, of the chairman of its greatest railroad corporation and the president of an express company, is cited by critics as indicating a reason why the Post Office Department is not authorized by the law to obtain better rates from railroads·and to compete with express companies in sending parcels.

Since 1878 there has been no reduction in the rate provided by law for railroad transportation of mails, which figures out, per ton-mile, $1.17 on a minimum of 200 pounds per day, 18.7 cents on a daily average of 5,000 pounds, and 5.8 cents on each additional 2,000 pounds average; though an express company will carry for other patrons a hundred pounds a thousand miles for $3.50, being 7 cents per ton-mile (involving scarcely half that payment for railroad transportation), and the railroads themselves carry a hundred pounds of freight a thousand miles for from $1 down to 35 cents, being from 2 cents down to .7 cent per ton-mile. A passenger is individually ticketed and 100 pounds of baggage individually checked at the mileage rate of 2 cents per mile, equivalent to 16 cents per ton-mile, while commuters are carried as low as $\frac{1}{2}$ cent a mile, or 4 cents per ton-mile. These figures suggest the need of a revision of contracts, which would largely offset the postal deficit and fully justify and make possible a proper parcels post.

There is now pending in Congress a bill promoted by the Postal Progress League, establishing a parcels post at the rate of 1 cent for each three ounces, 5 cents for a single pound, and 2 cents for each additional pound, making a maximum of 25 cents for an 11-pound parcel. The British parcels post insures a parcel up to $10 without charge, and for a registration fee of 4 cents up to $25, with 2 cents additional fee for each $50 up to $600; and in some countries packages may be mailed C. O. D. for an additional fee, the valuation being collected and returned through the post office.

The proposed consolidation of third and fourth class matter into a new third class at 1 cent for two ounces, or 8 cents per pound, would furnish a domestic parcels post to the limit of four pounds, and the objection that the cost of the possible 3,000 miles of land transportation in this country would involve loss on heavier parcels might be obviated by the adoption of a zone system corresponding to the standard time zones, under which a single rate might prepay within a single zone or between two adjacent zones; a once-and-a-half rate to a third zone, and a double rate to a fourth zone; so that a parcel might be sent from New York to Chicago for 8 cents, to Denver for 12 cents, and to San Francisco for 16 cents, a pound.

We have for some time had parcels-post arrangements with Mexico, the West Indies, and certain Central and South American states, and with Newfoundland, New Zealand, and Hong-kong at a price of 12 cents per pound (to Chile and Bolivia, 20 cents). A parcels post with Germany has been experimentally established, and the arrangement with the American Express Company, to which the British Government was driven by the attitude of the United States, will presently be replaced by parcels-post arrangements with Great Britain and France. To all the countries of the Postal Union, an American may send commercial papers for 5 cents for the first ten ounces and 1 cent for each additional two ounces, being 8 cents per pound, and samples of merchandise at 2 cents for the first four ounces and 1 cent for each additional two ounces, being also 8 cents per pound.

Free–Delivery Service

The city free-delivery system, established in 1863, is now extended to 1,100 letter-carrier post offices, and the special-delivery system, established in 1885, by which the special-delivery 10-cent stamp insures immediate delivery by messenger, is now in use at all post offices. But the great boon to the country has been the rural free-delivery service (described and illustrated in this magazine for January, 1903), which, with the electric trolley, the telephone, the telegraph, and the traveling library, has done so much to relieve the isolation of that third of our population connected with agricultural pursuits, and to bring to them the comforts and conveniences of city life. This service, which began experimentally in 1897 with 44 routes and an appropriation of $40,000, has increased until in 1904 there were 24,566 routes, in every State of the Union, delivering over 900,000,000 pieces of mail matter, at a cost of $12,640,070, or about 1⅓ cents each. This cost is more than the receipts from such matter, and in itself exceeds the postal deficit, but its value to the community is such as to render it one of the best investments that the post office can make, if any service whatever is to be conducted below cost.

The proposal of last year to prohibit rural carriers from carrying merchandise has been wisely replaced this year by a recommendation for a low postage rate on packages not exceeding five pounds in weight mailed from a local post office for delivery on a rural-delivery route from the same office, to be paid by a special stamp at three cents per pound or fraction thereof. An even rate of one cent for four ounces might be more in line with other postal rates and of greater convenience to the people. The new plan will be of further benefit to the rural community, and though for some years there will be an increase of expense over return, the growth of rural population and this new source of revenue may be expected to make the rural free-delivery system almost if not quite self-sustaining, and its full development may prove a chief credit of the present administration. An additional convenience has been suggested, by the use of a special telephone stamp which would authorize a rural postmaster to telephone a message to any telephone subscriber.

The registry service (first authorized by Congress in 1855), for a fee of 8 cents in addition to regular postage, prepaid with ordinary stamps, insures the registration of a letter at each point of its journey, a receipt to the sender and one from the addressee, and insurance up to $25 value. Post office money orders, first in use in 1865, can now be obtained at the 35,094 money-order offices for payment at any specified money-order office, for from 3 cents within $2.50 to 30 cents for $100, these rates covering also Hawaii, Porto Rico, the Philippine Islands, Canada, Newfoundland, Cuba, and the United States Postal Agency at Shanghai, China. In 1904, there were issued 50,392,554 domestic money orders, to the amount of $378,511,407, paying the Government $2,089,250 profit.

FOREIGN POSTAL FEATURES

Foreign postal systems have gone much further than our own in some respects. Great Britain, as well as several other countries, makes a postal monopoly of its telegraph, at the rate of a halfpenny, or 1 cent per word, address counted, with a minimum rate of sixpence, or 12 cents, for each telegraph. But the 90,000,000 telegrams sent in 1904 involved an operating loss of over £300,000, or $1,500,000. Great Britain has also recently taken over the telephone service as part of the postal system, but, as in Sweden and other countries, the competitive private systems seem to give more satisfactory results. Postal savings-banks exist throughout Great Britain as well as in other countries, that country having at last report 14,362 post-office savings-bank offices, with 9,403,852 accounts, aggregating £146,000,000, or over $700,000,000, an average of $75 each, on which $17,000,000 interest was paid during the year. A system of postal annuities and life insurance is connected with the British post-office savings-banks, but the use of this system at last report was confined to about 2,500 persons in a year, and its chief value seems to have been in keeping down the rates of friendly societies and regular life insurance companies.

Among other foreign features are the "blow-post," or pneumatic-tube service for quick delivery, as in Berlin and Paris, — a system less desirable here in these days of the telephone and our special-delivery service. Our own Post Office Department, however, uses pneumatic tubes for the transmission of mail matter between main and branch offices in the cities of New York, Brooklyn, Philadelphia, Boston, Chicago, and St. Louis. In France, Italy, and elsewhere, local deliveries are expedited by the use of automobiles. Switzerland has a library post, by which packages can be sent from or to a public library at about three cents for four pounds; and in Italy, the Scandinavian countries, and elsewhere, books may be sent between the officially recognized libraries, for the use of students, free of postage. A bill for a library post at one cent per pound, promoted by the American Library Association, is now before Congress. Belgium has a curious stamp, with a detachable coupon reading, "Not to be delivered on Sunday," which is left on the letter when Sunday delivery is not required, but otherwise detached.

DEPARTMENT ORGANIZATION

The Post Office Department, though it does a wonderful business in the interest of the people, is handicapped by a traditional and bureaucratic internal administration. The Postmaster General, who has been a cabinet officer since 1829, and has a salary of $8,000 only is mostly occupied in affixing to unread documents the perfunctory personal signature required by law, and in listening to political applicants, though civil service reform has much mitigated the political misuse of the Post Office. His immediate staff includes First, Second, Third, and Fourth Assistant Postmasters General, the ranking Assistant on duty becoming Acting Postmaster General in the absence of the chief. Among these, the several functions of the department are divided, mostly without method, illogically and inconveniently, and a bureaucracy has grown up, without a real administrative head, which fact has been an obstacle in the way of postal progress. The House Committee on Postal Affairs holds the purse-strings, and its chairman becomes, in fact, an outside executive of the department, while the many associations of post-office employees, of which the United National Association of Post-Office Clerks of the United States is a leading organization, though of excellent purpose, have devoted themselves to "influencing" Congressmen and punishing those who prove refractory.[1]

The Post Office Department needs, at the hands of Congress, an organization which shall bring its administration up to the standard of private corporations, with a well-paid executive of the highest ability as the right-hand of the cabinet officer; with competent superintendents of transportation; urban offices and delivery; rural offices and delivery; special delivery and registry; money orders; supplies, equipment and repairs; correspondence and records; dead letters; inspection; accounting and legal relations; making together an administrative council for the executive, as in the French post-office system.

Meantime, the spirit of bureaucracy, especially exemplified in the petty treatment of periodical publishers, under restrictions not required by law, should be replaced by common-sense business policy. The department also needs from Congress legal authorization to require from the railroads transportation rates not greater than those made to express companies, and it might not be unwise to remove the drastic restrictions in the law which forbid the use of private service for transmitting correspondence. The American public, in its righteous indignation at the uneven and often excessive rates of the telephone, telegraph, express, and railroad services, often forgets how wonderfully and effectively organized are these corporate administrations; and a comparison between these and governmental postal administration would be wholesome to both.

A Reformed System of Rates

To represent the interests of the public, the Postal Progress League and other organizations have been formed. In 1878, the Post Office

---

[1] Under the control and pay of the department are postmasters at 71,131 offices, 1,654 assistant postmasters, 25,410 clerks in first and second class offices, 11,621 clerks in the railway mail service, 20,761 city letter-carriers, and rural carriers on 24,566 routes; in all, over 155,000 employees, without counting others partially or indirectly employed.

Department took the wise course of calling a conference of publishers and other large users of the mails for consultation with the officers of the department in devising what became the Act of 1879. The time has come when there should be a revision of postal arrangements with the public, not in the shape of piecemeal legislation, but in a well-considered and unified plan of reform which should command the respect of Congress and the people. The country needs a simple system of rates, a parcels post, a postal check, and the better arrangements with foreign post offices which they are eager to make. A useful pamphlet of "General Postal Information for the Public," recently issued by the Third Assistant Postmaster-General, and to be had free at the post offices, illustrates too well the present complexity. Perhaps the simplest system of postal rates, of most convenience to the Government and the people, would be somewhat as follows: For letters, 2 cents per ounce, drop-letters 1 cent; for postal cards, 1 cent; for periodicals from the office of publication and books from public libraries, in bulk, 1 cent per pound without local free delivery, and 2 cents per pound with local free delivery; for periodicals and books otherwise mailed, 1 cent for four ounces, 4 cents per pound and 1 cent for each added half pound; for all else, a simple parcels-post system, including local free delivery, at 1 cent for two ounces, 8 cents per pound, and 1 cent for each added half pound, with half-rate for rural free delivery from the local office and extra rates on the zone system for extreme distances on packages above four pounds; the abolition of the "county fee" system and the restriction of the franking privilege to distinctly official correspondence; and a foreign post, uniform to all countries of the Postal Union, in accordance with the general practice, comprehensive of the best features of the postal service of other countries. Such a scheme, reforming rather than revolutionizing present methods, classification, and rates, would greatly reduce the cost of the department, possibly increase its revenue to the self-supporting point, and permit in the future successive reductions of rates. The possibilities of the Post Office as an agent for the people's good are indeed great, and the present is a favorable time for giving to our own country a postal system which shall in no respect be behind those of less-favored nations.

POST OFFICE DEPARTMENT: MAIL FRAUD ORDERS

[The post office department is the agency through which the federal government comes into closest contact with the body of citizens. The efficiency of its operations as compared with those of private companies gives the citizens a general criterion for testing the effectiveness of public administration. The use of the mails is a valuable privilege, the withdrawal of which by the government may be made the instrument for punishing and preventing wrong. The postal authorities refuse to allow the mailing facilities to be used for the purpose of practicing schemes of fraud and deception. Controversy has recently arisen about the procedure of the department in the matter of mail fraud orders, which will be illustrated by the following extracts.]

FRAUD ORDERS ISSUED BY THE POST OFFICE AUTHORITIES [1]

NEW schemes of deception invite new measures of prevention. This seems as apparent from a study of the Government's fraud-order business, as the history of burglary shows the growth of safety appliances. The Government has steadily tightened its rein over concerns using the postal service apparently for the purpose of cheating the public. This forms a valuable agency for the purification of advertising pages.

Uncle Sam has already issued 2,180 fraud orders. Assuming that each concern with a get-rich-quick scheme had 20,000 victims — and this estimate of the average number seems modest — a number equal to one-half of the entire population of the country has been victimized within the last fifteen years. There is no knowing how many innocent lambs have been saved by the postal shepherds from these postal wolves of small finance. A respectable minority of the American people might be placed under the designation "an easy mark." It is practically certain that the same fish must have risen repeatedly to the same shining bait, and fed fat the get-rich-quick fraternity. Otherwise there could not have been so many of them.

At first the executive departments of this Government dealt tenderly with persons having get-rich-quick schemes. "Fraudulent" lotteries only were under the ban of the law of 1872. The statute referred vaguely to false-pretense schemes, but executive officers ignored this part of it. The president of the famous Louisiana lottery company was No. 1 on the list of banned enterprise-managers, accessible in the dockets of the department. But a new law was necessary to put his undertaking out of business. "Fraudulent" was dropped in designating lotteries which were not to be permitted. The beneficent was added to the evil. After that all lotteries looked alike to the Government. Under the law which proved the beginning of the end for the gigantic Louisiana swindle, which for a generation had filched large sums from Americans with a speculative turn of mind, only registered letters and money-orders could be withheld. Subsequently the law was extended to include all mail matter.

The Louisiana Lottery people took the case to the Court of Appeals of the District of Columbia, attacking the constitutionality of the law. Judge Cox in a long opinion upheld the law, taking the ground that the right of the citizen to use Government postal facilities for the transmission of mail, was not a constitutional right, but a legislative privilege, which must be utilized according to the conditions placed upon it by Congress.

[1] *New York Evening Post*, April 25, 1905.

Lotteries, after the downfall of the Louisiana, have had a hard time in this country.

Judge Thomas, in President Cleveland's second Administration, had fraud orders issued against a number of persons whom he believed to have been acquiring money in tortuous ways. His practice was to issue the fraud order and have the mail held up on plausible complaint. Investigation came afterward. If the fraud order was found unwarranted, it was cancelled. This method was a trifle more summary than that of Judge Thomas's successors. Fraud orders are not now issued until the persons involved have had an opportunity to be heard.

As lotteries became scarce, the Post Office Department looked about for other game. It found some in the case of a patent-procuring concern. Would-be inventors, it seems, are almost as numerous as plain every-day "suckers." In many respects it is difficult to distinguish between these classes. The inventor furnished food for the patent concern. Putting it out of business by holding up its mail marks one of the earliest important cases decided on the ground of alleged fraud, or false-pretense, aside from the lottery element. This case was decided in 1897. Even that case was complicated by the disbarment of the head of the concern as a patent attorney.

Another famous case, turning upon alleged fraud and false pretense, was that of a concern, having headquarters at Fairfield, Me., which sold its victims materials and taught them to make artificial flowers. The flowers promised to be sources of great income to the victims, but they never quite arrived. Some defects appeared which could be cured by taking instruction in other lines, which the company would give for a consideration. After the victim discovered that the corn was musty and refused to follow further, he was dropped. A Federal judge, in passing upon this case, cast doubt upon the constitutionality of the whole Fraud-Order law, but the company had come into an equity court with hands so unclean that he would not attack the law for its benefit.

Still another step in advance was taken in the case of a New York concern which had a scheme for selling fountain pens for $2.50 each, and employing at $8 a week in advertising letter-writing everybody who bought a pen. It was an endless-chain scheme, growing constantly wider. All revenues were derived from the sale of the pens. This inverted financial pyramid was not thought stable by the Post Office people, and the concern was put out of business by a fraud order, in October, 1902, after having secured 19,000 patrons.

A most gentlemanly scheme, having no end of imitators, started by a diamond company in San Francisco, came to grief about a year ago, through the squeamishness of the postal authorities. This was such a beneficent scheme, and the men behind the "graft" showed such pious good faith, that the Department actually apologized for being obliged to attack it, and point out its financial fallaciousness. It was proposed to

give a $160 diamond to everybody who would pay $80 in weekly instal-
ments, thus putting each investor almost in the position of the chattel
loan man. The company depended upon lapses to "make good." Postal authorities said that was impossible, and the honest promoters went
under the shadow of the ban. All its fellows have followed suit. This
seems the lineal descendant of certain bond-investment schemes, which
at one time promised great possibilities.

Having gone to the limit in hunting down schemes of an alleged fraudulent character, the postal authorities swung back toward the lottery idea,
as it invaded guessing enterprises. This included guessing for prizes as
to the attendance at the St. Louis Fair, and guessing the number of
ballots cast for Roosevelt or for Parker. These cases brought out last
November an opinion by Attorney-General Moody, holding the Fraud-
Order law constitutional. Before that, attorneys-general held almost
uniformly the opposite view. Mr. Moody followed the United States
Supreme Court in the case of Public Clearing House against Coyne, and
the New York Court of Appeals in the Lavin case. A formal judicial
opinion had held that a cigarette guessing contest was legitimate. But
Mr. Moody and the courts he followed found elements of lottery in guessing contests. He also found that the term "due process of law," in the
Constitution, may mean hearing and action by an executive department,
when the parties have recourse to the courts, if aggrieved.

As it now stands, the powers of the Post Office Department are most
broad and sweeping. Racing schemes, bond investment schemes, employment schemes on the endless-chain plan, guessing schemes, and all
other such devious devices for getting into the private pocket of the public, are banned. Not only are advertisers of such schemes in danger, but
even the periodicals which run the advertisements may be excluded from
the mails. It is not necessary for the Department to prove actual fraud,
but it may act on proof of advertising a scheme of finance not feasible.
Newspapers must look carefully at their circulation schemes. The
Woman's World came to grief after landing $500,000 good American
dollars.

Fraud orders grow by seasons. The harvest time is between September
and May, when the good American, surrounded by his household gods,
reads the alluring advertisements and becomes impromptu a financier.
In 1899 fraud orders numbered 99; in 1901, 62, and in each of the years
1902 and 1904 they numbered 247. If one has visions of high finance,
before plunging he may do well to ponder the warning: "The fraud
order man will get you if you don't watch out."

SPEECH OF HON. EDGAR D. CRUMPACKER ON THE POST-OFFICE APPROPRIATION BILL [1]

MR. CRUMPACKER said:

Mr. Chairman: I will take advantage of the opportunity afforded by the debate upon this bill to submit some additional remarks upon the bill providing for a judicial review of fraud orders issued by the Post-master-General, which passed the House some weeks ago. There seems to be some misunderstanding respecting the scope and purpose of that bill, based, as far as I am able to learn, upon a careless or willful mis-representation of its provisions by individuals who seem to have little regard for the truth. It has come to be quite the fashion when any legislation is proposed that curtails or modifies power that is being exercised by a bureau officer in one of the Departments, however wise and just the measure may be, for some dilettante reformer who is long on theory and short on practical wisdom, and who has no faith in the common people nor respect for the integrity of the courts, to open up a tirade against the measure and to asperse the Representative who may propose it and all those who give it support.

I have observed, also, that some of the chiefs of bureaus in the Departments stubbornly resist every attempt to reduce or modify the power they exercise or to reduce in any measure the appropriations for the administration of their bureaus. It is not always a question of patriotism or public good with them, but often a question of personal and official aggrandizement. Some bureau chiefs have gone so far in their opposition to just and prudent measures as to inspire unjust attacks upon Members advocating them and to recklessly, at least, misrepresent their purpose and effect. These officers seem to have no difficulty in securing means of communicating their opposition to the public. There are individuals engaged in newspaper and magazine work who are willing to believe anything that may be told them by a bureau chief in disparagement of the ability and integrity of a representative of the people, and without inquiry or investigation they send out broadcast over the country gross misstatements concerning the provisions and purposes of proposed legislation. Those individuals seem to be imbued with the idea that this is a government of the bureaus, by the bureaus, and for the bureaus, and that any proposition, however wise or salutary, that in any degree minimizes the dignity or power of a bureau chief must of necessity be against the public good. It is human nature for one who is in the enjoyment of autocratic authority to resist every attempt made to limit or modify the exercise of that authority.

The House has a most salutary rule that prohibits legislation upon general appropriation bills. The object of the rule is to prevent "riders"

[1] *Congr. Record*, Feb. 19, 1907.

from being attached to appropriation bills and to secure the consideration of each measure independently upon its own merits.

Recently a newspaper correspondent, prompted by personal enmity or a general malicious instinct, assailed a Member of the House for making a point of order against an item of legislation that was contained in a general appropriation bill in violation of the rules of the House. The fact that the point of order was sustained and the action of the Member upheld by the presiding officer made no difference to the correspondent. He wanted a story. Intelligent and fair criticism of proposed legislation is of great good, but unjust and dishonest criticism is destructive of confidence in public men and even in government, and it does incalculable harm. Members of Congress must always be free to propose and support measures they honestly believe to be for the public good, and no Department officer should, under any circumstances, feel justified in misrepresenting measures or in imputing bad faith to Representatives who propose or support them.

THE FRAUD–ORDER LAW AND ITS ADMINISTRATION

The criticism of the bill for a judicial review of fraud orders has been chiefly a misrepresentation and perversion of its provisions. Under the existing law the Postmaster-General may issue a fraud order against any person whom he believes is using the mails for criminal or fraudulent purposes, and the law provides for no notice to the person to be effected and no opportunity for him to appear and defend himself. A fraud order is an order issued by the Assistant Attorney-General of the Post Office Department, in the name of the Postmaster-General, to the postmaster where the accused receives his mail, directing him to pay no money orders to the accused and to deliver no mail to him, but to stamp all mail that comes to him with the word "fraudulent" and return it to the writer where the envelope bears a return card; otherwise to forward it immediately to the Post Office Department, to be disposed of through the dead-letter office. The order covers all mail, business or social, without discrimination. In many and perhaps in most instances, as a matter of favor, the Department notifies the person to be effected by a fraud order and gives him an opportunity to appear and show cause, if he can, why the order should not be issued. The hearing is voluntary, and is conducted by the Assistant Attorney-General, who is bound by no rules and follows no fixed course of procedure. In some cases no notice is given at all. The law does not require it, and the Assistant Attorney-General decides when notice shall be given and when not. In numerous instances fraud orders have been issued upon the mere confidential report of a post-office inspector, without any notice whatever to the person affected or any opportunity to disprove the charges against him.

CHARACTER OF EVIDENCE UPON WHICH FRAUD ORDERS ARE ISSUED

Now, I want to say a few words in regard to the evidence upon which the Assistant Attorney-General acts in issuing fraud orders. I stated a moment ago that his action was based, in the main, upon confidential reports which were the result of secret investigations by post-office inspectors. They constitute the bulk of the evidence. The Assistant Attorney-General for the Department is himself first convinced, and then he notifies the person affected by the proposed action to appear and show cause, without allowing him to see the report or know what it contains. He is at once the prosecuting attorney, judge, and executioner, and the privilege of appearing before that officer, who has already made up his mind, to refute evidence that he can know nothing about is one without any practical value.

The Supreme Court has held that the fraud-order power may be conferred upon the Postmaster-General because the right to the mail is a privilege and not a vested right and that the proceeding is not criminal in its character. While this may be the correct constitutional theory, yet the party against whom a fraud order is issued is branded as a criminal and stigmatized as a perpetrator of fraud. It makes him an outlaw as far as one of the most important branches of the Government is concerned. The issuance of such an order covers all his mail and deprives him of the right to communicate with his friends, his wife, or his mother, or to receive any communication from them by means of the mails.

All of this is done upon confidential reports, the result of secret investigations based upon ex parte statements of persons whose motives can not be known, who may be responsible or who may be irresponsible, who may not be competent witnesses, and who are not sworn and do not carry the responsibilities of ordinary witnesses. Their names and identity are not disclosed, and their evidence does not contain one single safeguard against fraud or one single test of credibility. Such evidence would not be received in the humblest magistrate's court of the country in a case involving the investigation of the most inconsequential right of person or property.

The confidential nature of such reports and the statements they contain, including the names of persons giving information, is such that they are never made public or disclosed to the parties vitally affected by them. About a year ago this House adopted a resolution requesting the Postmaster-General to furnish it with the facts upon which a certain fraud order was issued and copies of the inspector's reports in the case, and that officer politely and respectfully returned the resolution to the House with the statement that it would not be compatible with the public interest to comply with the request.

The investigation and decision of fraud-order cases under the practice in the Department is necessarily made by the Assistant Attorney-General. During the two years ending June 30 last 660 fraud orders were issued and a number of cases investigated where the accused agreed to modify his advertising matter so that it would conform to the ideas of propriety of the Assistant Attorney-General, thereby obviating the issuing of an order excluding him from the mails. Over one case a day had to be examined and decided, and it would be out of the question for the Postmaster-General to give his personal attention to the examination and decision of these cases and attend to the other arduous and multifarious duties of his office. The Assistant Attorney-General devotes the bulk of his time to the fraud-order business. He refers complaints to post-office inspectors, examines reports, decides questions of law and fact, hears matter in defense, and practically has the decision of the ultimate question as to whether a fraud order shall be issued or not, although the work is done in the name of the Postmaster-General. It is a matter of common experience that men who represent the Government in hunting down and ferreting out fraud and in conducting prosecutions become imbued with an official prejudice to such an extent as to unfit them to deal justly between their own client and paymaster and one whose interests may be adverse. I do not say this in disparagement of this class of officials, but a man who has the zeal and enthusiasm necessary to make a success of the work in which he is engaged, unless he be exceptionally even tempered and well poised, is most apt to become inoculated with that official bias that will prevent his dealing justly with those whose interests he may have in charge.

The Assistant Attorney-General is a detective in a large sense, to hunt down frauds, and is the prosecutor to convict the perpetrators, and in the fraud-order practice he is the judge and jury to pass upon their guilt or innocence. In view of the vital questions that are involved directly and impliedly in the fraud-order practice, it is a most unsafe thing to intrust an officer of this kind with such unlimited power. This Government is said to be a Government of law and not of men. The personal and property rights of the citizens should not be vitally affected by any Department of Government, excepting in pursuance of law. In the execution of the fraud-order law much may depend upon the temperament and the ideals of the Assistant Attorney-General. One person occupying that position may have peculiarly high notions of business ethics and little or no patience with men who do not deal absolutely fairly with their fellows. On the other hand, another may have lax ideas respecting these matters and much sympathy for wrongdoers. Under a practice where the result must of necessity be largely colored by the temperament and sentiment of a departmental official, the vital concerns of the citizens ought not to be reposed.

I desire to impress upon the House, in addition, the dangerous character of the method of presenting proof on the part of the Government in fraud-order cases. The same zeal that I have referred to in connection with the Assistant Attorney-General characterizes the action of the post-office inspectors. There seems to be a belief or feeling on the part of these functionaries that unless they are able to discover official irregularities or individual delinquencies in connection with the mails their records as efficient officers will suffer. Their investigations are made secretly and contain, largely, interviews with citizens in various communities which are always private, and the names of the citizens who give information are to be kept inviolate.

How many men, prompted by feelings of envy or jealousy against a business rival, with the understanding that their names will not be disclosed under any circumstances, will be prompted to give information that may be largely colored by business jealousy or personal envy — information that as citizens carrying the responsibilities of a witness in public they would under no circumstances feel at liberty to give. Such testimony is a positive menace to the safety of person, reputation, and property under any system of administration. It is contrary to the commonest notions of justice and fair dealing. Due process of law, as is commonly understood in our system of government, means that process of law that is administered in the open, where the accused party may have a right to confront his accusers; where those who give testimony on either side must carry the solemn responsibilities of their conduct before the public.

I have no sympathy with or respect for the policy that affects the important rights of person, reputation, or property by means of confidential reports of secret emissaries of the law. Reports containing evidence respecting the rights of the citizen should always be made public. No consideration of delicacy or embarrassment should justify the Government in blasting the reputation and ruining the business of a citizen without giving him an opportunity to know exactly who has testified against him and to what he has testified. The reports of inspectors under any practice should be open to the person who may be affected by the fraud order. He should be allowed to know who have given information or testified against him, and citizens who are interviewed should understand that their names and statements would be open to inspection by the person against whom they testify or give information. This would have a most wholesome and salutary influence. Men would see that the statements that were written up by the post-office inspectors and credited to them were fair and just and absolutely true. There should be no inducement or opportunity for men to attempt to stab the business or reputation of rivals in the dark.

Even under the present law the investigation of fraud-order questions should be conducted in as open a manner as possible. Star-chamber procedure has no place in the administration of rights in this Government. It is contrary to the spirit of the age. The whole fraud-order practice in the Post Office Department, however honest and pure the intentions and purposes of its administrators may be, is out of harmony with the principles of individual liberty, and it ought to be discontinued. There is no adequate excuse for it. It is claimed, I know, that if reports were made public and the names of men who give information were disclosed it would be difficult, if not impossible, for post-office inspectors to secure necessary information in this class of cases. I make the assertion that a citizen who will not give testimony except upon condition that his name be withheld from the public, and particularly from the individual against whom he testifies, as a rule is not worthy of credence. His testimony is to be suspected and should not be regarded as sufficient to deprive any citizen of any substantial right.

The Federal criminal code imposes penalties for almost every act that would justify the issuing of a fraud order. If post-office inspectors, in investigating crimes and frauds, would investigate them with a view of detecting the perpetrators and their reports should be immediately transmitted to the Department of Justice, where instructions could be sent to arrest the criminals, it would largely tend to stop the practice of debauching the mails. The Postmaster-General, in his recent report, claims that under the fraud-order practice lotteries and other criminal concerns have almost been driven out of existence. In my humble judgment, if there were no penalty excepting that of a fraud order, the country would be overrun with lotteries, "green-goods" institutions, and other criminal concerns to-day. The criminal laws have suppressed lotteries and "green-goods" dispensers. They have been the efficient power in purifying the mails and protecting them against the schemes and devices of evil doers.

In making these criticisms of the fraud-order practice, it is not my intention to reflect in any degree upon the Postmatser-General, the assistant attorney-general for the Post Office Department, or of any other official. The result is the necessary and logical outcome of the arbitrary system of investigation authorized by the statutes. It is not the fault of the officers personally, but the fault of the system, and it is the system that I am complaining about and which I believe ought to be materially modified.

EXPANSION OF FRAUD–ORDER POWERS

If the fraud-order law were now administered according to its original purpose and intention, I would be the last man to raise my voice against it, arbitrary and despotic though it seems. I have no use for criminals and swindlers who seek to debauch the mails for unlawful purposes, but where men who honestly believe they are innocent of violations of law are denied the right of the mails and branded with infamy I believe they should be accorded the privilege of going into court and proving their innocence if they can.

The fraud-order law was originally intended to enable the Postmaster-General to withhold mails from the promoters of lotteries, "green-goods" institutions, get-rich-quick concerns, and fly-by-night affairs that were essentially and palpably fraudulent and criminal. It was not intended that it should interfere with old established business institutions that could be reached through the civil and criminal courts, but during the last two or three years a surveillance has been instituted over old establishments using the mails in a mail-order business, and numerous concerns of that kind have been brought before the Assistant Attorney-General and subjected to all manner of embarrassment and humiliation, and in some instances fraud orders have been issued against them and their business and reputations forever ruined. It is the ambitious policy of the Assistant Attorney-General for the Department in the fraud-order line during the last few years that has subjected this salutary power to the criticism that it is receiving all over the country at this time.[1]

[1] Opinion expressed by a Writer in the North American Review, April, 1907:

In administering the present law the Department has been so consistently reasonable that there is little apparent occasion for recourse to the courts. There is no opposition on the part of the Department to such an amendment as will give court review, if it does not deprive the Department of its present immediate effectiveness and therefore of its entire usefulness in this means of public protection. There can be no objection to every man having the right of appeal to the courts against any possible or apparent injustice; but to carry that right so far as to take away the force of the order, to vitiate its effectiveness, or remove the matter from the jurisdiction of the Department during court review, would obviously render the position of the Department unreasonably embarrassing; as by law it would be expected to protect the public while handicapped by an amendment rendering it powerless to do so.

The present statutes overcome conditions with which the ordinary machinery of the law is inadequate to deal. The convenient and almost necessary facility of communication afforded by the Post Office Department and the freedom of communication from inspection obviously lay the service open to grave abuse. Without this authority which enables the Postmaster-General to act quickly and effectively when unlawful use of mails is established, the public would be constantly at the mercy of hordes of rascals who have become expert inventors and promoters of devices to defraud.

It is not the law, but the law's delay, which the operators of fraudulent methods would be glad to obtain. For it must be borne in mind that many, if not most, of the schemes to defraud are of the fly-by-night order; of the kind whose methods and base of operations are constantly changing; who shift from name to name and city to city, for the express purpose of avoiding too close scrutiny; who are often hard to locate for the deeds of the present and harder to convict for the deeds of the past.

In New York, recently, a dozen different names were successively used by one concern, a change being made immediately on the discovery that it was attracting attention — made for the express purpose of escaping the detrimental effect of a fraud order. This plan would obviously be much more successful if the restriction came from the slowly moving courts.

THE DEPARTMENT OF AGRICULTURE

[The United States Department of Agriculture carries on extensive services for the purpose of investigating the conditions of agriculture, of improving methods of introducing new plants and animals. The developmental work of this department is illustrated by the following selections.]

FROM PRESIDENT ROOSEVELT'S MESSAGE, DECEMBER 6, 1904

Agriculture. The Department of Agriculture has grown into an educational institution with a faculty of two thousand specialists making research into all the sciences of production. The Congress appropriates, directly and indirectly, six millions of dollars annually to carry on this work. It reaches every State and Territory in the Union and the islands of the sea lately come under our flag. Coöperation is had with the State experiment stations, and with many other institutions and individuals. The world is carefully searched for new varieties of grains, fruits, grasses, vegetables, trees, and shrubs, suitable to various localities in our country· and marked benefit to our producers has resulted.

The activities of our age in lines of research have reached the tillers of the soil and inspired them with ambition to know more of the principles that govern the forces of nature with which they have to deal. Nearly half of the people of this country devote their energies to growing things from the soil. Until a recent date little has been done to prepare these millions for their life work. In most lines of human activity college-trained men are the leaders. The farmer had no opportunity for special training until the Congress made provision for it forty years ago. During these years progress has been made and teachers have been prepared. Over five thousand students are in attendance at our State agricultural colleges. The Federal Government expends ten millions of dollars annually toward this education and for research in Washington and in the several States and Territories. The Department of Agriculture has given facilities for post-graduate work to five hundred young men during the last seven years, preparing them for advanced lines of work in the Department and in the State institutions.

The facts concerning meteorology and its relations to plant and animal life are being systematically inquired into. Temperature and moisture are controlling factors in all agricultural operations. The seasons of the cyclones of the Caribbean Sea and their paths are being forecasted with increasing accuracy. The cold winds that come from the north are anticipated and their times and intensity told to farmers, gardeners, and fruiterers in all southern localities.

We sell two hundred and fifty million dollars' worth of animals and animal products to foreign countries every year, in addition to supplying our own people more cheaply and abundantly than any other nation is

26

able to provide for its people. Successful manufacturing depends primarily on cheap food, which accounts to a considerable extent for our growth in this direction. The Department of Agriculture, by careful inspection of meats, guards the health of our people and gives clean bills of health to deserving exports; it is prepared to deal promptly with imported diseases of animals, and maintain the excellence of our flocks and herds in this respect. There should be an annual census of the live stock of the Nation.

We sell abroad about six hundred million dollars' worth of plants and their products every year. Strenuous efforts are being made to import from foreign countries such grains as are suitable to our varying localities. Seven years ago we bought three-fourths of our rice; by helping the rice growers on the Gulf coast to secure seeds from the Orient suited to their conditions, and by giving them adequate protection, they now supply home demand and export to the islands of the Caribbean Sea and to other rice-growing countries. Wheat and other grains have been imported from light-rainfall countries to our lands in the West and Southwest that have not grown crops because of light precipitation, resulting in an extensive addition to our cropping area and our home-making territory that can not be irrigated. Ten million bushels of first-class macaroni wheat were grown from these experimental importations last year. Fruits suitable to our soils and climates are being imported from all the countries of the Old World — the fig from Turkey, the almond from Spain, the date from Algeria, the mango from India. We are helping our fruit growers to get their crops into European markets by studying methods of preservation through refrigeration, packing, and handling, which have been quite successful. We are helping our hop growers by importing varieties that ripen earlier and later than the kinds they have been raising, thereby lengthening the harvesting season. The cotton crop of the country is threatened with root rot, the bollworm, and the boll weevil. Our pathologists will find immune varieties that will resist the root disease, and the bollworm can be dealt with, but the boll weevil is a serious menace to the cotton crop. It is a Central American insect that has become acclimated in Texas and has done great damage. A scientist of the Department of Agriculture has found the weevil at home in Guatemala being kept in check by an ant, which has been brought to our cotton fields for observation. It is hoped that it may serve a good purpose.

The soils of the country are getting attention from the farmer's standpoint, and interesting results are following. We have duplicates of the soils that grow the wrapper tobacco in Sumatra and the filler tobacco in Cuba. It will be only a question of time when the large amounts paid to these countries will be paid to our own people. The reclamation of alkali lands is progressing, to give object lessons to our people in methods by which worthless lands may be made productive.

The insect friends and enemies of the farmer are getting attention. The enemy of the San Jose scale was found near the Great Wall of China, and is now cleaning up all our orchards. The fig-fertilizing insect imported from Turkey has helped to establish an industry in California that amounts to from fifty to one hundred tons of dried figs annually, and is extending over the Pacific coast. A parasitic fly from South Africa is keeping in subjection the black scale, the worst pest of the orange and lemon industry in California.

Careful preliminary work is being done towards producing our own silk. The mulberry is being distributed in large numbers, eggs are being imported and distributed, improved reels were imported from Europe last year, and two expert reelers were brought to Washington to reel the crop of cocoons and teach the art to our own people.

The crop-reporting system of the Department of Agriculture is being brought closer to accuracy every year. It has two hundred and fifty thousand reporters selected from people in eight vocations in life. It has arrangements with most European countries for interchange of estimates, so that our people may know as nearly as possible with what they must compete.

Irrigation. During the two and a half years that have elapsed since the passage of the reclamation act rapid progress has been made in the surveys and examinations of the opportunities for reclamation in the thirteen States and three Territories of the arid West. Construction has already been begun on the largest and most important of the irrigation works, and plans are being completed for works which will utilize the funds now available. The operations are being carried on by the Reclamation Service, a corps of engineers selected through competitive civil-service examinations. This corps includes experienced consulting and constructing engineers as well as various experts in mechanical and legal matters, and is composed largely of men who have spent most of their lives in practical affairs connected with irrigation. The larger problems have been solved and it now remains to execute with care, economy, and thoroughness the work which has been laid out. All important details are being carefully considered by boards of consulting engineers, selected for their thorough knowledge and practical experience. Each project is taken up on the ground by competent men and viewed from the standpoint of the creation of prosperous homes, and of promptly refunding to the Treasury the cost of construction. The reclamation act has been found to be remarkably complete and effective, and so broad in its provisions that a wide range of undertakings has been possible under it. At the same time, economy is guaranteed by the fact that the funds must ultimately be returned to be used over again.

Forests. It is the cardinal principle of the forest-reserve policy of this Administration that the reserves are for use. Whatever interferes with the use of their resources is to be avoided by every possible means.

But these resources must be used in such a way as to make them permanent.

The forest policy of the Government is just now a subject of vivid public interest throughout the West and to the people of the United States in general. The forest reserves themselves are of extreme value to the present as well as to the future welfare of all the western public-land States. They powerfully affect the use and disposal of the public lands. They are of special importance because they preserve the water supply and the supply of timber for domestic purposes, and so promote settlement under the reclamation act. Indeed, they are essential to the welfare of every one of the great interests of the West.

Forest reserves are created for two principal purposes. The first is to preserve the water supply. This is their most important use. The principal users of the water thus preserved are irrigation ranchers and settlers, cities and towns to whom their municipal water supplies are of the very first importance, users and furnishers of water power, and the users of water for domestic, manufacturing, mining, and other purposes. All these are directly dependent upon the forest reserves.

The second reason for which forest reserves are created is to preserve the timber supply for various classes of wood users. Among the more important of these are settlers under the reclamation act and other acts, for whom a cheap and accessible supply of timber for domestic uses is absolutely necessary; miners and prospectors, who are in serious danger of losing their timber supply by fire or through export by lumber companies when timber lands adjacent to their mines pass into private ownership; lumbermen, transportation companies, builders, and commercial interests in general.

Although the wisdom of creating forest reserves is nearly everywhere heartily recognized, yet in a few localities there has been misunderstanding and complaint. The following statement is therefore desirable:

The forest-reserve policy can be successful only when it has the full support of the people of the West. It can not safely, and should not in any case, be imposed upon them against their will. But neither can we accept the views of those whose only interest in the forest is temporary; who are anxious to reap what they have not sown and then move away, leaving desolation behind them. On the contrary, it is everywhere and always the interest of the permanent settler and the permanent business man, the man with a stake in the country, which must be considered and which must decide.

The making of forest reserves within railroad and wagon-road land-grant limits will hereafter, as for the past three years, be so managed as to prevent the issue, under the act of June 4, 1897, of base for exchange or lieu selection (usually called scrip). In all cases where forest reserves within areas covered by land grants appear to be essential to the prosperity of settlers, miners, or others, the Government lands within such proposed forest reserves will, as in the recent past, be withdrawn from sale or entry pending the completion of such negotiations with the owners of the land grants as will prevent the creation of so-called scrip.

It was formerly the custom to make forest reserves without first getting definite and detailed information as to the character of land and timber within their boundaries. This method of action often resulted in badly chosen boundaries and consequent injustice to settlers and others. Therefore this Administration adopted the present method of first withdrawing the land from disposal, followed by careful examination on the ground and the preparation of detailed maps and descriptions, before any forest reserve is created.

I have repeatedly called attention to the confusion which exists in Government forest matters because the work is scattered among three independent organizations. The United States is the only one of the great nations in which the forest work of the Government is not concentrated under one department, in consonance with the plainest dictates of good administration and common sense. The present arrangement is bad from every point of view. Merely to mention it is to prove that it should be terminated at once. As I have repeatedly recommended, all the forest work of the Government should be concentrated in the Department of Agriculture, where the larger part of that work is already done, where practically all of the trained foresters of the Government are employed, where chiefly in Washington there is comprehensive first-hand knowledge of the problems of the reserves acquired on the ground, where all problems relating to growth from the soil are already gathered, and where all the sciences auxiliary to forestry are at hand for prompt and effective coöperation. These reasons are decisive in themselves, but it should be added that the great organizations of citizens whose interests are affected by the forest reserves, such as the National Live Stock Association, the National Wool Growers' Association, the American Mining Congress, the National Irrigation Congress, and the National Board of Trade, have uniformly, emphatically, and most of them repeatedly, expressed themselves in favor of placing all Government forest work in the Department of Agriculture because of the peculiar adaptation of that Department for it. It is true, also, that the forest services of nearly all the great nations of the world are under the respective departments of agriculture, while in but two of the smaller nations and in one colony are they under the department of the interior. This is the result of long and varied experience and it agrees fully with the requirements of good administration in our own case.

The creation of a forest service in the Department of Agriculture will have for its important results:

First. A better handling of all forest work, because it will be under a single head, and because the vast and indispensable experience of the Department in all matters pertaining to the forest reserves, to forestry in general, and to other forms of production from the soil, will be easily and rapidly accessible.

Second. The reserves themselves, being handled from the point of view of the man in the field, instead of the man in the office, will be more easily and more widely useful to the people of the West than has been the case hitherto.

Third. Within a comparatively short time the reserves will become self-supporting. This is important, because continually and rapidly increasing appropriations will be necessary for the proper care of this exceedingly important interest of the Nation, and they can and should be offset by returns from the National forests. Under similar circumstances the forest possessions of other great nations form an important source of revenue to their governments.

Every administrative officer concerned is convinced of the necessity for the proposed consolidation of forest work in the Department of Agriculture, and I myself have urged it more than once in former messages. Again I commend it to the early and favorable consideration of the Congress. The interests of the Nation at large and of the West in particular have suffered greatly because of the delay.

SPEECH OF HON. FRANKLIN E. BROOKS ON THE AGRICULTURAL APPROPRIATION BILL [1]

MR. BROOKS of Colorado said:

Mr. Chairman: I listened yesterday with considerable interest to the fervid and sometimes rather hysterical eloquence of the gentlemen who were rushing in rapid procession to express allegiance to the interests of the farmers and the men who toil; and, incidentally, to express their appreciation of the work of this Department. Now, gentlemen, I realize that the period of nominating conventions is at hand, and therefore I trust that all the remarks of all the gentlemen may be as seed sown in good ground; that they may bring forth fruit, and that the result may abundantly justify the expectation at the time of harvest.

I yield to no man in my interest in the agricultural industries of this country, in the great forces that are making for national prosperity. These gentlemen do not say anything on behalf of those interests in general, that I would not say if I could. But I am bound to take issue with them on some of the conclusions that they draw. I recognize as thoroughly as they do that agriculture is the great primary source of productive wealth. I recognize more, that its prosperity is the necessary and essential condition of national prosperity, advancement, and growth. I recall that the classic and Chinese mythologies gave to agriculture a divine origin, and that, in order further to dignify the subject, they

[1] *Congr. Record*, May 1, 1906.

brought from the heavens a god to teach its mysteries to mankind. I am inclined to think, however, that our latter-day, twentieth century, practical point of view gives even more distinct recognition, when it devotes to the study of agricultural problems, as it does, this body of trained scientists who for the last twelve years have been shedding so much luster on the Department of Agriculture and giving so much of reputation and distinction to it.

I believe in the Department of Agriculture. I believe thoroughly in its work. I believe in its great Secretary, who started it on its career of advancement and growth and who for nearly ten years has so ably directed its progress. I believe in the men who are under Secretary Wilson, the able heads of departments, and in the faithful and energetic men who are working under them. The work fascinates me. It appeals to me. It appeals to my imagination. It appeals to my hopes of the future of this country. It appeals to my sense of duty to the people and the constituents whom I have the honor to represent. I am not afraid of the man with the hoe, and I have no fears of the militant farmer. I am not alarmed at the size of these appropriations. They seem very small, comparatively, and entirely reasonable. They seem abundantly justified by the work the Department has been doing.

Without going too much into detail, I should like to call the attention of the committee briefly to a few of the results of this work before saying anything on this question of free garden seeds which we are discussing.

The American farmer is by no means a babe in swaddling clothes. Given a fair start and an open field he can take care of himself; but his work can be vastly facilitated, his efficiency tremendously increased, and the highest interests of every citizen of the country promoted by the guidance, suggestion, and helpful advice of such bureaus as have been established in the last twelve years.

It was Mark Twain who said that the cauliflower was a cabbage with a college education, and it has been the function of the national Department of Agriculture to give college educations not only to the cabbage, but to the orange and the sugar beet, the wheat of Minnesota and the tobacco of Connecticut, to the cotton of Texas and the apple of New York and Michigan, to the horses of the mountains and the dairy cows of Iowa. True, they say that the Department reeks with paternalism, but there is paternalism and paternalism, and there is nothing in the helpful work of these bureaus which would disturb the shades even of Jefferson.

I wish it had been in the power of every Member of this House to listen to the statements made before the committee by the heads of the various executive branches of the Department. Failing in that, I wish that each might find time to read the reports of these hearings. They are a liberal education in applied science in the field of agriculture, and if anyone has had the bad taste to recall the earlier designation of the Department in semi-derision as the "cow bureau," I think he will be heartily ashamed of it before he gets through with his studies. The work is not only theoretical, and it is not purely educational, although it is, and should be in the main, experimental and suggestive. It is distinctly practical and is more than justified by direct returns.

There is not one field of governmental activity where a dollar spent brings a tenth of the return in actual good to the people that does the little expenditure which we give, more or less grudgingly, to this Department. It covers a wide field in national life, and in every line of its activities it demonstrates every year in a cold matter of dollars and cents its increasing financial importance.

The Weather Bureau saves in a month in the spring floods many times its entire cost since its institution in the saving of property and life, and its researches in the field of meteorological science are both wonderful and fascinating.

If the Bureau of Animal Industry had done nothing else in its whole career but to save the domestic animals of the country from the scourge of the hoof-and-mouth disease, it would have abundantly justified every dollar that it has cost, but that is only one small portion of its work. Its daily routine is made up of the protection of the people's food supply — increasing its volume and decreasing its cost; protecting the farmer and stock grower from diseases and adding enormously to our national wealth. It has done and is doing in its meat-inspection work perhaps more than any one single agency to develop and hold a foreign market for our agricultural productions, and our meats to-day find an entrance into Germany, France, Belgium, and other European centers solely because they are viséed by this Bureau.

The Department has recently taken over the immense forests on our public lands, and forested areas to-day aggregating more than 100,000,000 acres are being cared for, preserved, and developed by the Department of Agriculture. While there is a possibility for difference of opinion as to the wisdom or some phases of this work, its importance and its possibilities of good in the preservation of the forest and the conservation of the water supply, in the development of the arid regions, and the making possible of steady and successful irrigation are absolutely beyond computation, and the tact and skill with which this work has been done under its present management has gone far toward removing any possible ground for complaint.

It is useless to enumerate in detail the individual bureaus with their almost spectacular work, but while we are talking of dollars and cents let us bear in mind that the experiment stations in all the States and Territories have cost the Government until now only $790,000 a year, and the additional work in connection with the stations in Washington increases these figures by only $200,000. That is a large sum of money, but a Minnesota experiment station alone has added more than this sum per annum to the value of the wheat crop of the country in improving the type and character of the wheat grown. Figures are dry and meaningless things in the abstract, but in the concrete they tell their story.

The addition of a single kernel of wheat per head means an addition of more than $5,000,000 per annum to our national wealth, and the methods of seed selection introduced and practiced by these experiment stations have far more than equaled this increase.

We are spending about $30,000,000 in building vast reservoirs, canals, monumental dams, and structures, which we hope shall last to the end of time, to conserve and preserve the waters in the semiarid regions. We are doing this through the agency of trained and technical engineers whose work is exciting the admiration of every beholder. A hundred thousand dollars hardly pays for the reconnoissance for one of the gigantic projects undertaken by the national Reclamation Service, but the Reclamation Bureau spends not one cent of its millions in solving, or attempting to solve, any of the myriad questions relating to the application of water to the soil, relating to irrigation as an art, relating to the economic use of the water it has cost these millions to save.

It remains for one of the bureaus of the Office of Experiment Stations, with a sum of only $102,000 altogether, to work along these lines and to achieve results which the western farmer regards as the most important of anything connected with the work of reclamation. There is no part of the work of the Department that meets with readier welcome at the hands of those for whom it is done than does this work of the Bureau of Irrigation and Drainage Investigation, and yet with this $102,000 that has been given to this Bureau there is carried on not only the irrigation work, but drainage development and experimentation in twenty States and the reclamation of millions of acres of land rendered useless by alkali and similar mineral elements.

I am very glad that the bill before us carries above $27,000 increase for this work.

With a total expenditure of less than $5,000 the Department last year located and detected the poison that, under the name of "loco," has cost the stockmen of this country, speaking conservatively, $10,000,000, and this was done although scientist after scientist and expert after expert had declared the poison a myth.

No one of all these phases of this work is more beneficial than is that of the particular Bureau which we have under contemplation in this item — the Bureau of Plant Industry. None is more ably officered and directed. Its costs, according to the figures of this bill, about $575,000. That is the equivalent in cost of a thousand rounds of ammunition for a 12-inch gun, and the results of the work of the Bureau of Plant Industry simply can not be computed. These results are not only a benefit to the rural population, not only to the men for whom we plead so earnestly, but they are a benefit to the whole people; they increase our food supply;

they promote our commerce; they help our people in every particular. Because they are so far-reaching, and because they are so beneficent and important, I protest against men of the character and caliber of those who are at the head of this Department having their time and energies and opportunities frittered away in sending out these absurd little donations of ordinary garden seeds to the farmer, to men who do not want them. I do not want this important work interfered with. I do not want this great bureau to continue under our direction doing something that seems to me ignoble and unworthy — unworthy of the Congress, unworthy the Department of Agriculture, and, most of all, unworthy the American farmer.

I do not think the committee intended to take anything from the farmer. I know that I did not. I do not believe that that was the thought at all. What we wanted to do was to substitute something that was of value for something that was unimportant and inconsiderable; something that really amounted to something, that would accomplish something, and was of practical utility.

When the Department was first organized, Congress very aptly and very properly made a part of its duty the distribution of rare and valuable seeds, but they were to be rare and valuable seeds, not the kinds that had been known for three centuries; not the variety that our forbears brought with them to Jamestown and Plymouth. They were to be rare and valuable seeds; something that would add to the productive power and wealth of the country and advance the interest of the farming population.

What the committee, if I understand it, attempted to do is simply this: they attempted to confine this work to the legitimate field of the distribution of rare and valuable seeds. There was no thought, I am sure, of dealing either illiberally or parsimoniously with it. On the other . hand, they believe that we have appropriated sufficiently so that that work may be carried on with success according to its legitimate purpose.

There are endless instances of the importance of the distribution if properly directed. The seedless orange was developed and introduced by the Bureau of Plant Industry, and afterwards distributed through this very appropriation. This one fruit has been worth more to the people of this country than all the radishes, pumpkins, lettuce, and beans that have been sent out through the Department of Agriculture since this distribution began. The statisticians tell us that the California crop of seedless orange alone is worth from $7,000,000 to $8,000,000 annually.

In the same way and through the same distribution the Government has been sending out macaroni wheat. The Bureau of Plant Industry introduced it from Russia and Asia and distributed it freely to our farmers, and to-day it is adding to the income-bearing possibilities of the country infinitely more than all of these ordinary seeds that they are sending out for us under our franks. This is something the farmer can not get at the corner grocery, and the cash value of the work is to be figured in millions of dollars. Last year it is estimated that we produced in this country from $10,000,000, to $15,000,000 in this product alone, and the beauty of it is that it fills a new field and positively adds that amount to our productive wealth.

Mr. WADSWORTH. And they have done that within the last three years.

Mr. BROOKS of Colorado. And the chairman calls my attention to the fact that this work has all been done within the last three years. The same thing is true of the Kaffir corn, emmer, and brome. Those are things that are of real value, and they are sent out under the appropriation for the Congressional free-seed distribution, but they are not the ordinary garden seeds that you can buy anywhere for 1 or 2 cents a package.

I was much interested yesterday in the remarks of the gentleman from South Carolina [Mr. Ellerbe]. They seemed to be very apt, very sound, and very sensible. What he said about the wilt-resisting cotton is all true. It has added enormously to the receipts of the cotton growing States and the cotton growing section has not yet begun to reap the full returns, but I did not notice any plea for free beans in the gentleman's remarks or any argument for rhubarb or radishes or anything of that sort. All that the gentleman said was the strongest possible argument for the work of the Department in sending out rare seeds and against garden seeds.

The wilt-resisting cotton was a rare and valuable thing that was developed by the Bureau and sent out under this form of seed distribution. Now, the committee has attempted to still provide for the rare and valuable plants and seeds. There is no disposition to leave out the wilt-resisting cotton, there is no disposition to leave out the further production of the seedless orange, or the Kaffir corn, or the macaroni wheat. There will be an amendment offered by the committee that will make that matter thoroughly clear, and will secure the continuance of the work without any restrictions. What the committee attempted to do was to leave in the bill all the appropriation that hitherto had been devoted to the rare and valuable seeds, and to eliminate and leave out of the bill this indefensible donation of no value which is, in many cases, regarded with ridicule, and justly so, by the very men to whom it is sent.

There is an ample field for work with rare seeds and plants. There are hundreds of localities all over the world where we still can get just such plants as those which that Bureau has been finding for us in the last years. The scientists from the Department are now searching in Asia, in Turkey, in India, in Africa, in northern Russia, and in Australia, and from those sections we are getting things that our farmers can use and render available from one end of this country to the other. It is true that many of them are semi-tropical and will interest mainly the

South, like the orange, the mango, the fig, the grape fruit, and date, but it is also true that many of them are hardy and will interest the North, like the hardier kind of wheat, and the hardy crops that will grow clear to the Canada line and in altitudes of 6,000 or 7,000 feet — grains and fruits from Siberia and northern Russia, which thrive wonderfully when brought to our warmer sections. That is the kind of work I plead for and have interest in.

We expend something like $500,000 a year in one single drug — opium — and we import that from foreign countries, and our total importation of foreign drugs and medicinal plants amounts to more than $5,000,000 annually.

The CHAIRMAN. The time of the gentleman has expired.

Mr. WADSWORTH. Mr. Chairman, I ask unanimous consent that the gentleman may be allowed to conclude his remarks.

The CHAIRMAN. The gentleman from New York asks unanimous consent that the gentleman from Colorado may be permitted to conclude his remarks. Is there objection?

Mr. FINLEY. Mr. Chairman, I understand that the gentleman is discussing the seed proposition. I would like to know if we have reached that provision in the bill.

Mr. WADSWORTH. Oh, yes; we have.

Mr. FINLEY. Then I have no objection.

The CHAIRMAN. The Chair hears no objection.

Mr. BROOKS of Colorado. Mr. Chairman, I think I shall take only a few minutes, for I shall very briefly conclude with one or two things that I want to call attention to. As I was saying, we are expending $500,000 a year for a single drug. That drug and many others can be grown with profit, and great profit, in Maine, in New Hampshire, in Vermont, and in the Northern States. Crops like these can be made a kind of by-product to the farmer and ought to be introduced, and this Department is trying to do it through this Bureau. Now, the committee proposes to extend the usefulness of the Bureau along those lines and to substitute in its distribution digitalis and stramonium and plants like those for peas and beans and such plants as you can get anywhere. Only last week there was a very apt illustration of what I am saying. There is one concern engaged in the manufacture of celluloid in this country that pays $500,000 a year for camphor. Camphor, as we all know, is a monopoly of the Japanese Government in the island of Formosa. Probably the other uses of camphor in this country amount to about $2,000,000 a year.

Last year down in Florida one of the experts of this Department in going around found a man who was trimming some ornamental camphor trees. He got the clippings from those trees and experimented with them in the Bureau. He found that he could get a higher content of camphor oil and a better quality of camphor than they could in the island of

Formosa, where they cut down and kill the tree. He further found that large tracts of land in Florida which were comparatively valueless for other purposes were admirably adapted for growing these trees. He went immediately to the celluloid people, showed them the result of his work, and explained to them the possibility of introducing the growth of these trees into this country, and last week they concluded the purchase of lands in Florida for the investment of $150,000 in the growing of American camphor. How does that work compare with our donations of 2-cent packages of cabbage and rhubarb and rutabaga?

We pay $500,000 a year to Germany and France for our beet-sugar seed. The Department of Agriculture is developing a beet-sugar seed to-day in this country that is superior in saccharine content, in hardness and availability to anything that the Germans or French can produce; and I prefer to see my Colorado farmers get this improved sugar-beet seed than these common seeds that they do not want, and I know my Michigan and Utah and Minnesota friends feel the same way. I believe that Department can assist the gentleman from Tennessee [Mr. Gaines] to find some rare seeds of this sort, that his people will think just as much of as they do of the peas and beans which he says they prize so highly, and if he does, he will accomplish a substantial result in developing new agricultural possibilities for his section.

. I do not agree with the gentleman from Maryland [Mr. Mudd], and I do not believe that he got at the real point of this situation in his remarks yesterday. Shortly after I was first elected to Congress and before I knew some of the mysteries of the work of a Congressman which I have since learned, I was awakened in the dead vast and middle of night by a telegram from a very enthusiastic rural constituent, and it read like this:

Send seeds at once; no Republican seeds in this county.

I complied with that urgent demand as soon as I could, and the returns at the succeeding election, in the Republican crop, were amply satisfactory and highly commendable from my point of view. My enthusiastic rural friend had gotten at the real gist of this question. It is an attempt to secure a little, petty, unworthy, ignoble influence for ourselves as Congressmen in a way that we ought to be ashamed of, and it is a way that I hope will be abandoned.

The American farmer is not a babe in swaddling clothes. He can see through this little gift very easily. The man with the hoe is not what he was even when Millet painted him or when Markham maligned him into fame. In America he is not only a tiller of the soil; he is a mechanic, manufacturer, and business man, and in these later days he is a chemist, physicist, bacteriologist, and entomologist as well. I think he understands and values this 2-cent contribution at its real worth.

I want to make myself entirely clear, and, at the risk of repetition, let me repeat that I believe in proper and legitimate seed distribution. It is only the kind of seeds that I object to. I do not and can not believe that the sending out of ordinary common garden seeds is a proper or legitimate distribution, and I shall oppose it. I will, however, vote any reasonable sum for the work of sending out new, rare, and valuable seeds and plants, and believe this would result in great good in the future, as it has in the past.

For work such as I have described in some twenty bureaus we provide this year $7,250,000. It reclaims our land; it renders fertile our exhausted reaches; it improves our crops; it increases, cheapens, improves, and diversifies the food supplies of our toiling millions; it protects our forests, our flocks, and our herds; it increases by billions of dollars annually our foreign and domestic commerce; it furnishes the most wholesome, safest, and most elevating form of employment to the people; it injures no one; it is beneficent, helpful, and unobtrusive. Its total cost represents an expenditure of a million dollars a day for a single week. For the arts of war, including therein, as we properly should, our pension budget, we spent this year, in round numbers, a million dollars a day for the days of a whole year, and I venture to say that no man on the floor of this House will begin to compare the usefulness, beneficence, and far-reaching results of the work of the Department of Agriculture with that of our Army and Navy combined.

I join with our friends of the Military and Naval Committees heartily, cheerfully, and enthusiastically in every effort that they make to protect this country at home and abroad, to advance its prestige, to make its name and its flag honored, respected, and revered; I yield to no one in my support of everything which makes for our national honor and advantage; I will vote battle ships as long as there is a real need. The scare head of rampant militarism has no terrors for me, but in the name of the thirty millions of farming population who make up the great producing element of our body politic I protest against any cheeseparing or restrictive economies as applied to the work of this Department. We talk about the stupendous balance of trade in our favor. On this side of the Chamber we point with pride, and justly point with pride, to an aggregate balance for the twelve years of Republican ascendance amounting to something like $4,000,000,000, but we should go further and pay our respects and distinguished consideration to the farmers of this country who have not only made that balance possible, but in order to do so have wiped out an adverse balance against us for the same period of over $890,000,000.

As the work grows it is necessary that comparatively new fields from time to time be entered upon, and this bill and the two previous bills have carried one item in itself somewhat novel, of which I wish to speak very briefly. In 1904 we appropriated $25,000 for experiments in animal feeding and breeding. The appropriation was continued last year, and it is carried in the bill before us. Under that appropriation, small and meager as it is, the Department has inaugurated two small experiments in the developing of an American type of horse, one in the East and one in the West; has made instructive and valuable experiments in sheep breeding in coöperation with the Iowa station; has already done a great work in the development of the poultry industry, which, although tremendous in its returns, has never received the attention it deserved; has been carrying on a series of most valuable and interesting experiments in calorimetric tests of the heat and flesh producing power of different food elements in connection with the Pennsylvania experiment station, and in several places in the South has started, or has under contemplation, similar work in feeding and breeding.

The field that this work opens upon is vast and important and has been hitherto almost neglected by the Government. We have lagged far behind the work of the other leading powers. We spend annually hundreds of thousands of dollars in importing foreign stock. Our horses, with the exception of two strains of trotting stock, which are really families rather than types, are Percheron, Belgian, Oldenburg, and Clydesdale; our cattle are Holsteins, Ayrshires, Swiss, Jerseys, or Herefords; our sheep are Cotswolds, Southdowns, and Merinos, and our swine are foreign in their origin and names; only two breeds of chickens proudly flaunt an American name and are the result of American breeding. It is high time that the genius and energy of the American breeder should be turned to the growth and development of native strains and American types. We can learn much from our foreign friends on this subject. We frequently hear how one or another phase of modern progress is due in some direct or indirect manner to the Corsican first emperor of the French.

It is interesting to know that the great Hungarian breeding stable at Lipitza was started by an Arabian stallion captured from Napoleon at the battle of Leipzig. With that beginning the Austro-Hungarian Government has gradually developed, until to-day it spends over $800,000 a year in its maintenance of its horse-breeding establishments, with immense advantage to the individual horse breeders and without any encroachment upon or interference with individual enterprises. There is a single breeding station — Mezöhegyes — extending over 50,000 acres, which employs 6,000 civil and military employees and obtains the finest breeding stock available in the markets of the world, and to-day the Imperial Government makes no more proper or beneficial use of its funds.

One of the Austrian royal stables at Kis Ber was headed by an old-time English thoroughbred, "Buccaneer." The winner of the Derby and the winner of the Grand Prix in 1876 both came from this stable, and the descendants of Buccaneer from this stable had won in 1902 $1,100,000, in prizes.

After the fall of the second empire t? French found their agricultural industries terribly crippled, and none r.re than their breeding of horses, caused largely by the terrible losses sutred in the Franco-Prussian war. The French department of agricultui immediately took up this work with tremendous activity, and it has :own to such an extent that the budget of 1902, the last figures obtaizble, carried an appropriation of $1,600,000 for horse-breeding station and no one, to my knowledge, has suggested that the French were otlr than frugal, careful, and businesslike in their governmental expensc The work is a fixture in French system and has demonstrated its great nd increasing value.

The Prussian Government spent in)x a quarter of a million dollars, and that is for Prussia alone. The Cind Duchy of Oldenburg for a hundred years has been growing and dreloping a strain of coach horses, until the name of Oldenburg is know. not for any statesmanship nor for military prowess, but for the supcor excellence of its horses, from Australia to Siberia, from Germany ι Japan, and from Lapland to Cape Town and back.

With all their lack of initiative an sluggishness in many regards, the Russian Government spends near a million dollars a year in its breeding of remounts and domestic hocs.

The Italian budget for 1900 carrie nearly $100,000. In 1904 the Government embarked upon a mucl nore extensive scheme and, in addition to its previous work. in roun numbers, $50,000 was devoted to the purchase of new animals, about ι much for prizes and subsidies to different organizations of breeders, $5z:00 for veterinary surgeons, and corresponding amounts for other purːses. Not long ago the Italian Government paid $17,000 for a Derby inner to put in one of its breeding establishments. The people are .uch interested and regard the work with marked approbation.

The English Government, through pzes and subsidies, spends about $30,000 a year, and its lack of initiatʋ in this work is the subject of general regret. For many years the ʋyal commission appointed to investigate the subject has pleaded with Parliament for larger appropriations and has pointed out the fact that the English were falling behind the other countries in this work. Som ιf the Canadian provinces have just started, and the press reports a :w days ago contained an item that $25,000 had been paid for a singl norse to start a stable at Truro, Nova Scotia.

We have invested, all told, a little ver $10,000 in horses, and the State of Colorado, where the experimıt was first tried, added almost as much for stables and similar expenιtures connected with the work. We have to-day the beginning of an exʝriment which competent judges consider of the greatest promise. Theı is no field to which the American farmer can more safely direct hiːnergies with greater hope and certainty of return than the breeding of ιe horses, and there is no place in which the Government can more roperly and more effectively render him assistance than by putting the work on a systematic and scientific basis. I do not mean breeding racig horses alone, but an average horse of superior speed, courage, strength and endurance, which is demanded in increasing numbers by our domeic trade and by the foreign markets; of the kind for which there is a costantly increasing demand and relatively decreasing supply.

The cost of carriage horses has icreased in this country since 1891 in the average sum of over $100. he same fact is observed elsewhere. The export value is given now at $3c, as against $174 then. In 1900, and the year was by no means extrardinary, Germany imported 90,000 horses, and for years Germany has ient from $17,000,000 to $20,000,000 abroad for horses annually. Englad in the ten years from 1891 to 1900 purchased abroad 342,000, at a tou cost of about $100,000,000, and the demand is steadily growing. Frar:, on the other hand, from its greater breeding facilities, had large numirs to sell.

As I understand it, it is not propsed to imitate the Italian or Austrian systems, with their tremendous tablishments of government-owned horses, but rather, with small natnal expenditure, to direct and assist cooperative circles of breeders, locing to the establishment of an available native type and to raising th general average of excellence of the American road stock.

Rather something more or less sembling the French system, which is essentially coöperative breeding nder Government supervision. The expenditure is large, but the retms are proportionately even larger. As long ago as 1887, with a yearly aintenance charge and expenses for renewals and new stock amountin to some 1,400,000 francs, there was an income to the State, outside c sales, of 815,000 francs, and the statistics show that if this were is primary object, the returns could have been largely increased.

The real benefit has been the wiespread general improvement in the common stock — the half-breeds the work horse, and the ordinary driving horses — exactly the fiel: in which we have done very little systematic work. What France aa Hungary and the Grand Duchy of Oldenburg have done we certainly can, and should do.

At first the American breeders wre inclined to look with some question upon this venture, but as it has egun to work itself out it now meets with almost universal approval, aa I believe that a few years will demonstrate that this is one of the wist ventures that the Department has undertaken. Similar work in the improvement of strains of dairy and beef cattle, swine and poultry and jeep, instituted in response to a very general request and demand, shos the importance of the work undertaken.

I have devoted considerable atntion to the work of two particular bureaus, not because they excel ne work of the other bureaus, but

After the fall of the second empire the French found their agricultural industries terribly crippled, and none more than their breeding of horses, caused largely by the terrible losses suffered in the Franco-Prussian war. The French department of agriculture immediately took up this work with tremendous activity, and it has grown to such an extent that the budget of 1902, the last figures obtainable, carried an appropriation of $1,600,000 for horse-breeding stations, and no one, to my knowledge, has suggested that the French were other than frugal, careful, and businesslike in their governmental expenses. The work is a fixture in French system and has demonstrated its great and increasing value.

The Prussian Government spent in 1900 a quarter of a million dollars, and that is for Prussia alone. The Grand Duchy of Oldenburg for a hundred years has been growing and developing a strain of coach horses, until the name of Oldenburg is known, not for any statesmanship nor for military prowess, but for the superior excellence of its horses, from Australia to Siberia, from Germany to Japan, and from Lapland to Cape Town and back.

With all their lack of initiative and sluggishness in many regards, the Russian Government spends nearly a million dollars a year in its breeding of remounts and domestic horses.

The Italian budget for 1900 carried nearly $100,000. In 1904 the Government embarked upon a much more extensive scheme and, in addition to its previous work, in round numbers, $50,000 was devoted to the purchase of new animals, about as much for prizes and subsidies to different organizations of breeders, $50,000 for veterinary surgeons, and corresponding amounts for other purposes. Not long ago the Italian Government paid $17,000 for a Derby winner to put in one of its breeding establishments. The people are much interested and regard the work with marked approbation.

The English Government, through prizes and subsidies, spends about $30,000 a year, and its lack of initiative in this work is the subject of general regret. For many years the royal commission appointed to investigate the subject has pleaded with Parliament for larger appropriations and has pointed out the fact that the English were falling behind the other countries in this work. Some of the Canadian provinces have just started, and the press reports a few days ago contained an item that $25,000 had been paid for a single horse to start a stable at Truro, Nova Scotia.

We have invested, all told, a little over $10,000 in horses, and the State of Colorado, where the experiment was first tried, added almost as much for stables and similar expenditures connected with the work. We have to-day the beginning of an experiment which competent judges consider of the greatest promise. There is no field to which the American farmer can more safely direct his energies with greater hope and certainty of return than the breeding of fine horses, and there is no place in which the Government can more properly and more effectively render him assistance than by putting the work on a systematic and scientific basis. I do not mean breeding racing horses alone, but an average horse of superior speed, courage, strength, and endurance, which is demanded in increasing numbers by our domestic trade and by the foreign markets; of the kind for which there is a constantly increasing demand and relatively decreasing supply.

The cost of carriage horses has increased in this country since 1891 in the average sum of over $100. The same fact is observed elsewhere. The export value is given now at $308, as against $174 then. In 1900, and the year was by no means extraordinary, Germany imported 90,000 horses, and for years Germany has spent from $17,000,000 to $20,000,000 abroad for horses annually. England in the ten years from 1891 to 1900 purchased abroad 342,000, at a total cost of about $100,000,000, and the demand is steadily growing. France, on the other hand, from its greater breeding facilities, had large numbers to sell.

As I understand it, it is not proposed to imitate the Italian or Austrian systems, with their tremendous establishments of government-owned horses, but rather, with small national expenditure, to direct and assist cooperative circles of breeders, looking to the establishment of an available native type and to raising the general average of excellence of the American road stock.

Rather something more or less resembling the French system, which is essentially coöperative breeding under Government supervision. The expenditure is large, but the returns are proportionately even larger. As long ago as 1887, with a yearly maintenance charge and expenses for renewals and new stock amounting to some 1,400,000 francs, there was an income to the State, outside of sales, of 815,000 francs, and the statistics show that if this were the primary object, the returns could have been largely increased.

The real benefit has been the widespread general improvement in the common stock — the half-breeds, the work horse, and the ordinary driving horses — exactly the field in which we have done very little systematic work. What France and Hungary and the Grand Duchy of Oldenburg have done we certainly can, and should do.

At first the American breeders were inclined to look with some question upon this venture, but as it has begun to work itself out it now meets with almost universal approval, and I believe that a few years will demonstrate that this is one of the wisest ventures that the Department has undertaken. Similar work in the improvement of strains of dairy and beef cattle, swine and poultry and sheep, instituted in response to a very general request and demand, shows the importance of the work undertaken.

I have devoted considerable attention to the work of two particular bureaus, not because they excel the work of the other bureaus, but

27

because of the particular interest which attaches to their work at the present time. The whole Department of Agriculture is serving the people in a most admirable way. It is increasing, cheapening, and improving our food supply; it is increasing the fertility of our country; it is supplying the enormous demands of our growing commerce; it is furnishing the best and safest kind of employment to the people. There is no other form of governmental activity that receives, or should receive, a more liberal degree of support at the hands of Congress than does the Department of Agriculture.

There is every reason why that should be so. The latter-day problems which are pressing on this country for solution are almost without exception problems which come from, and are the result of a change of the type of development over great areas of this country. A change from an essentially rural and agricultural type to an essentially industrial and manufacturing type. We view with alarm the great and disproportionate growth of our industrial centers. We view with alarm the influx of alien hordes, the growth of socialistic ideas, the growing urban discontent and the strife of wage-earners and the masses. We regret and deplore the drift from the country to the city, the passing of the saner forms of rural life, the simpler form of living which characterized generations that have gone, and thus far we have only deplored and only viewed with regret. We have not done one single thing for a remedy.

Mr. Chairman and gentlemen, the remedy, if remedy there exists, in my judgment, lies along the very line on which the Department of Agriculture is working. It lies in making the work of the American farmer more elevating, more pleasant, more attractive and more profitable. It lies in elevating his occupation to a proper plane of dignity, in recognizing the importance of his pursuit as a profession as well as a means of livelihood. It lies in teaching young men they can devote to this work just as much intelligent preparation, just as much thoughtful earnestness, just as much ability, as to railroad problems or finance or any other form of industry that occupies the human mind. It lies in keeping the young men on the farms and preventing their crowding into the less desirable, but apparently more attractive occupations.

And we can best do this, gentlemen, by liberally and generously supporting these men, who for years, without flourish of trumpets and without any accessories of military parade, have quietly, but with an efficiency equaled by no other similar body of men in the world, been bringing before the farmers of this country the richest fruit of all the ages and the highest results of scientific investigation when applied to the field of agricultural science, and we can not do it by this petty little distribution of free garden seed. [Applause.]

THE SCIENTIFIC WORK OF THE GOVERNMENT [1]

By S. P. LANGLEY [2]

ANY attempt to make a survey of the distinctly scientific activities of the Government must necessarily be brief in a series which has already elsewhere considered the numerous incidental agencies for scientific work in bureaus attached to one or another of the Executive Departments. How numerous these are may be inferred from the subjoined list, which is confessedly incomplete, being confined to those bureaus which have a certain number of distinctly scientific employees:

Under the Department of the Treasury:

Supervising Architect's Office	Coast and Geodetic Survey
Director of the Mint	Marine Hospital Service
Light-House Board	Bureau of Standards

Department of War:

Surgeon-General's Office	Bureau of Ordinance
Chief of Engineers	Chief Signal Officer

Department of the Navy:

Hydrographic Office	Nautical Almanac
Naval Observatory	Bureau of Medicine and Surgery

Department of the Interior:

Patent Office	Geological Survey

Department of Agriculture:

Weather Bureau	Bureau of Forestry
Bureau of Animal Industry	Bureau of Soils
Bureau of Chemistry	Division of Biological Survey
Office of Experiment Stations	Bureau of Plant Industry
Division of Entomology	

Commission of Fish and Fisheries.

Smithsonian Institution:

National Museum	National Zoölogical Park
Astrophysical Observatory	Bureau of American Ethnology

[1] Part of an article in *Scribner's Magazine*, January, 1904. Reprinted by permission Copyright.

[2] Secretary of the Smithsonian Institution.

The newly created *Departmentof Commerce and Labor* will include, after July 1, 1903, the following beforementioned bureaus:

National Bureau of Standards   Commission of Fish and Fisheries
Coast and Geodetic Survey   Light-House Board

*   *   *   *   *   *   *

Jefferson's interest in scienc made his administration an especially noteworthy one from a point ofriew both scientific and educational, and explorations and surveys whichultimately resulted in the establishment both of the Geological Survey nd of the Coast Survey, were initiated under his presidency.

The Geological Survey, wkch was originally a topographic one, practically originated in the exeditions of Lewis, Pike, and Lewis and Clark, but was especially develbed by the surveys for a Pacific railway, followed by a long list of exploutions which became systematized under King, Hayden, and Wheeler, ad definitely organized as the U. S. Geological Survey on March, 3 187, with Clarence King as its first director, Major J. W. Powell being hi immediate successor, and Prof. C. D. Walcott its present incumbent

The Geological Survey has : present an extensive organization under the Interior Department, devong its energies to geological investigation of the United States, to topogrohic surveys conducted on a large scale, to a certain amount of paleontogical work growing out of such scientific activities in connection with geogical investigations, and, more recently, has had placed under its direcon the initiation and carrying out of a vast scheme for the irrigation othe arid regions of the West, which it is expected will add to the fruitfu soil of the United States many millions of acres. This Survey is in frndly coöperation with other branches of the Interior Department, notaly the Land Office, and with each State in the Union; with the Forest· Bureau of the Department of Agriculture, and with the various Ste geological and hydrographic surveys, exhibiting a highly intelligent cganization of importance to science and of utility to the people, givin to and deriving help from individual geologists connected with manof the large and even small universities and colleges of the country, ad presenting altogether the most perfect system of geological investigtion, combined with topographic· and economic work known to any cuntry. It has produced a body of most capable men who are original i both their economic and scientific work· It has earned the confidence of 'ongress and the people, and its requirements both for research and pblication are being met with a generous hand.

The credit for the inceptio of the Coast Survey is divided among various persons, though it woul appear to have early enlisted the interest of President Jefferson an Secretary Gallatin, and to have been powerfully stimulated by the rival in this country of Ferdinand Rudolph Hassler, a Swiss, who virtually made the plans upon which the subsequent operations of this Survey were prosecuted.

The Survey dates its origin from an act of Congress passed in 1807 for surveying the coasts of the United States. It had a checkered and somewhat intermittent career until 1832 when it was reorganized, though its control has from time to time alternated between various departments. It was attached to the Navy Department for a brief period; then for many years it was under the Treasury, and by Act of Congress of this year has been transferred to the new Department of Commerce. It has had as its Superintendents after Hassler such eminent men as Bache, Peirce, Patterson, Hilgard, Mendenhall, Pritchett and its present incumbent, Tittman. It has now over one hundred field officers, and a fleet of twelve steamers and six sailing vessels, besides many launches and small craft. In addition to topographic work it carries on geodetic and magnetic surveys, it has had an office of weights and measures, and has been custodian of the National standards. The development of this last function recently, and with the fullest coöperation of the Coast Survey, has resulted in the establishment of an independent Bureau of Standards of large scope.

Superintendent Tittman, in a recent description of its work, stated that it had since its inception made about 30,000 square miles of topographic surveys, sounded minutely nearly 300,000 square miles of water, and made deep-sea soundings over little less than a million square miles. It has completed a first survey of the Atlantic, Gulf, and Pacific Coasts of the United States, and its triangulation cover between 300,000 and 400,000 square miles. It has published over 500 charts besides the Coast Pilot volumes of the Atlantic and Pacific coasts; and carefully studied the laws of the earth's magnetism (these latter being now investigated through magnetic observatories in coöperation with foreign governments), and its geodetic work is also being carried on with international coöperation.

The Coast Survey, moreover, is frequently called upon to serve, through its officers as experts, in the determination of boundaries, whether between the States or in matters involving disputes with other nations holding territory adjacent to the United States. Since the Spanish-American War, important labors have devolved upon the survey in Porto Rico and in the Philippines, where coast surveys are urgently needed and are of high importance for military and commercial purposes.

The difference between the unscientific and the scientific idea of the order of this world, already alluded to, can hardly be emphasized more than in the conception which made a meteorological bureau rational and possible. "The wind bloweth where it listeth" was the conception of ancient times, but the eighteenth century had already reached the idea that the movements of the winds, from the Trades which blew across the planet to the eddy that whirls the dust in the street, are as much subject to law as are the courses of the stars.

The Weather Bureau is now a highly equipped organization under a Chief, Willis L. Moore, the officer third in rank in the Department. The country is covered with its stations. Its reports, issued twice daily, have come to be looked for in every portion of the United States by all the people, whose daily life is to a certain extent influenced by them, and the value of its work in the saving of life and shipping on the coasts by its prediction of storms and floods, as well as the saving to the crops through timely notice of sudden changes, such as frosts, etc., is incalculable.

The work which the people know best is the general forecasts of the weather, which are conducted on the best obtainable system; forecasts which, though founded on an order of things as subject to law as the courses of the stars, are far from having yet reached the precision of astronomical science, though the results obtained are unrivalled in their excellence by those of any other nation. The preparation of the weather map involves the daily sounding of the heights of the aërial ocean above, simultaneously by observers all over the country, and the joining of these sounding stations on the map by contour lines which indicate the direction of that great aërial ocean's flow. This direction can not of course be dete:mined with anything like the certainty attainable in the deduction of the path of a star, yet the result, though still a probability only, is a very useful one by which we all guide our daily lives. Will it be greatly better for us if it is ever otherwise, and we come to the time when we know long in advance what the weather will be, and this and many other like uncertainties are wiped out from the variety of our daily life?

These general maps are prepared in the office at Washington, from despatches sent by local offices, and the Bureau's use of the telegraph service alone costs $300,000 per annum. It distributes in the shape of cards, maps, and publications nearly 55,000,000 pieces yearly, and in cases of special agricultural industries, particularly susceptible to destruction through changes in weather, special services have been established, notably for cotton, sugar, and rice, in the Southern States, and for fruit and wheat in California.

Meteorology is a science which, in the main, can only be prosecuted successfully through the Government, owing to the fact that deductions must be based upon a great number of observations carried on for long periods and over wide areas; so that incidentally to, and prerequisite for, the conduct and improvement of its practical and economic work, scientific investigations of the highest moment have been from time to time carried on under the auspices of this branch of the service. The most notable of these in recent years has been the aërial research of studying meteorological phenomena at high altitudes through the use of kites, experiments in wireless telegraphy, and in other fields relating to atmospheric phenomena. A scientific man whose name has long been honorably associated with this original work is Cleveland Abbe, who has been connected with the service since 1867, and who still continues active as a prosecutor of it, and as Editor of the Bureau's publications.

* * * * * * * *

Historians and philosophers have not infrequently remarked that the stress of war results in the advancement of science and learning. Napoleon's invasion of Egypt carried in its train the unlocking of the mysteries of the hieroglyphs and the production of the great work "Description de l'Egypte." More recently the foundation of the University of Strassburg signalized the close of the Franco-Prussian War, while the establishment of the Johns Hopkins University was a direct resultant of the war between the States, and was intended, at least in the mind of the founder, to assist in healing the breaches this had created.

It was during the darkest days of this same war that Congress established the National Academy of Sciences, whose creation, foreshadowed by the organization of such private societies as the American Association for the Advancement of Science, had been long in the minds of public men. The actual need of scientific organization was shown during the war, when this nation apparently first awakened to the fact that in every department of activity, and more especially in the military and naval establishments, the services of scientific experts were required. During the war period, Joseph Henry, the Secretary of the Smithsonian Institution, was in almost constant intercourse with President Lincoln; and in that era, before the days of specialization, he was called on to give advice on the most diverse subjects.

It was then that the idea of a nonresident National Academy, without localization, like the National Academy of Paris or the Royal Society of London, but composed of eminent men, whose services might be called into requisition by the Government, was created. This body continues in existence, as the most generally representative and dignified aggregation of American men of science, and while suffering under the disadvantages of not having a permanent home, nor officials whose time can be exclusively devoted to its work, has in special cases when called upon rendered valuable service to the Government by its advice.

The Department of Agriculture has become a large factor in the scientific life of the Government, so large as to render possible in a brief article only the barest enumeration of its activities.

As noted above, it acquired the weather service, which had been successfully carried on through various agencies. In the distribution of seeds already alluded to, its work has grown to vast proportions.

The systematic investigations in nearly every department of biological science directly or remotely connected with the life and health and diseases of animals and plants, the observations of the life habits of all forms which may be either helpful or noxious to agriculture, investigations into the origin and spread, the restriction and the cure of contagious diseases among domestic animals, are but a part of its work. These are carried on in highly equipped laboratories by great numbers of investigators, whose work is welded by excellent organizers into a uniform, compact, and intelligent whole, together with a system of distribution of information of a popular and untechnical character through suitable publications. This is aided by a most efficient support on the part of Congress, and all these and more have been the care of this Department, which has rendered service of incalculable importance, not only in the spread of ascertained knowledge of economic value, but in the enlargement in all domains of such knowledge, presenting the most signal success of such scientific organization yet undertaken by the National Government.

In 1902 a partial reorganization was effected, the most conspicuous advance being the establishment and greater enlargement of the Department of Forestry, which is seriously grappling with the most interesting and important problem of the control of timberlands, not only upon the public reserves, but even in the vast acreage in private hands; and to such work the new division under the present charge of Gifford Pinchot is devoting itself.

The surgeons of the Army and the Navy from early days exhibited their interest in scientific work, a number of them being among the pioneer naturalists and ethnologists in America. As a result of the important professional labors of the surgeons in the Army and again, as an outgrowth of the War between the States, the Army Medical Museum was established, with the Surgeon-General's Library, which is believed to be the most complete medical library in the world, and which, under the direction of John S. Billings, aided by Robert Fletcher, not only collected a unique library, but issued the most comprehensively arranged and useful catalogue known in any department of learning. It has added to it a medical and surgical collection of the highest importance to the profession and has stimulated the growth within the last few years of a military medical college.

The United States Fish Commission, established in 1871, has illustrated in a most gratifying manner the great possibilities of applying earnest scientific work to the wants of the people, and these have brought about results of vast importance and of great economic value. It was established as an outgrowth of the Smithsonian Institution under its Secretary, Spencer F. Baird, who is credited with the statement that a mile of ocean along our coasts can furnish more food products than ten miles of fertile land. During his lifetime it was to a certain extent carried on in connection with the Smithsonian Institution, and has done a great work for the advancement of our knowledge of the life of every description of creature inhabiting the fresh waters of our country and the oceans surrounding it. It has increased to a degree hardly to be believed the quantity of fish available for our people, and has put within the reach of the poor, healthful and nourishing food, at one time only possible for the rich to enjoy.

The general work of the Commission as administered is under three divisions, which are known as:

(1) Division of Inquiry respecting food fishes.

(2) Division of Fisheries.

(3) Division of Fish Culture.

The principal part of its scientific work is under the first division, ordinarily known as the Division of Scientific Inquiry, and comprises:

1. The investigation of the fishing-grounds of the Atlantic, Gulf, and Pacific Coasts and the inland waters of the United States, with the view of determining the food resources and the developing of the commercial fisheries.

2. The investigation of the causes of the decrease of food fishes in the waters of the United States.

3. The study of the waters of the coast and interior to determine the feasibility of increasing their natural resources.

4. The dissemination of information concerning the distribution and habits of marine animals and their capture, and their preparation for the markets.

5. Examination into the adaptability of sites for fish-cultural stations and investigation of the diseases incident to fishes at such stations and at large.

The second division, known as the Division of Fisheries, deals with the economic phases of the fisheries themselves, such as the collection of statistical data, the study of the apparatus and methods of capture with special reference to their utility and their effect on the fisheries, the best methods of utilizing the products, the effect of fishery legislation, international fishery relations, and all other matters affecting the economy of aquatic resources.

The work of the Division of Fish Culture consists in the hatching and distribution of marine and fresh-water fishes for the purpose of maintaining existing fisheries, restocking grounds that have been depleted by over-fishing or injurious methods, and creating new fisheries either by the introduction of foreign fishes in the waters of the United States or transplanting native fishes as, for example, the establishment of the shad and striped bass fishery on the Pacific Coast. The results of the work of this division have been most gratifying. Millions of pounds of fish are now captured in waters where they were originally unknown, and equally valuable results have been secured not only in maintaining the various important fisheries of the Atlantic and Pacific Coasts, but grounds which had become depleted are now supporting valuable fisheries. This work is carried on at thirty-five hatching stations established by Act of Congress in the various States, and four railroad cars are in constant use in distributing their products, besides a number of small boats, launches, and vessels.

Entirely new avenues of scientific research have been opened by the Commission, with which the name of G. Brown Goode will ever be associated, most notably in the discovery of the deep-sea forms of the North Atlantic basin. His work, with the coöperation of such men of distinction as Alexander Agassiz and David Starr Jordan, aided by the faithful and efficient labors of a large staff of ichthyologists and fish-culturists, has resulted in securing a systematic investigation of the waters of the United States, and the biological and physical problems which they present. By a study of the methods of fisheries past and present, the causes of deterioration of fish in various waters have been discovered and remedies applied, and useful food fishes have been enormously multiplied throughout the country; whilst important international problems dealing both with sea and fresh-water fisheries, and with the problem of the fur seals, have been powerfully aided by this Commission and by the experts connected with it.

And yet the expense of the Commission is inconsiderable when compared with the increase of wealth and the means of livelihood it affords the American people.

It is not so very long, as nations count years, since the length of a king of England's arm, marked rudely on an iron bar by a blacksmith's chisel, was made a national standard of lengths; and this was a real advance over a condition of things existing when almost every country had its own measures.

In contrast to this, we have now in Washington the Bureau of Standards, alluded to above in connection with the Coast Survey, which is intended for the purpose of the standardization of machines for measurement and other service, together with the instruments used in everyday life, as well as for philosophical apparatus. It is under the charge of a capable physicist and administrator, S. W. Stratton. Its work will comprehend researches in the domain of physics, extending both into chemistry and engineering, and Congress has appropriated funds for the erection of buildings and the purchase of apparatus. A mechanical laboratory costing about $125,000 and a physical building costing about $200,000 will be erected. This bureau is so new that its results can hardly yet be spoken of, but in a country like ours, in which so much of the national wealth and progress is due to inventive genius and improvement of machinery, any steps tending to the further introduction of exactness in this important branch of our national life can not fail to be productive of most useful results.

The Marine Hospital Service and the Department of Public Health, which among other things has under its care all federal supervision of these departments of sanitation, and so far as possible without conflicting with state laws, the control of all persons suffering from contagious diseases, has rendered a great service to the country by its intelligent handling of the various contagious diseases and plagues which from time to time have invaded our shores. Under this service a laboratory has been recently established where constant and successful experiments are being made in that most important branch of medical science, preventive medicine.

The Bureau of Labor, established in 1885, has, incidentally to its practical functions, done much valuable research work and in the collection and publication of statistics bearing upon social and economic problems, and has been effective in bringing about a better understanding of the conditions of human labor.

Many agencies remain unspoken of, but among these, two, the National Library, known to the law as the Library of Congress, and the Smithsonian Institution, must have separate mention.

Scientific research in the modern sense is impracticable without access to books, since it is incumbent upon each investigator to examine the works of his predecessors, and in announcing his results to state the extent of his dependence upon those who have preceded him in the field.

The Library of Congress was not established, of course, with any such purpose in view. It was at first strictly what its name implies, and its need was felt even as early as the Continental Congress. The origin of the present library goes back to the removal of the Capitol to Washington, but in the very beginning, as early as 1806, it was recognized that Congress itself required something different from mere law books or important books of reference, and the general subjects which might now be termed polite literature and "the humanities" began to be incorporated in the Library at that early date. This policy, which has been kept up and extended, has made the Library in fact, if not in name, a National Library.

From the Capitol it was removed in 1897 to its splendid new building, one certainly better adapted to library purposes than any other in the world. This Library contained, in 1902, nearly 800,000 books and over 300,000 pamphlets, a total of over 1,000,000 titles, this being exclusive of the law library and manuscripts, maps, pieces of music, and prints, which together make a total considerably over half a million. It is now virtually a general library, and while it bears some special relation to the needs of Congress, and of necessity devotes itself as one of its main features to Americana, is still a library universal in scope, and in it there is represented every department of human knowledge. Upon it the men of science connected with the Government may draw freely.

By judicious expenditure of its enlarged means for the purchase of books within recent years. It has added materially to its collections in the physical and natural sciences. It is engaged in the publication of special lists and bibliographies which, while not directly intended for scientific purposes, yet have much value to science, and are a most efficient aid to the prosecution of the scientific work of every branch of the Government.

Of necessity special libraries also exist: that of the Surgeon-General's Office, the most notable, has already been alluded to, but the others, maintained by the Geological Survey, the Department of Agriculture, and indeed in every scientific bureau and office of the Government, are of increasing value and utility to persons engaged in special work. These are conducted and added to in harmonious relations with each other, and with the Library of Congress; so that without a common organization, there has grown up an understanding which avoids unnecessary duplication, and which arranges for the interchange of books among the various libraries, and altogether furnishes a most efficient system for procuring and using scientific works.

I come last to speak of the Smithsonian Institution. I have endeavored in the little space allotted, to briefly review the scientific activities of the United States Government. Every administrator is prone to the natural risk of magnifying the work of his own department, but the Smithsonian Institution, occupying a unique position in that it is a kind of ward of the Nation, has secured for itself so firm a hold upon the interest of the people of this country, and so distinguished a position abroad, that it may be spoken of objectively.

The Smithsonian Institution, as is known to all men, originated in the bequest of an Englishman. James Smithson, who died in 1829, and left his fortune to the United States to found at Washington an establishment under the name of the Smithsonian Institution "for the increase and diffusion of knowledge among men." Congress after much discussion passed a law in 1846 founding the Institution. It created the "Establishment" or corporate body, consisting of the President of the United States, the Vice-President, the Chief Justice and the members of the Cabinet. It provided for a Board of Regents for its government, and for a Secretary who, as Secretary to both of these Boards, should be the executive officer. It named as the principal purposes to which the Institution was to be devoted, the establishment of a library, of a museum, of a gallery of art, the giving of lectures, and other cognate methods in carrying out the will of its founder.

At the time of its organization, the Institution was relatively the best endowed scientific establishment in America. Its various purposes enumerated in its charter have been carried out. It formed a library (now to a great extent deposited in the Library of Congress) which is the best collection of transactions of learned societies and of scientific periodicals in the United States, and one of the great collections of the world. It began a museum, now known as the National Museum, and still under its charge, which in everything that pertains to the fauna and flora, the ethnology and geology of North America, is the most considerable in existence, and which bears within itself the nuclei of most important collections in American History in the progress of mechanic arts and in all the departments of learning which go to make up a museum of universal scope.

The Institution exists for two main purposes:

1. The Increase, and
2. The Diffusion, of Knowledge.

In addition to carrying on the objects in furtherance of these purposes enjoined upon it by its fundamental law, it has published from its private fund contributions for the increase of human knowledge of almost every description, resulting from explorations, the study of collections, original investigations, and experiment.

It has established also a system of international scientific exchanges which has become a recognized means of bringing the learned institutions and learned men of all countries into closer relations.

The income of this original fund has been in later years supplemented by annual appropriations from the Government, for extending and carrying on the work of the Museum, the Exchanges, the maintenance of a Zoölogical Park, an Astrophysical Observatory, and a Bureau of American Ethnology. The relation of the Institution, as such, to these various agencies, is that of a trustee for the National Government, entrusted with their direction and supervision, and bearing the responsibility for their proper and effective administration.

The National Museum, under the direction of the Smithsonian Institution, does not consist solely of objects for entertainment, but is rather a vast organized collection of the ideas and works of man on this continent, beginning with primitive man, and showing how his simple arts and his simple faith grew into complex culture and organized religions. It is impossible here to give an adequate conception of the range of this collection, which includes with the material products of this continent, relics of the Nation's history in war and peace, and perhaps the finest existing collection of personal relics of Washington and other historic Americans. It is the place of deposit of the collections of the Bureau of Ethnology, which, under the care of the late Major Powell, has described and published the history of primitive American man. Congress has just appropriated three and one-half millions of dollars for the adequate housing of these great collections.

The Bureau of International Exchanges is rather for the convenience of scientific men in the matter of diffusing their researches than a work of science in itself, though it spreads its operations over the whole world and has 30,000 correspondents outside of the United States.

The National Zoölogical Park grew from a small collection maintained in the rear of the present building of the Institution to the occupancy of its present picturesque grounds of 167 acres, now embraced in the ever-growing city. Its fundamental object is the preservation of our North American game. It is not supposed that it can in this small space alone keep from extinction the races which are fast following the buffalo, but it can offer a city of refuge for them and an object-lesson under the immediate eye of Congress.

The Astrophysical Observatory is dealing with man's relations to the sun and with problems which affect his welfare in a material sense. It has extended the known spectrum, through the invisible infra-red, to an extent many times that known to Sir Isaac Newton.

The establishment of the Smithsonian Institution at the time when it came into existence was a matter of supreme importance for the development of science in America. Sixty years ago, the funds for research were small and the avenues of publication inconsiderable. Two or three important scientific societies were in existence, but their funds were limited. No body of scientific men anywhere acknowledged a leader, and at a time, too, when most important investigations both in the physical and natural sciences were being made.

The acceptance by the Government of the trusteeship of this fund of Smithson's gave a national center for American science to gather about. It brought into existence, too, an organization which in Joseph Henry found a man strong enough to take up uninvestigated problems which had not yet been moulded into definite practical shape, and to advance their solution to a point where others might avail themselves of the Institution's work.

This, in brief, was the early policy of the Institution, and continues so to the present day. As indicated in the preceding portions of this article, the Smithsonian Institution has had much to do with originating work in other Government scientific departments. The importance of its early contributions to meteorology and to the establishment of what is now the weather service is universally acknowledged. It gave aid to those explorations which in a large measure resulted in the formation of the Geological Survey. The Fish Commission, the Bureau of Ethnology and the National Herbarium originated here. The system of international exchange of scientific publications, projected by the Smithsonian, found no one to take it up until the Institution organized its work, and this system both of Governmental exchanges and scientific exchanges, it continues to administer. Not so well known are its relations to such remote matters as the acoustics of the Hall of the House of Representatives, the methods by which vessels signal in fogs and the work of the Light-House Board.

In pursuance of its motto "Per Orbem," it has aided by grants not only in the United States but in other parts of the world, investigators engaged in original scientific work. It has published treatises containing new information of great value to students, and it has distributed among the people probably more than a half million volumes containing accurate scientific information in popular form. Ethnological researches among the American Indians were powerfully stimulated by it from its inception, and the first volume of its well-known series of "Smithsonian Contributions to Knowledge" was upon this subject. The researches made here in connection with the problem of aërial navigation have been largely instrumental in taking this work, heretofore derided and considered impracticable, into the realms of respectable and active scientific investigation.

Through a special fund, known as the Hodgkins Fund, a portion of which is devoted to the investigation of atmospheric air in relation to the welfare of man, our knowledge of the composition and properties of the atmosphere has been greatly extended. The Institution laid the foundation of methods of scientific library work in cataloguing, which so distinguishes American libraries from others, it originated the project of cataloguing all scientific papers by international coöperation and is at present, in default of any action by Congress, acting as the representative of the United States in the present International Catalogue of Scientific Literature published by a bureau with its seat at London. Under its auspices, and through it, such organizations as the American Historical Association have issued many works of value to historians and public men.

It remains in conclusion to point out the fact not usually recognized, that it was through the gift of Smithson and its acceptance by the Government that the steps for Governmental science, which were deemed difficult under constitutional limitations, were gradually made easy after the Institution was founded. Direct appropriations for science were, and continue to be, resisted upon constitutional grounds, but when the Smithson Fund was finally accepted by the Government and provision for carrying out the will of its founder was made, and Congress imposed upon the Institution obligations which its fund was not sufficient to meet, notably the establishment of a museum for the reception, care, and exhibition of the results of Government exploring expeditions, the step was made easy for Congress to provide through the Institution for carrying out its own behests; and much easier than if the different organization of such establishments outright and upon an independent basis had been attempted.

It is difficult to get practical men to provide for projects which are still in the experimental stage. The work necessary to the creation of the Weather Bureau and the Fish Commission would probably never have been accomplished but for the existence of an agency which provided for the initial and experimental stages of these two important National scientific projects. Indeed, so obviously practical a thing as scientific agriculture was promoted by the Smithsonian Institution in conjunction with the Commissioner of Patents, in the days when Congress had not yet seen its way clear to take this up.

It is not to be doubted that the philosophical workers of the United States will in the future recognize as the two dominant factors which produced the National scientific activity, first, the practical need of the Government for expert work in every department, and second, the establishment of the Smithsonian Institution, which, without violating the political consciences of our statesmen, enabled them to provide the means for scientific work whose ultimate economic importance has proven of the highest value to the Nation.

Such and so numerous are the scientific bureaus of the Government that it has seemed impossible, in this brief space, to do more than catalogue them, though each would become an interesting study if treated in detail, which would occupy a volume rather than an article.

SPECIAL AGENTS

[The numerous new functions which the federal administrative departments have recently been undertaking call for a body of highly trained and able officials. Although the rank and file of the clerical force in the departments must chiefly be relied on for the performance of this work, there have also been employed a great number of special agents for the purpose of conducting investigations and supplying specific information. This matter is discussed in the following speech of Mr. J. A. Tawney.]

Speech of Representative James A. Tawney on the Legislative Appropriation Bill [1]

Mr. Tawney said:

Mr. Chairman: This bill carries appropriations for the expenses of the legislative, executive, and judicial branches of the Federal Government for the next fiscal year. It abolishes 308 places now provided for by law, carrying salaries aggregating $360,360.25. It creates 243 new places and appropriates salaries therefor aggregating $276,324. It reduces 64 salaries for positions now provided and appropriated for by law aggregating $8,400, and increases 104 salaries, the aggregate increase equaling $16,930. In a word, therefore, the net reduction, as will be seen from these figures, made by this bill on account of positions and salaries abolished and reduced is $76,506.25.

These facts and figures ought to convince this House that your Committee on Appropriations has not neglected its duty in respect to inquiring into the condition of the public service in the respective Departments

[1] *Congr. Record*, March 19, 1906.

of the Government, and also into the necessity for positions now existing or which the Departments ask to have created and the salaries which ought to be provided for the positions thus created.

I listened with much interest to the remarks of the gentleman from Maine [Mr. Littlefield] last Friday, when he presented to the House and to the country facts tending to show the marvelous increase in the salaries and in the number of positions during the last eight years.

From his statement it appears that from 1888 up to and including 1898 the average annual increase in salaries aggregates about $2,000,000, and that the average annual increase in salaries since that time has been about $11,000,000. While the gentleman from Maine [Mr. Littlefield] did not seek to convey to the House the impression that the Committee on Appropriations was responsible for these increases, both in salaries and in positions, I fear that his remarks may have left upon the minds of many Members the impression that such is the case.

I therefore desire, Mr. Chairman, to call attention to the fact that there are two principal causes for these increases. One is the creation of the Department of Commerce, with an aggregate expenditure for salaries for the fiscal year 1905 of $2,142,739.84. The other is the establishment of the rural free-delivery service, increasing salaries annually to the extent of $20,480,000. Both of these causes have occurred since the date mentioned by the gentleman from Maine. When you deduct the increases made necessary by these two facts, together with some increases demanded by laws enacted by Congress, you will find that the average increase in both positions and salaries since 1898 created and carried in the appropriation bills does not exceed to any material extent the average increase in both positions and salaries prior to that time.

But, Mr. Chairman, it is nevertheless a fact, one that is well known to every Member of this House who has had any extended service, that in the enactment of legislation by Congress there is altogether too little attention paid to the consequent increase in both salaries and positions for which appropriations must thereafter be made. It is Congress, therefore, and not the Committee on Appropriations that must assume responsibility for originating practically all the increases in the past, for when a law passed by Congress authorizes any of the Executive Departments to undertake a new work or to undertake a new investigation which involves a vast amount of labor and a large number of Government employees, there is thereby created a necessity for additional expense, additional positions and increases in salaries for which that Department will submit to Congress its estimates, and thereupon the Committee on Appropriations has no alternative except to report appropriations for the purpose of meeting this additional expense.

I am glad, sir, that, as I have heretofore said, the present appropriation bill is not open to this criticism. It is the first one I believe that the Committee on Appropriations has reported in about ten years which has not carried an aggregate increase in salaries and positions greater than the last preceding appropriation bill or the current law.

I was therefore very glad to observe the independent investigation and inquiry which the gentleman from Maine [Mr. Littlefield] has given to the subject-matter of the appropriation bill now under consideration and to the subject-matter of the same bill reported and enacted in previous Congresses. If other Members would exercise their right and their privilege in a similar way, and devote time to the investigation and inquiry into the expenditure of public money and into the estimates submitted by the Departments, I feel confident that it would be of material benefit to the House and of great advantage to the Government and to the people. It would tend to prompt committees having jurisdiction of appropriation bills to be more careful in their investigation, more searching in their inquiries into the estimates submitted, and when their bills come before the House there would be less occasion and less justification for the superficial criticism which is so frequently indulged in upon this floor.

Mr. Chairman, I have realized for some time that the Federal Government was rapidly increasing its police supervision throughout the entire country. I have realized to some extent that we were rapidly assuming control and general supervision of the domestic affairs of the people of the States in the doing of that which belongs peculiarly to the States. But, sir, not until I came to examine the estimates of the several Departments of the Government for appropriations for the next fiscal year did I have any conception of the rapidity with which this extension of the Federal policing and Federal supervision of the domestic affairs of the people of the States was growing and being extended. For the purpose of ascertaining with some degree of certainty the extent to which the power of the Federal Government in this respect has been extended, I have ascertained from all the Executive Departments of the Government the growth of the inspection and general agents service during the past decade. I selected this branch of the public service for the purpose of ascertaining the extent of the growth of the centralization of Federal power and the extent to which the Federal Government is engaging to-day in the work of doing that which belongs peculiarly to the States. I have done this because it is through that service that this power is exercised to a greater extent than through any other branch of the public service. In the statement I have prepared and will submit as a part of my remarks I have separated this service and given each branch of the inspection and special-agent service of each Department separately.

An examination of this statement shows the total number of inspectors and special agents employed in the public service in 1896, the aggregate amount appropriated for that service, and also the aggregate number who were employed in that service in 1906 and the aggregate appropria-

DATA CONCERNING AGENTS, INSPECTORS, EXAMINERS, ETC.

Title	Where employed	1896		1906	
		Number	Compensation	Number	Compensation
Special agents, etc.	Bureau of Labor	20	$28,400.00	40	$57,200.00
Special agents	Census Office	..	....	735	500,000.00
Examiners and special agents	Department of Justice	11	27,500.00	20	45,220.00
Special agents and inspectors	Treasury	149	257,027.00	168	315,827.50
Suppressing counterfeiting and other crimes	Treasury	..	65,000.00	..	125,000.00
Mine inspectors	Interior Department	3	6,000.00	2	4,000.00
Inspectors, examiners, and special agents	do.	67	96,985.00	120	180,728.50
Special examiners	Pension Office	150	105,000.00	125	162,500.00
Inspectors	Indian Affairs	32	72,260.00	38	85,075.00
Inspectors, mail depredations	Post Office Department.	108	176,400.00	226	368,150.00
Agents	Alaskan seal fisheries.	4	12,950.00	4	12,950.00
Do.	Salmon fisheries	..	....	2	7,000.00
Do.	Rural free delivery	..	....	167	227,100.00
Special agents	Department of Commerce and Labor.	..	....	4	12,520.00
Do.	do.	..	....	31	62,152.00
Inspectors	Bureau of Immigration.	91	128,504.00	454	664,665.00
Do.	Steamboat-Inspection Service.	132	242,200.00	165	311,800.00
Assistant superintendents and agents.	Post Office Department.	4	6,400.00	39	70,200.00
Agents, inspectors, etc.	Agricultural Department.	160	....	773	1,355,640.00[1]
Total		931	1,315,526.00	3,113	4,567,728.00

[1] Amount from which authority is given to employ agents, inspectors, etc.

tions therefor. From this statement it will be observed that since 1896, or in the last decade, the number of special agents and experts in the Bureau of Labor has increased 100 per cent, and the amount expended for this service has likewise increased about 100 per cent. It will also be observed that the increase in the number of inspectors, examiners, and special agents of the Interior Department during the last decade has increased 79 per cent, and the amount of the expenditure for that service has increased 86 per cent, while we have increased the number of examiners, inspectors, etc., by the establishment of the Department of Commerce and Labor, in addition to the increases in the bureaus which were taken into that Department, to the extent of thirty-five.

The most notable increase, perhaps, will be found in the Department of Agriculture, where in 1896 they had only 160 inspectors, special agents, etc., and in 1906 they have 773. The total number of special agents and inspectors employed by the Government in the field and outside of the District of Columbia in 1896 was 931, while the total number in 1906 employed for that service is 3,113, an increase of 383 per cent. In 1896 we were expending for this special-agent and inspection service only $1,315,526, while to-day, ten years thereafter, we are appropriating $4,567,728.

Another remarkable fact which will be observed from this statement and which proves the rapid growth and extension of Federal control over the domestic affairs of the people of the States is the fact that although our revenue increased during the past decade 74 per cent the increase in the number of revenue agents, inspectors, and customs collectors and agents has been only 13 per cent and the amount appropriated for this service has increased only 22 per cent. The same small increase is true in all of the other Departments of the Government where this inspection service is employed legitimately for the benefit of the Government and for the purpose of collecting the revenue and protecting from fraud the interests of the Government when those interests require protection. The enormous increase in this service, as shown by this statement, is in those Departments of the Government which, under authority of law, have to deal with the affairs of the States or the people of the States, and much of this Federal service is rendered in conjunction with the States, or, as it is so commonly called, "Federal coöperation with the States," in the doing of that which belongs exclusively to the States. It must be borne in mind, too, that when a service of this kind is established or extended it at the same time involves a very large increase in the administrative force of the Department which is charged with the duty and responsibility of conducting the work or carrying on the service thus required.

I call attention to these facts, Mr. Chairman, in the hope of arresting the attention of Congress and the country to the marvelous growth during the past decade of a service which, if continued on the demand of the people as they have demanded in the past, will in the near future necessitate the expenditure of enormous sums from the Federal Treasury, pauperize the power of the States, obliterate the rights of the States, leaving the question only of State dependence or independence.

Mr. Chairman, we are directly responsible to the people for the money we are authorizing administrative officers to expend. It is theirs, not ours. These officers may justify their failure to comply with the law on the ground of sympathy, influence, or because of political pressure, but that excuse does not serve to relieve any Member of this House from his individual responsibility in respect to the appropriation of money for the public service or for any other purpose. The discharge of this duty demands labor, time, and thorough investigation into all the intricate and minute details of departmental administration. The Committee on Appropriations devoted five weeks to the investigation of this service and to a most careful inquiry into the estimates of the respective departments concerning their needs for the coming fiscal year. I am free to say, Mr. Chairman, not having had any previous experience on the Committee on Appropriations, and like most Members, having paid less attention to the subject than perhaps I ought to have done, that I was amazed at many of the disclosures revealed by that investigation. I do not insinuate or intimate that there is to-day or that there has been any corrupt practices on the part of any administrative officer of the Government; but I was surprised to find that the heads of the administrative departments of the Government pay so little attention to the details of the service in their respective Departments. I realize that they all have grave and enormous responsibilities in connection with the work of their Departments and the policies they must inaugurate and carry out, but at the same time the discretion necessarily vested in them by law is delegated to subordinate officers and clerks, who are not directly responsible to Congress, to a degree utterly inconsistent with good administration. The investigation shows that these heads of bureaus and chiefs of divisions, in almost every instance, are as susceptible to sympathy and influence as their superiors. The result is that when Congress says that a clerk, who is inefficient for any cause, shall be dismissed, the duty of reporting the fact of inefficiency has been delegated to the chief of the division in which that clerk is employed. Because of his intimate relation to the clerk or because of favoritism that chief is not so apt to enforce the law as he would be if it were practical for the departmental head himself to ascertain the question of efficiency or inefficiency. Hence we are told that one reason why this provision of law is not enforced is the fact, first, that they have not ordinarily the heart to turn these old people out, and, second, if they had, they are not reported to them as being inefficient, and therefore the evidence is not before them which requires them to do so.

In the Library of Congress the Librarian informed the committee that there was one man there over 70 years of age, totally, or almost totally, incapacitated for the discharge of his duties. When the Librarian was asked why he did not dismiss him he informed the committee that he could not. Well, why not — who is behind him? And immediately the answer came, "Chief Justice Taney." Further inquiry elicited the fact that out of respect for the memory of Chief Justice Taney, who appointed this man in the Library many years ago, the Supreme Court of the United States insists upon his retention.

The Secretary of the Interior cited several instances of a similar character. The Secretary of War informed the committee that it was practically impossible for any head of a Department to enforce that law, not alone because of his sympathy for the clerk who had arrived at that age when he or she was no longer capable of rendering efficient services, but also because of the pressure brought to bear by Members of Congress and Senators and other public officials in order to continue the employment of that particular clerk. This is not a condition, gentlemen, peculiar to this Administration. It is a condition that has obtained in all Administrations, and it will always obtain under our present system. It is for this reason that the Congress of the United States must enact an arbitrary law, whereby presumptive inefficiency resulting from age must be accepted as sufficient cause for separation from the public service.

In this investigation, Mr. Chairman, there are several matters of administration that the committees thought ought to be remedied. First let me call your attention to the fact disclosed in the hearings, that the Departments of Government are competing with one another for clerical service, a condition that has grown out of the increases in salaries of certain clerks in certain Departments doing identically the same character of work. One chief of a bureau, the Bureau of Standards, informed us that in the last two years it has been impossible for him to keep a stenographer and typewriter in his Bureau much more than six months. Why? He informed the committee that by the time the clerk had served six months, or a little more, he discovered that in the Treasury Department they were paying higher salaries for clerks doing identically the same work, and as soon as there was a vacancy in the Treasury Department he would ask for a transfer. The chief of that Bureau says he has not the heart to refuse to consent to his transfer when he is told the clerk can better his condition by transfer to the extent of from three to four hundred dollars a year.

This practice, Mr. Chairman, leads to a demoralization of the public service. The complaint is so universal on the part of the heads of Departments that your committee has deemed it necessary to report a provision prohibiting the transfer of clerks from one Department to another until the clerk has served in the Department from which he asks to be transferred at least three years. I am informed by the heads of Departments and bureau chiefs that from the standpoint of the public service this provision will, be of great value. It will not only tend to produce greater contentment among the clerks, but will also tend toward an equalization of compensation for the same general character of work.

The other provision which has been reported, and which has been commented on more or less in the general debate and in the public press of this city, is the provision respecting super-annuation in the Executive Departments and governmental establishments in the District of Columbia. That some legislation is necessary on this subject I think every Member of this House admits. It is a subject that has commanded more or less of attention on the part of Congress ever since I have been a Member of this body.

THE WORK OF THE KEEP COMMISSION [1]

IN constituting the Committee on Departmental Methods, somewhat more than two years ago, President Roosevelt chose five of the younger officials of the civil service, each one of whom already had a reputation for administrative ability and breadth of view. These men were named: Hon. Charles A. Keep, Assistant Secretary of the Treasury; Hon. Frank H. Hitchcock, First Assistant Postmaster-General; Hon. Lawrence O. Murray, Assistant Secretary of Commerce and Labor; Hon. James R. Garfield, at that time chief of the Bureau of Corporations, but since appointed Secretary of the Interior, and Hon. Gifford Pinchot, Chief of the Forest Service.

The Commission was directed by the President to ascertain where and in what respects our present Government methods fall short of the best business standards of to-day and to recommend measures of reform.

The commission carefully selected seventy employees of the Government, with varied experience, and formed them into sub-committees, which were used as probes to search the innermost recesses of the administrative machinery and discover the actual existing conditions. The committees made close inquiry into every condition and every phase of work connected with the service, and the resultant reports and recommendations exhaustively cover the ground, from sanitation of offices to making of Government contracts.

The remedial recommendations of the commission have almost all met with the approval of the President, and, where the authority of legislation is not necessary, they have been put into effect with as little delay as possible, so that this reform movement has been in active operation for two years and has advanced a long way toward the contemplated consummation. When the desired action of Congress has been secured the executive branches of our Government will be by far the most efficient and economical of any in existence.

[1] From an article by C. H. Forbes-Lindsay in the *Review of Reviews*, Febr., 1908.

A brief review of a few of the subjects treated by the commission will afford an idea of the scope and direction of the inquiry and of the measure of improvement likely to result from it.

Personnel and Salaries of the Service

The salaries now paid in the departmental service in Washington are based upon a classification of the clerks made by acts of Congress of 1853 and 1854, which graded the entire clerical force (except the departments of State and Justice) into four classes. To-day there are individual bureaus that have more employees than the entire departmental service had in 1853, and the responsibilities of their chiefs are incalculably greater than were those of the men who held similar positions fifty years ago. Nevertheless, there has never been any attempt to reclassify the positions, or to adjust the salaries with reference to these changed conditions, so that, at the present time, the most startling anomalies and inequities exist. Not only is there a great diversity of compensation for the same kind of work, but persons receiving the higher salaries are in many cases rendering the simplest routine service, while others in the lowest grades are performing duties of the most exacting character. Throughout the entire service the relation of the easier position, the more difficult position, and the responsible supervisory position has not for many years been adequately distinguished by the salary grades.

The lower grades of clerical employees in the Government service are better paid than the same class in private employment. Nevertheless, these positions have been the hardest of all to fill with competent persons. In the last fiscal year, 1462 eligibles were offered positions at less than $900 a year in the departments at Washington. More than 30 per cent declined, with the serious consequence that it was necessary to appoint in their stead individuals of distinctly inferior qualifications. The effect of this condition is far-reaching, since it is from the lower grades that the service is built up. It may be inferred that the young man of parts, who is confident of his ability to rise in the world, can not be tempted by the higher salary at the outset of his career, when it is accompanied by prospects of promotion decidedly limited as compared with those offered by commercial corporations.

On the other hand, the difficulty experienced in securing properly qualified clerks for positions paying from $1000 to $1500, and the great number of resignations from these grades, clearly indicate that the same character of service commands higher compensation in the business market. As to the supervisory, professional, and technical positions, they have long been recognized as very much underpaid in our departments.

These conditions have the effect of attracting to the Government service two distinct classes of men: First, those who have little ambition and no stomach for the struggle of the strong, and who find in a Washington clerkship a peaceful haven and a modest competence for life. Second, men actuated by public spirit, hope of political preferment, or desire to do big things, who are willing to sink monetary considerations for the sake of exceptional opportunities. Illustrations of this class are: Assistant Secretary of State Robert Bacon; Mr. Gifford Pinchot, of the Forest Service; Dr. Charles D. Walcott, of the Smithsonian Institution; Mr. Frederick Newell, of the Reclamation Service. In such instances we find men of the highest administrative ability directing interests equivalent to the management of a great railroad, on salaries of $4000 or $5000 a year.

The recommendations of the commission, which will require Congressional approval, contemplate a complete reclassification of the service and a corresponding readjustment of salaries. The proposed system aims to attract a higher grade of recruits, by doing away with the $50 and $60 a month clerks and making the salary for the lowest grade $900 a year. Frequent promotion is provided for, favoritism is guarded against, and the ultimate prospect is improved by a suggested long-service pension and life insurance. In the upper grades the salaries are placed sufficiently high to develop and retain the best executive and expert service.

The commission estimates that these increases in remuneration will entail no more than 10 per cent addition to the appropriations for salaries, which would represent an amount trivial in comparison with the sum that will be saved as a result of the economies already effected by the investigation, and would be further justified by the higher class of entrants to the Government service and the enhanced standard of efficiency that will be maintained in every grade.

Introducing Up-to-date Commercial Methods

One of the most important features of latter-day commercial accounting is the analytical form of bookkeeping, which is styled "cost-keeping." Manufacturing establishments employ it to ascertain in detail the cost of articles produced; railroads use it in the analyses of their operating expenses, and insurance companies depend upon it for statistics of the general costs of management and agency operation. States and municipalities are adopting the system with marked effect, and it has proved to be of no less assistance in government work than in commercial business. It will make comparison possible between the operations of establishments doing the same class of manufacturing, such as mints, arsenals, and navy yards. It will enable the head of a department or bureau to determine where economies may be effected by introducing new arrangements in organization, or new methods in practice, to estimate more intelligently on the probable cost of future operations, to make contracts with closer calculation, to fix selling prices on products transferred to other branches of the Government, or sold to foreign governments, or to private concerns.

Cost-keeping, heretofore practiced in only two or three recently organized government bureaus, will in future be employed wherever benefit can be derived from it, and the resultant advantages in mere dollars and cents must amount to millions every year.

In the matter of accounting, the commission found even the Treasury deplorably behind the times. This was one of the first subjects investigated, and reforms have been in force long enough to show the most markedly beneficial effects. As examples: The Treasury, which formerly only balanced its books once a year, at the expenditure of a great deal of time and trouble, now has a double-entry system of bookkeeping in force which enables it to strike a true balance at the close of each day's work. The account of the disbursing officer at New York, which used to take six months to make out, is now completed in two weeks. In a certain branch of the Government, where large and numerous financial transactions are carried on, the officials, who were accustomed to take ninety days to render an account, are now ready to do so daily. If a disbursing officer makes his last payment, for instance, at ten o'clock in the morning, he can give a complete account of his affairs at noon of the same day. The Auditor of the Treasury, who has been in the habit, — and necessarily so under the old system, — of settling disbursing officers' accounts largely on faith, now has all the checks and vouchers before him with which to verify them.

These improvements, be it understood, have not been achieved by any increase of the machinery. They are simply the results of better system, attained with less labor than was expended on the antiquated and cumbersome methods which have been abolished.

Needed Reforms in the Purchase of Supplies

It would naturally be supposed that in an institution purchasing supplies in such enormous quantities as does our Government the patent opportunities for economy and standardization would be embraced. Such has not, however, been the case. Each department, — and, in cases, a separate bureau or division, — advertises independently for what it needs, and contracts at a price without knowledge or regard for what the same goods are costing other branches of the Government or private corporations. A certain mucilage costs one department $1.84 per dozen quarts and another $3 per dozen quarts. The prices of the same make of pencils range from $2.27 per gross to $3.36 per gross. The cost of ice varies from 13 to 30 cents per 100 pounds, and no two departments contract for coal at the same figures. It should be borne in mind that articles of small unit value are consumed in quantities that represent hundreds of thousands of dollars, and the aggregate bills of the Government for such ordinary supplies run into the millions yearly.

No attempt whatever has been made to standardize supplies, so that 133 varieties of pencils, 28 kinds of ink, 263 different styles of pen-points, and all sorts of typewriter ribbon, are used in the various government offices. Hardly any check is placed upon waste or peculation. It would seem that every employee of the Government in Washington, from cabinet minister to colored messenger, uses twenty-three pencils each month, or, say, a total of 7,000,000 pencils a year, at a cost of $150,000.

A bill to provide for the betterment of these conditions was introduced at the last session of Congress, but it was blocked in the Senate. However, in case the opposition to the measure continues in the present Congress, the Keep Commission has devised a plan which will make for a great improvement in the purchase of supplies. An inter-department committee is suggested which shall insure uniformity in prices, and, with the coöperation of the Bureau of Standards, shall establish standards of quality and test goods furnished under contract.

Results in Efficiency and Economy

There are many phases of the commission's work, and highly important ones, which it is impossible to notice in the limits of this article. The changes effected and suggested seem to be in almost every case adequate and practicable. They must result in vast improvement of service and enormous economy of administration. These are more than ever important considerations in this day, when modern civilization demands of Government an ever increasing service and the exercise of entirely new functions.

Of course, it is impossible to make a precise statement of the amount of saving in money, or of the degree of improvement in service that may be expected to result from the labors of the Keep Commission, but a few concrete illustrations will afford the basis for a general idea on both points. Careful inquiry among chiefs of bureaus and divisions elicited the assurance that in a great majority of cases they anticipate at least doubled efficiency, and economies averaging 30 per cent of former expenditures.

The Interior Department has almost completed a thorough reorganization. There were formerly a number of divisions through which all correspondence and matters for the consideration of the Secretary passed and were prepared for his action. The system involved serious delays and a great amount of unnecessary labor. There were other divisions, — one to furnish documents, another stationery, a third furniture, and so on, — which have all been consolidated, with important saving in work and expense. In the Land Office the increase in efficiency is incalculable, —

certainly several hundred per cent, — and the saving in administration will be $500,000 a year. The estimate for the Secretary's office proper is $40,000 less than last year, despite the fact that the business to be done is greater. The work of the department is performed in less than half the time it used to consume, and the task of improvement is still in progress.

Public printing offers a good illustration of decrease in expenditures accompanied by improved service. A member of the cabinet once said to the writer: "If an official wants to hide something effectually from the public he cannot do better than put it in his annual report. No one will ever see it." This jest is almost a literal truth. The reports have been cumbersome and repellent. They contained repetitions of the same matter, scientific treatises, general discussions, philosophical reflections, biographies and eulogies, and, in short, irrelevant and redundant matter of all kinds, and illustrations that had no excuse for their presence. In compliance with an executive order, the current reports have been restricted to pertinent subjects and are free from the objectionable features. They are, in consequence, much more useful, and have cost $200,000 less than usual.

An enormous quantity of utterly useless printed material for which no demand existed has been issued by the Government yearly. In the past ten years 800,000 duplicate volumes have been returned to the Superintendent of Documents, and he has, for lack of storage facilities, declined the return of several hundred thousand more. And these figures relate solely to duplication in distribution to libraries and take no account of similar waste in the distribution to individuals. How great that has been may be inferred from the experience gained in the issue of two recent publications where the usual method was departed from. By taking care to prevent more than one copy going to the same individual a saving of 85,000 volumes was effected in these cases alone.

ADMINISTRATIVE TRIBUNALS AND REGULATIONS[1]

[As the administration of the United States government comes in closer touch with the people and as the functions of the administrative departments increase, the citizens will be more directly affected by the adjudications of the administrative bodies and by the regulations which are imposed by administrative authorities. The whole movement is indicative of a general change of American attitude toward government in its relation to the general life of the country and to the individual. From the spirit in which our earlier constitutions were framed, with their explicit restriction of governments, to the present readiness for supervision, regulation, and general administrative expansion is a significant change.]

IN the United States we have a body of administrative tribunals, not courts, whose decisions are in many instances as final as those of the regular judicial establishments. They limit liberty and control property; and in the matters in which their decisions are final, the day in court becomes a day in the presence of administrative authorities only. And numerous as are our courts, the body of our administrative tribunals is perhaps larger. Under a strict definition they may be numbered by the scores, under a more liberal definition by the hundreds. Though they are not dignified by the formal recognition which has been accorded to the administrative tribunals of France, Germany and Austria, their power is in some matters even more substantial.

The administrative tribunals. — The administrative authorities in the United States which have powers of adjudication, or of discretionary determination, have usually been termed tribunals rather than courts. This term has been employed by the president, the circuit court of appeals, officers of the department of justice and writers on administrative law here and abroad. But the American administrative tribunal, because of the rank growth of the law on which it depends, is generally a thing of indefinite outlines. In a broad — and, it must be confessed, loose — sense the term "tribunal" may be, and has been, applied to all administrative officers exercising discretionary powers. If we use the term in this sense, then the administrative tribunals in the state and national governments are manifold in number and type. But there is a narrower usage — yet still an indefinite usage — which applies it only to administrative authorities which either in their procedure, their constitution or their powers, or in one or more of these matters, closely resemble courts of general jurisdiction. It is rather with the latter class that we are here concerned, for while the former is well known, in connection with the law of public officers, the latter has scarcely a niche in our accepted legal classification.

[1] "American Administrative Tribunals," by Harold M. Bowman, in *Political Science Quarterly*, 21, 609. Reproduced in part, by permission.

The administrative tribunals of the states and of the nation are even more distinct, each from the other, than are the state and national judicial courts. They form two separate systems. Though the federal judges have displayed a tactful policy of non-interference, the national courts may in some cases control the state courts, directly or indirectly. But the national administration seldom or never interferes with the state administration by administrative as distinguished from judicial process. Their remoteness is even more emphasized by their diverse characters and by the difference in the matters with which they have to deal.

The state boards, bureaus, or offices which have the power of adjudication or discretionary determination, and which are assimilated in their procedure, constitution, or powers to the judicial courts, are of many kinds. They range from dairy commissions up to boards of health and superintendents and boards of education; and of recent years they are to be found in almost every branch of commonwealth administration. One of the most remarkable tendencies in commonwealth administration at the present time is the rapid multiplication of such authorities. In 1903 alone, about 140 new permanent state boards and offices were created, as well as some 75 temporary commissions and 39 special investigating committees.[1] Of course many of these organs of government are not tribunals even in the loose sense in which the term is here employed, but are more properly merely administrative authorities.

The administrative tribunals of the national government are more highly developed than those of the states, one of them being so like a court in its organization and procedure as to have received that designation. The more conspicuous among them are the boards of general appraisers, the comptroller of the treasury, the interstate commerce commission, the court of claims, the commissioner of internal revenue and the secretary of the interior. There are in addition many minor and inferior tribunals. Their number is accounted for not so much by the variety of subjects which fall under the national administration as by the hierarchical organization of that administration. This has resulted in a system of appellate jurisdiction which is seldom found in the states. Among these minor tribunals are the commissioner of pensions, the board of pension appeals, the patent office's board of examiners-in-chief, the register and receiver of the general land-office.

French writers on administrative law, such as M. Laferrière, whose attitude is adopted by M. Jacquelin, refuse to consider our federal court of claims as in any sense an administrative court, because, "like all the federal courts," it is subject to the control of the supreme court. It is, says Laferrière, a judicial tribunal, deciding administrative causes. These two writers seem to take the position that if the court of claims can not be considered an administrative tribunal, much less can any other board or office that is found in the United States. For this reason,

---

[1] *New York State Library Bulletin*, "Review of Legislation for 1903."

perhaps, they do not examine the other tribunals in any detail. And seemingly they fail in due appreciation of the fact that many acts of our administrative tribunals may not be reviewed by the courts.[1] The courts may entertain jurisdiction to ascertain whether these tribunals are competent to act in the particular case, but this is far different from actual control.

It is also to be noted that the interstate commerce commission has generally received little or no consideration in the scanty literature of American administrative law. The reason for this is not clear, but the most plausible explanation seems to be found in the fact that the commission, except in so far as it may be deemed an arm of the criminal courts, does not have to do with the relations between the government and natural or artificial persons, but rather with the relations between such persons themselves. From this point of view it is like the ordinary civil courts. In the judgment of the present writer the interstate commerce commission is sufficiently peculiar to be placed in a category by itself; but it should not be excluded from the list of administrative tribunals, in any broad consideration of this subject, especially as its activity seems likely to develop important principles of administrative law. It should finally be noted that, to make the consideration of the subject complete, the activity of the ordinary courts in their employment of the injunction and other extraordinary legal remedies would have to be considered, but this topic is beyond the limits of the present article.

Powers and Organization. — It is in the powers and organization of the administrative tribunals that their chief interest lies. What are the extent and limits of their powers of "administrative adjudication"? The decisions of the state courts and of the United States supreme court indicate that the United States constitution and the constitutions of the states do not bar the grant to administrative authorities of the power to make a final determination after a hearing. Even when the determination seriously affects property rights, its finality has in many cases been upheld, though of course the administrative authority, like a court, must be careful to keep within its jurisdiction. Thus some of the state courts have admitted the finality of the determinations of boards of health in respect to nuisances. It is true that certain of these cases preserve a judicial review of such determinations through the writ of *certiorari;* but the review does not extend over the findings of fact but is limited to the jurisdiction of the board and the regularity of its proceedings. The law of some states affords even less protection from arbitrary action in this matter than the French law, though a bill of rights is unknown

---

[1] How strong the statement of the American situation with respect to this matter may be made will be suggested by an extract from a recent book on American administrative law: "Within the scope of its jurisdiction the adjudication of the administration is final unless there be a provision to the contrary." Wyman, Administrative Law, sec. 115. But it is evident from other passages in this book that the author would qualify this statement somewhat. It is too general.

to the French constitution. The United States supreme court has held that the finding by administrative officers of the amount of a tax to be paid (the tax being a license tax) was final, even though the complainant had no opportunity to be heard before the assessment of the tax.[1] The same court has held that the determination of an administrative authority is final as regards the admission into this country of Chinese who claim that they are American citizens.[2] An administrative tribunal may thus in effect deprive a man of his citizenship. And these findings will not be reviewed by the courts — at least in the absence of complaint of abuse of discretion — even on the writ of *habeas corpus*. The conclusion from this must be either that an administrative tribunal will protect the liberties of the individual as scrupulously as a judicial court, or that the citizen has been deprived of one of his greatest historic rights.[3] Perhaps the former is the true conclusion. In any event, these decisions indicate the great power that may be granted to the administration.

The determination of the board of general appraisers upon a question of valuation is final, and it is stated that only upon allegation of fraud will a rehearing be granted. The decisions of state educational authorities are often not subject to review by the courts. The authority of the New York commissioner of education in the decision of appeals from lower school authorities is final. The code of Iowa provides that the decision of the state superintendent of public instruction on appeal shall be final, and the supreme court of the state has refused to interfere with such decision when the superintendent has acted within his jurisdiction. It is curious to note that in an early case this court described this function of the superintendent as "ministerial." Later it called it "judicial"; then "*quasi*-judicial." The terms "administrative," "*quasi*-administrative," "discretionary," etc., have been applied elsewhere. Such are the mutations of the judicial mind. And how well they illustrate the pains with which anything like a scientific nomenclature for the administrative law is born! The existing nomenclature has all the defects of a fortuitous development.

[1] *McMillen* v. *Anderson*, 95 U. S. 37, and *Cary* v. *Curtis*, 3 Howard, 236, cited in Goodnow, *op. cit.*, p. 336.

[2] *United States* v. *Ju Toy*, 198 U. S. 253.

[3] Mr. Justice Brown, with whom Mr. Justice Peckham concurred, said in dissenting: "It has been seen that under these rules [concerning immigration] it is the duty of the immigration officer to prevent communication with the Chinese seeking to land by any one except his own officers. He is to conduct a private examination with only the witnesses present whom he may designate. . . . If this be not a star-chamber proceeding of the most stringent sort, what more is necessary to make it one? I do not see how any one can read these rules and hold that they constitute due process of law for the arrest and deportation of a citizen of the United States. . . . Such a decision is to my mind appalling. By all the authorities the banishment of a citizen is punishment, and punishment of the severest kind. . . . This petitioner has been guilty of no crime, and so judicially determined. Yet in defiance of this adjudication of innocence, with only examination before a ministerial officer, he is compelled to suffer punishment as a criminal and is denied the protection of either a grand or petty jury." *Ibid.*, pp. 268, 269, 273.

Not only may the jurisdiction of the administrative tribunal be final; in some cases it is also exclusive. In others it is concurrent or alternative with that of the courts. Some decisions by these tribunals are binding upon the administration, but are subject to review and modification by the courts. And if the authority in some cases is of great importance, in others it is shadowy. The interstate commerce commission was at first believed to have very material powers, but to-day it is characterized as merely "an investigating and prosecuting administrative body, whose findings are given a *prima facie* force in judicial proceedings." Justice Jackson in the Kentucky and Indiana Bridge case, the first important decision under the act to regulate commerce, described the commission as the referee of each and every circuit court of the United States. It may also institute proceedings in the courts, "and thus be a prosecutor in the same cases wherein it has acted as judge."

The incidental powers of the administrative tribunals vary quite as widely as their determinative authority. The power to subpœna witnesses and in effect compel them to testify is possessed by some tribunals and is totally denied to others. It is of course true that in those instances where this power is possessed, the actual punishment for contempt — with rare exceptions, if any — will be imposed by a court. In some cases the administrative tribunal is so constituted and its powers are of such a nature as to admit of self-execution of its orders. A board of health may thus not only order a quarantine but, in the exercise of its police power, it may enforce it. The judgments of the federal court of claims are of themselves mandatory upon the secretary of the treasury. But for the actual enforcement of its orders the administrative tribunal must very generally depend upon the assistance of a court. The scope of the order which may be issued by the administrative authority is determined by common law or statute, as indeed is the extent of its powers generally. Thus the definition of nuisances and the scope of an order of abatement are largely matters of common law. The statute may give an administrative tribunal power to issue an order so general in scope as in effect to amount to legislation. In the American Warehousemen's Association case the interstate commerce commission, in reliance upon the statute and a decision of the supreme court, while expressly negativing its intention "to make any order in this case as such," issued a general order requiring carriers to state in their tariffs what free storage was granted and the terms and conditions under which it was granted. Instructed by the abuses in the particular instances the commission thus made a regulation to meet the general situation.[1]

It is apparent from the preceding discussion that even the property and liberty of the individual are in some measure subject to administrative tribunals, and that the review of the action of these bodies by

[1] *American Warehousemen's Association* v. *Illinois Central R. R. Co. et al.*, 7 I. C. C. Rep. 556, at 591 and 592.

the courts is frequently no more than a review for regularity. But on these points the courts are sensitive. Liberty and property are their special wards, just as the private law is their peculiar demesne. This explains the contention of some lawyers that power to make a rate could not be given to the interstate commerce commission because the exercise of such a power would amount to a taking of property, and the milder contention that the courts must be allowed to step in whenever they deem the rate confiscatory. One of the most tangible expressions of this jealous devotion to the authority of the courts in the United States is found in the extent to which contracts are kept under judicial control. Even when the power of the administrative tribunal is plenary with respect to other matters, it may be denied any shred of authority over contracts. On the other hand, in those countries, notably France, where the administration is more scientifically organized, there is a division of authority. In France the administration may act in three different capacities in making contracts: first, in connection with its functions as superintendent of the private domain; second, in connection with its administration of public services; and third, in connection with its action as *puissance publique*, for example in connection with its concessions of certain franchises or privileges. In the last case the contract is said to be administrative in its nature, and the administrative tribunals therefore almost necessarily have jurisdiction over it. In the first and second cases the contract is administrative only when the law declares it to be so; hence in these cases the ordinary courts have sole jurisdiction, subject to exceptions, the exceptions being more frequent in the first case than in the second. Many of the American administrative tribunals indeed have jurisdiction in respect to contracts, but it is a ragged, uncertain, and in some cases almost accidental jurisdiction. The comparative precision of the French law is absolutely wanting. This is not to say that the French law is without defects. Certain of the complexities which have resulted from the separation of its administrative and judicial courts have at least the factitious character and the superficial absurdity of some of the fictions of our common law.

Administrative procedure. — The administrative tribunals of the United States differ as much in their processes as in their powers. In some of them the procedure has much of the formalism of the regular courts. In general, while they have their own peculiar make of red tape, they are impatient of the punctilious give-and-take of plea, demurrer, replication, motion, and amendment.[1] They aim at expedition and economy. They are primarily executive agents and as such prone to take the substance and let the shadow go. The very spirit of adminis-

[1] "Things are done in administrative adjudication which could never be done in judicial process. Principles are violated in administrative process which are fundamental in the courts. Often the whole solemn procedure is upset so that there may be prompt administration." Wyman, *op. cit.*, sec. 119.

tration is the accomplishment of things. This may and no doubt does at times result in the sacrifice of rights. But safeguards are established. For example, in the case of pension claims, after the preliminary adjudication of fact and law there may be a reference to the commissioner of pensions, and then an appeal to the secretary of the interior which is in effect decided by a special board of pension appeals. Safeguards in the way of administrative appeal in cases of interference in applications for a patent and in cases of protest before the land office are even more detailed and conservative of rights. Still the administrative tribunals incline toward the laxer rules of *ex parte* proceedings. These tribunals are often as well satisfied by written as by oral testimony. The rules of evidence are little known to them and even less employed. The court of claims acts without a jury, the court itself being judge of both the law and the facts. Indeed, it may be said that the jury system is foreign to the administrative tribunals. Parties whose names do not appear on the record are often allowed to intervene with little or no formality. The interstate commerce commission, in its more important investigations, frequently extends a general invitation to all interested to appear and testify before it. In numerous cases it has allowed the attorneys of special interests to displace its own attorneys, and this has generally been much to the advantage of the inquiry. Examination of the testimony in some of the commission's inquiries reveals that at times "a voice" has asked a question and "a voice" has made reply. The evidence given by such mediums in the commission's seances appears as a part of the printed record and no motion for its exclusion seems to have been made.

Some further light is thrown upon the methods of administrative tribunals by an examination of their respect for their own previous decisions. The influence of that sovereign principle of the common law which bids the court to follow precedents prevails even here. It could not well be otherwise in a country whose jurisprudence is Anglo-Saxon. Thus the school tribunals in the states frequently publish extensive reports or copious digests of their decisions for the guidance of their successors. The decisions of the court of claims, of the treasury, of the comptroller of the treasury, of the interstate commerce commission and of other administrative authorities are published. The comptroller of the treasury has held that a decision of a comptroller should not be reversed by a successor upon the presentation of a case involving the same state of facts unless there was a manifest error in the interpretation of the law. Many other illustrations of this attitude might be given. The interstate commerce commission has manifested a keen sense of the importance of continuity in its interpretation of the law. But after all, the application of the rule which dictates adherence to established principles is quite different from its application in the courts of law. Administrative tribunals are not careful to make due distinctions between the dicta and the rulings in preceding cases. Often their findings are based so distinctly upon the special facts of the single case that precedent can hardly be said to exist. An instructive and amusing illustration of an attempt to reconcile a decision with alleged precedents is found in a case decided by the interstate commerce commission. In maintaining that the shipper of petroleum in barrels should not be charged for the weight of the barrel, since the shipper in tanks was not charged for the weight of the tank, the commission stoutly protested that it was following its precedents. The contrary had been contended with much vigor by those who opposed this ruling. And on the face of the cases it fully appears that the commission's language, although it was not as clear as it might have been, gave much warrant for this contrary assumption. The commission, after having asserted at many pages' length that its decisions were consistent and that it had followed its own precedents, wound up with the assertion that it was an administrative body and was therefore not obliged to follow precedent when it saw fit to do otherwise.[1] It would of course arrest the necessary development of law in the new fields in which these tribunals are working if they observed the rule of *stare decisis* in anything like the degree in which it is observed in the ordinary courts.

The fact that the procedure is so largely untechnical and often expeditious, if not summary, conduces to a result which affords one of the best arguments for the maintenance and extension of these tribunals. This is the comparative inexpensiveness to private individuals of proceedings before them. Frequently the expense is borne almost entirely by the government, and the cost to the government is much less than that of prosecutions in criminal courts.

GOVERNMENT BY EXECUTIVE RULINGS [2]

By Albert Dean Currier

The recent extensive exercise of the power of Congress "to regulate commerce," etc., under the provisions of the Constitution, has revived, at this time, a close scrutiny and study of the letter and spirit of our national Constitution, not only by our statesmen, but also by all persons who are interested in good government. The rapid growth of Federal power involves not only the power of Congress, under some attempted constructions of the Constitution, to enact general laws which frequently clash with the laws of the States, but also involves the rapidly increasing practice by Congress of delegating to the executive heads of govern-

---

[1] *Rice, Robinson and Witherop* v. *W. N. Y. & Penna. R. R. Co.*, 4 I. C. C. Rep. 131, at 155.
[2] *North American Review*, September, 1907. Reproduced in part, by permission.

mental departments the power to exercise functions which properly belong to the legislative and judicial branches of the Government.

The people of the United States are a very busy people, interested in the progress of their individual affairs. They are so busy that they are inclined to leave the study and enforcement of those principles which make for good government to those who make politics their business. So great has become this *laissez-faire* policy of the people, and so great has been their faith in the executive officials of the Government, that they have not fully realized the rapid growth of the executive branch of our Government, which is silently and surely usurping many of the functions of government that properly belong to the legislative and judicial branches. This growth of power in the executive branch appears to be due, principally, to the tendency of the legislative branch of the Government, as heretofore mentioned, to delegate to the executive heads of departments the power to make "Rules and Regulations" under general laws enacted by Congress, with power to interpret such laws wherein they may appear ambiguous or silent upon specific matters.

* * * * * * * *

The Constitution vests the executive power of the Government in the President of the United States, but, inasmuch as it is physically impossible for one person to perform all the executive duties and functions of the Government, Congress has prescribed by statutory laws (Secs. 158 to 161, inclusive, of the United States Statutes) that the executive functions shall be distributed among "executive departments"; and it is also prescribed (Sec. 161, United States Statutes) that "the head of each department is authorized to prescribe regulations, not inconsistent with law, for the government of his department, the conduct of its officers and clerks, the distribution and performance of its business, and the custody, use, and preservation of the records, papers, and property appertaining to it." The direction of the President is to be presumed in all the instructions and rules issuing from the competent departments.[1]

Although the Constitution and the statutes creating such executive offices do not anticipate or legally permit the promulgation of regulations except for the purpose of enforcing such rights, duties and obligations as are clearly defined by statute, yet, in those specific matters upon which the Federal statutes are ambiguous or silent, by virtue of the discretionary power vested in the executive heads of departments by Congress and the authority delegated to such executive officers by certain acts of Congress, portions of the laws are interpreted by executive officials, and the deficiencies in such laws are supplied by executive rulings thereon. Such executive rulings are often based upon forced and strained constructions of the statutory laws.

[1] See *Wilcox* v. *Jackson*, 13 Pet. (U. S.) 513; *Confiscation Cases*, 20 Wall. (U. S.) 92; *Wolsey* v. *Chapman*, 101 U. S. 769; *U. S.* v. *Fletcher*, 148 U. S. 89, and other legal authorities.

In recent years, the extensive and rapid growth of all sorts of industries and business pursuits in the United States has imposed, both upon the State Legislatures and Congress, duties which require much expert knowledge in the framing of just laws. Congressional Committees rely greatly for recommendation and advice upon departmental officials, who are often inclined to recommend the delegation of more authority and greater discretionary power to the executive heads of departments. The public too often fails in properly advising its representatives in Congress, especially upon matters which require technical knowledge, and the experts who represent various industries before Congressional Committees are frequently regarded as being prejudiced in favor of private interests. Thus, many specific questions which should be determined by Congress and which should be adjusted by proper Congressional Acts, are, by the terms of the Acts themselves, left to the executive heads of departments to be determined and enforced by them.

The exercise of such discretionary power by the executive heads of departments involves, *first*, a legal interpretation of the laws, which is a judicial function, and, *second*, the preparation and adoption of rules and regulations thereunder, which are properly legislative functions.

Such rulings by the executive head of any department may have the effect of destroying one class of industries and the building up of another class.

As an example of such power, a commission of the executive branch of the Government consisting of the Secretary of the Treasury, the Secretary of Agriculture and the Secretary of Commerce and Labor, may, by virtue of the extraordinary discretionary powers vested in it under the Food and Drugs Act of 1906, in any ruling which it may see fit to promulgate, prohibit the manufacture and sale of some articles of food which it considers adulterated, but which many food experts may have decided to be wholesome and free from deleterious substances. It may prohibit the use of a label bearing the name by which such article has for many years been known to the public, if it considers such label to be false or misleading, although the majority of the people, and even the minority of the commission who have had a more extensive experience and knowledge in connection with the same, may dissent from its opinion. The same executive commission may, by virtue of its authority, under the same law, prohibit the use of labels which are duly registered trade marks, thereby destroying the use of properties which, by reason of long use, have become valuable assets of the parties which have so used them.

Under the Congressional Appropriation Act of 1907, the Secretary of Agriculture may, "whenever he has reason to believe that any articles are being imported from foreign countries which are dangerous to the health of the people of the United States," request the Secretary of the Treasury to refuse delivery of such articles to the consignee; and such request is mandatory upon the Secretary of the Treasury. It is true that these specific Acts now referred to provide that manufacturers and importers of food who may be accused of violations of such rules and regulations shall be granted hearings before the executive head of the Agricultural Department, but the decision of the question of criminal prosecution lies wholly with such executive official. On the other hand, the Secretary of Agriculture may, in his discretion, neglect or refuse to enforce the manifest purpose and intent of the laws above referred to, if he so desires.

Similar conditions prevail to a greater or less extent in nearly all executive departments of the Government, and the Federal courts cannot issue a writ of mandamus to compel an executive head of a department to perform his duties in accordance with the manifest purpose of an Act of Congress, as to those specific matters in which discretionary power has been delegated to such executive by such Act.[1]

A certain condition of affairs, alleged to have arisen under the powers granted to the executive head of the Post-office Department to make "rules and regulations," is well described in a memorable speech delivered by the Hon. Edward Dean Crumpacker, a member of Congress from Indiana, before the House of Representatives on April 11th, 1906, in discussing the Post-office Appropriation Bill then before the House, from which speech, as it appears in the *Congressional Record*, the following extracts are quoted:

"Mr. CRUMPACKER. 'I understand there is a system of penalties imposed by the regulations of the Post-office Department. The gentleman must remember that that Department has legislative, executive and judicial powers combined. It exercises all the powers of the Government over the postal business of the country. . . .

"'The criticism that I am making is of the law and not of the officers, because I assume that they are performing their duties in accordance with postal regulations or the law. I do not know which it is; possibly it may be both. . . .

"'There is a system of postal espionage in this country that is absolutely inconsistent with the spirit of free institutions, and it is not what should be expected in a land of law and liberty.

"'Post-office inspectors may lodge complaints with the Postmaster-General that the business of an individual is fraudulent. The Postmaster-General may be satisfied from the secret reports of the inspectors that there are some irregularities in the character of the business the particular individual is conducting, and he may peremptorily enter a fraud order and withhold from that individual the privileges of the mails, absolutely ruining his business and blasting forever his business reputation. When that citizen calls upon the Postmaster-General, asking permission to see the charges that have been made against him, he is informed that they are confidential and is refused the privilege.'"

---

[1] See *U. S.* v. *Blaine*, 139 U. S. 306; *U. S.* v. *Guthrie*, 17 How. (U. S.) 284 and other citations thereunder.

There have also been many bitter complaints from a large number of citizens as to alleged unjust rulings by the executive officials of the Department of the Interior as to the methods of the disposition of certain Government lands, concerning which Congress has given to the Secretary of the Interior discretionary powers.

Recently a ruling issued by the Secretary of Agriculture proclaimed, in apparent contradiction to the intent and purpose of the Food and Drugs Act of 1906, that butter is exempt from certain provisions of the Act referred to, while other articles of food and drink are not favored with such exemption. This ruling is alleged to have been based upon a technical definition of the term by which the product referred to is usually known, created in a Congressional Act of a radically different nature and purpose over twenty years ago, which definition was so created by the words of that Act itself "for the purpose of this Act." Although often requested so to do, the executive head of the department referred to has refused to submit the legal phase of this question to the Department of Justice for an opinion thereon.

Congress frequently delegates to executive officials authority not only to make rules and regulations as to the conduct of the general *executive* business of their departments, but also delegates discretionary power in the promulgation of rules and regulations under certain statutory laws with reference to matters which are not specifically mentioned in such laws.

And the rules and regulations promulgated by executive heads of departments are endowed with the full force and effect of law, and are to be so regarded until the courts shall have decided that they are inconsistent with the statutory laws. Where the language in a statute is ambiguous and open to different interpretations, the construction put upon it by the executive department is regarded as decisive.[1]

Moreover, violations of the rules and regulations promulgated by the executive heads of departments, thus having the force and effect of law, are frequently punishable by severe penalties prescribed in general statutory Acts. Generally there is no provision for direct appeal by the accused person to the courts from such executive rulings. Persons who may believe that injustice has been done, that they have been discriminated against by such rules and regulations and that such rulings are not consistent with the statutory laws, must submit to the injustice, by compliance, or to the only alternative, which is an indictment and criminal prosecution for an alleged violation of such rules and regulations. Again, the rules and regulations prescribed to-day by an executive official may be stricken out and a new set of rules and regulations promulgated by him to-morrow, concerning the same subject. This may be done without any alteration whatever of the statutory laws, but simply by

[1] See *Brown* v. *U. S.*, 113 U. S. 568; *St. Paul, Minnesota, etc., Ry. Co.* v. *Phelps*, 137 U. S. 528, and other citations thereunder.

reason of a new interpretation of the law by the executive officer to whom the power to make rules and regulations is delegated by Congress.

In one division of the Treasury Department, the Division of Customs, the exercise of discretionary power by executive officials formerly worked so much injustice in the appraisal of importations under the tariff schedule that Congress found it necessary, under pressure of a popular demand, to create by the act of June 10th, 1890, a Board of General Appraisers, from whose decisions the importer may, under certain conditions, apply to the Circuit Court of the United States for a review of the questions of law and fact involved. However, there appears to be no such provision for appeal to the courts from the rulings of the Commissioner of Internal Revenue, when approved by the Secretary of the Treasury; and it was only after a gigantic struggle in Congressional Committees and upon the floors of both Houses of Congress that the Act of Congress for the enlargement of the powers of the Interstate Commerce Commission, approved June 29th, 1906, was so amended as to provide an appeal to the courts, under certain conditions, from the decisions of the Interstate Commerce Commission, which Commission is practically a part of the executive branch of the Government.

In accepting delegated powers to construe Congressional acts which are general in their scope, and to make rules and regulations thereunder, the executive branch of the Government assumes great responsibilities and arbitrary power. Yet the Chief Executive of our Government is apparently requesting that Congress shall delegate still greater discretionary powers to the executive heads of Government departments.

It was, perhaps, with a sense of such responsibility that the Hon. John W. Yerkes, Commissioner of Internal Revenue, when his advice was requested by the Committee on Ways and Means in the House of Representatives on February 7th, 1906, in consideration of the House Bill relating to free alcohol in the arts and manufactures, said: "I do not want a general bill, leaving everything to be determined as to methods, modes, processes, rules and regulations by the Department." In connection with the same bill, when he appeared before the Senate Committee on Finance on May 5th, 1906, he repeated the same statement, and further said: "There was my view with regard to the bill, and it indicates clearly that I did not want the scope of power and authority that is given under the House Bill."

It may, therefore, be noted that not all the executive officials of the Government are seeking greater discretionary powers in their respective departments.

The foregoing paragraphs are probably sufficient to indicate the general tendency of the executive branch of our Government to usurp the powers and functions of the legislative and judicial branches.

It is the belief of many of our best statesmen that the true intent and spirit of the Constitution are thus being thwarted, and that the fundamental principles of our Government are thus being gradually undermined.

Congress, as a body, appears to be slow to recognize the evils which result from the delegation of its powers to the executive branch of the Government. The judiciary conservatively guards against encroachments upon the legislative and executive branches of the Government and generally refrains from interfering with the discretionary powers delegated by Congress to the executive heads of departments.

Upon a review of these conditions, questions naturally arise as to the proper remedy for the evils which thus appear. Is Congress, burdened with its multiplying duties, able to enact all the laws demanded by the people in forms so clear and specific, as to all the new problems of our rapidly growing industries and general business interests, that rulings by executive heads of departments shall be unnecessary, except as to the conduct of the persons working under them and the purely executive business of their respective departments? Is the executive branch of our Government exercising functions in excess of its constitutional powers? Are the citizens of our country performing their civic duties in fully and properly advising their representatives in Congress, and insisting upon proper legislation? Are the people of the various States neglecting the studies of political science and the practice of those civic virtues which make for good government? Are we to give the constitutional powers of the legislative and judicial branches of our Government, wholly or in part, into the hands of the executive?

The Hon. Elihu Root says, in his recent admirable book on "The Citizen's Part in Government":

"More than all, our hopes must depend upon the general and active participation of the whole governing body of the American democracy in working out the problems and applying the principles of government with wisdom, with integrity, with just and kindly consideration for the rights of others — every citizen doing his full and manly duty for his country."

The sovereignty which is vested in the people may be maintained only by its proper exercise. Should we not, therefore, in the interests of personal rights and civil liberty, strive to abolish the evils of our political system as they appear, to the end "that the Government of the people, by the people, and for the people, shall not perish from the earth"?

GOVERNMENT PRINTING [1]

THE article in the September *Atlantic* on "The Problem of Federal Printing," by W. S. Rossiter of the Census Bureau, is a quiet, mostly statistical account of the enormous development and great cost of this branch of governmental activity. The Public Printer of the United States, in a word, directs the greatest printing office in the world, it being in capacity and output five or six times as large as the Imprimerie Nationale.

Mr. Rossiter's figures show strikingly how the Government at Washington has become more and more adrip with printer's ink. In 1790 the total cost of Federal printing was $8,785; in 1904, $7,080,906. By the graphic chart illustrating the expansion of this business, it appears that there have been ups and downs in it, but that since about 1892 the curve has swept upward continuously and portentously — the total outlay having nearly doubled in that period. Mr. Rossiter estimates that the cost of Government printing in the decade 1900–1909 will exceed $60,000,000 — or more than had been spent on it from 1790 to 1880. It is not surprising that alarm has been taken at this making of many books in the Government Printing Office. President Roosevelt has discovered a superfluity here, much of the sort that Baring-Gould denounced in German printing, and has called for retrenchment, though it has not been observed that he himself has furnished the Government printers less "copy" than before. Congress has appointed a joint committee to inquire into the matter. On all sides it seems to be agreed that the public printing has increased, is increasing, and ought to be diminished.

But to discover the *vestigia retrorsum* is always the rub, in such matters. Everybody is willing that everybody else should leave a report or monograph inedited, but as for his own — why, the machinery of Government could scarcely go on unless it were got up handsomely with charts and plates. The truth is that the printing habit has grown upon us immensely. It is not confined to the Government at Washington. The various States show an increase in public printing almost as marked as that voted by Congress. Their total outlay on this item, Mr. Rossiter informs us, has nearly doubled in twenty years — rising from $1,561,350 in 1880 to $2,740,323 in 1900. Five or six States, and those in general the most backward, have been able to curtail this expense, but the others have pushed it to higher and higher figures. New York's printing bill, for example, was $145,610 in 1880; in 1900, it was $654,330. Doubtless there has been extravagance in State work of this kind, though most of the States let it by contract; yet there can be no question that the great

[1] *New York Evening Post*, 1905.

increase in Government publications has met a popular demand. The people have been rather proud of the elaborate State and Federal reports on forests and fisheries, on mines and water-supplies, on insect pests and improved grains and better methods of cultivation — in short, on every topic or entity in the heavens above or the earth beneath that could interest a village Solomon. And we Americans are, in this respect, the envy of foreigners. More than once has the London *Spectator* sighed over some elaborate volume *de luxe* issued by our Printing Office, of a scientific or social interest, and regretted that such work could so seldom be matched in Great Britain.

No utility, however, no æsthetic gratification can justify waste; and that the Government Printing Office at Washington is extravagantly conducted, Mr. Rossiter's showing leaves one in no possible doubt. The cost of printing is "decidedly higher than the charge for similar commercial work." Indeed, asserts the writer we follow, if this Government plant doing a business of $7,000,000 a year were transformed into a private concern, "the owners would discover that the charges for product, although they do not include the usual and important items of rent, interest, and profit, are nevertheless from one and one-half to ten times as high as the prices charged for similar work by printers who include the omitted items." Let prescribers of the Government ownership panacea take due note of this. It is the ugliest symptom of the disease they are treating.

Mr. Rossiter's explanation of the fact that "it is practically impossible to secure from Government employees the work — clerical or manual — that is expected and exacted from employees of private concerns," is, to say the least, engagingly simple. The reason is not, he protests, politics. It is not wrapped up in the nature of public administration. No; the trouble is with "the climate of Washington." He must mean moral climate, for printers certainly do the average amount of work in far hotter cities; Kipling describes a scene of almost demonic activity in the office of the *Pioneer* of Allahabad. But in Washington, avers Mr. Rossiter, there is a "lack of commercial excitement," and that "rush and bustle" which keys up workers elsewhere. Yes; and there is also, as every one knows, the feeling that Uncle Sam is the sleepiest and most lenient of employers; that there are Representatives and Senators to keep you in your job, no matter how worthless you are; and all the other complex of motive and influence which makes Government work notoriously more costly and less efficient than private. If a really competent Public Printer were employed, paid what his services were worth (not the mere $4,500 now assigned to the superintendent of a $7,000,000 business), and given an absolutely free hand, with a warning to the politicians not to meddle, he could doubtless effect great economies and tone the Printing Office up as it needs; but short of some such radical reform we are likely to see small improvement.

SPEAKER CANNON'S MAIDEN SPEECH, ON PUBLIC DOCUMENTS [1]

MR. CANNON said:

"Suppose, however, that it really will cost to send these public documents through the mails free as much as the postage at full rates would be if it were prepaid, still I think it would be wise to distribute them. In this Republic of ours the people are sovereign, and to govern properly they must have not only patriotism and honesty, but also intelligence and a knowledge of the principles of the Government and the manner in which the Government is administered, and therefore they have established free schools all over the country for the instruction of the people at the public expense; and the temper of our people is to make that instruction compulsory, and properly so, for each citizen practically is as much interested in the proper exercise of the right of franchise by the humblest and poorest citizen of the Republic, as he is in his own proper action; and as the different executive officers of the Government, as well as persons constituting the legislature, are only for the time being acting as the agents of the people, it is important, aye, not only important, but indispensable, if the genius of our institutions is preserved and the Government properly administered, that the people should keep track of the acts and doings of their agents. It is true that now news is given very generally to the people through the newspapers of the country; but when we consider the hurried manner in which it is prepared, as well as in which it is read, and that the papers frequently, I may say generally, contain a mere digest of the proceedings of Congress, of the transactions of the different Departments connected with the Executive, and that from the very nature of things the reports, as digested and published, frequently contain errors, and are warped by partisan feeling, the necessity of a correct and complete record of the proceedings of the legislative and executive branches of the Government being published in convenient form for use and preservation, and distributed to the people for their information, is at once seen.

* * * * * * * *

"The truth is, the people get valuable information concerning the administration of the Government in all its departments and branches from these documents, and my observation is that information obtained therefrom passes orally from man to man; and while I am proud of our great cities, and many of the citizens who reside therein, noted for their proficiency in their respective callings and their great energy and industry in accomplishing that which they undertake, yet in the country, among

[1] *Congr. Record*, Feb. 18, 1874.

the producers, the men who earn bread by the sweat of their faces, you find equally as great industry, and I dare say more general intelligence and patriotism; and this class of men especially are anxious to receive public documents and read them."

A MEMBER. "The gentleman must have oats in his pocket."

"I understand the gentleman. Yes; I have oats in my pocket and hay seed in my hair [great laughter]; and the Western people generally are affected in the same way; and we expect that the seed, being good, will yield a good crop, I trust tenfold; and the sooner legislation is had, not only as proposed by this bill, but in all other respects as the people desire and equity and justice shall dictate, the better it will be in the long run for all people in this country, whatever may be their calling or wherever they may reside."

* * * * * * * *

In closing he said:

"And last, but not least, we are told that the city press of the country oppose this bill, or any other measures that will give the people free public documents, for the reason, as alleged, that the individuals or incorporated companies conducting the same are desirous of monopolizing the means of information touching the affairs of the Government, at least to the exclusion of information to be furnished by the Government at the general expense. And it is also claimed by some that Members can not afford to advocate and vote for this bill, for the reason that the city press will declare war upon them and continue the same until they lose standing with their constituency. I do not believe that the city press will as a unit oppose this bill. A portion of it may from selfish motives, in some instances, and honestly in others. I certainly have no desire to call upon myself the assaults of the city press, or any portion of it. Nor do I fear it as long as I truly represent my constituents and act, in my representative capacity, for the interest of the people generally. Nor would I change the power of the press to assail my acts or those of anyone else. On the contrary, every Member of Congress, or other agent of the people, should court a fair criticism of his acts, and if he vitally misrepresents the people, they should, and no doubt would, fail to continue him in places of trust. But no man is a proper person to represent the people unless he has the honesty and the backbone to stand and do what is right and for the interest of the people, without reference to what anyone may say of him, or what the action of the press may be in the premises."

INSTRUCTIONS TO THE PHILIPPINE COMMISSION

[After the Philippine Islands had been acquired under the Treaty of Paris, the administration of the Islands was for a while carried on by military authority. President McKinley, however, sent a commission to the Islands to report on conditions and to make recommendations for future action. In 1900 a Civil Commission was appointed for the government of the Islands. The instructions which were issued by the President to this commission are given below.]

"In the message transmitted to the congress on the 5th of December, 1899, I said, speaking of the Philippine Islands: 'As long as the insurrection continues the military arm must necessarily be supreme. But there is no reason why steps should not be taken from time to time to inaugurate governments essentially popular in their form as fast as territory is held and controlled by our troops. To this end I am considering the advisability of the return of the commission or such of the members thereof as can be secured to aid the existing authorities and facilitate this work throughout the islands.'

"To give effect to the intention thus expressed, I have appointed Hon. William H. Taft of Ohio, Prof. Dean C. Worcester of Michigan, Hon. Luke E. Wright of Tennessee, Hon. Henry C. Ide of Vermont, and Prof. Bernard Moses of California, commissioners to the Philippine Islands to continue and perfect the work of organizing and establishing civil government already commenced by the military authorities, subject in all respects to any laws which Congress may hereafter enact.

"The commissioners named will meet and act as a board, and the Hon. William H. Taft is designated as president of the board. It is probable that the transfer of authority from military commanders to civil officers will be gradual and will occupy a considerable period. Its successful accomplishment and the maintenance of peace and order in the meantime will require the most perfect coöperation between the civil and military authorities in the island and both should be directed during the transition period by the same Executive department. The commission will therefore report to the secretary of war and all their action will be subject to your approval and control.

"You will instruct the commission to proceed to the city of Manila where they will make their principal office and to communicate with the military governor of the Philippine Islands whom you will at the same time direct to render to them every assistance within his power in the performance of their duties. Without hampering them by too specific instructions, they should in general be enjoined, after making themselves familiar with the conditions and needs of the country to devote their attention in the first instance to the establishment of municipal governments, in which the natives of the islands both in the cities and in the rural communities shall be afforded the opportunity to manage their own local affairs to the fullest extent of which they are capable and subject to the least degree of supervision and control which a careful study of their capacities and observation of the workings of native control show to be consistent with the maintenance of law, order and loyalty.

"The next subject in order of importance should be the organization of government in the larger administrative divisions corresponding to countries, departments or provinces in which the common interests of many of several municipalities falling within the same tribal lines, or the same natural geographical limits may best be subserved by a common administration. Whenever the commission is of the opinion that the condition of affairs in the islands is such that the central administration may be safely transferred from military to civil control they will report that conclusion to you, with their recommendations as to the form of central government to be established for the purpose of taking over the control.

"Beginning with the first day of September, 1900, the authority to exercise subject to my approval, through the secretary of war, that part of the power of government in the Philippine Islands which is of a legislative nature is to be transferred from the military governor of the islands to this commission to be thereafter exercised by them in the place and stead of the military government under such rules and regulations as you shall prescribe, until the establishment of the civil central government for the islands contemplated in the last foregoing paragraph, or until congress shall otherwise provide. Exercise of this legislative authority will include the making of rules and orders, having the effect of law for the raising of revenue by taxes, customs duties, and imposts; the appropriation and expenditure of public funds of the islands; the establishment of an educational system throughout the islands; the establishment of a system to secure an efficient civil service; the organization and establishment of courts; the organization and establishment of municipal and departmental governments and all other matters of a civil nature for which the military governor is now competent to provide by rules or orders of a legislative character.

"The commission will also have power during the same period to appoint to office such officers under the judicial, educational, and civil service systems and in the municipal and departmental governments as shall be provided for. Until the complete transfer of control the military governor will remain the chief executive head of the government of the islands and will exercise their executive authority now possessed by him and herein expressly assigned to the commission, subject, however, to the rules and orders enacted by the commission in the exercise of legislative powers conferred upon them. In the meantime the municipal and departmental governments will continue to report to the military governor and be subject to his administrative supervision and control, under your direction, but that supervision and control will be confined within the narrowest limits consistent with the requirements that the powers of government in the municipalities and departments shall be honestly and effectively exercised and that law and order and individual freedom shall be maintained.

"All legislative rules and orders, establishments of governments and appointments to office by the commission will take effect immediately or at such time as they shall designate, subject to your approval and action upon the coming in of the commission's reports, which are to be made from time to time as their action is taken. Wherever civil governments are constituted under the direction of the commission such military posts, garrisons, and forces will be continued for the suppression of in-. surrection and brigandage and the maintenance of law and order as the military commander shall deem requisite and the military forces shall be at all times subject under his orders to the call of the civil authorities for the maintenance of law and order and the enforcement of their authority.

"In the establishment of municipal governments the commission will take as the basis of their work the governments established by the military governor under his order of Aug. 8, 1899, and under the report of the board constituted by the military governor by his order of Jan. 29, 1900, to formulate and report a plan of municipal government, of which his honor, Cayetano Arellano, president of the audienca, was chairman and they will give to the conclusions of that board the weight and consideration which the high character and distinguished abilities of its members justify.

"In the constitution of departmental or provincial governments they will give especial attention to the existing government of the island of Negros, constituted, with the approval of the people of that island, under the order of the military governor of July 22, 1899, and after verifying, so far as may be practicable, the reports of the successful working of that government they will be guided by the experience thus acquired so far as it may be applicable to the condition existing in other portions of the Philippines. They will avail themselves to the fullest degree practicable of the conclusions reached by the previous commission to the Philippines.

"In the distribution of powers among the governments organized by the commission the presumption is always to be in favor of the smaller subdivision, so that all the powers which can properly be exercised by the municipal government shall be vested in that government and all the powers of a more general character which can be exercised by the departmental government shall be vested in that government and that in the governmental system, which is the result of the process, the central government of the island, following the example of the distribution of the powers between the states and the national government of the United States, shall have no direct administration except of matters of purely general concern and shall have only such supervision and control over local governments as may be necessary to secure and enforce faithful and efficient administration by local officers.

"The many different degrees of civilization and varieties of custom and capacity among the people of the different islands preclude very definite instructions as to the part which the people shall take in the selection of their own offices, but these general rules are to be observed; that in all cases the municipal officers who administer the local affairs of the people are to be selected by the people, and that wherever officers of more extended jurisdiction are to be selected in any way natives of the islands are to be preferred, and if they can be found competent and willing to perform the duties, they are to receive the offices in preference to any others.

"It will be necessary to fill some offices for the present with Americans which after a time may well be filled by natives of the islands. As soon as practicable a system for ascertaining the merit and fitness of candidates for civil office should be put in force. An indispensable qualification for all offices and positions of trust and authority in the islands must be absolute and unconditional loyalty to the United States and absolute and unhampered authority and power to remove and punish any officer deviating from that standard must at all times be retained in the hands of the central authority of the islands.

"In all the forms of government and administrative provisions which they are authorized to prescribe the commission should bear in mind that the government which they are establishing is designed not for our satisfaction, or for the expression of our theoretical views, but for the happiness, peace, and prosperity of the people of the Philippine Islands, and the measures adopted should be made to conform to their customs, their habits, and even their prejudices, to the fullest extent consistent with the accomplishment of the indispensable requisites of just and effective government.

"At the same time the commission should bear in mind, and the people of the islands should be made plainly to understand that there are certain great principles of government which have made the basis of our governmental system which we deem essential to the rule of law and the maintenance of individual freedom, and of which they have, unfortunately, learned by experience possessed by us; that there are also certain practical rules of government which we have found to be essential to the preservation of these great principles of liberty and law and that these principles and these rules of government must be established and maintained in their islands for the sake of their liberty and happiness, however much they may conflict with the customs or laws of procedure with which they are familiar.

"It is evident that the most enlightened thought of the Philippine Islands fully appreciates the importance of these principles and rules and they will inevitably within a short time command universal assent. Upon every division and branch of the government of the Philippines, therefore, must be imposed three inviolable rules:

"That no person shall be deprived of life, liberty, or property without due process of law; that private property shall not be taken for public use without just compensation; that in all criminal prosecutions the accused shall enjoy the right to a speedy and public trial, to be informed of the nature and cause of the accusation, to be confronted with the witnesses against him, to have compulsory process for obtaining witnesses in his favor, and to have the assistance of counsel for his defense; that excessive bail shall not be required, nor excessive fines imposed, nor cruel and unusual punishment inflicted; that no person shall be put twice in jeopardy for the same offense, or be compelled in any criminal case to be a witness against himself; that the right to be secure against unreasonable searches and seizures shall not be violated; that neither slavery nor involuntary servitude shall exist except as a punishment for crime; that no bill of attainder or *ex post facto* law shall be passed; that no law shall be passed abridging the freedom of speech or of the press or the rights of the people to peacefully assemble and petition the government for redress of grievances; that no law shall be made respecting an establishment of religion or prohibiting the free exercise thereof; and the free exercise and enjoyment of religious profession and worship without discrimination or preference shall forever be allowed.

" It will be the duty of the commission to make a thorough investigation into the titles to the large tracts of land held or claimed by individuals or by religious orders; into the justice of the claims and complaints made against such land holders by the people of the island or any part of the people and to seek by wise and peaceable measures a just settlement of the controversies and redress of wrongs which have · caused strife and bloodshed in the past. In the performance of this duty the commission is enjoined to see that no injustice is done; to have regard for substantial rights and equity, disregarding technicalities so far as substantial right permits and to observe the following rules:

"That the provision of the treaty of Paris pledging the United States to the protection of all rights of property in the islands and as well the principle of our own government which prohibits the taking of private property without due process of law, shall not be violated; that the welfare of the people of the islands which should be a paramount consideration shall be attained consistently with this rule of property right; that if it becomes necessary for the public interest of the people of the islands to dispose of claims to property which the commission finds to be not lawfully acquired and held disposition shall be made thereof by due legal procedure in which there shall be full opportunity for fair and impartial hearing and judgment; that if the same public interests require the extinguishment of property rights lawfully acquired and held due compensation shall be made out of the public treasury therefor; that no form of religion and no minister of religion shall be forced upon any community or upon any citizen of the islands; that upon the other hand, no minister of religion shall be interfered with or molested in following his calling, and that the separation between state and church shall be real, entire, and absolute.

"It will be the duty of the commission to promote and extend and as they find occasion, to improve, the system of education already inaugurated by the military authorities. In doing this they should regard as of first importance the extension of a system of primary education which shall be free to all and which shall tend to fit the people for the duties of citizenship and for the ordinary avocations of a civilized community. This instruction should be given in the first instance in every part of the islands in the language of the people. In view of the great number of languages spoken by the different tribes, it is especially important to the prosperity of the islands that a common medium of communication may be established and it is obviously desirable that this medium should be the English language. Especial attention should be at once given to affording full opportunity to all the people of the islands to acquire the use of the English language.

"It may be well that the main changes which should be made in the system of taxation and in the body of the laws under which the people are governed, except such changes as have already been made by the military government, should be relegated to the civil government, which is to be established under the auspices of the commission. It will, however, be the duty of the commission to inquire diligently as to whether there are any further changes which ought not to be delayed, and if so, they are authorized to make such changes, subject to your approval. In doing so they are to bear in mind that taxes which tend to penalize or repress industry and enterprise are to be avoided; that provisions for taxation should be simple so that they may be understood by the people; that they should affect the fewest practicable subjects of taxation which will serve for the general distribution of the burden.

"The main body of the laws which regulate the rights and obligations of the people should be maintained with as little interference as possible. Changes made should be mainly in procedure, and in the criminal laws to secure speedy and impartial trials, and at the same time effective administration and respect for individual rights.

"In dealing with the uncivilized tribes of the islands the commission should adopt the same course followed by Congress in permitting the tribes of our North American Indians to maintain their tribal organization and government and under which many of those tribes are now living in peace and contentment surrounded by a civilization to which they are unable or unwilling to conform. Such tribal governments should, however, be subjected to wise and firm regulation, and, without undue or petty interference, constant and active effort should be exercised to prevent barbarous practices and introduce civilized customs.

"Upon all officers and employees of the United States both civil and military, should be impressed a sense of the duty to observe not merely the material, but the personal and social rights of the people of the islands, and to treat them with the same courtesy and respect for their personal dignity which the people of the United States are accustomed to require from each citizen."

The articles of capitulation of the city of Manila on the 13th of August, 1898, concluded with these words: "This city, its inhabitants, its churches and religious worship, its educational establishments and its private property of all descriptions, are placed under the special safeguard of the faith and honor of the American army." I believe that this pledge has been faithfully kept. As high and sacred an obligation rests upon the government of the United States to give protection for property and life, civil and religious freedom, and wise, firm, and unselfish guidance in the paths of peace and prosperity to all the people of the Philippine Islands. I charge this commission to labor for the full performance of this obligation, which concerns the honor and conscience of their country, in the firm hope that through their labors all the inhabitants of the Philippine Islands may come to look back with gratitude to the day when God gave victory to American arms at Manila and set their lands under the sovereignty and the protection of the people of the United States.

ADMINISTRATION OF CUBA, PORTO RICO AND THE PHILIPPINE ISLANDS [1]

THE master mind in the work of administering the Government of Porto Rico, Cuba, and the Philippine Islands under military occupation, and in building up civil government in those islands, was that of the Secretary of War. He was obliged to construct even the tools with which he worked. The War Department had no bureau or administrative organization for disposing of the vast amount of department work occasioned by the acquisition and government of our new possessions, yet such organization was necessary to keep the Secretary of War from being overwhelmed in hopeless confusion; thereupon, what is now the Bureau of Insular Affairs was created. With reference thereto Secretary Root, in his report for 1901, said: "It performs, with admirable and constantly increasing efficiency, the great variety of duties which, in other countries, would be described as belonging to a colonial office, and would be performed by a much more pretentious establishment."

[1] From an article on the War Department by Governor Charles E. Magoon, in *Scribner's Magazine*, 1903.

The responsibility of determining the problems which arose, devolved upon the Secretary of War, and practical necessities required a determination in advance of Congressional action or judicial decision. Many problems raised new or long forgotten questions as to the character of the Federal Government, the nature and extent of the Nation's sovereignty, the division of its powers, and the extent of its authority at home and abroad. It was necessary to ascertain and observe precedents in dealing with unprecedented situations, and duly regard a long line of judicial decisions touching but not meeting the issue involved. Different civilizations, different systems of law and procedure, and different modes of thought brought into contact evolved a great crowd of difficult questions. New facts and changed conditions called for the interpretation and application of our own rules of policy and the establishment of further rules. Different views as to the scope of authority under the distribution of powers required reconciliation. The application of the law of military occupation to rights and practices existing under the laws of Spain, and the process of overturning inveterate wrongs brought about frequent appeals to the highest authority, which, being made in the name of justice, compelled consideration. At the same time the work of construction of civil government was carried to successful completion. A delicate and difficult task was that of transferring the public powers from the military to the civil organization, to bridge the chasm between the military camps and the forums of peace. In Cuba the change was effected by means of a constitutional convention which adopted a form of government and a constitution therefor; officials were elected thereunder at elections held under the auspices of the Military Government. The necessities of the public service being provided for, the military authorities withdrew from place and power, the civilian officials entered upon the discharge of their duties, and the Republic of Cuba took its place in the family of nations.

At this stage in the affairs of Cuba it became necessary for Secretary Root to solve the far-reaching problem of fixing the general principles for the permanent regulation of the relations between Cuba and the United States, so as to preclude the possibility of complications which might interfere with the amity essential to the welfare of both countries. Cuba is so situated, geographically, that it must be either the steadfast ally or the natural enemy of the United States. Internationally, the United States is bound to see that the Government of Cuba is conducted with due regard to the standards erected by modern civilization and the obligations devolving upon a member of the family of nations. Nationally, the United States is bound to promote its own industrial welfare, military defense, and domestic tranquillity, and especially to prevent the recurrence of yellow fever, that in the past periodically ravaged our shores. The measures adopted necessarily must be projected into the period when Cuba would be an independent State; mutuality was essential to their continuance, if not to their adoption; the inhabitants of the island were eager to exercise the powers of independent sovereignty; and, therefore, the task presented was that of permitting the exercise of the powers of the on-coming Government of Cuba, in respect of these matters, and at the same time insure that said powers would not be employed in an unwarranted or ill-advised manner, so as to embarrass or delay the accomplishment of the laudable purposes of the United States. The plan adopted by Secretary Root was to make the general relations to be sustained by the Republic of Cuba to the United States part and parcel of the basic structure of the Republic of Cuba; the declaration of those relations to be a condition precedent to the establishment of independent government in the island, and the surrender thereto of the powers and authority acquired by the United States by the war with Spain and the Treaty of Paris. The order of the Military Government dated July 25, 1900, authorizing the election and assemblage of the delegates to the Constitutional Convention, declared the purpose of the convention to be "to frame and adopt a constitution for the people of Cuba, and, as a part thereof, to provide for and agree with the Government of the United States upon the relations to exist between that Government and the Government of Cuba." When the Convention assembled the Military Governor, pursuant to instruction, admonished them as follows:

It will be your duty, first, to frame and adopt a constitution for Cuba, and when that has been done, to formulate what, in your opinion, ought to be the relations between Cuba and the United States. When you have formulated the relations which, in your opinion, ought to exist between Cuba and the United States, the Government of the United States will, doubtless, take such action on its part as shall lead to a final and authoritative agreement between the people of the two countries to the promotion of their common interests.

The wisdom of this course was soon manifest. The Cuban convention formulated a constitution, but omitted action with reference to the relations to exist between Cuba and the United States; whereupon Congress took the initiative and adopted what is known as the "Platt Amendment," specifically setting forth the general characteristics of such relations. The provisions of that amendment were adopted by the Constitutional Convention, and thereby became as much a part of the governmental organization and polity of the Cuban State as is the Constitution of Cuba.

The construction and maintenance of popular government in the Philippines presented no problem more serious than how to accomplish the transition from military to civil government, for the change was to be made "under fire" and in the presence of a formidable insurrection. The task set before Secretary Root was to devise a plan which would enable civil government to keep abreast with the success of our arms and at the same time continue available at all times the authority and organization of the Military Government to meet possible emergencies. The task was nearly as difficult as the impossible proposition of causing two bodies to occupy the same space at the same time. The plan adopted and successfully carried out was that set forth in the instructions to the Philippine Commission, dated April 7, 1900. These instructions were prepared by Secretary Root. They constitute the Magna Charta of the Philippines, and will contest with the Emancipation Proclamation for the rank of first of American State documents.

It is remarkable and gratifying that the work of developing civil government in Porto Rico, Cuba, and the Philippines was accomplished by exercising the military powers of the United States. The army, organized, trained, and equipped for the work of destruction, was utilized by the President and the Secretary of War as an instrument of construction. That which was fashioned to overthrow and expel one government was devoted to the purpose of erecting another. The war powers of this nation, although outside of the limitations of our laws and Constitution, knowing nothing of their restrictions, bound only by the discretion of the Commander-in-Chief and the practices of civilized warfare, were effectively used to construct, out of and for a people ignorant of our form of government and the principles on which it is founded, a government incorporating and inculcating the principles and theories which have made the United States foremost among the nations of the earth.

X

LEGISLATIVE AND ADMINISTRATIVE PROBLEMS

[The article by Mr. Samuel W. McCall, Member of Congress from Massachusetts, on the Fifty-ninth Congress, gives an excellent account of the legislative problems before the nation at that time. The matters upon which action was then taken do not yield in importance even to the great structural activities at the beginning of our national life. Then it was the framework of the state that was to be fitly planned and carefully erected, now it is the conditions of social and economic life themselves that are to be given legislative form. The first session of the Fifty-ninth Congress thus becomes a turning point in our national development.]

THE FIFTY–NINTH CONGRESS [1]

By Samuel W. McCall

It is easy to overestimate the historical importance of our contemporary politics, although it is far from being the worst fault that we should treat them too seriously. Questions that are discussed with a vast deal — I will not say of passion, for there is little genuine passion in our current politics — but with a vast deal of noise, are somehow quickly displaced by other questions no more important nor more closely related to the real life of the nation, and permanently disappear. We have witnessed in the last decade the sudden rise of statesmen, almost purely the creatures of executive favor, who have in a moment blazed from the horizon to the zenith, whose greatness has been established by executive proclamations and solemnly ratified by university degrees conferred with academic eloquence, and we are already asking ourselves what they really said or did that history will trouble itself to recall. Its verdicts we may be sure will not be greatly influenced by the extravagance of contemporary censure or contemporary praise. Whether or not a President really said not long ago, as reported, "In Mr. —— I have a great Secretary of State, in Mr. —— a great Attorney-General" — and so on throughout nearly the whole Cabinet list — and then, "in Mr. —— I have the greatest war minister that has appeared on either side of the ocean in our time," there are plenty of contemporary utterances to prove amply that now, not in the troubled times that try men's souls, but in the fat era

---

[1] *The Atlantic Monthly*, Nov. 1906. Reprinted with permission. Copyright.

of a gross material prosperity, the real golden age of statesmen has at last dawned.

All this leads to caution in expressing emphatic opinions concerning contemporary politics, although the extreme of censure is more often met with than that of praise in dealing with Congress, except when it suits the whim of the moment to treat that department of the government as the mere organ of the executive. It is somewhat the fashion to rank the present Congress, in the importance of its work, with the congresses immediately following the Civil War. I think this opinion may safely be treated as an exaggerated one; and that it has done nothing that can equal in constitutional importance the first act for the government of Porto Rico, or, in point of industrial importance, the Wilson or the Dingley Tariff Act, or that can approach in the logical response to a critical condition of the country the repeal of the silver-purchasing clause of the Sherman Act. And if one ventured farther back he would find other legislation of equal importance this side of the period of Reconstruction.

But the record of the first session of the Fifty-ninth Congress is very notable both for what was done and what was not done, although the balance is strongly in favor of actual achievement. It failed to pass the bill granting free trade to the Philippine Islands, and the tariff escaped that judicious revision which it has so often been proclaimed to be the peculiar prerogative of its friends to bestow; but it passed the bills for untaxed industrial alcohol, for meat inspection, for pure food, for the admission of the territories, and for a form of government railroad rate-making. It also displayed a remarkable capacity for spending money, and granted a total of appropriations of almost fantastic proportions.

The membership of the two houses in point of character and ability will compare not unfavorably with the best congresses that have ever been sent to Washington. Although they lacked the very few overshadowing figures associated with the congresses of past times, they contained men of rare talent, while their average membership was of a character scarcely to encourage those who delight in disparaging their own time in comparison with the past, or with the future their imaginations paint.

It would not be difficult to name a score of senators who in debate or in some other important feature of the work of a senator will be likely to be remembered at least by the next generation. "There does not seem to be a quorum in the divine presence," Mr. Reed once sarcastically observed, as he entered the Senate Chamber when a senator was delivering an elaborate and carefully prepared speech to a small number of sleepy colleagues. But Mr. Reed, who signalized his speakership by his daring way of counting a quorum, and who always went to the heart of the subject himself, rarely making a speech in the House over fifteen minutes long, did not regard with favor the average set speech. The set speech of a senator is usually one of portentous length. Senatorial dignity seems to demand the quality of length as a tribute to the importance of the rule for unlimited debate. Many long speeches were spoken in the Senate during the late session, some of them unnecessarily long doubtless, and devoted to the elaboration of points that were not always of the first magnitude, but on the whole the debates in that body, especially that upon the railroad rate bill, displayed a very high order of ability. Some of the strongest men in the Senate had previously been members of the House, where they had passed unrecognized by the public at anything like their real value. Men who had served in the House with Mr. Bailey, for instance, knew that he was a man of rare talent; but the newspapers, which generally employed themselves in ridiculing him at that period of his career, made the discovery after he became a member of the Senate that he was a debater of commanding ability.

The House did not lack in able men. It chose as Speaker the most picturesque character in current American politics, a very efficient presiding officer, but seen at his best in debate upon the floor of the House. The floor leaders of the majority were Payne, the chairman of Ways and Means, and Dalzell and Grosvenor of the Committee on Rules; and when to these are added Hepburn, Hitt, Williams, Littlefield, Burton, Clark, Cockran, Russell, and others whom space forbids to name and whom not to name seems invidious, there is presented a variety of talent that would add strength to any legislative chamber in the world. Ninety men, the number of the membership of the Senate, might be chosen from the House, and in aggregate of ability they would equal the present Senate.

The bill for free trade with the Philippine Islands passed the House, but failed in the Senate. It was supported by the Democrats generally and by a majority of the Republicans, but it encountered the opposition of a formidable contingent of Republican members who came chiefly from the agricultural states, and feared that the unrestricted competition of Philippine sugars would have an adverse effect upon our beet sugar industry. As an economic measure simply, little could be said in its favor save from the standpoint of absolute free trade, for no people in the world differ from us more widely in their social system, standard of wages and of living, and in industrial conditions generally. From considerations of commerce and industry alone, there is scarcely a country in the world with which we should not more quickly have free trade than with the Philippine Islands. And as to their importance to us as customers, the grandiloquent prophecies so freely indulged in, in 1898 and 1899, about the markets for our products that we were about to conquer, become for the first time impressive when we read them to-day in the light of that magnificent total of $6,000,000 of exports, which we have at last been able to attain after eight years of benevolent assimilation, to say nothing of reconcentration and war. But from the stand-

point of justice the measure was irresistible. Having forcibly taken from them and arrogated to ourselves the power of deciding what taxes those people should pay, having levied in all their ports our own high duties against other nations, and especially against those nations with which they would naturally trade, it would not merely be unjust, it would be inhuman, for us to deny them the benefits of the system of which we had imposed upon them all the burdens. They should have nothing less than free trade with this country until we shall again remember our own history and reëstablish the principles upon which our government was founded. When that time shall come, the people of those islands will decide for themselves what taxes they shall pay.

The most important measure of the session from an industrial stand-point was the "denatured" alcohol bill, so called, as if the prime object of nature in making alcohol was to provide a beverage. The bill removed the entire tax from alcohol which had been rendered undrinkable, so that this important agent in the arts might be used with comparative freedom. The tax remains as it was before upon alcohol which might be used for drink. Free alcohol in the arts was a feature of the tariff act of 1894, but Mr. Carlisle, then Secretary of the Treasury, found difficulty in preparing regulations which would clearly separate alcohol used in the arts from that used as a beverage, and prevent frauds upon the treasury; and the provision, although the law of the land, was never put in force. But some foreign countries have successfully employed the device of mingling with the alcohol substances that would render it poisonous or revolting to the human stomach, and have thus baffled the ingenuity of those who would sell it for drink. The legislation of the last session was based upon the experience of those countries, and it cannot fail to have a most important effect. Free alcohol in the arts lies almost at the basis of industrial Germany, which employs it to the extent of 75,000,000 gallons a year. Our own tax of $2.18 on each gallon was practically prohibitive, and in those important manufactures which depended upon its use we were at the mercy of our rivals. The possibilities of the employment of alcohol in producing light, heat, and power are also enormous, as gallon for gallon it has a far greater potency than the best grade of refined petroleum, and need not much, if at all, exceed it in price. The only opposition to the bill came from the wood alcohol interests, but as the use of that article even in the arts is attended with danger to life and health, no reason appeared for taxing for its benefit a more efficient and safer rival product, and the bill passed by a nearly unanimous vote.

The pure food bill was designed to prevent the transportation across state lines of adulterated, deleterious, and misbranded foods, and the chief instrumentality created to accomplish this purpose was a system of federal inspection supported by penalties of varying degrees of severity. The bill was based upon an enlarged, and possibly an unjustifiable, construction of the commerce clause of the Constitution, just as the taxing power has been amplified and often employed, not to provide revenue, but for purposes essentially foreign to it, and to regulate, suppress, and promote business and industry. The passage of the bill was largely due to Mr. Hepburn, chairman of the Committee on Inter-State and Foreign Commerce, under whose leadership it had, in a modified form, passed the House of Representatives in a previous congress. The most valuable portion of the legislation is that aimed at the traffic in patent medicines containing deadly poisons covered by false and attractive labels, — a form of industry which all the resources of federal and state law might well be employed to suppress.

Of the same general character as the pure food law was the meat inspection amendment to the Agricultural Appropriation Bill. The methods of preparing animal food even in the best regulated home kitchens would not always seem appetizing, if reported with a too close attention to detail, lit up by a sufficient play of fancy. But the colossal slaughter houses of Chicago, however well conducted, would inevitably afford a field for the higher imagination, which, if properly exercised, would turn the stomach of an Esquimau. But it is sufficient to say with regard to this amendment that it was not at all necessary to nauseate a nation, and strike down for the time an important foreign trade, in order to obtain an enactment which the great packers themselves may well have been eager to secure. For, in addition to the benefit of the certificate of purity, placed upon their product at the expense of the Government, the law will tend to drive out of the interstate and foreign trade some of those establishments which are too small to occupy an inspector, and will thus still further centralize the industry.

The legislation to which I have just been referring illustrates very well the striking principle dominating the work of the entire session. Congress was apparently animated by a profound faith in the infallibility of federal supervision. That the federal inspector was made of the same stuff as the state inspector, that some of the most sweeping financial swindles of the age, some of the most appalling disasters upon the ocean, occurred under a system of direct federal supervision, were facts that either were lost sight of entirely or were not regarded of the first consequence. And it is probably correct to say that Congress was responsive to the popular opinion of the moment. It is a most attractive way of dealing with an evil, not for one to fight it himself and face the disgusting details, nor for the community which is immediately affected to combat it, but to call upon the great central deity at Washington. What more powerful fulmination can there be against crime than a federal statute? Against this magnificent device the old-fashioned notion of keeping power near the people has little weight. The inhabitant of a city sees the water works which have been stolen, he knows the aldermen who helped to carry them away, and within fair limits he can reach a just conclusion upon the questions of guilt or innocence, and whether the law has been justly enforced. But the distance of the Washington stage is suited to sleight-of-hand and the red fire of the tableaux, and it matters not that the guilty may be dramatically absolved and the innocent attacked, and that mere suspicion or laudation may more easily take the place of proof, if only the central performer on the stage is willing to work the machinery of justice for political ends. The unknown and the distant have an obvious advantage over the near and the commonplace, for they strongly appeal to the imagination.

Excessive federal supervision of course disregards the boundaries that have been established between the national and state governments, and by centralizing authority more and more at a greater distance from the mass of the people it causes power when exercised to strike with a heavier incidence, just as a falling body acquires momentum and strikes the harder the farther it has fallen. But still worse, it tends to establish a relation between the government and the individual which ought never to exist, and which leads him to rely upon the government to do those things which he should do for himself. The debate upon the appropriation for the geological survey well illustrates this tendency. When once an executive bureau has been established it is the well-settled rule for it, not merely to "grow up with the country," but to expand with far greater rapidity than the country's growth. In reaching out for an enlarged jurisdiction it not infrequently duplicates the work already performed by some other bureau. If a special appropriation is granted it for a temporary work, the temporary appropriation is apt to grow into a fixed or an increasing annual charge upon the Treasury. The splendid proportions to which the appropriations for the geological survey have grown showed that that excellent bureau was no exception to this rule. A few years ago a special work of testing such substances as fuels and building materials was put in the charge of this bureau. This special work was established in connection with the St. Louis Exposition, which, of course, has passed into history. But it was proposed on an appropriation bill at the last session to continue this work, which was not the testing of materials and fuels upon the public domain, but of materials and fuels belonging to private individuals. It proposed to have the government do something at its own expense which the individual had in times past done for himself and done very successfully. But from the debate one would perceive the greatly superior way in which a private work could be performed by men holding an office under the government, — and at its cost; he would wonder that we had on the whole made some progress upon individual initiative, and that the telephone, the telegraph, and the other marvels of invention had not first been brought to light by men in the classified service or wearing a federal uniform; and listening to the debate, he would have marveled still more when he recalled some government institution, — the naval observatory for instance, with its wonderful equipment of telescopes and other instruments, its large and talented staff paid by the government to explore the heavens, and its magnificent appropriation, — and remembered that — omitting one rare man — its discoveries would not compare in importance with those of some half-starved college professor in charge of a meagre and poorly equipped observatory upon some New England hillside. A noteworthy feature of the incident was that the appropriation was favored by conspicuous members of the party claiming as its own the time-honored creed that the government which governs best governs least.

I have referred to the efficiency of the present Congress in the expenditure of public money. The total appropriations of the session amounted to $880,000,000, and if the appropriations for the Panama Canal and on account of the public debt are deducted, there will still remain nearly $800,000,000, as the cost of running all the departments of government for a single year, including the post office. It may perhaps be urged that appropriations amounting in all to $35,000,000, to cover deficiencies in previous years, should also be deducted; but deficiency has become a regular feature of our budget, and, if we may judge from the precedents, Congress at a future time will be called upon to provide for the deficiencies of the current fiscal year. This total of $800,000,000 of annual expenditure is about $300,000,000 greater than the corresponding expenditures for the first fiscal year of the McKinley administration. This astounding increase of about sixty per cent in the period of nine years demands some scrutiny and explanation.

An analysis of the appropriations will show that much the larger part of the entire increase is due to our vastly greater expenditures for military purposes. That our appropriations for these purposes might be somewhat lessened with safety is doubtless true, but the greater part of the increase is the necessary consequence of the policy of empire and glory upon which we entered at the conclusion of the Spanish War. That policy affected the United States no more profoundly in the principles of its government than in its military problem. In 1898 a great ocean separated our territory from every nation that might make itself formidable to us in war. If prior to that year Japan, for instance, had desired to attack us she would have been compelled to bring her war ships, with their limited steaming radius, and her armies, across the Pacific, and to fight us upon the American side of that sea — a task she could not hope successfully to perform. And the hopelessness of the undertaking would have made it practically certain that she would never attempt it. But to-day, if she determined to attack us, all she would need to do would be to seize some little island of ours lying at her own doors, and we should be compelled to cross the Pacific to give her battle; for as a practical question, I think no one doubts that the United States in the present temper of its people would defend the least of its possessions from forcible capture. In other words, our "world power" statesmen at a stroke of

the pen converted this superb ocean rampart into a rampart for a possible foe, which it would be necessary for us to cross for the purposes of
defending our own territory.   Since then we have rendered ourselves so
vulnerable to attack, it would scarcely be the part of wisdom to rely
entirely upon the pacific intentions of other nations and permit an abject
military weakness to appeal too strongly to their warlike ambition.

A further scrutiny of the appropriations will also bring to light the
fact that there has been a very considerable increase in the cost of running
the machinery of civil government, made necessarily large by the steady
encroachment of the national government.   The plea that our national
expenditure on the basis of population is less than that of some of the
other great powers contains an obvious fallacy.   It does not take into
the account the federated character of our system.   Our state and municipal governments support the weight of public education, of constructing and maintaining roads, furnishing protection against fire, providing
the courts which decide the great mass of controversies, and maintaining
the internal peace and order.   The people of Massachusetts, for instance,
tax themselves each year about $25 per capita in order to carry out these
great purposes of government which are partly or wholly performed by
the more centralized governments of foreign nations.   When all our
governmental expenditures are taken into account there is not more than
one great foreign power, if, indeed, there is a single one, that can vie with
us in amount of taxation.

Undoubtedly the most important enactment of the session, judged by
the effort expended to secure its passage, and by that feature of the legislation from which it took its name, was the Railroad Rate Bill.[1]   No
subject in our recent politics has been talked about more vaguely nor
been less understood than the precise form of the railroad question involved in the bill.   It would not be an exaggeration to say that public
opinion, the argument upon the subject in the first presidential message,
and the body of the debate, were directed to a point which was absolutely
unrelated to the controverted principle of the bill.   Every feature of the
legislation which might tend to prevent or punish discrimination by
railroads could have been passed without debate and by unanimous
consent; but when government rate-making was put forth as a cure for
discrimination there was presented an economic non-sequitur, so palpable as not to stand the test of a moment's serious thought.

To understand the situation more clearly, and to discover how far,
if at all, the rate-making provision of the bill responded to any evil
related to it and to any well-developed public opinion, it will be necessary to revert to the session before the last, when the subject first engaged the attention of Congress.   In his annual message in December,
1904, the President dealt at length with the evils of discrimination and
the giving of rebates by railroads, and concluded by proposing as a

---

[1] Mr. McCall was one of the few Congressmen who voted against this bill.

remedy that authority be conferred upon the interstate commission, when a given rate was complained of, to establish a new rate which should have effect immediately and stand until set aside by the courts. There was undoubtedly a strong public sentiment at that time against railroad discrimination, but such sentiment as existed in favor of giving the commission authority to fix rates was confined to the commission itself or to isolated utterances of a few individuals. Certainly, if one looks for the manifestation of a public opinion in favor of government rate-making prior to the last presidential election, in the important news-papers, the platforms of the great parties, or the utterances of their candidates, he will look in vain.

It was pointed out very early in the debate that followed the introduc-tion of a rate bill in the preceding congress, that there was no logical relation between the fixing of rates by the government and the giving of rebates or secret rates by the railroads. If a governmental agency should set aside a rate established by a railroad and substitute another for it, the railroad could as easily give a secret rebate from the new rate as from the one that had been set aside. The making of rates by the commission would do no more to prevent rebates, as was said by Mr. Ackworth, a leading British authority, than would the reënactment of Magna Charta. Senator Dolliver, the leading Republican supporter, in the Senate, of government rate-making, formally admitted during the debate at the last session that it would not prove a remedy for rebates.

But the recommendation had been made by a Republican president, and it at once became party policy; it was enthusiastically supported by the Democratic party, with the modern principles of which it was precisely in line; every known instance of railroad favoritism, the graft-ing of insurance officials, the magnitude of swollen fortunes, almost every financial and economic evil of the times very naturally served the pur-poses of argument in favor of a measure the inception of which had vio-lated every logical rule, and government rate-making finally passed with only seven dissenting votes in the House and three in the Senate.

The debate upon the bill will rank among the notable congressional debates of the generation. In the House, where the rules and the practice make it easy to limit discussion, it was much more brief than in the Senate and for that reason perhaps the speeches were devoted much less to detail and dealt more broadly and comprehensively with the important features and the vital policy of the bill. If the volume of the debate in the House is reduced one half by rejecting the glowing anti-corporation sentiments which might perhaps be expected in a body whose members were about to come before the people for reëlection, there will remain a thorough and informing discussion of the bill.

Most of the speeches in the Senate ignored the broad economic and constitutional grounds of debate, and there was an imposing display of technical but rather irrelevant learning. This scrutiny of detail resulted

from the rules of the Senate, which secure the unlimited right of amendment and debate. But with the exception of the court-review amendment and that prohibiting common carriers from engaging in other forms
of business, the contributions of the Senate to the bill were not of the first
importance. Great legal skill was shown in debating whether the bill
would be constitutional if it did not contain an express and broad provision for a court review, as if the courts would not protect all constitutional rights without the express direction of Congress. Whether the
bill attempted to delegate legislative power was a much more robust
constitutional point. This point received little attention in the Senate
outside of the masterly speech of Senator Foraker, which in its luminous
treatment of the broad legal and constitutional questions involved was
the incomparable speech of the senatorial debate. Admitting for the
purpose of argument that the making of railroad rates was within the
power of Congress to regulate commerce between the states, Congress
itself would have to exercise the power and could not delegate it to any
other body. But it was asserted by the friends of the bill that in giving
the commission authority to fix only such rates as were just and reasonable, Congress established the rule of rates, and that nothing was left
for the commission but to perform a merely ministerial act without the
exercise of any legislative discretion. This would seem equivalent to
asserting that Congress itself does not exercise legislative discretion unless
in such acts as are unjust and unreasonable. If Congress can confer
the power to fix just and reasonable railroad rates upon a commission,
then it can in the same way confer any of its other great powers, and
commissions may be created to establish reasonable tariff rates or to
declare just wars, or to make just and reasonable regulations upon any
federal subject. The principle of the bill would thus seem to involve
nothing less than congressional abdication.

The opponents of the bill contended that the law should require all
rates to be just and reasonable, and that under such a provision the individual could always secure redress in the courts for any extortion by the
railroad. Judging by the readiness of juries to award round verdicts
against railroads for damages to persons and property, it cannot be
doubted that the railroads would maintain a system of unjust or preferential rates at the peril of bankruptcy if the individual should proceed
in the courts, which are the forum where rights are made practical, and
a government by law is secured. If the commission were endowed with
greater power to initiate proceedings where upon investigation it believed
a rate to be unjust, the practical remedy against excessive charges would
be more effective than in the Hepburn bill. The power of testing every
rate exercised by judges scattered over the whole country would in no
degree tend to centralization, but the fixing of rates by a central commission at Washington, whose members were appointed by the President,
and were subject to removal by him at any time, would mean centraliza-

tion of the worst character. For what greater power could an ambitious president, seeking reëlection, ask than the power, by his coercive authority over the commission, to fix every freight rate between the two oceans, and to discriminate in favor of a community whose vote he was attempting to secure as against a community which was hopelessly antagonistic.

Fifteen years ago Chief Justice Cooley, then the chairman of the commission, declared that the task of fixing freight rates for the whole country would be a superhuman one for the commission to perform. To-day the task would be twice as great, owing to the expansion of our railroad system. Instead, then, of the flexible American system of adjusting rates to the demands of business and the competition of railroads and localities, any material interference by the commission in the making of rates would be likely to give us the unyielding and wooden schedules characteristic of bureau rate-making abroad; and instead of the low long-distance rate which has enabled the most remote parts of our country to trade with one another and has been responsible for the settlement of the interior portions of the Union, we should need to prepare ourselves, if foreign experience is of any weight, to witness a rate based upon distance which would be fatal to the long-distance traffic. An important practical safeguard against the chief evils of commission rate-making so far as the railroads are concerned will be found in the fact that their task, as Chief Justice Cooley said, is superhuman, and therefore impossible of performance, and in the sweeping provision for a court review.

So far as the prevention of discrimination is involved it is noteworthy that there is nothing in the bill which approaches in its definite and sweeping terms the Elkins Law, which had been upon the statute books nearly two years before the rate-making programme was proposed, and which had never been seriously enforced. There was nothing of mystery about this statute. It required no profound legal knowledge, but only the ability to read, to discover in its provisions the most comprehensive remedy for rebates, both against the railroad which gave and the shipper who received them. The effective proceedings against discrimination instituted under the Elkins Act during the last six months, which have almost uniformly been upheld by the courts, make it certain that if that act had been enforced prior to the President's first recommendation for commission rate-making, the recommendation, if made at all, would have been based upon some other ground than the prevention of rebates and discrimination. And as there was at that time no general complaint that railroad charges were excessive, the recommendation would probably never have been made at all.

The work of the Congress is, of course, not yet complete, although it is not probable that important legislation of a general character will be secured at the short session. The Immigration bill, which has passed both houses in different forms and is now in conference, may be enacted. The situation in Cuba may demand legislative action, which it is to be hoped will not destroy the independence of the little republic, in line with those flamboyant speeches which were made for Philippine annexation, and are now being repeated. But almost the whole time of the ten weeks' session will be required for the passage of the great annual supply bills.

I have referred to those features of the record of the session which seemed to me of the chief importance. It remains for me to suggest an obvious question of a general character, and not related to any particular measure. Did the course of legislation show that enlarged participation of the executive in the work of Congress, the tendency towards which had been witnessed in recent years? To this question I imagine only a single answer will be given. The influence of the executive upon legislation is to-day by no means confined to those common constitutional methods of expression, the veto and the message recommending legislation, but it is chiefly shown by an influence exerted upon the individual members, upon the legislative machinery of the two houses, and even by special messages upon amendments proposed to particular bills, which in effect amount to written speeches upon the mere details and phraseology of measures, and are read in that House in which the debate is proceeding. There are concentrated in the person of the President the great authority of the party leadership and the far greater practical authority which results from the vast powers of his office, of which by no means the least important, and certainly the most corrupting, is the control of the patronage. Unless there is a scrupulous and restrained exercise of these enormous powers, the presidential office becomes a formidable engine for throwing the whole mechanism of the Constitution out of gear. The practical absorption of the great prerogatives of Congress has gone as far as it can be permitted to go with safety to our system of government.

After all the laudations upon mere rapidity of motion without regard to direction, and the supreme importance of "doing things," with discrimination as to the character of the "things" a secondary matter, something still remains to be said in favor of parliamentary institutions, which in Great Britain and in this country have furnished the world with the best models of free government. One representative will be slow, over-cautious, and never disposed to action; another will be all impulse, and in reaching his conclusions will scorn to indulge in the process of thought; but in a great body of representatives the influence of extremes will be largely nullified and a comparatively safe average will be struck. But where you have a government of one man, it is apt to be a government by fits and starts, depending rather upon individual traits than upon the law. If your ruler is ultra-conservative, your government may never move at all. If he is erratic and emotional, ready to settle over night the problems that have vexed the ages, you will have a government of instability, and the great ship will be sailed, not by the charts and the settled currents of opinion, but like a cat-rigged boat, trimmed to catch every whiff of wind that may at the moment be blowing. At a time when Parliamentary institutions are becoming more powerful in Europe, and our people are looking with extreme sympathy upon the attempt in Russia to establish a duma, it is significant that we should be regarding with silence and apparent unconcern a movement in the direction of the practical obliteration of the Congress of the United States, and that we should apparently be turning our faces away from those nations with which we are most closely allied in civilization and ranging ourselves by the side of those South American countries where congresses and even courts employ themselves in registering executive decrees. And although it must be confessed that executive government is likely to afford a loftier stage for the exhibition of those arts with which the rapidly increasing breed of political acrobats and sword-swallowers may thrill the galleries of the country, the American people are not yet ready consciously to adopt such a system however entertaining it might be. The clear and general understanding of the danger will provide a certain remedy.

FEDERAL CONTROL OF CORPORATIONS

[When the government of the United States was founded, business was carried on almost entirely by individuals acting singly or in partnerships. The government then dealt practically only with natural persons, corporate action being rather the exception. In our own age important business matters are carried on almost entirely through corporations. The relation of the government to these artificial creations of the law, which have nevertheless developed an exceedingly strong vitality, is one of the most important problems of the day. This is true especially since corporations have through the process of concentration extended their field of activity over the entire national territory, so that the states can not effectively control their action. The problems thus arising are dealt with in the following selections.]

FROM PRESIDENT ROOSEVELT'S MESSAGE OF DECEMBER, 1906

THE present Congress has taken long strides in the direction of securing proper supervision and control by the National Government over corporations engaged in interstate business — and the enormous majority of corporations of any size are engaged in interstate business. The passage of the railway rate bill, and only to a less degree the passage of the pure food bill, and the provision for increasing and rendering more effective national control over the beef-packing industry, mark an important advance in the proper direction. In the short session it will perhaps be difficult to do much further along this line; and it may be best to wait until the laws have been in operation for a number of months before endeavoring to increase their scope, because only operation will show with exactness their merits and their shortcomings and thus give opportunity to define what further remedial legislation is needed. Yet in my judgment it will in the end be advisable in connection with the packing-house inspection law to provide for putting a date on the label and for charging the cost of inspection to the packers. All these laws have already justified their enactment. The interstate commerce law, for instance, has rather amusingly falsified the predictions, both of those who asserted that it would ruin the railroads and of those who asserted that it did not go far enough and would accomplish nothing. During the last five months the railroads have shown increased earnings and some of them unusual dividends; while during the same period the mere taking effect of the law has produced an unprecedented, a hitherto unheard-of, number of voluntary reductions in freights and fares by the railroads. Since the founding of the Commission there has never been a time of equal length in which anything like so many reduced tariffs have been put into effect. On August 27, for instance, two days before the new law went into effect, the Commission received notices of over five thousand separate tariffs which represented reductions from previous rates.

.It must not be supposed, however, that with the passage of these laws it will be possible to stop progress along the line of increasing the power of the National Government over the use of capital in interstate commerce. For example, there will ultimately be need of enlarging the powers of the Interstate Commerce Commission along several different lines, so as to give it a larger and more efficient control over the railroads.

It can not too often be repeated that experience has conclusively shown the impossibility of securing by the actions of nearly half a hundred different State legislatures anything but ineffective chaos in the way of dealing with the great corporations which do not operate exclusively within the limits of any one State. In some method, whether by a national license law or in other fashion, we must exercise, and that at an early date, a far more complete control than at present over these great corporations — a control that will among other things prevent the evils of excessive overcapitalization, and that will compel the disclosure by each big corporation of its stockholders and of its properties and business, whether owned directly or through subsidiary or affiliated corporations. This will tend to put a stop to the securing of inordinate profits by favored individuals at the expense whether of the general public, the stockholders, or the wageworkers. Our effort should be not so much to prevent consolidation as such, but so to supervise and control it as to see that it results in no harm to the people. The reactionary or ultraconservative apologists for the misuse of wealth assail the effort to secure such control as a step toward socialism. As a matter of fact it is these reactionaries and ultraconservatives who are themselves most potent in increasing socialistic feeling. One of the most efficient methods of averting the consequences of a dangerous agitation, which is 80 per cent wrong, is to remedy the 20 per cent of evil as to which the agitation is well founded. The best way to avert the very undesirable move for the governmental ownership of railways is to secure by the Government on behalf of the people as a whole such adequate control and regulation of the great inter-state common carriers as will do away with the evils which give rise to agitations against them. So the proper antidote to the dangerous and wicked agitation against the men of wealth as such is to secure by proper legislation and executive action the abolition of the grave abuses which actually do obtain in connection with the business use of wealth under our present system — or rather no system — of failure to exercise any adequate control at all. Some persons speak as if the exercise of such governmental control would do away with the freedom of individual initiative and dwarf individual effort. This is not a fact. It would be a veritable calamity to fail to put a premium upon individual initiative, individual capacity and effort; upon the energy, character, and foresight which it is so important to encourage in the individual. But as a matter of fact the deadening and degrading effect of pure socialism, and especially of its extreme form communism, and the destruction of individual character which they would bring about, are in part achieved by the wholly unregulated competition which results in a single individual or corporation rising at the expense of all others until his or its rise effectually checks all competition and reduces former competitors to a position of utter inferiority and subordination.

In enacting and enforcing such legislation as this Congress already has to its credit, we are working on a coherent plan, with the steady endeavor to secure the needed reform by the joint action of the moderate men, the plain men who do not wish anything hysterical or dangerous, but who do intend to deal in resolute common-sense fashion with the real and great evils of the present system. The reactionaries and the violent extremists show symptoms of joining hands against us. Both assert, for instance, that if logical, we should go to government ownership of railroads and the like; the reactionaries, because on such an issue they think the people would stand with them, while the extremists care rather to preach discontent and agitation than to achieve solid results. As a matter of fact, our position is as remote from that of the Bourbon reactionary as from that of the impracticable or sinister visionary. We hold that the Government should not conduct the business of the nation, but that it should exercise such supervision as will insure its being conducted in the interest of the nation. Our aim is, so far as may be, to secure, for all decent, hard working men, equality of opportunity and equality of burden.

The actual working of our laws has shown that the effort to prohibit all combination, good or bad, is noxious where it is not ineffective. Combination of capital like combination of labor is a necessary element of our present industrial system. It is not possible completely to prevent it; and if it were possible, such complete prevention would do damage to the body politic. What we need is not vainly to try to prevent all combination, but to secure such rigorous and adequate control and supervision of the combinations as to prevent their injuring the public, or existing in such form as inevitably to threaten injury — for the mere fact that a combination has secured practically complete control of a necessary of life would under any circumstances show that such combination was to be presumed to be adverse to the public interest. It is unfortunate that our present laws should forbid all combinations, instead of sharply discriminating between those combinations which do good and those combinations which do evil. Rebates, for instance, are as often due to the pressure of big shippers (as was shown in the investigation of the Standard Oil Company and as has been shown since by the investigation of the tobacco and sugar trusts) as to the initiative of big railroads. Often railroads would like to combine for the purpose of preventing a big shipper from maintaining improper advantages at the expense of small shippers and of the general public. Such a combination, instead of being forbidden by law, should be favored. In other words, it should be permitted to railroads to make agreements, provided these agreements were sanctioned by the Interstate Commerce Commission and were published. With these two conditions complied with it is impossible to see what harm such a combination could do to the public at large. It is a public evil to have on the statute books a law incapable of full enforcement because both judges and juries realize that its full enforcement would destroy the business of the country; for the result is to make decent railroad men violators of the law against their will, and to put a premium on the behavior of the wilful wrongdoers. Such a result in turn tends to throw the decent man and the wilful wrongdoer into close association, and in the end to drag down the former to the latter's level; for the man who becomes a lawbreaker in one way unhappily tends to lose all respect for law and to be willing to break it in many ways. No more scathing condemnation could be visited upon a law than is contained in the words of the Interstate Commerce Commission when, in commenting upon the fact that the numerous joint traffic associations do technically violate the law, they say: "The decision of the United States Supreme Court in the Trans-Missouri case and the Joint Traffic Association case has produced no practical effect upon the railway operations of the country. Such associations, in fact, exist now as they did before these decisions, and with the same general effect. In justice to all parties, we ought probably to add that it is difficult to see how our interstate railway could be operated with due regard to the interest of the shipper and the railway without concerted action of the kind afforded through these associations."

This means that the law as construed by the Supreme Court is such that the business of the country can not be conducted without breaking it. I recommend that you give careful and early consideration to this subject, and, if you find the opinion of the Interstate Commerce Commission justified, that you amend the law so as to obviate the evil disclosed.

From President Roosevelt's Message of December, 1907

"In order to insure a healthy social and industrial life, every big corporation should be held responsible by, and be accountable to, some sovereign strong enough to control its conduct. I am in no sense hostile to corporations. This is an age of combination, and any effort to prevent all combination will be not only useless, but in the end vicious, because of the contempt for law which the failure to enforce law inevitably produces. We should, moreover, recognize in cordial and ample fashion the immense good effected by corporate agencies in a country such as ours, and the wealth of intellect, energy, and fidelity devoted to their service, and therefore normally to the service of the public, by their officers and directors. The corporation has come to stay, just as the trade union has come to stay. Each can do and has done great good. Each should be favored so long as it does good. But each should be sharply checked where it acts against law and justice.

". . . The makers of our National Constitution provided especially that the regulation of interstate commerce should come within the sphere of the General Government. The arguments in favor of their taking this stand were even then overwhelming. But they are far stronger to-day, in view of the enormous development of great business agencies, usually corporate in form. Experience has shown conclusively that it is useless to try to get any adequate regulation and supervision of these great corporations by State action. Such regulation and supervision can only be effectively exercised by a sovereign whose jurisdiction is coextensive with the field of work of the corporations — that is, by the National Government. I believe that this regulation and supervision can be obtained by the enactment of law by the Congress. . . . Our steady aim should be by legislation, cautiously and carefully undertaken, but resolutely persevered in, to assert the sovereignty of the National Government by affirmative action.

"This is only in form an innovation. In substance it is merely a restoration; for from the earliest time such regulation of industrial activities has been recognized in the action of the lawmaking bodies; and all that I propose is to meet the changed conditions in such manner as will prevent the Commonwealth abdicating the power it has always possessed, not only in this country, but also in England before and since this country became a separate nation.

"It has been a misfortune that the National laws on this subject have hitherto been of a negative or prohibitive rather than an affirmative kind, and still more that they have in part sought to prohibit what could not be effectively prohibited, and have in part in their prohibitions confounded what should be allowed and what should not be allowed. It is generally useless to try to prohibit all restraint on competition, whether this restraint be reasonable or unreasonable; and where it is not useless it is generally hurtful.. . . . The successful prosecution of one device to evade the law immediately develops another device to accomplish the same purpose. What is needed is not sweeping prohibition of every arrangement, good or bad, which may tend to restrict competition, but such adequate supervision and regulation as will prevent any restriction of competition from being to the detriment of the public, as well as such supervision and regulation as will prevent other abuses in no way connected with restriction of competition."

I have called your attention in these quotations to what I have already said because I am satisfied that it is the duty of the National Government to embody in action the principles thus expressed.

No small part of the trouble that we have comes from carrying to an extreme the national virtue of self-reliance, of independence in initiative and action. It is wise to conserve this virtue and to provide for its fullest exercise, compatible with seeing that liberty does not become a liberty to wrong others. Unfortunately, this is the kind of liberty that the lack of all effective regulation inevitably breeds. The founders of the Constitution provided that the National Government should have complete and sole control of interstate commerce. There was then practically no interstate business save such as was conducted by water, and this the National Government at once proceeded to regulate in thoroughgoing and effective fashion. Conditions have now so wholly changed that the interstate commerce by water is insignificant compared with the amount that goes by land, and almost all big business concerns are now engaged in interstate commerce. As a result, it can be but partially and imperfectly controlled or regulated by the action of any one of the several States; such action inevitably tending to be either too drastic or else too lax, and in either case ineffective for the purposes of justice. Only the National Government can in throughgoing fashion exercise the needed control. This does not mean that there should be any extension of Federal authority, for such authority already exists under the Constitution in amplest and most far-reaching form; but it does mean that there should be an extension of Federal activity. This is not advocating centralization. It is merely looking facts in the face, and realizing that centralization in business has already come and can not be avoided or undone, and that the public at large can only protect itself from certain evil effects of this business centralization by providing better methods for the exercise of control through the authority already centralized in the National Government by the Constitution itself. There must be no halt in the healthy constructive course of action which this

Nation has elected to pursue, and has steadily pursued, during the last six years, as shown both in the legislation of the Congress and the administration of the law by the Department of Justice. The most vital need is in connection with the railroads. As to these, in my judgment there should now be either a national incorporation act or a law licensing railway companies to engage in interstate commerce upon certain conditions. The law should be so framed as to give to the Interstate Commerce Commission power to pass upon the future issue of securities, while ample means should be provided to enable the Commission, whenever in its judgment it is necessary, to make a physical valuation of any railroad. As I stated in my message to the Congress a year ago, railroads should be given power to enter into agreements, subject to these agreements being made public in minute detail and to the consent of the Interstate Commerce Commission being first obtained. Until the National Government assumes proper control of interstate commerce, in the exercise of the authority it already possesses, it will be impossible either to give to or to get from the railroads full justice. The railroads and all other great corporations will do well to recognize that this control must come; the only question is as to what governmental body can most wisely exercise it. The courts will determine the limits within which the Federal authority can exercise it, and there will still remain ample work within each State for the railway commission of that State; and the National Interstate Commerce Commission will work in harmony with the several State commissions, each within its own province, to achieve the desired end.

Moreover, in my judgment there should be additional legislation looking to the proper control of the great business concerns engaged in interstate business, this control to be exercised for their own benefit and prosperity no less than for the protection of investors and of the general public. As I have repeatedly said in Messages to the Congress and elsewhere, experience has definitely shown not merely the unwisdom but the futility of endeavoring to put a stop to all business combinations. Modern industrial conditions are such that combination is not only necessary but inevitable. It is so in the world of business just as it is so in the world of labor, and it is as idle to desire to put an end to all corporations, to all big combinations of capital, as to desire to put an end to combinations of labor. Corporation and labor union alike have come to stay. Each, if properly managed, is a source of good and not evil. Whenever in either there is evil, it should be promptly held to account; but it should receive hearty encouragement so long as it is properly managed. It is profoundly immoral to put or keep on the statute books a law, nominally in the interest of public morality, that really puts a premium upon public immorality, by undertaking to forbid honest men from doing what must be done under modern business conditions, so that the law itself provides that its own infraction must be the condition precedent upon business success. To aim at the accomplishment of too much usually means the accomplishment of too little, and often the doing of positive damage.

As I have elsewhere said:

"All this is substantially what I have said over and over again. Surely it ought not to be necessary to say that it in no shape or way represents any hostility to corporations as such. On the contrary, it means a frank recognition of the fact that combinations of capital, like combinations of labor, are a natural result of modern conditions and of our National development. As far as in my ability lies my endeavor is and will be to prevent abuse of power by either and to favor both so long as they do well. The aim of the National Government is quite as much to favor and protect honest corporations, honest business men of wealth, as to bring to justice those individuals and corporations representing dishonest methods. Most certainly there will be no relaxation by the Government authorities in the effort to get at any great railroad wrecker — any man who by clever swindling devices robs investors, oppresses wage-workers, and does injustice to the general public. But any such move as this is in the interest of honest railway operators, of honest corporations, and of those who, when they invest their small savings in stocks and bonds, wish to be assured that these will represent money honestly expended for legitimate business purposes. To confer upon the National Government the power for which I ask would be a check upon overcapitalization and upon the clever gamblers who benefit by overcapitalization. But it alone would mean an increase in the value, an increase in the safety of the stocks and bonds of law-abiding, honestly managed railroads, and would render it far easier to market their securities. I believe in proper publicity. There has been complaint of some of the investigations recently carried on, but those who complain should put the blame where it belongs — upon the misdeeds which are done in darkness and not upon the investigations which brought them to light. The Administration is responsible for turning on the light, but it is not responsible for what the light showed. I ask for full power to be given the Federal Government, because no single State can by legislation effectually cope with these powerful corporations engaged in interstate commerce, and, while doing them full justice, exact from them in return full justice to others. The conditions of railroad activity, the conditions of our immense interstate commerce, are such as to make the Central Government alone competent to exercise full supervision and control.

"The grave abuses in individual cases of railroad management in the past represent wrongs not merely to the general public, but, above all, wrongs to fair-dealing and honest corporations and men of wealth, because they excite a popular anger and distrust which from the very nature of the case tends to include in the sweep of its resentment good and bad alike. From the standpoint of the public I cannot too earnestly say that as soon as the natural and proper resentment aroused by these abuses becomes indiscriminate and unthinking, it also becomes not merely unwise and unfair, but calculated to defeat the very ends which those feeling it have in view. There has been plenty of dishonest work by corporations in the past. There will not be the slightest let-up in the effort to hunt down and punish every dishonest man. But the bulk of our business is honestly done. In the natural indignation the people feel over the dishonesty, it is all essential that they should not lose their heads and get drawn into an indiscriminate raid upon all corporations, all people of wealth, whether they do well or ill. Out of any such wild movement good will not come, can not come, and never has come. On the contrary, the surest way to invite reaction is to follow the lead of either demagogue or visionary in a sweeping assault upon property values and upon public confidence, which would work incalculable damage in the business world and would produce such distrust of the agitators that in the revulsion the distrust would extend to honest men who, in sincere and sane fashion, are trying to remedy the evils.".

The antitrust law should not be repealed; but it should be made both more efficient and more in harmony with actual conditions. It should be so amended as to forbid only the kind of combination which does harm to the general public, such amendment to be accompanied by, or to be an incident of, a grant of supervisory power to the Government over these big concerns engaged in interstate business. This should be accompanied by provision for the compulsory publication of accounts and the subjection of books and papers to the inspection of the Government officials. A beginning has already been made for such supervision by the establishment of the Bureau of Corporations.

The antitrust law should not prohibit combinations that do no injustice to the public, still less those the existence of which is on the whole of benefit to the public. But even if this feature of the law were abolished, there would remain as an equally objectionable feature the difficulty and delay now incident to its enforcement. The Government must now submit to irksome and repeated delay before obtaining a final decision of the courts upon proceedings instituted and even a favorable decree may mean an empty victory. Moreover, to attempt to control these corporations by lawsuits means to impose upon both the Department of Justice and the courts an impossible burden; it is not feasible to carry on more than a limited number of such suits. Such a law to be really effective must of course be administered by an executive body, and not merely by means of lawsuits. The design should be to prevent the abuses incident to the creation of unhealthy and improper combinations, instead of waiting until they are in existence and then attempting to destroy them by civil or criminal proceedings.

A combination should not be tolerated if it abuse the power acquired by combination to the public detriment. No corporation or association of any kind should be permitted to engage in foreign or interstate commerce that is formed for the purpose of, or whose operations create, a monopoly or general control of the production sale, or distribution of any one or more of the prime necessities of life or articles of general use and necessity. Such combinations are against public policy; they violate the common law; the doors of the courts are closed to those who are parties to them, and I believe the Congress can close the channels of interstate commerce against them for its protection. The law should make its prohibitions and permissions as clear and definite as possible, leaving the least possible room for arbitrary action, or allegation of such action, on the part of the Executive, or of divergent interpretations by the courts. Among the points to be aimed at should be the prohibition of unhealthy competition, such as by rendering service at an actual loss for the purpose of crushing out competition, the prevention of inflation of capital, and the prohibition of a corporation's making exclusive trade with itself a condition of having any trade with itself. Reasonable agreements between, or combinations of, corporations should be permitted, provided they are first submitted to and approved by some appropriate Government body.

The Congress has the power to charter corporations to engage in interstate and foreign commerce, and a general law can be enacted under the provisions of which existing corporations could take out Federal charters and new Federal corporations could be created. An essential provision of such a law should be a method of predetermining by some Federal board or commission whether the applicant for a Federal charter was an association or combination within the restrictions of the Federal law. Provision should also be made for complete publicity in all matters affecting the public and complete protection to the investing public and the shareholders in the matter of issuing corporate securities. If an incorporation law is not deemed advisable, a license act for big interstate corporations might be enacted; or a combination of the two might be tried. The supervision established might be analogous to that now exercised over national banks. At least, the antitrust act should be supplemented by specific prohibitions of the methods which experience has shown have been of most service in enabling monopolistic combinations to crush out competition. The real owners of a corporation should be compelled to do business in their own name. The right to hold stock in other corporations should hereafter be denied to interstate corporations, unless on approval by the proper Government officials, and a prerequisite to such approval should be the listing with the Government of all owners and stockholders, both by the corporation owning such stock and by the corporation in which such stock is owned.

To confer upon the National Government, in connection with the amendment I advocate in the antitrust law, power of supervision over big business concerns engaged in interstate commerce, would benefit them as it has benefited the national banks. In the recent business crisis it is noteworthy that the institutions which failed were institutions which were not under the supervision and control of the National Government. Those which were under National control stood the test.

National control of the kind above advocated would be to the benefit of every well-managed railway. From the standpoint of the public there is need for additional tracks, additional terminals, and improvements in the actual handling of the railroads, and all this as rapidly as possible. Ample, safe, and speedy transportation facilities are even more necessary than cheap transportation. Therefore, there is need for the investment of money which will provide for all these things while at the same time securing as far as is possible better wages and shorter hours for their employees. Therefore, while there must be just and reasonable regulation of rates, we should be the first to protest against any arbitrary and unthinking movement to cut them down without the fullest and most careful consideration of all interests concerned and of the actual needs of the situation. Only a special body of men acting for the National Government under authority conferred upon it by the Congress is competent to pass judgment on such a matter.

Those who fear, from any reason, the extension of Federal activity will do well to study the history not only of the national banking act, but of the pure-food law, and notably the meat inspection law recently enacted. The pure-food law was opposed so violently that its passage was delayed for a decade; yet it has worked unmixed and immediate good. The meat inspection law was even more violently assailed; and the same men who now denounce the attitude of the National Government in seeking to oversee and control the workings of interstate common carriers and business concerns, then asserted that we were "discrediting and ruining a great American industry." Two years have not elapsed, and already it has become evident that the great benefit the law confers upon the public is accompanied by an equal benefit to the reputable packing establishments. The latter are better off under the law than they were without it. The benefit to interstate common carriers and business concerns from the legislation I advocate would be equally marked.

Incidentally, in the passage of the pure-food law the action of the various State food and dairy commissioners showed in striking fashion how much good for the whole people results from the hearty coöperation of the Federal and State officials in securing a given reform. It is primarily to the action of these State commissioners that we owe the enactment of this law; for they aroused the people, first to demand the enactment and enforcement of State laws on the subject, and then the enactment of the Federal law, without which the State laws were largely ineffective. There must be the closest coöperation between the National and State governments in administering these laws.

PRESIDENT ROOSEVELT AND THE TRUSTS [1]

BY S. J. McLean

THE framers of the Constitution of the United States, fearing to place wide powers and unlimited sovereignty in the hands of the Federal Gov-

[1] *The Quarterly Review*, July, 1907.

ernment, specified the powers granted to the central authority, the powers not so granted being reserved either to the States or to the people. Under this arrangement the most important powers possessed by Congress in regard to industry are conferred by the interstate commerce clause, which empowers Congress "to regulate commerce with foreign nations, and among the several States, and with the Indian tribes." Supplementary authority is derived from the power to levy taxes, to establish post offices and post-roads, and to coin money. The right "to make all laws which shall be necessary and proper for carrying into execution the foregoing powers" must also be read as indicating the scope of the Federal jurisdiction.

The commanding position of the Supreme Court, which is the final judge of all Federal legislation, claims for its decisions the closest attention. In the famous series of judgments given, at an early period in the Court's history, by Chief Justice Marshall, the principle of giving a broad construction of the powers conferred on the Federal Government was adopted. Although there has from time to time been an ebb and flow, dependent on the personnel of the Court, the precedents set by Marshall have on the whole been followed. It may therefore be said that it has been the policy of the Court to construe broadly the constitutionality of the powers exercised by Congress, while at the same time a technical legal interpretation has been given to the terms of the statutes under which such powers are exercised. Under a rigid written Constitution — for the process of amendment provided is so cumbrous as to be practically unavailable — the Supreme Court is the elastic portion of the Constitution which provides, by implication, for the broadening of power to meet new exigencies. In the definition of constitutionality, questions of policy, as well as of strict law, have their weight.

However correct in theory, from an historical standpoint, the strict-construction theory of the Constitution may have been, it received a deathblow from the Civil War. Though it was not wholly true that the laws were silent while arms were being borne, it was no time for niceties of construction; and a national support was given to the broad-construction tendencies of the Court. In the Legal-Tender cases, which upheld the constitutionality of the issue of inconvertible paper with a legal-tender attribute, a broad justification was found in the necessities of war. In the exercise of the power to tax Congress has a wide discretion. A tax may be levied either for revenue or for prohibitive purposes. When Congress, in 1869, excluded State bank-notes from circulation by imposing upon them a tax of 10 per cent, the Court upheld this as a legitimate exercise of power, and stated that "the judicial department can not prescribe to the legislative department of Government limitations upon the exercise of its acknowledged powers." [1]

---

[1] *Veazie Bank* v. *Fenno*, 8 Wallace, U. S., 532.

The breadth of construction of the interstate commerce clause is especially noteworthy. Marshall's decision in 1824, that commerce includes not only traffic but intercourse as well, gave a trend to more recent decisions; but interstate commerce was of minor importance in the earlier days. During the first forty years of the Supreme Court's existence, only five cases came before it in which the construction of this clause was involved. With the expansion of the railway system and the general industrial development of the country, questions arising under this head have become increasingly frequent. In 1895, in a case which arose out of the aggression of organized labor during the Chicago strike, it was stated:

The constitution has not changed. . . . But it operates to-day upon modes of interstate commerce unknown to the fathers; and it will operate with equal force upon any new modes of such commerce which the future may develop.[1]

When the need of railway regulation was appreciated, it was under the interstate commerce clause that regulative legislation was passed. This legislation was stoutly opposed by the railway interests, which stigmatized it as an unwarrantable interference with private industry. One pessimistic critic contended that it was a movement towards centralization, and that "the next natural step must be the purchase and absolute control by the same power of all this vast railroad property." There were others who argued that this legislation was an unjustifiable interference with State activity.

The next exercise of power under this clause was concerned with an attempt to regulate industrial combinations. In two years one hundred and thirty-eight Bills dealing with this subject were introduced in Congress. Finally, in 1890, the anti-trust legislation known as the Sherman Law was passed. This was a compromise measure, and, like so many of the compromise measures passed by Congress, was inexact in phraseology. It is entitled "an Act to protect trade and commerce against unlawful restraints and monopolies." This implies that there are lawful restraints and monopolies. But the Act states that "every contract, combination, in the form of trust or otherwise, or conspiracy in restraint of trade or commerce among the several States . . . is illegal." While "monopolizing" is prohibited, no definition of this term is given; and it must be remembered that "monopolizing" is not a word of legal precision.

The regulation of Trusts is complicated by the fact that there is no Federal corporation law. Corporations engaging in interstate commerce do so under a State charter. The difficulty thus presented is well exemplified by the United States Steel Corporation. This organization attracts attention, not only because of its huge capitalization, but also because of the wide sweep of its business and of its resources. This giant

[1] *In re Debs*, 158 U. S., 564.

corporation, which is well described by Dr. Gutmann in the book mentioned in our list, is chartered under a law of New Jersey. Congress has
no power over manufacture as such. In 1895, in a decision in an action
against the Sugar Trust, the Supreme Court held that, although a combination had been formed controlling 98 per cent of the sugar-refinery
of the country, this did not come within the scope of the anti-trust legislation. Only the consequences of combination, not the combination
itself, could be dealt with.

Although it was generally supposed that railways were exempt from
the anti-trust legislation, since they were already covered by the Act to
regulate commerce, some of the most signal decisions have been those
concerned with railways. In 1897 and in 1898, in the Traffic Association
cases,[1] organizations formed to maintain "reasonable " rates were declared to be combinations to maintain rates, and therefore prohibited
by the anti-trust legislation. Railways were declared to be "instruments
of commerce," and their business is commerce itself. This was carried
further in the Northern Securities decision in 1904. In this case a
"holding company " of exceedingly wide powers was formed under a
New Jersey charter. By control of majority stock-holdings in the Great
Northern and the Northern Pacific, it controlled these railways and their
subordinate lines. Not one mile of the railways concerned was situated
in the State from which the charter was obtained. The holding company
did not operate the railways; it simply controlled them through its
majority holdings. By deciding that this company was a combination
in restraint of trade, the Court, while avoiding a direct expression of
opinion on the subject, in reality decided that ownership of property
falls within the scope of the legislation whenever such ownership, if
allowed to continue, might result in restraint of interstate commerce.

The powers of Congress over Trusts under existing legislation, as
established by court decisions, are substantially as follows. The power
to regulate gives the power to prohibit; this may be exercised either
under the taxing power or under the interstate commerce clause. Every
combination which directly or necessarily operates in restraint of trade
or commerce among the several States is illegal. Railways engaged in
interstate commerce are subject to the anti-trust Act. Congress has established the rule of free competition among those engaged in interstate
commerce; every combination which would extinguish competition
between otherwise competing railways engaged in interstate commerce,
and which would in that way restrain such commerce, is illegal. The
provisions of the anti-trust Act apply to private manufacturers or dealers
as well as to corporations. The natural effect of competition is to
increase commerce; and an agreement whose direct effect is to prevent
this play of competition restrains instead of promoting trade and commerce. The legislative prohibitions are not limited to "unreasonable

[1] 167 U. S., 290, and 171 U. S., 505.

restraints," but are directed against all restraints, whether reasonable or unreasonable; therefore the Court will not consider evidence in regard to the reasonableness of the restraint. It is not necessary to show that a combination results or will result in a complete monopoly; it is only essential to show that by its necessary operation it tends to restrain inter-state commerce or to create a monopoly in such commerce, and to deprive the public of the advantages that flow from free competition.

In his message to Congress in 1901, President Roosevelt said:

In the interest of the whole people the nation should, without interfering with the powers of the States in the matter, itself also assume powers of super-vision and regulation over corporations doing an interstate business.

In annual messages and in addresses he has from time to time returned to the subject, and in stronger terms. A large part of the rising tide of opposition to the Trusts and desire for their adequate regulation, arises from the appreciation of their evils which his educational campaign has evoked. At the same time, when the question of remedies arises, the limitations due to his political connections appear. To those who urge that the Trust problem is to be settled by depriving monopolized prod-ucts of protection through duties, President Roosevelt, in his letter to Congressman Watson, of Indiana, August 20, 1906 — a letter intended to be used as a campaign document — replied as follows:

The cry that the problem can be met by any changes in the tariff, represents, consciously or unconsciously, an effort to divert public attention from the only method of taking regulative action.

The protective tariff is not so important a factor in Trust preservation as some, including Mr. Bryan, think; nor is it a negligible quantity, as President Roosevelt contends. While he has become more radical in his attitude towards domestic industry, he has become more conserva-tive in regard to the tariff. He has inclined more and more to the reactionary attitude of the "stand pat" section of the Republican party — a section which fears that the pillars of the existing edifice will be pulled down if repairs are made on the roof. This attitude was apparent in the President's speech at Milwaukee on April 3, 1903, when he said that to regulate Trusts through the tariff would be to put an end to the prosperity of the Trusts by putting an end to the prosperity of the nation. The speech of Mr. Roosevelt's lieutenant, Mr. Taft, Secretary of War, at Bath, Maine, on Sept. 5, 1906 may be taken as summarizing the President's position.

It is impracticable, by a revision of the tariff, to destroy Trusts. The effect which a protective tariff has in aid of Trusts is a partial exclusion or hampering of foreign competition in articles manufactured by Trusts, thus narrowing the competition to be met and overcome by illegal Trust methods; but the principle of excluding or burdening foreign competition with home competition is the protective system. . . . The question presented is whether it is wiser to maintain the benefits of the protective system, and deal with the evils of the management of Trusts by specific legislation directed to those evils, or, in an attempt to curb Trusts, to pull down the whole protective system.

To the President the Trust problem is one of domestic policy. The policy favored by him and accepted by the Republican party, although not without protest, is summed up under the words publicity and regulation. In his message to the Legislature of New York in 1900, President (then Governor) Roosevelt said:

Supervision and publicity are needed quite as much for the sake of the honest corporations as for the sake of the public. The corporation that manages its affairs honestly has a right to demand protection against the dishonest corporation. . . . The first essential is knowledge of the facts — publicity.

Under legislation enacted in 1903, on the recommendation of the President, provision was made for publicity in regard to corporate affairs by the establishment of a Bureau of Corporations, a sub-department of the new department of Commerce and Labor. Mr. James R. Garfield, a son of the late President Garfield, was appointed Commissioner of Corporations. He was given power to investigate the business of corporations, joint-stock companies, or corporate combinations engaged in interstate commerce; and to gather information to enable the President to make recommendations to Congress in regard to the regulation of interstate commerce. The reports made to the President are to receive such publicity as he may direct. Under this legislation investigations of the conditions existing in the beef and oil industries have been conducted by Mr. Garfield. The work of the Bureau of Corporations is primarily an inquiry into the industrial and legal methods used by the agencies engaged in interstate and foreign commerce; and the purpose of such inquiry is to afford accurate knowledge of the industrial conditions upon which there may be based intelligent legislative action.

The power in regard to regulation has been exercised under the interstate commerce clause. While Mr. Bryan, in his recent speech at Louisville, Kentucky, held that strict regulation of the railways is advisable, he at the same time holds that the country must ultimately accept government ownership in order to escape not only the corrupting effect of the railway in politics, but also the evils arising from extortionate rates and rebates. To President Roosevelt government ownership is a last resort. He believes in railway regulation; and he has been successful in getting the Railway Commission legislation strengthened. He has throughout held that, if rebating were abolished, much of the strength of the Trusts would disappear.

Though the Interstate Commerce Commission has contended almost from the outset that the power to establish a reasonable rate, when a rate has been found unreasonable in an action before the Commission, is essential, its contention was not taken seriously until President Roosevelt, in his annual message in 1904, said:

As a fair security to the shipper, the Commission should be vested with the power, when a given rate is challenged, and after full review found to be unreasonable, to decide, subject to judicial review, what will be a reasonable rate to take its place.

As a result of his urgent advocacy, both in 1904 and in 1905, amendatory legislation was passed in the last session of Congress. In addition to conferring the amendatory rate-making power, the abuses of the "midnight tariff" system are prevented by requiring thirty days' notice of changes in rates, instead of the shorter period formerly demanded. Rebating in any form is forbidden; and stringent penalties are provided. The railway company which shall "offer, grant, or give" a rebate is subject to a fine varying from $1000 to $20,000 for each offense; and railway officials participating in such an arrangement are punishable by fine, or by fine and imprisonment. The shipper who shall "solicit, accept, or receive" a rebate is liable to similar penalties. To ascertain whether rebates are given, the Interstate Commerce Commission is empowered to appoint examiners to inspect the books of the railway companies. Further, in an action dealing with rebates, all rebates received during a period six years prior to the commencement of the action may also be dealt with. Private cars are also placed under the supervision of the Commission.

Though the scope of the anti-trust Act was not extended during the last session of Congress, additional powers of regulation under the interstate commerce clause were granted in regard to other matters. Under the new meat-inspection law, which became effective on October 1, 1906, meat and meat-products can not enter into interstate commerce unless they are marked "inspected and passed." The purpose of the Act is to prevent the use in interstate or foreign commerce of meat and meat-products which are unwholesome or otherwise unfit for human food. The determination of these conditions is delegated to the Bureau of Animal Industry, a sub-department of the Department of Agriculture, under whose immediate authority more than six hundred inspectors have been assigned to places in half as many packing establishments and railway shopping points in the meat-producing districts. As the result of many years agitation, a "pure food" law was passed, which applies to food, drink, and drugs. For the breach of the law fines and imprisonment are provided.

The present is a period of great activity in the prosecution of Trusts, not only in the Federal field, but also in the States. In New York the local ice combination has been prosecuted because of artificial enhancement of prices. In the District of Columbia and in the city of Philadelphia actions have also been initiated against local ice combinations. In Toledo, Ohio, the Circuit Court recently upheld a decision whereby three ice-dealers, who were convicted of violating the State anti-trust Act, were sentenced to fines of $2500 and six months' imprisonment in the work-house. In the same State, on October 19, the Standard Oil Co. was found guilty of infractions of the State anti-trust Act under which fines totalling $5,000,000 may be imposed. An appeal has been lodged against this decision.

But, while in the States some action has been taken against the Trusts, it is in the Federal field that the greatest activity is shown. This activity has been especially noteworthy since President Roosevelt's accession to office. In 1903 a special appropriation of $500,000 was made by Congress to aid in the enforcement of the anti-trust law and the Act to regulate commerce. By legislation of the same year provision was made that in suits under these Acts, when the United States is the complainant and there is a sufficient public interest involved, the case may, on the certificate of the Attorney-General, take precedence on the docket. This power was exercised in the Northern Securities case. The increased activity under these laws is shown in the following table of original proceedings begun and prosecuted:

Periods	For violation of anti-trust Act	For violation of Act to regulate commerce
Under Pres. Harrison	7	17
" " Cleveland	6	32
" " McKinley	3	12
" " Roosevelt	16	60

In the prosecutions arising under the interstate commerce clause there has been a coöperation of the various agencies. Investigations and proceedings have been conducted by the Interstate Commerce Commission; prosecutions under the anti-trust Act have been made by the Department of Justice; while investigations on which actions have been based have been made by the Commissioner of Corporations. Without attempting an exhaustive list, we may mention some of the more salient actions.

In the year 1905 a perpetual injunction was obtained from the Supreme Court against the principal packing companies, restraining them from combining and agreeing on prices at which their products were to be disposed of in States other than those of manufacture. In 1902 an injunction was obtained against the Federal Salt Company. This company had made arrangements whereby other companies agreed neither to import, buy, nor sell salt except from and to the Federal Salt Company, and not to engage in or assist in the production of salt west of the Mississippi River during the continuation of this contract. This arrangement had enhanced the price of salt 400 per cent.

The decision in the Northern Securities case frustrated the attempt to centralize through a holding company the control of competing railways. Proceedings under the rebating section of the railway legislation led on June 22, 1906, to the imposition of fines totalling $75,000 on four of the packing companies and the Chicago, Burlington, and Quincy Railway. Two individual defendants in New York, who had received rebates, were punished by fines and imprisonment, the penalty being $6000 and four months' imprisonment in the first case, and $4000 and three months' imprisonment in the second. This is the first time that rebating has actually been punished by imprisonment; and Attorney-General Moody hopes that it will have "the most potent effect in checking the widespread practice of unlawful discriminations." Early in October the New York Central Railway was found guilty of granting rebates on shipments made by the Sugar Trust. An arrangement had been entered into in 1904 whereby a rebate of five cents per hundred pounds was to be made. The information which led to this action being taken was collected in the first instance by the lieutenants of Mr. W. R. Hearst, and was handed over by him to the Attorney-General. The railway was fined $108,000, or about two dollars in fines for every dollar which it has recently received in rebates. The result is excellent; there is a stability in railway rates that has long been absent. So far, the suits instituted by the Attorney-General have led to the collection of over $300,000 in fines, and the imprisonment of two freight brokers who conspired to get rebates. President Roosevelt's administration claims that the enforcement of the law has greatly improved the situation; and that, to quote the words of Secretary Taft, "the fear of the law has been put into the hearts of the members of these great corporations."

The most important of the actions the Government now has in hand is that against the Standard Oil Co. It is intended to proceed against this company on the ground that it has, contrary to law, been receiving discriminative rates. Investigations have been conducted by Federal grand juries in Ohio, New York, Kansas, and Illinois. In August the grand jury at Chicago returned ten indictments, covering 6428 counts against the Standard Oil Co. for receiving rebates. These investigations are simply preliminary to more general action by the Government. In addition to the proceedings in the Federal courts, the Interstate Commerce Commission is conducting investigations under a resolution of Congress passed at its last session. In November last, Attorney-General Moody instituted an action against the Standard Oil Co. under the anti-trust Act. The stock at once fell from about 700 to 512. A favorable outcome in such a case will mean a very significant expansion of Federal power. In the prohibitions of the anti-trust legislation no provision is made for a company or a corporation which by mere accretion has come to control a dominating part of a particular industry. The Standard Oil claims to be a company, not a combination. In an action against it there will be involved, if its contention that it is a company is upheld, the question whether a monopoly possessed by one company is forbidden; and the further question whether mere size, apart from any overt act, subjects a company to the provisions of the anti-trust legislation. It is probable that, even with an expedited procedure, two years will elapse before the case is decided by the Supreme Court.

There is a danger at the present time that the prevailing fear of Trusts may go too far. The opinion of M. Leroy-Beaulieu, in his "The United States in the Twentieth Century" (p. x), that "an unduly high opinion has been entertained of the dangers as well as of the strength of the Trusts, and of the part they have played in the development of American manufacture," is undoubtedly justified. Especial attention has been devoted to the public dangers arising from inflated capitalization; but time has shown that this is a weakness in the combinations. But the days of "hands off" have passed; and it is well that it is so. At the same time the division of power between the Federal Government and the States renders difficult the work of regulation — a work which, apart from any question of constitutional limitations, has inherent difficulties — and attracts attention to the limitations of the constitution. The State Governments, which were intended to be bulwarks of private right, have too often been the protectors of private greed. Regulation through the individual States is, in default of concerted action, futile; it means irritation, not control.

It may be argued that it is within the power of Congress to pass an incorporation Act, and to grant to corporations so chartered the right to produce. But such corporations would carry on their manufacturing within the confines of some State or States; they would therefore be subject to local regulation and taxation. This would involve radical industrial and political changes. It is the expediency, rather than the legality, of a Federal corporation law which presents a difficulty. The President said, in his Harrisburg speech,

It is the narrow construction of the powers of the national government which in our democracy has proved the chief means of limiting the national power to cut out abuses, and which is now the chief bulwark of the great moneyed interests which oppose and dread any attempt to place them under efficient governmental control.

It is on this ground that he has favored the placing of insurance under national control, although the Courts have repeatedly decided that insurance is not commerce. But in the extension of powers, which he favors, the Government will have to proceed indirectly. The most that can be expected in the way of more thorough control of corporations is that they shall be required to take out licenses before engaging in inter-state commerce. Under such an arrangement the granting of licenses could be made conditional on submission to regulation. Substantially this arrangement is involved in the provisions of the recent meat-inspection law, whose rigid provisions must be met, under penalty of exclusion from interstate commerce.

The weakness of the legislation passed under the interstate commerce clause is patent. The anti-trust law, a hurried compromise measure, in its sweeping prohibitions, makes no distinction between predominating industrial influence due to illicit favors or improper combinations and that due to legitimate economic conditions. The Act to regulate railways has, by its prohibition of pooling (*i. e.* joint-purse arrangements), accelerated the movement towards consolidation. The Supreme Court has held that the rule of free competition laid down in the anti-trust Act applies to railways as well. By declaring illegal all agreements to maintain rates it laid down a technical doctrine which, if upheld in its entirety, would be subversive of business. Whether established formally or informally, agreements as to rates are absolutely essential. Such agreements exist to-day, and must of necessity exist; and, in acting under them, the railways are in technical disobedience to the law.

In his message to the New York Legislature in 1900, Governor Roosevelt said:

Much of the legislation not only proposed but enacted against Trusts is not one whit more intelligent than the medieval Bull against the comet, and has not been one particle more effective.

As President, in his annual message to Congress in 1905, he said:

It is generally useless to try to stop all restraint on competition, whether this restraint be reasonable or unreasonable; and, when it is not useless, it is generally hurtful.

In his message of Dec. 1906 he reiterated the warning.

It is not possible completely to prevent it [consolidation]; and, if it were possible, such complete prevention would do damage to the body-politic.

Though the Supreme Court has said that Congress has established the rule of free competition, and that it is not for the Court to question the industrial expediency of such legislation, there are some signs of a modification of this position. The Circuit Court of Appeals has held [1] that

---

[1] *Whitwell* v. *Continental Tobacco Co.*, 60 C. C. A. Reports, 290.

the Act must have a reasonable construction, and that it could not be the true meaning of the law that every attempt to monopolize any part of interstate commerce was illegal. Somewhat greater strength is given to this position by the decision of Mr. Justice Brewer in the Northern Securities case. This decision was rendered by a bare majority, four judges, including the Chief Justice, dissenting. Though Justice Brewer was of the majority, he filed a separate decision, in which he said that

Congress did not intend to reach and destroy those minor contracts in partial restraint of trade which the long course of decisions at common law had affirmed were reasonable, and ought to be upheld.

This line of reasoning would cause the Court to look to the intent, not to the mere fact, of combination. It is abundantly manifest that, if the movement for Trust regulation in the United States is to be efficiently regulative, not simply prohibitory, it must recognize that the beneficial effect of untrammeled competition — even if it were possible to obtain it — is an outworn sophistry; and that the public is interested not in the mere limitation of competition, whatever be the cause of such limitation, but its effect on national prosperity.

In the enforcement of the laws against combinations, the punitive methods have been prohibitions and fines. Mr. Bryan asks "how many of the Trust magnates are in jail?" He contends that "safety lies not in futile attempts at the restraint of Trusts, but in legislation which will make a private monopoly impossible." As to what constitutes a "private monopoly" he is extremely vague. "The plan of attack," he continues, "must contemplate the total and complete overthrow of the monopoly principle in industry." Again: "The man who is in favor of regulating it [the private monopoly] might just as well take off the mask and declare himself; for you can not regulate a private monopoly; it regulates you."

While President Roosevelt stands for such regulation as will, to quote his favorite phrase, "give a square deal," he is, as the size and intricacy of the problem grow upon him, becoming more radical. The investigations of the Bureau of Corporations (whose latest reports appeared in May) show that illicit railway favors have done much to build up the Standard Oil monopoly. The President holds that railway control is the central matter. The Government must possess full power to supervise and control the railways engaging in interstate traffic — power as thorough as that which it already exercises in regard to the banking system. But it appears that he is at times doubtful of the successful outcome of the regulative policy. To him the problem is becoming twofold — the regulation of the Trusts and the regulation of large fortunes. Recently he has shown that he regards these as a complementary phase of the problem. In his "muck-rake" speech, April 13, 1906, he said that ultimately the nation would have to consider the imposition of progressive taxation with a view to preventing the owners of enormous fortunes handing on more than a certain amount to any one individual. To most this was a mere statement of his beliefs in regard to ultimate tendencies. But in his Harrisburg speech, on October 4, 1906, he stated his position in stronger language.

It is our clear duty to see . . that there is adequate supervision and control over the business use of the swollen fortunes of to-day, and also to determine the conditions upon which those fortunes are to be transmitted, and the percentage they shall pay to the Government whose protecting arm alone enabled them to exist. Only the nation can do this work. . . . I maintain that the national Government should have complete power to deal with all of this wealth which in any way goes into the commerce between the States — and practically all of it that is employed in the great corporations does thus go in.

Had the proposition been simply one to obtain increased revenue through an inheritance tax it would, no doubt, have obtained a generous support. But the ultra-radicalism of a plan whereby social policy, not revenue, is to be the end in view is far in advance of public opinion. The connection between the large fortunes and the illicit phases of the Trust problem is assumed, not proven. If the regulation and limitation of private wealth is to be undertaken, and if the Government is, in its discretion, to determine when a fortune is dangerous to the public — such determination being dependent upon the size of the fortune, not upon its use — such a course will not only be a dangerous invasion of private rights, but will also, of necessity, entail upon the Federal Government a systematic redistribution of wealth — a task for which it is manifestly unsuited.

REPRESENTATIVE COCKRAN ON CORPORATE POWER [1]

Mr. Speaker, it is a stupendous issue — this between the President and the mighty forces of corruption whose challenge of battle he has accepted. The elements arrayed against him are the most formidable that ever did battle in a struggle for privilege. The powers they can invoke are stronger in many respects than the powers exercised by government itself. I wonder if Members of this body realize the extent of the powers these embattled interests can put in motion.

In a lecture delivered in my own State a few weeks ago, I undertook to say that our political system had undergone a silent but radical revolution during the last few years, that the greatest powers in the community were no longer exercised in legislative bodies, in the council chambers of cabinets, or in the offices of a chief executive, but in the rooms where a few men direct the administration of great corporations or plan new corporate enterprises. True, there has been no change in

[1] *Congr. Record*, Feb. 15, 1908.

the outward structure of our institutions, but the most profound revolutions have been those that affect not the form but the substance of government. All the forms of republican government survived in Rome long after the Republic itself had been replaced by absolute despotism. The atrocities of Caligula and Nero and Domitian, perpetrated under the authority of a republic, show that forms the most venerable may be preserved to perpetration of oppressions the most atrocious. And so, sir, the outward structure of our Government remains wholly unchanged. Not merely does our Constitution survive in form, but all our constitutional formulas are still acknowledged universally and invoked exclusively.

Constitutionally each man has the right to go where he pleases, to work when he pleases for whom he pleases and for what he pleases, but between him and the exercise of these privileges lie formidable powers which the Constitution never contemplated and which government does not control. Practically no man can take one step from his own door to engage in the ordinary competitions of life except on conditions and terms fixed by some corporation operating a transit system, controlled by a few persons — generally by one — with whose selection government has nothing to do, whose orders and regulations, though binding on a whole community, government hardly pretends to regulate. What avails it a citizen that legally, constitutionally, theoretically he can sell his labor for what he pleases when the value of the wages he may earn is fixed absolutely by a few men in whose selection he has no voice, whose course he can not control or even influence? The cost of implements necessary to his calling, of the clothes that cover him, the food he eats, the fuel he burns, the materials used in constructing the house that shelters him, are all determined absolutely and even arbitrarily by some half a dozen men, who are also believed to control the chief highways of commerce throughout the country, and, therefore, the immense capital necessary to their operation. With the vast banking deposits which the control of production and transportation places at their disposal these same men dominate the financial institutions of every great city. And thus they govern not merely the volume of production and the means of transportation by which commodities are exchanged, but also, through control of the banks, they regulate credit, which is the very lifeblood of commerce.

Compared with these enormous powers exercised in secret by men clothed with no official authority, subject to no public supervision, acknowledging no responsibility, how trivial are the powers exercised by the nominal or constitutional government, whether State or Federal, or both combined. The National Government never comes in contact with me except when it delivers my letters or examines my baggage at the dock on my return from a foreign trip. These men affect closely every act of my life, every exercise of my muscular energy, every effort that I make for the improvement of my own condition, every plan that I contemplate for the employment of my resources and my talents. While I refrain from crime I have no reason to be conscious that government, Federal or State, exists. But I can not take a step about my daily affairs without paying tribute to these forces, whose authority is undisputable, yet whom it is often impossible to locate, whose power is boundless, yet whose very identity is unknown. [Applause on the Democratic side.]

Sir, the powers wielded by these forces must be controlled by law or they must themselves become actually the government. It has been said that these powers are necessary and inevitable products and features of a highly organized industrial system. The President's message does not discuss the extent of these powers nor the justification of them. It merely insists that whatever they be they must remain subordinate and subject to the law of the land. When we consider the influences they exercise, their power to reward the public man who serves them and to assail the one who obstructs their plans or assails their privilege, it would seem as if the outcome of a conflict between them and the constitutional government might be doubtful. Certain it is that the rewards in their power to bestow are preferred by many men of great talent to the highest honors of public life.

Twenty years ago a seat in the Senate was considered the supreme reward of political success, ample compensation for a lifetime of arduous labor, fitting crown for the most splendid career. Have we not recently seen the toga surrendered by one of the most distinguished Senators to become the adviser of financiers? And it is widely suspected that there are others ready, aye, eager, to follow his example if opportunity offer.

In New York — I speak here of that which is within my own knowledge — there was a time, and that not long ago, when a seat on the bench was the prize toward which every lawyer aspired, the success for which he labored, the fulfillment of his highest ambition. Within a few years we have seen one judge after another quitting that exalted post to accept the retainers of financiers, and it is quite generally believed that those who remain on the bench are straining their eyes for an opportunity to quit the severe atmosphere of the courts for the profitable though less honorable service of corporations.

Sir, this is a spectacle which may well cause thoughtful men the gravest apprehension. The very life of the Republic is involved in maintaining the vigor and independence of the courts. We have restricted the powers of legislature and no injury has followed to the body politic. We may reduce the scope of Executive authority, and no serious harm may ensue. But there must be in every system of government some depository of ultimate power, some department that can fix limits to the authority of all others. In a republic that power must always remain with the courts. It is a significant fact that whenever one of these judges exchanged the judicial ermine that is honorable for the livery of corporations that is profitable he invariably became a mouthpiece and exponent of the apprehensions entertained by his new employers — that the President is inclined to carry his love of justice too far.

Sir, not even when the doubts proceed from the mouths of ex-judges transformed into corporation attorneys can it be admitted that love of justice, however strong, in any public servant is incompatible with the material interest of the people.

Never, at least, sir, will that be admitted on this side of the Chamber. Here we believe that justice is the true fountain of prosperity. [Applause.] So long as justice governs any enterprise it can have no fear of injury from enforcement of the law. Law can never be the foe of industry, but always its companion and handmaiden. Through law it enjoys peace, which is the essential condition of its efficiency. By law its fruits are defended and its prosperity promoted. It is crime which fattens on wrong, and its beneficiaries — the dishonest in commerce, the rotten in morals, the corrupt in politics — that can have any reason to fear the light of publicity or the sword of justice, and against these may that light never be obscured, may that sword never be sheathed. [Applause.]

Sir, if the rewards bestowed on their adherents, advocates, advisers, and apologists by these forces of intrenched wrong be so large that they are preferred to places of highest honor in the public service, so are the penalties formidable that they seek to inflict on their opponents, critics, or prosecutors. It would seem as if the man who incurs their resentment must be prepared to renounce hopes of the most profitable professional employment or of admission to the charmed circle of high finance with its opportunities for enormous profit. He must risk even his hopes of public approval. The storm which has raged round the ears of the President ever since he dared to take up the challenge thrown down by these great interests shows strikingly the extent to which they can affect public opinion by poisoning the sources of public information through their ownership of many leading newspapers. The public man whom they pursue will find his words misquoted or suppressed, if distortion be impossible, his motives assailed, purposes attributed to him which are furthest from his own conception, a thousand difficulties created in his way when he returns to the constituents whom he tried to save from spoliation. The corrupt need no incitement to hostility against the honest. But hitherto many of the well disposed were cajoled into serving these interests by appeals cunningly directed to their fears and prejudices.

When we measure the enormous powers wielded by these interests whose gage of battle the President has now picked up, controlling, as they do, every avenue of success in the professions, in politics, and in commerce, we must realize that hitherto opposition to their unlawful privileges by a public man demanded qualities little short of heroic. Here, sir, is the capital value of the President's message, which all good men must applaud, however they may have criticised or reflected on any former acts of the. Administration. It states in unmistakable terms the exact nature of the contest before the country. Whoever reads it will see that the issue is between enforcing the law against all men and suspending the law in favor of a few men. On that issue, once stated, it will be impossible to divide the American people. The demand for justice embodied in this message neither party will undertake to ignore or deny in its platform — the Republican party because it will not dare and this party of ours because it will not want to evade it. [Applause on the Democratic side.] It results, sir, that the campaign now opening will not be a contest between conflicting principles, but a choice of the champion who will do most effective battle for a cause which all will cherish, or at least profess to cherish. While no one will openly antagonize the President's position, the prospect of their being loyally maintained will turn entirely on the character of the man chosen to enforce them during the next four years.

Sir, it is no ordinary political contest, but a crusade to which the President invites us. The man to make the fight successfully must be animated by the spirit, the courage, and the unselfishness of a crusader. But, sir, the qualities of heroism are not common. The stuff of which crusaders are made is not to be found on every side. These qualities were described vividly more than eight hundred years ago, when Pope Urban II preached the first crusade to the great gathering at Clermont. You remember, sir, that while urging his hearers to take up arms for the delivery of the Holy Land from impious domination he told them they must not expect prizes of any earthly value, but they must renounce all hopes of gain or fortune. They must turn their backs upon the homes they loved; in frail barks they must cross seas wide and stormy; they must walk with bleeding feet over burning sands; they must face with dauntless breasts the scimiter of the Saracen; they must even, if need be, with naked hands climb the walls surrounding the city of the Holy Sepulcher profaned by the infidel's possession, and all these sacrifices must be made, all these fatigues undergone, all these perils incurred without any hope of reward or return, except the consciousness of a high duty loyally done. And as that vast assemblage, moved by his words, cried out with one mighty voice "It is God's will!" "It is God's will!" the Pope added, "Be those words your motto: Id Deus vult — It is God's will! Go forward in His name!"

Mr. Chairman, that spirit of readiness to face all difficulties for the sake of justice because it is God's will is the spirit which must animate the man fit to lead this campaign. Whoever undertakes the burden of this contest hoping for personal reward will very probably be disappointed. With all the avenues to success — professional, financial, and political — guarded, patrolled, policed by sentries of the enemy whom he must fight, he must be ready to suffer, if need be, pecuniary embarrassment, misrepresentations of his motives and conduct, seduction of his allies, betrayal by men he trusts, defeat of his policies by treason even if he be successful at the polls. But, sir, though he be forced to taste all the bitterness of hopeless conflict, his sacrifice will not be in vain, his defeat will not be final. Sooner or later his cause will triumph. Though both parties be complaisant, though legislatures be corrupt, though courts be subservient, though judges may prefer to win the favor of powerful interests than do justice upon wealthy criminals, none the less the cause of the people will prevail, because it embodies that justice against which no organization of men has ever yet been able to make a successful stand. [Applause.]

But, sir, where is this champion to be found who, animated by the spirit of a crusader, will cheerfully face disappointment or disaster rather than compromise a principle, resting his hope of success not upon political finesse, but on devotion to an ideal? There is no crusader on the Republican side except one [applause on the Democratic side], and he is disqualified from the fray. His acceptance of a nomination by either party, or by both parties, would not be elevation, but abasement, almost dishonor. He has renounced the field of politics, and through that renunciation he has been lifted to a nobler plane by the spontaneous judgment of civilization. [Applause on the Democratic side.] Never before in the history of this country has a President, while still in office, succeeded in embodying so completely and voicing so emphatically the conscience of the people that a message of his will be embodied in the platforms of both political parties. And this domination of the whole political field has been accomplished in the face of a rancor fiercer than ever was evoked by any of his predecessors, not while he enjoys even a prospect that his official term may be prolonged, but after he has openly and finally renounced every chance of remaining in office. That, sir, is a position no President has ever before achieved, at least not till long after he had passed from the scenes of contentious politics and the grasses had been growing for many seasons above his breast. [Applause.] The position reached by this man no party success could improve, but any partisan affiliation must lower. For him to become the nominee of a party, whatever the outcome, would be to put on a duller armor, to enlist in a baser cause, to fight behind a meaner banner. [Applause on the Democratic side.] No friend would tempt him to such a descent; no patriot would deem him capable of contemplating it. [Applause.]

THE RAILWAY RATE ACT OF 1906 [1]

Summary by George R. Peck

By the act approved June 29, 1906, and made effective sixty days after its passage, Congress has increased the membership of the Inter-

[1] This summary is taken from the annual address of the President of the American Bar Assoc., 1906.

state Commerce Commission to seven; increased the salary of the office to ten thousand dollars, and made the term of appointment seven years. The law has been extended to include interstate carriage by pipe lines; the term "common carrier" to include "express companies and sleeping car companies"; the term "railroad" to include "all bridges and ferries used or operated in connection with any railroad," all switches, spurs, tracks and terminal facilities of every kind, as also all freight depots, yards and grounds used or necessary in transportation or delivery of property; and the term "transportation" to include cars and other vehicles and all instrumentalities and facilities of shipment or carriage, irrespective of ownership, and all services in connection with the receipt, delivery, elevation and transfer in transit, ventilation, refrigeration or icing, storage and handling of property so transported. Every carrier subject to the act is required to provide and furnish such transportation upon reasonable request and to establish through routes and just and reasonable rates applicable thereto.

All carriers subject to the act must on application construct, maintain and operate on reasonable terms switch connections with any lateral branch line of railroad or shipper tendering interstate traffic where such connection is reasonably practicable, can be safely made, and will furnish sufficient business to justify it. The Commission is empowered to order such connection on complaint of any shipper if the carrier refuses voluntarily so to construct, maintain and operate the demanded connection.

Tariffs must be filed with the Commission and conspicuously posted "in every depot, station or office of such carrier where passengers are received for transportation, in such form that they shall be accessible to the public and can be conveniently inspected," showing all local, through, interstate and interforeign rates and charges of every kind relating to the transportation. Where through lines do not provide through rates, the separate rates of each carrier must appear, and if through rates on freight shipped from the United States through a foreign country into the United States are not so made, public customs duties, "as if said freight were of foreign production," are imposed. No changes in such tariff rates can be made except after thirty days notice, unless the Commission shall, in its discretion, in particular instances, or under special or peculiar circumstances or conditions permit. The names of all carriers, parties to any tariff, must appear thereon and each must file with the Commission express concurrence therein, and copies of all agreements between carriers in respect to transportation covered by the act must be filed with the Commission.

The Commission is authorized to prescribe the form of the schedules or tariffs the carriers are required to keep posted for public inspection. All carriers are forbidden to engage in any transportation of any freight or passenger not covered by such published schedules or to charge "a greater or less or different compensation" than shown by the published schedules, for any service, or extend to any shipper "any privileges or facilities" not specified in such tariffs.

After May 1, 1908, interstate or foreign transportation by any carrier is forbidden of any article or commodity "other than timber and the manufactured products thereof," which has been manufactured, mined or produced by it or under its authority, or which it may own or be interested in, whether in whole or in part, except where necessary and intended for its own use as a common carrier.

Passes and reduced rates are forbidden after this year, except to railroad men and their families, ministers and persons engaged in religious and charitable work, inmates of soldiers' and sailors' homes, and a few other classes.

The act requires that all charges shall be "just and reasonable," and prohibits all others.

The Commission may, *sua sponte*, or on complaint, investigate any rate, charge, regulation or practice, and may determine whether such rate or practice is "unjust or unreasonable, or unjustly discriminatory, or unduly preferential or prejudicial, or otherwise in violation of any of the provisions of this act"; may prescribe a maximum "just and reasonable rate or rates, charge or charges," and "what regulation or practice in respect to such transportation is just, fair and reasonable to be thereafter followed." Its orders (except for the payment of money) shall take effect in such reasonable time, not less than thirty days, and shall continue in force not exceeding two years, as the Commission may prescribe, unless "suspended or modified or set aside by the Commission or be suspended or set aside by a court of competent jurisdiction."

Whenever carriers, parties to a joint tariff, fail to agree as to the division thereof, the Commission may determine for them.

The Commission may, on complaint and hearing, establish through routes and joint rates; determine the proportions of division of rates among them where the carriers refuse or neglect to establish such through routes and joint rates, "provided no reasonable or satisfactory through route exists, and this provision shall apply when one of the connecting carriers is a water line."

Where the shipper renders any service or furnishes "any instrumentality" used in the transportation, the Commission may hear and determine what is a reasonable maximum charge to be paid by the carrier therefor.

The Commission may, on complaint, after hearing, order the defendant carrier to pay complainant the sum of any "award of damages" for a violation of the act. Refusal to pay may be followed by suit by the party entitled, in a Federal Court, wherein the findings and order of the Commission "shall be *prima facie* evidence of the facts therein stated." If the petitioner prevails, costs, including "a reasonable attorney's fee," shall be taxed against the carrier. The complaint must be filed with the Commission within two years from the time "the cause accrues," and court proceedings to enforce any order of the Commission awarding damages within one year from the date of the order. Claims accrued prior to the act may be presented within one year. Where money damages are awarded, a single order may embrace joint plaintiffs and joint defendants, and suit may be brought in any federal judicial district for its enforcement, "where any one of such joint plaintiffs could maintain such suit against any one of such joint defendants."

Process may also be served in any other district where any other joint defendant has its principal operating office.

Service of the Commission's orders are to be made by sending copy thereof through registered mail "to any one of the principal offices or agents of the carrier at his usual place of business," and the registry mail receipt shall be *prima facie* evidence of the "receipt of such order by the carrier in due course of mail."

On failure or neglect of any carrier to obey any order of the Commission. (other than for the payment of money) the injured party or the Commission may apply "to the Circuit Court in the District where such carrier has its principal operating office or in which the violation or disobedience of such order shall happen for an enforcement of such order." Such application is to be by petition and the Court may enforce the order by any proper process. Appeals go direct to the Supreme Court and have precedence over all cases except criminal ones, but do not vacate or suspend the order. These suits are to be brought in the District where the carrier has his principal office.

In time of actual or threatened war and upon demand of the President, preference must be given over all other traffic to the transportation of troops and materials of war, and the carriers are required to adopt every means within their control to facilitate and expedite the military traffic.

The act provides that anything done or omitted by any officer or agent of the carrier constituting a misdemeanor under the interstate Commerce acts shall also subject the carrier corporation to like penalties, and if any official shall knowingly offer and give, or any shipper ask or receive any rebate or discrimination, they shall severally be fined from one thousand dollars to twenty thousand dollars or imprisoned not exceeding two years, or be both fined and imprisoned.

The Commission may require and the carriers must furnish under prescribed penalties annual reports for the preceding year ending June 30th, as well as monthly reports of earnings and expenses, "or special reports within a specified period and subject to like penalty for default." The annual reports are to be in great detail and show nearly everything concerning the financial condition and physical operation of the road.

The Commission may also prescribe forms "of any and all accounts, records and memoranda to be kept by carriers subject to the provisions of this act, including the accounts, records and memoranda of the movement of traffic as well as the receipts and expenditures of moneys," to which the Commission shall at all times have access by its agents, and it is made unlawful under drastic penalties for the carriers to deny such access thereto or "to keep any other accounts, records, or memoranda than those prescribed or approved by the Commission." False entries thereon by any person is made a misdemeanor punishable by fine not less than one thousand dollars or more than five thousand dollars, or by imprisonment for not less than one nor more than five years, or by both fine and imprisonment.

Any examiner who divulges any information, except upon judicial direction, is made subject to a fine not exceeding five thousand dollars or imprisonment not exceeding two years, or both.

On interstate shipments carriers may no longer limit their liability to their own line, but are responsible for loss or damage on the lines of connecting carriers.

All existing laws relating to attendance of witnesses, production of evidence, and compelling testimony are made applicable to all proceedings and hearings under the new act.

By a separate act approved on the same date (June 30, 1906), it is provided that in respect to proceedings under the interstate commerce and related acts "immunity shall extend only to a natural person who, in obedience to a subpœna, gives testimony under oath or produces evidence, documentary or otherwise, under oath."

By an act approved June 20, 1906, the time for continuous interstate transportation of cattle, sheep, swine or other animals has been extended from twenty-eight to thirty-six hours where the owner or custodian so requests the carrier in writing, and requiring unloading, water and feeding under prescribed penalties.

By an act approved June 11, 1906, all interstate carriers are made liable to all employees for injury or death caused by negligence of any of the employees or the defect or insufficiency due to negligence in track equipment, machinery or works. Negligence is made a question of fact for the jury, and slight negligence of the injured employee shall not bar recovery when the negligence of the employer was gross in comparison. No contract of employment nor benefit agreements shall constitute a bar or defense to actions for death or personal injury.[1]

By an act approved June 12, 1906, the importation, exportation or carriage in interstate commerce of falsely or spuriously stamped articles of merchandise made of gold or silver or their alloys is forbidden, and all persons found guilty of violating the act are to be punished as therein prescribed. The act is made effective one year after its passage.

[1] [This act was held unconstitutional by the Supreme Court in 1907. A new act was passed in 1908. See *infra*, p. 527.]

EXTRACTS FROM THE REPORT OF THE INTERSTATE COMMERCE COMMISSION, DECEMBER 23, 1907

To the Senate and House of Representatives:

The Interstate Commerce Commission has the honor to submit its twenty-first annual report for the consideration of the Congress.

Little more is attempted in this report than a general statement of the work performed by the Commission during the past year in the discharge of its official duties. A considerable part of the time has been occupied in giving administrative construction to various provisions of the law for the guidance of both shippers and carriers. To secure the best results of legislation with the least possible delay there was obvious need of a correct and uniform interpretation of the statute. Therefore, without reference to questions arising in particular cases, and to avoid unnecessary controversy, it has seemed our duty to construe the law in advance wherever it appeared obscure or ambiguous, so that the obligations of the railroads and the rights of the public might be promptly understood. This has resulted in numerous rulings explaining our view of the meaning and application of different sections and paragraphs of the statute. These rulings have in practically every instance been accepted by the carriers, even in cases where their legal advisers were not entirely in accord with the opinion of the Commission. The rulings and regulations already promulgated will be revised and printed in a separate document.

The benefits of this course are beyond question. The Commission has endeavored to adopt a workable construction of the law in all cases, and has as a rule announced its conclusions in matters of importance only after conference and discussion with representative shippers and traffic officials. This is especially true with reference to tariff regulations, a subject which is treated at some length in a subsequent part of this report. This matter is fundamental in any scheme of public regulation. There is scarcely a complaint or controversy which is not based upon the schedules of rates and charges established by the carriers. If those schedules are clear and definite in their statements, there is no excuse for disregarding them. If the rates and regulations are reasonable and plainly announced, the shipper knows his rights and the railway official knows the obligations of his company. If the charges are claimed to be excessive or discriminatory, the question can be intelligently determined after the full hearing which the statute provides. It is believed that the efforts of the Commission in this direction have already been fruitful of good results and that they will prove of increasing value in the future.

The amended law has now been in force for upwards of fifteen months, and some opinion may be expressed as to its operation and effects. The substantive provisions of the original act, forbidding the exaction of unreasonable charges and prohibiting discriminations between persons and places, were unchanged by the legislation of 1906. The main purpose of that legislation was to provide more adequate means for the enforcement of rights and duties already declared to exist. The vital principle of a right is found in the obligation to respect it. Without remedial procedure the declaratory portion of any law is little more than the statutory expression of a sentiment, but when efficient machinery for securing observance is provided the performance of definite duties and the recognition of definite rights may be expected to follow in ordinary conduct without resort to litigation. That this is true in regard to the amended act, and to an extent not generally appreciated, is confidently asserted. Just as the value of criminal laws is measured by the peace and security of society rather than the occasional conviction of offenders, so the salutary effects of the present statute are shown in the more general enjoyment of previously existing rights rather than by the number of cases in which the authority of the Commission has been invoked or the list of decisions and prosecutions which makes up the record of administration.

It is likewise true that the substantial and permanent benefits of this law are indirect and frequently unperceived even by those who in fact profit by its observance. It means much for the present and more for the future that the principles of this law have gained greatly in general understanding and acceptance. The injustice of many practices which were once almost characteristic of railway operations is now clearly apprehended, and an insistent public sentiment supports every effort for their suppression. By railway managers almost without exception the amended law has been accepted in good faith, and they exhibit for the most part a sincere and earnest disposition to conform their methods to its requirements. It was not to be expected that needed reforms could be brought about without more or less difficulty and delay, but it is unquestionably the fact that great progress has been made and that further improvement is clearly assured. To a gratifying extent there has been readjustment of rates and correction of abuses by the carriers themselves. Methods and usages of one sort and another which operated to individual advantage have been voluntarily changed, and it is not too much to say that there is now a freedom from forbidden discriminations which is actual and general to a degree never before approached. As this process goes on, as special privileges disappear and favoritism ceases to be even suspected, the indirect but not less certain benefits of the law will become more and more apparent.

An incidental respect in which equality of treatment has been greatly promoted is in such matters as switching, terminal, demurrage, reconsignment, elevation, and other charges making up the aggregate cost of transportation. In the past it was often within the power of a carrier to waive charges of this nature in favor of particular shippers while collecting them from business rivals. Now the law and the rules of the Commission require all charges of this description to be plainly stated in the tariffs and to be applied with the same exactness and uniformity as the transportation rate itself. This is only one of the ways in which distinct advance has been made toward placing competing shippers in each locality upon a basis of equality in the enjoyment of a public service.

It is this general and marked improvement in transportation conditions that the Commission observes with special gratification. The amended law with its enforceable remedies, the wider recognition of its fundamental justice, the quickened sense of public obligation on the part of railway managers, the clearer perception by shippers of all classes that any individual advantage is morally as well as legally indefensible, and the augmented influence of the Commission resulting from its increased authority have all combined to materially diminish offensive practices of every sort and to signally promote the purposes for which the law was enacted.

This results in the voluntary adjustment by the parties without resort to the Commission of a vast number of controversies which otherwise would ripen into complaint and litigation, while in numerous instances a settlement is effected by the friendly intervention of the Commission, through correspondence or personal interviews, between the shipper and carrier directly concerned. The nature and extent of the Commission's efforts in this direction are summarized in another part of this report.

Where formal proceedings were necessary the Commission has generally been able to afford prompt relief when the facts disclosed appeared to warrant a corrective order. Between August 28, 1906, and November 4, 1907, the Commission rendered decisions, after full hearing upon complaint and answer, in 107 contested cases, a list of which appears in a subsequent chapter of this report. In 46 of these cases orders were made against the defendant carriers; in 46 the complaints were dismissed; in the remaining 15 no orders were made, for reasons stated in each proceeding. With a single exception every order made by the Commission in these cases was promptly complied with by the carrier or carriers against which it was directed. In one case a bill was filed to restrain the enforcement of an order, mainly on the ground that the Commission had no authority to make it, and a preliminary stay granted. But the motion for an injunction *pendente lite* was denied, with the result that the order became effective and is now being complied with by the carrier in question. The case has not yet been tried in the Circuit Court.

Two subjects are discussed in subsequent chapters of this report to which, and the recommendations made in connection therewith, special attention is invited. One is the matter of advances in rates, which the

Commission is wholly without power to prevent; the other, the dreadful destruction of life in railway accidents, which are not now the subject of official investigation under Federal authority. Other recommendations are made in connection with various matters which are deemed of sufficient importance to require consideration in this report.

In our last annual report mention was made of the car shortage prevailing at that time and the consequent distress in certain parts of the country. The inability of the Commission to afford any effective relief was pointed out, and it was further stated that the Commission was not prepared to recommend a definite scheme of legislative action. While the car shortage is not at present so acute as a year ago, it still exists in some sections, and the general question of the provision of adequate transportation facilities unquestionably merits serious consideration by the Congress. The whole problem, involving insufficient car and track capacity, congested terminals, slow train movement, and other incidents, may be said to be due to the fact that the facilities of the carriers have not kept pace with the commercial growth of the country. One eminent railroad president has estimated that during the period from 1895 to 1905 the traffic offered for carriage in the United States increased 110 per cent, while during the same period the instrumentalities for handling this traffic increased only 20 per cent.

During the past decade the commercial condition of the country has been one of increasing prosperity. If business undertakings proportionately increase during future years, the railroads of the country must add to their tracks, cars, and other facilities to an extent difficult to estimate. The ability of the carriers to transport traffic measures the profitable production of this vast country, with its ninety millions of people, abundant capital, and practically unlimited resources. Manifestly, it is an economic waste for the farm, the mine, or the factory to put labor and capital into the production of commodities which can not be transported to market with reasonable despatch. If the present output can not in many instances be transported except after ruinous delays, it is not reasonable to presume that capital will readily seek investment in new undertakings. It may conservatively be stated that the inadequacy of transportation facilities is little less than alarming; that its continuation may place an arbitrary limit upon the future productivity of the land, and that the solution of the difficult financial and physical problems involved is worthy the most earnest thought and effort of all who believe in the full development of our country and the largest opportunity for its people.

Under the operation of the Interstate Commerce Act the right to initiate interstate rates rests entirely with the railway, which may, by giving thirty days' notice, put into effect any rate or any regulation or practice affecting a rate which it sees fit. The Commission is not required to approve these rates and has no authority whatever to condemn them. It can only act upon a rate so established by the railway in case a formal complaint is filed attacking that rate and after a full hearing. This is the express provision of the statute.

RATE SCHEDULES AND APPLICATION OF RATES

Definiteness, clearness, and simplicity in stating transportation charges, uniformity in applying the rates so stated, and stable conditions are ends aimed at in the law and sought by the Commission in administering it. ·

Prior to the enactment of the amended law the time of notice of changes in rates required by the act was too short to give stability to conditions of transportation, even if the terms of the law had been carefully observed. Tariffs were issued upon statutory notice and upon no notice at all. Opportunities to get business were met by issuing a tariff "expiring with this shipment;" by quotation of rates found in some other carrier's tariffs and applicable via another route; by quotation of rates not found in any tariff; by forwarding under regular tariff rates and refunding an agreed-upon portion thereof and by forwarding under regular tariff rates and agreeing to "protect" any rate of any competing carrier. Some carriers openly published declarations of which the following is a sample:

"Tariffs published by connecting lines to competitive points on this road, or to points beyond, which do not read in connection with this road, will be protected by this road, if the rates in such tariff are less than those published by originating line in connection with this road."

As a necessary outcome of such practices the official files of tariffs were very voluminous and contained an endless number of contradictions and conflicts. To bring order out of this condition and at the same time have all the carriers conducting transportation to the utmost extent of their overtaxed facilities was an important, a delicate, and a large undertaking.

This work was approached by the formation, after exhaustive conferences with traffic officials of carriers, of a code of regulations governing the construction of tariffs, which was promulgated to become effective May 1, 1907, and June 1, 1907, as to freight and passenger tariffs, respectively.

This code has been supplemented from time to time, as occasion demanded, by administrative rulings of the Commission, by which many misunderstandings and differences of opinion have been harmonized. It is pleasing to note that such rulings have, very generally, been cheerfully accepted by carriers and shippers.

As an aid to elimination of the objectionable, contradictory, and conflicting features which were contained in the tariffs that were on file and in use when the amended act became effective, and for the purpose of permitting carriers to promptly adjust interstate rates in harmony with interstate rates that were changed by State authorities, the Commission has exercised its discretion to permit changes in rates and schedules on less than statutory notice more freely than it would under different conditions.

Many of the features that have been eliminated affected the interests of so many shippers and localities that considerable time was necessarily consumed in arranging for and providing superseding rates and regulations which would not work severe or irreparable injury to innocent parties. Much has been done along this line, much is now being done, and much remains to be done. The task is by no means hopeless and, now that a good foundation is laid for it, more progress will be apparent on the surface in the future. In this work the Commission has insisted upon all of the progress that was possible within the limits of the ability of the carriers' tariff and rate forces and the capacity of the available printing facilities. In the twelve months ended November 30, 1907, there were filed with the Commission 220,982 tariff publications, all containing changes in rates and rules governing transportation, and about 400,000 notices of concurrence in tariffs.

Under former practices, adopted and followed by the carriers, no provision was made for definite concurrence by a carrier in tariffs issued by another carrier. The general, if not universal, understanding was that a carrier accepted any rates published by another carrier if it did not file specific notice of nonconcurrence therein. This liability was not, however, always accepted, and numerous complications and controversies arose from a carrier denying responsibility under a tariff on the ground that it had not specifically concurred therein. The tariff regulations adopted by the Commission require affirmative, definite concurrence from a carrier before it may be named as a party to a joint tariff.

Much traffic is moved under joint tariffs, participated in by many carriers, and issued by joint agent, who acts under powers of attorney given by his several principals. This plan commends itself strongly. It operates to reduce the number of tariff publications and assists greatly in avoiding conflict between tariffs of a given carrier in two or more of which conflicting rates upon the same commodity, between the same points and at the same time are, under old practices, not infrequently found.

The unrestrained and run-mad competition which has been resorted to in the past has resulted in the establishment of some conditions, privileges, contracts, and allowances in connection with the furnishing of transportation by carriers, which created, or which contain the elements of, the discriminations which the law condemns. Many of these are of long standing, are far-reaching in their effects, and involve some fine questions of law. The requirement that every privilege or charge in connection with the transportation offered by a carrier shall be plainly stated in a duly published, filed, and posted tariff will, no doubt, eliminate the discriminatory practices, except such as may be the subject of litigation before this Commission or in the courts.

* * * * * * * *

DIVISION OF PROSECUTIONS

Early in the present year the Commission organized a new division known as the "division of prosecutions," to take full charge of investigations into criminal violations of the act to regulate commerce. On receipt of information of any violation of the act amounting to a criminal infraction of the law, it becomes the duty of this division to make such investigations as may be necessary to determine whether or not the matter is one proper to be brought to the attention of the Department of Justice. In any case where it is finally determined by the Commission that a criminal prosecution is proper, it is the duty of the division to prepare the case for presentation to the United States attorney in the district having jurisdiction.

In connection with this work of enforcement of the law by means of criminal prosecutions, the Department of Justice and its various district attorneys have, throughout the year, been active and effective. Almost without exception those prosecutions brought to trial have resulted in convictions; also a number of highly important cases have been won in the appellate courts.

Investigations during the year by the division of prosecutions give warrant for the statement that rebating by the direct payment of money or by billing at less than the published rates is now far less common than ever before. The amendments to the act to regulate commerce and to the Elkins Act, made in June, 1906, by which imprisonment as a possible penalty was restored, are chiefly responsible for this cessation in rebating by direct methods.

Preferences are undoubtedly enjoyed by some shippers by which they are given a substantial advantage over their unfavored competitors. The means by which the bulk of these preferences are given are so plainly devices to evade the law that no new legislation is necessary for their suppression.

OPERATING DIVISION OF THE COMMISSION

Since the twentieth annual report of the Commission was submitted to Congress, 5,156 complaints have been filed with the Commission for consideration and action. These cases include both formal and informal complaints, as well as proceedings and investigations instituted by the Commission upon its own motion and under resolutions of the Congress. The number of formal cases and investigations instituted during the year was 415, relating directly to the rates and practices of 2,236 carriers. This shows a very great increase over previous years, as the number of such complaints filed in 1905 was 65 and 82 in the year 1906, while the total number filed during the six years previous to 1907 was 350, or 65 less than in the present year. A detailed statement of the formal complaints docketed during the year, with a brief statement of the provisions of the law claimed to be violated, will be found in Appendix C of this report. In addition to these formal complaints, 359 petitions for reparation have been filed and served on more than 2,500 carriers as a result of the decisions of the Commission in the cases of H. H. Tift and others against the Southern Railway Company and others, and Central Yellow Pine Association against the Illinois Central Railroad Company and others, which decisions were sustained by the Supreme Court of the United States. Accompanying these petitions were thousands of pages of tabulated statements showing the shipments of lumber upon which reparation is claimed, adding materially to the work necessary to the filing and serving of these petitions.

The work of the Commission in all its branches has increased to such an extent that it seems almost impossible to prepare a statement that will show the relative yearly increase with any degree of accuracy. Take, for example, the increase in the number of complaints filed, which, of course, means a corresponding increase in the amount of work performed in the Operating Division alone. In the year 1905, when only 65 complaints were filed, it required in the service of the complaints and the assignment of the cases for hearing the preparation of 2,500 letters and notices, while during the present year this branch of the work, not counting general correspondence in regard to the cases, amounted to more than 15,000 letters and notices. In addition to this something like 2,500 answers and other pleadings were filed, each one of which had to be filed, docketed, and acknowledged.

As shown in a detailed statement further on in this report, 276 hearings were held during the year at various places in the United States, at which more than 35,000 pages of testimony were taken, amounting to something like 88,000 folios. A comparison with the hearings of former years shows an increase of 350 per cent, as 79 hearings were held in 1905 and 73 in 1906. Some of these hearings occupied the attention of one or more Commissioners or special examiners from one day to a week. In one instance eighteen days were occupied in the hearing of one complaint, while a number required more than a week each.

In the matter of informal complaints filed during the present year an even greater increase is found. During the present year 4,382 complaints of this character were filed with the Commission, as against 503 in the year 1905, and 1,002 in the year 1906, showing an increase of more than 400 per cent over the preceding year. It is found impracticable to give a more detailed statement of these informal proceedings in this report, but it may safely be stated that they allege violations of every section of the law.

During the year informal reparation claims were awarded to injured shippers by the Commission in 561 cases, aggregating about $104,700. A synopsis of these cases appears in Appendix F of this report, which shows the causes for which the money damages were allowed. About 200 reparation claims were denied. So important has this branch of the work become that it has recently been made a special division and transferred to the Division of Statistics and Accounts.

In the matter of the correspondence of the Commission this steady yearly increase is still further manifested. During the year 1905 the Commission received 23,720 letters and in 1906, 29,966 letters, while during the present year 66,933 letters were received, briefed, filed, and answered, averaging more than 218 letters for each working day in the year. This statement relates entirely to the operating branch of the Commission.

The increased power vested in the Commission by the recent amendments to the act has naturally led to the multiplication of the number of complaints presented by letter, and these complaints relate to every conceivable subject connected with the rates, methods, practices, and service of interstate carriers.

A fair conception of the work performed by the Commission in the field of regulation is not possible without reference to the results attained in respect to these cases in which formal complaint is not filed, nor proceedings of a formal nature pursued by the complainant. The public is not advised of the full extent of the work accomplished in securing, through correspondence, the voluntary adjustment by carriers of questions in dispute relating to interstate transportation, nor is the public cognizant of the extreme importance and value of the results attained.

Through the medium of correspondence is secured the settlement of many matters extremely vexatious to shippers. The questions thus amicably adjusted are not alone questions affecting the interest of individuals; on the contrary, the effect of the action taken by carriers in the adjustment of these complaints is often of widespread interest and advantage to large communities, if not indeed of vital importance to considerable sections of country. Controversies arising out of the relations between the carriers themselves are likewise, in many instances, presented to the Commission for arbitration. The Commission is also called upon frequently by traffic officials of carriers to indicate what is considered to be the proper and lawful course to be pursued in respect to the application of rates or regulations affecting transportation. Thus it will be seen that many great benefits result from the adjustment or settlement through correspondence of questions informally submitted for investigation.

The traffic officials of the carriers have manifested to a commendable degree a disposition and willingness to fairly and carefully consider the merits of complaints thus called to their attention by the Commission, and have voluntarily reduced their rates and applied corrective measures in numerous cases.

Naturally many of the informal complaints presented, while involving grievances growing out of conditions related to interstate transportation, are yet not within the purview of the provisions of the statute or the jurisdiction of the Commission. Of the total number of complaints filed almost one-half were cases of this nature. In approximately 2,500 cases the informal complaint made had relation to matters within the jurisdiction of the Commission, and in nearly 1,400 cases relief has been secured and amicable adjustment effected through correspondence, without the necessity or expense of formal proceedings. In respect to 600 of these cases, including those in which special reparation orders were granted upon submission of claims to the Commission by the consignee, consignor, or by the carriers themselves, the remedy thus applied by the carriers involved the reduction of rates.

The adjustment of more than 600 cases, including those claims in respect to which authority was granted to carriers to make special reparation, resulted in refund to shippers of a portion of the charges previously collected. Relief has also been secured through the intervention of the Commission in respect to many other miscellaneous matters, among which may be specially mentioned the securing of improved service in cases where shippers complained of being subjected to inconvenience and loss owing to the failure or refusal of carriers to furnish equipment for the transportation of their commodities; also through expediting the settlement of claims filed against railroad companies in cases where unreasonable delay in making final disposition is charged.

The carriers declined to take action for the removal of the cause of complaint in 875 cases, basing their refusal upon the contention that the rates or practices in regard to which complaint related were just and reasonable. Quite a large number of the informal complaints filed during the year are still pending, awaiting further information or advice from the complainant or action by the carrier.

Two hundred and seventy-six hearings and investigations of alleged violations of the act to regulate commerce, including several investigations under joint resolutions of Congress, have been had at general sessions of the Commission at its office in Washington and at special sessions held in New York, and other cities throughout the United States.

THE EMPLOYERS' LIABILITY BILL [1]

WASHINGTON, April 10. — By far the most important bill of the present session of Congress has passed the two houses, with only one dissenting vote recorded against it. Political exigencies demanded that the Republicans enact an employers' liability law to replace the one recently shattered by a Supreme Court decision. The terms and provisions of the law were, in a manner of speaking, unimportant. The main thing was to enact a law which could bear the title of an employers' liability measure.

Therefore, it has come to pass that the measure of largest general consequence passed by Congress at this session, affecting thousands of people, was enacted after forty minutes of restricted discussion in the House, and a brief afternoon of superficial and perfunctory debate in the Senate. Many of the able lawyers in both branches of Congress believe the act will not stand the test of the Supreme Court. If an employers' liability law is finally to take its place on the statute book, they believe, all of the work will have to be done over again. Indeed, so widely prevalent is this belief that the bill, which has been sent to the President for its approval, is in several of its features so clearly unconstitutional that in the House Mr. Parker of New Jersey, Mr. Payne of New York, Mr. Keifer of Ohio, openly said as much. Nevertheless, they voted for the bill, leaving Mr. Littlefield of Maine the sole dissenter in either branch against the bill.

The conditions in the Senate, under which the bill was hurriedly passed yesterday afternoon, caused Senator Teller to make earnest protest. Senator Teller was not the only person who confessed to a lack of information about the bill. Many Senators said privately yesterday afternoon that they had not even read the House bill, which the Senate passed without amendment. It is absurd on the face of it that there should be unanimous agreement in both Houses of Congress on a bill involving important Constitutional questions. In so small a body as the Supreme Court, the proverbial division of the justices is five to four on all cases involving grave Constitutional problems. This was the division on the previously enacted employers' liability law.

The Senate's hasty action yesterday afternoon came as a surprise. It is no uncommon thing for the members of the House to follow, sheep-like, in a trail blazed for them by their so-called leaders. Observers of legislation in Washington have become accustomed to seeing the House passing up undigested legislation to be properly whipped into shape after thorough and intelligent discussion in the Senate. It is also no uncommon sight to see one of the great annual appropriation bills authorizing an expenditure of $20,000,000 or more yawned through the

[1] *The New York Evening Post*, April 10, 1908.

Senate on a dreary afternoon, and practically without debate. But it does cause comment and surprise when a bill involving Constitutional rights is rattled through the Senate without deliberation and without any debate worthy of the name.

Senator Knox was so confident that the employers' liability law, which recently failed to meet the Supreme Court test, was unconstitutional, that, before the court had handed down its decision, he had ready for introduction in the Senate another measure intended to meet the objections which he felt sure the court would raise. He precisely foreshadowed the court's decision, and immediately introduced his bill. This is the measure that Senator Teller referred to as "the Senate bill."

On January 6 last the Supreme Court declared the previously enacted employers' liability act unconstitutional upon the one main ground that it undertook to apply its provisions to all common carriers engaged in interstate commerce, regardless of the fact that injuries may often happen to employees of such carriers who are not at the time of the injury engaged in forwarding interstate commerce. The decision, in which the court was divided — four to five — held that the failure of Congress to separate the employees who are engaged in interstate commerce at the time of the injury from the mass of the employees of the common carrier, was sufficient to destroy the validity of the act.

Senator Dolliver, in explaining the enactment which now awaits the approval of the President, asserted that it contained four substantive propositions, which he outlined.

First, it modifies the old law of the negligence of coemployees. The old law, which took root in the United States two generations ago, was to the effect that an employee injured by the negligence of a fellow-workman could not recover. This bill abolishes that doctrine, and gives the employee the right to recover for injuries arising from the negligence of his fellow-workman.

The second proposition modifies the law whereby, in other generations, workmen were held by the court to assume the risks arising from defective machinery.

In the third place, the present enactment modifies radically the law of contributory negligence. As administered by our courts it has been uniformly held that an employee suffering an injury to which his own negligence contributed can not, by reason of that participation in the injury, have any recovery at law. This act liberalizes that doctrine of the law. It is based upon the theory that where an injury occurs partly by reason of the negligence of the employer and partly by reason of the negligence of an employee, the jury ought to determine what part of the injury arises from the negligence of the plaintiff and take away from the sum total of his damages allowed that part which can properly be apportioned to his own negligence. That principle has been called in some of the books the "doctrine of comparative negligence."

In the fourth place, the present bill undertakes to modify somewhat the common law applicable to certain agreements or contracts made between employers and their workmen, in which the latter agree, in consideration of some form of insurance or indemnity fund, to give up the right to sue in the courts.

THE BUREAU OF CORPORATIONS

[The newly created Department of Commerce and Labor numbers among its subdivisions the Bureau of Corporations. ·The nature of the work of this bureau is set forth in the following synopsis of the first report of the bureau and by extracts from the report of December, 1906.]

The Report of December, 1904

THE first general report of the Commissioner of Corporations, James R. Garfield, covering the period from the organization of the bureau to June 30, 1904, shows that the work of the bureau up to that date had been almost entirely the laying of a foundation of accurate knowledge of the legal and general business conditions with which the bureau must deal and a clear definition of the problems for the consideration of which it was created. The result of the work is summarized as follows:

(1) Commercial and industrial conditions present the foremost problems of to-day. There exists a deep-rooted general feeling of dissatisfaction with existing conditions. Some causes of dissatisfaction are apparent, and the evils very real and great.

(2) The present legal conditions under which corporate business is carried on are extremely unsatisfactory. They admit of, and invite, extreme abuse. They are the result of forced growth under divergent pressures, and in their present anomalous state represent the needs or demands of special interests and are not a permanent body of law adopted to provide properly for all the interests involved. Furthermore, the "State system," applied to interstate businesses, has developed additional and peculiar evils; a diversity so great as to amount in operation to anarchy; an inevitable tendency toward the lowest level of lax regulation, and the unequal and disastrous contest between State Legislatures and commercial forces of national size and power.

(3) No satisfactory reform is to be expected under the "State system" of incorporation.

(4) The Federal Government has at its command sufficient power to remedy these conditions in its control of interstate commerce, supplemented by subsidiary and incidental powers.

(5) So far the commerce clause of the Constitution has had a negative development only, both under Congress and by judicial interpretation. With

the exception of the interstate commerce act — the force of which has been seriously weakened by judicial interpretation — and the navigation laws, there has been no really affirmative attempt to regulate interstate commerce. The commerce clause has been chiefly used to prevent the interference by States with interstate commerce.

(6) The creation of this bureau affords a means for getting essential facts. In addition to the value to Congress of such information, the publication of facts, the dissemination of knowledge, will bring into existence the influence of an enlightened public opinion which properly applied would go far to develop the sense of public trust involved in the control of private wealth and the sense of personal responsibility on the part of officers or managers of corporations.

(7) The work of the bureau can proceed along the lines of inquiry and report, adding fact upon fact in proof of existing conditions, but no real remedy can be expected until Congress takes action by affirmative use of the great powers granted under the commerce clause of the Constitution.

(8) The possible Congressional actions are:

(a) Delegation to the States of control over interstate commerce. This is believed to be unconstitutional, and secondly subject to all the objections applicable to the present "State system."

(b) Compulsory Federal incorporation of interstate commerce companies. This is probably legally practicable, but it involves radical industrial and political changes by the centralization of power in the Federal Government, and presents serious difficulties because of its effect upon the authority of the States over such corporations in matters of taxation and local regulation. Any optional law of this character would not overcome these difficulties.

(c) Federal license or franchise for interstate commerce. Legally this is practicable; it avoids the legal difficulties of national incorporation as well as the practical one of centralization of power, and gives the national Government direct regulation of the agencies of interstate and foreign commerce.

(9) I therefore beg to suggest that Congress be requested to consider the advisability of enacting a law for the legislative regulation of interstate and foreign commerce under a license of franchise, which in general should provide as follows:

(a) The granting of a Federal franchise or license to engage in interstate commerce.

(b) The imposition of all necessary requirements as to corporate organization and management as a condition precedent to the grant of such franchise or license.

(c) The requirement of such reports and returns as may be desired as a condition of the retention of such franchise or license.

(d) The prohibition of all corporations and corporate agencies from engaging in interstate and foreign commerce without such Federal franchise or license.

(e) The full protection of the grantees of such franchise or license who obey the laws applicable thereto.

(f) The right to refuse or withdraw such franchise or license in case of violation of law, with appropriate right of judicial appeal to prevent abuse of power by the administrative officer.

This bureau, under the direction of the secretary of Commerce and Labor, affords the appropriate machinery for the administration of such a law. It is fully appreciated that this recommendation is not new, but has been the subject of most serious and exhaustive consideration by public officials and commissions, as well as private persons technically well qualified to speak. The Industrial Commission, in its final report on this subject, recommended, among other things, the adoption of a plan quite similar to this. It is neither necessary nor wise to attempt, in this report, to elaborate the details of such an act; but the bureau has upon its files abundant, and in many particulars, exhaustive information which would be immediately available for the use of Congress or any committee thereof which might have under consideration such a measure.

WORK OF THE BUREAU

The report begins with a recital of the law under which the bureau was created, followed by a description of its organization. Its first work was a thorough study of the purposes of its organic law and the jurisdiction and powers of the Commissioner. The report says that the work of the bureau falls naturally into the following divisions:

(a) Special investigations of particular corporations, joint stock companies, or corporate combinations engaged in interstate and foreign commerce. For this purpose the commissioner is given power to compel the production of testimony.

(b) The collection and publication of useful information regarding corporations engaged in interstate and foreign commerce.

(c) Insurance companies are included specifically under the work of obtaining useful information; but because of the decisions of our courts regarding insurance the question of the power of the commissioner over insurance companies requires special consideration. Federal control over insurance and the exercise over insurance corporations of the compulsory powers of the commissioner rest upon the same legal basis, raising at the outset the question whether insurance is in any of its forms interstate commerce. . . . The rapid development of insurance business, its extent, the enormous amount of money and the diversity of interests involved, and the present business methods suggest that under existing conditions insurance is commerce, and may be subjected to Federal regulations through affirmation action by Congress. The whole question is receiving most careful consideration upon both legal and economic grounds.

(d) Legal research — A most important branch of work is the determination of the entire legal situation applicable to the bureau, to its powers, and to its present and future work, developing the same along the following lines:

(1) Compiling and digesting court decisions applicable to the bureau, to its powers of investigation, its legal status and the means by which it shall perform its functions, and to the great questions and problems which are before the bureau.

(2) Compiling and digesting Federal and State statute laws relating to the purposes of the bureau.

(3) Compiling and comparing the laws of foreign countries upon kindred subjects.

(4) Compiling and digesting in summarized and available form facts showing the actual operation of such laws now in existence.

(5) Preparing in outline such possible and desirable modifications of existing laws relating to the subject-matter of the Bureau's work as may be from time to time indicated by development of that work.

(6) Determining the legal relations that would be established by the enactment of such possible modifications with especial reference to the effects thereof on State laws, and the interrelation of Federal and State jurisdictions.

(e) Economic and statistical work — In this work there will be the greatest possible use of all material available from other Government offices in order to avoid unnecessary duplication of effort, expense, and almost inevitable conflicts in results. Statistics will be compiled and published only for the purpose of properly presenting the special problems with which the Bureau is dealing. The economic work will necessarily be of vital importance in preparing and presenting the results of special investigations, and in rightly interpreting the mass of information obtained.

The commissioner's powers are defined as follows:

Subject to the direction of the secretary of commerce and labor, to investigate the organization, conduct, and management of corporations (other than common carriers) engaged in interstate commerce; to compel by subpœna the attendance of witnesses, and the production of books, papers, and documents for such purpose; to administer oaths; to obtain the aid of the Federal courts in the procuring of such testimony; to require reports from such corporations; to investigate the legal conditions applicable to such corporations, and the legal questions raised thereby; and to report to the President the information so acquired. The commissioner may determine the form of procedure in investigations, subject to the qualification that hearings may not be in public.

The commissioner has no judicial powers, nor can he make or enforce any orders against corporations or private individuals other than those directly necessitated in procuring information. He can impose no fines or penalties. Even within the scope of his duties, he must invoke the aid of a Federal court for the enforcement of his proper orders or requirements. . . . His entire compulsory powers of inquiry are further confined to the consideration of facts relating to corporations, joint stock companies, or corporate combinations.

The study of the law and industrial conditions, as above outlined, resulted in the adoption of the following general policy regarding the Bureau and the conduct of its work:

As the commissioner is not charged with the enforcement of any law nor with the prosecution of persons or corporations alleged to be or found to be violating any law, the work of the Bureau is primarily an inquiry into the industrial and legal methods used by the agencies engaged in interstate and foreign commerce, and the purpose of such inquiry to afford accurate knowledge of industrial conditions upon which there may be based intelligent legislative action.

In the investigation of special corporations the commissioner will necessarily acquire knowledge of business facts, the publication of which would be an infringement of private rights. The method of reporting and making public the results of these investigations affords a means, through the President, for protecting private rights. In this particular the method of procedure is similar to the action and reports of the comptroller of the currency regarding national banks. There will thus be presented to Congress all relevant facts except such as would afford to any corporation information which would injure the legitimate business of a competitor and destroy the incentive for individual superiority and thrift.

While the purpose of inquiries and special investigations is not to discover violations of Federal statutes, yet, if facts are found showing such violation, they will be reported as other facts to the President for such consideration and action as may be appropriate or necessary.

Under present industrial conditions, secrecy and dishonesty in promotion, overcapitalization, unfair discrimination by means of transportation and other rebates, unfair and predatory competition, secrecy of corporate administration, and misleading or dishonest financial statements are generally recognized as the principal evils. It is admitted that the chief difficulty in the way of providing ample remedies has been the conflict between Federal and State authority as to jurisdiction over many of the acts of great industrial agencies, and the uncertainty of the extent of regulation exercised or to be exercised by the Federal Government over agencies engaged in both State and interstate commerce.

The immediate work is, hence, not to prove the existence of such evils and difficulties, but to find possible remedies for them. The remedies must not be simply to destroy existing bad conditions — mere destruction affords only temporary relief — but they must provide something better to take the place of what is changed. The imposition of severe penalties will not end industrial evils. We must find and remove their cause, leaving only the extreme or exceptional cases to be dealt with by criminal statutes.

The Government should secure means for fair business competition, freedom from unjust discrimination, such publicity of corporate organization and management as will disclose real financial worth and methods, should provide a jurisdiction broad enough to meet existing conditions, and then should fully protect the person or corporation obeying the law and promptly punish the violator of the law.

The facts upon which remedial legislation must be based are in the possession of persons and corporations engaged in business — some have been given to the public, others have been incidentally furnished through judicial and legislative proceedings, and others have been held as business secrets. As to the first two classes, the Bureau has been systematically collecting them from all available sources; as to the last class, special inquiries have been made or are being made from particular corporations. In dealing with this class of facts it is recognized that there is a fair ground for discussion as to whether certain questions are infringements upon private rights; hence the following method of procedure has been adopted:

Inquiry is made directly from the persons or corporations under investigation; if it be determined that the Government is entitled to the information, it must be given voluntarily or the compulsory process of the statute will be invoked; if the Government is not entitled to the information, then no detective method will be used to discover it.

There has been no attempt to define the scope of the inquiry to be made, nor to limit it to certain classes of facts. All facts which will give information regarding interstate and foreign commerce, or will assist Congress in regulating such commerce, are subjects of legitimate inquiry.

One line of inquiry concerning which question has been raised is as to the cost of production of articles used in or subjects of interstate and foreign commerce. So far it has not been necessary to test this question in court, but it is believed that aside from any other reason the question is proper because of the power of Congress to impose tariff duties in the regulation of commerce. The ideal tariff duty is the difference between the cost of production at home and abroad; hence Congress has the right to know what is the cost of production. Furthermore, it is claimed that the tariff gives an unfair advantage to corporations and persons engaged in the manufacture and distribution of protected articles which are the subjects of interstate and foreign commerce. Congress has the right to know whether this be true or not, and this Bureau affords a most appropriate and efficient means for obtaining such information.

In brief, the policy of the Bureau in the accomplishment of the purposes of its creation is to coöperate with, not antagonize, the business world; the immediate object of its inquiries is the suggestion of constructive legislation, not the institution of criminal prosecutions. It purposes, through exhaustive investigations of law and fact, to secure conservative action and to avoid ill-considered attack upon corporations charged with unfair or dishonest practices. Legitimate business — law-respecting persons and corporations — have nothing to fear from the proposed exercise of this great governmental power of inquiry.

The report goes on to discuss corporation law, and the present system of incorporation by States; the various Federal and State anti-trust laws, tax laws, and laws against unfair competition; the constitutional powers of Congress over corporate business, concluding with remedial legislation.

Annual Report of the Commissioner of Corporations 1906

Sir: I have the honor to submit the report of the Commissioner of Corporations for the fiscal year ended June 30, 1906.

There have been no changes in the Act of Feburary 14, 1903, by which the Bureau was created. Certain important statutory changes, however, have taken place, which do affect the Bureau; first, the Act of Congress approved June 30, 1906, defining the extent to which immunity from prosecution shall be allowed to those giving information under the compulsory powers of the Commissioner, which act merely declares and makes unquestionable the clear intent of the existing law; and second, the so-called railway-rate law, which amends the Interstate Commerce Act and acts amendatory thereof.

The total appropriations for the Bureau for the said fiscal year were $217,879.40. The amount of $136,535.80 was expended. The appropriations for the fiscal year 1906 to 1907 are $185,920.

The number of persons employed by the Bureau on June 30, 1906, was 73. The estimates for the year ending June 30, 1908, are $248,220.

As the investigations conducted by the Bureau often expand in unforeseen directions it is impossible to estimate with accuracy the specific work which will be done in a given period. It has been, therefore, wise to keep the organization in a flexible condition, so that its force may be applied as the exigencies of the work develop; with the lump sum appropriation it has been possible to adapt the means to the end desired with comparatively little waste of time or money.

The legal work of the Bureau in the past year has been largely concerned with the interpretation of statutes relating to transportation, together with a consideration of numerous proposed forms of legislation on this subject. Considerable time also has been devoted to laws relating to railway discriminations. The report of the Commissioner on the Transportation of Petroleum, which dealt almost entirely with railway discriminations in favor of the Standard Oil Company, has led to a very careful consideration of the interstate commerce act, the Elkins Act, and various other laws affecting transportation. Pursuant to the letter of the President, submitting the said report to Congress, the Department of Justice has taken up the discriminations set forth in the said report and assistance has been given by this Bureau to the Department of Justice in preparing criminal cases in connection therewith.

Digests of the various State corporation laws in the Bureau have been kept up to date and compilations have been made of certain branches of such laws.

During the course of the investigation of the oil industry it was discovered that a very widespread system of railway discriminations existed in favor of the Standard Oil Company, affecting a very large proportion of the country and resulting substantially in giving to the Standard Oil Company an overwhelming advantage in transportation in almost all sections of the country; that this system had been in existence for a number of years, and that largely by virtue of it the Standard had been able to restrict or eliminate competition throughout many parts of the country and thereafter reap the benefits of monopoly. These railway discriminations took various forms, often very ingenious in their nature, and so skilfully concealed that their existence was very rarely suspected even by the active competitors of the Standard, although such competitors knew that in general they were doing business at a disadvantage. This system of discriminations was discovered by the agents of the Bureau when examining the oil-shipping records and accounts of the various railroads.

So important was the effect of these discriminations that it was deemed best to make a special report on the Transportation of Petroleum. This report was submitted to the President and by him transmitted to Congress on May 2, 1906. The regular adjournment of Federal Courts for the summer has made it impossible as yet to secure the trial of any of the criminal cases growing out of this investigation, but indictments containing 8,193 counts have been returned by the various grand juries. It is claimed that the various devices by which these discriminations were obtained are permissible under the law, but this contention seems untenable. The purpose of the law is to provide equality of opportunity and treatment to all shippers. The law deals with the result, not the device by which the result is accomplished. The more clever the device the more flagrant is the violation of the law, for wilful intent to evade is shown. If this be not the true interpretation of the law, it becomes worse than useless, because it offers false security and opens the door to fraud.

A most striking and important result immediately followed the investigation of the Bureau; the railroads canceled substantially all the secret rates, illegal or improper discriminations, and in many cases the discriminations in open rates. Thus a widespread system of railway discrimination was wiped out of existence because of the discovery by the agents of the Bureau and before any prosecutions were brought thereon. The shippers of oil advise the Bureau that for the first time in many years they are now rapidly obtaining equality of treatment from the transportation companies.

Work on the other phases of the oil industry and the investigations of the tobacco, steel, sugar, and coal industries are well advanced; special reports thereon will be made in due course. An inquiry into canal and water transportation has been started.

The work of the Bureau during the past year presents very strikingly the power of efficient publicity for the correction of corporate abuses wholly apart from the penal or remedial processes of the Courts. No more convincing illustration of this power has been given than the experience of the Bureau in connection with the above-mentioned system of railway discriminations in favor of the Standard Oil Company and the change of the system by its mere exposure. In most cases, as soon as the officers of a railroad were aware that the agent of the Bureau had discovered a discrimination, the improper rate was canceled or the discrimination removed. This action on the part of the railroad officers was all the more striking inasmuch as it could hardly have been taken with a view to escape from criminal liability, because that criminal liability, if existing at all, had already been incurred and could not be mitigated or evaded by cancellation of the discriminatory rate or regulation; and further, the fact of that voluntary action was a convincing admission of the unfairness of the rate or regulation. In short, the experience of the Bureau indicates that enforced publicity of facts is a most efficient means of putting an end to such discriminations.

A great advance toward publicity has been made by the new law increasing the powers of the Interstate Commerce Commission. All books and records of railroad companies are now open to the examination of agents of the Commission. The Government will no longer be hampered by being limited to search for single items, but every entry, every record will be scrutinized.

The meat-inspection and pure-food laws are the most recent examples of the extension of the principle of publicity. The meat-inspection law goes further by affirmatively establishing the principle of imposing a condition precedent upon the right to engage in interstate commerce. Meat products cannot be transported in interstate and foreign commerce until they have been subjected to Federal inspection and such inspection evidenced by labels. This is in effect the requirement of a license to engage in interstate commerce.

The investigations conducted by the Bureau, the effect of the interstate-commerce laws, the results of prosecutions under the anti-trust law, the reasons which compelled the enactment of the meat-inspection and pure-food laws, all lead me to earnestly urge again the desirability of and necessity for the establishment of Federal inspection and supervision of the greater industrial corporations engaged in interstate and foreign commerce, substantially as outlined in the license plan suggested in my annual reports for 1904 and 1905.

Such a plan is but the extension of a well-tried and efficient means for the proper regulation of business. It will not interfere with the power and authority of the States over the corporations created under State laws. It will be the exercise of direct affirmative power by the Federal Government over the actions of corporations when engaged in interstate and foreign commerce, which cannot be dealt with by State authority. It will give a simple and effective method of dealing with such corporations in a jurisdiction coextensive with their field of operation.

Such inspection is not an invasion of private rights. A corporation should not be treated as an individual; it has great powers and enjoys public rights which an individual cannot exercise; it is given some of the attributes of sovereignty, i. e., perpetual life, and in some instances the right of eminent domain; the unrestricted exercise of its powers may permit it to grow strong enough to unduly influence and in measure control the political life of the State which created it. Such a result would be intolerable. Hence, for reasons of public safety and self-preservation a government must retain and exercise proper regulation of and control over corporations. Such regulation and control can not

vestigations of law and fact, to secure conservative ...
considered attack on corporations charged with un-
tices. Legitimate business — law-respecting persons
have nothing to fear from the proposed exercise of this
power of inquiry.

The report goes on to discuss corporation law, and
of incorporation by States; the various Federal a:
laws, tax laws, and laws against unfair competition;
powers of Congress over corporate business, conclud:
legislation.

ANNUAL REPORT OF THE COMMISSIONER OF COR:

SIR: I have the honor to submit the report of the
Corporations for the fiscal year ended June 30, 1906.
There have been no changes in the Act of Febura
which the Bureau was created. Certain important st:
however, have taken place, which do affect the Burea:
of Congress approved June 30, 1906, defining the i(
immunity from prosecution shall be allowed to those
tion under the compulsory powers of the Commissic
merely declares and makes unquestionable the clear int(

ing law; and Interstate Commerce Act ...

The total ... $21,879 ... priations ... year ...

The number ... 73. ...

...

Digests of the various State corporation ... kept up to date and ...

of such laws.

During the course of the ... covered that a very widespread ... in favor of the Standard Oil Company ... tion of the country and reaching ... Oil Company an overwhelming ... all sections of the country, that ... a number of years, and that largely to ... been able to restrict or eliminate ... the country and thereafter reap the ... way discriminations took various forms ... nature, and so skillfully concealed that ... suspected even by the active ... competitors knew that ... vantage. This system of ...

be wisely exercised unless the government has full and accurate knowledge of the ownership, management, and properties of corporations. This knowledge can only be obtained by opening all the books and records of corporations to public inspection, but protecting, of course, the corporation from unreasonable examination or the injurious exposure of its legitimate business.

The suggested Federal license law will restore individual responsibility and prevent the corporation from being the hiding place of the irresponsible, dishonest, or corrupt manager. As long as the individual can hide behind a corporation, can conceal his acts upon the records of a corporation, can escape personal responsibility by means of the corporation, so long will the corporation be used as an agency for imposition, fraud, and corruption. The moment the books and records of a corporation are open to proper public inspection the danger of such wrongs will be reduced to a minimum. The corporation is not then soulless, for the individuals who control it are known, and personal responsibility for its actions can be instantly fixed upon them.

Such a law will afford a means for gaining accurate information, so that the people of our country may form an intelligent opinion of industrial conditions, and not be driven to extreme and unwise action by the clamor of those who assail all great corporate interests because some have done ill.

Above all, a license system will provide the most effective method for dealing with the corporation whose managers violate law, by providing that the penalty for such violation shall be the revocation of the license, and the consequent denial of the opportunity to engage in interstate commerce. Such a penalty should not, of course, be imposed without affording the corporation opportunity to appeal to the courts and obtain necessary protection against unjustifiable or improper executive action.

Respectfully,   JAMES RUDOLPH GARFIELD,
Commissioner of Corporations.
The SECRETARY OF COMMERCE AND LABOR.

PRESERVATION AND DEVELOPMENT OF NATURAL RESOURCES

[The natural resources of the United States appeared unlimited even in the last generation, but at the present time the nation and its leaders are coming to realize that the wasteful methods of exploitation which have thus far been employed can no longer be tolerated lest the county should lose its rich inheritance. In order to preserve and develop the natural resources, new administrative services have been established in the federal and state governments, and laws have been passed designed to protect the national wealth against wasteful methods of exploitation. The questions involved in this matter are illustrated by the following selections.]

FROM THE SECOND ANNUAL MESSAGE OF PRESIDENT CLEVELAND, DECEMBER, 1886

THE recommendations of the Secretary of the Interior and the Commissioner of the General Land Office looking to the better protection of public lands and of the public surveys, the preservation of national forests, the adjudication of grants to States and incorporations and of private land claims, and the increased efficiency of the public-land service, are commended to the attention of Congress. To secure the widest distribution of public lands in limited quantities among settlers for residence and cultivation, and thus make the greatest number of individual homes, was the primary object of the public-land legislation in the early days of the republic. This system was a simple one. It commenced with an admirable scheme of public surveys, by which the humblest citizen could identify the tract upon which he wished to establish his home. The price of lands was placed within the reach of all the enterprising, industrious, and honest pioneer citizens of the country. It was soon, however, found that the object of the laws was perverted, under the system of cash sales, from a distribution of land among the people to an accumulation of land capital by wealthy and speculative persons. To check this tendency a preference right of purchase was given to settlers on the land, a plan which culminated in the general Preemption Act of 1841.

The foundation of this system was actual residence and cultivation. Twenty years later the homestead law was devised more surely to place actual homes in the possession of actual cultivators of the soil. The land was given without price, the sole conditions being residence, improvement, and cultivation. Other laws have followed, each designed to encourage the acquirement and use of land in limited individual quantities. But in later years these laws, through vicious administrative methods and under changed conditions of communication and transportation, have been so evaded and violated that their beneficent purpose is threatened with entire defeat. The methods of such evasions and violations are set forth in detail in the reports of the Secretary of the Interior and Commissioner of the General Land Office. The rapid appropriation of our public lands without *bona fide* settlement or cultivation, and not only without intention of residence, but for the purpose of their aggregation in large holdings, in many cases in the hands of foreigners, invites the serious and immediate attention of Congress.

The energies of the land department have been devoted, during the present administration, to remedy defects and correct abuses in the public-land service. The results of these efforts are so largely in the nature of reforms in the processes and methods of our land system as to prevent adequate estimate; but it appears by a compilation from the reports of the Commissioner of the General Land Office, that the immediate effect in leading cases which have come to a final termination, has been the restoration to the mass of public lands of 2,750,000 acres; that 2,370,000 acres are embraced in investigations now pending before the Departments of the courts, and that the action of Congress has been asked to effect the restoration of 2,790,000 acres additional; besides which four million acres have been withheld from reservation, and the rights of entry thereon maintained.

I recommend the repeal of the Preëmption and Timberculture Acts, and that the homestead laws be so amended as better to secure compliance with their requirements of residence, improvement, and cultivation for the period of five years from date of entry, without commutation or provision for speculative relinquishment. I also recommend the repeal of the desert-land laws, unless it shall be the pleasure of the Congress so to amend these laws as to render them less liable to abuses. As the chief motive for an evasion of the laws, and the principal cause of their result in land accumulation instead of land distribution, is the facility with which transfers are made of the right intended to be secured to settlers, it may be deemed advisable to provide by legislation some guards and checks upon the alienation of homestead rights and lands covered thereby until patents issue.

ADDRESS OF PRESIDENT ROOSEVELT ON NATURAL RESOURCES, BEFORE THE MEETING OF GOVERNORS, 1908

GOVERNORS of the several States; and gentlemen: I welcome you to this conference at the White House. You have come hither at my request so that we may join together to consider the question of the conservation and use of the great fundamental sources of wealth of this nation. So vital is this question, that for the first time in our history the chief executive officers of the States separately, and of the States together forming the nation, have met to consider it.

With the Governors come men from each state chosen for their special acquaintance with the terms of the problem that is before us. Among them are experts in natural resources and representatives of national organizations concerned in the development and use of these resources; the Senators and Representatives in Congress; the Supreme Court, the Cabinet, and the Inland Waterways Commission have likewise been invited to the conference, which is therefore national in a peculiar sense.

This conference on the conservation of natural resources is in effect a meeting of the representatives of all the people of the United States called to consider the weightiest problem now before the nation; and the occasion for the meeting lies in the fact that the natural resources of our country are in danger of exhaustion if we permit the old wasteful methods of exploiting them longer to continue.

With the rise of peoples from savagery to civilization, and with the consequent growth in the extent and variety of the needs of the average man, there comes a steadily increasing growth of the amount demanded by this average man from the actual resources of the country. Yet, rather curiously, at the same time the average man is apt to lose his realization of this dependence upon nature.

Savages, and very primitive peoples generally, concern themselves only with superficial natural resources; with those which they obtain from the actual surface of the ground. As peoples become a little less primitive, their industries, although in a rude manner, are extended to resources below the surface; then, with what we call civilization and the extension of knowledge, more resources come into use, industries are multiplied, and foresight begins to become a necessary and prominent factor in life. Crops are cultivated; animals are domesticated; and metals are mastered.

Every step of the progress of mankind is marked by the discovery and use of natural resources previously unused. Without such progressive knowledge and utilization of natural resources population could not grow, nor industries multiply, nor the hidden wealth of the earth be developed for the benefit of mankind.

Rapid Pace of Present-Day Living

From the first beginnings of civilization, on the banks of the Nile and the Euphrates, the industrial progress of the world has gone on slowly, with occasional setbacks, but on the whole steadily, through tens of centuries to the present day. But of late the rapidity of the process has increased at such a rate that more space has been actually covered during the century and a quarter occupied by our national life than during the preceding six thousand years that take us back to the earliest monuments of Egypt, to the earliest cities of the Babylonian plain.

When the founders of this nation met at Independence Hall in Philadelphia the conditions of commerce had not fundamentally changed from what they were when the Phœnician keels first furrowed the lonely waters of the Mediterranean. The differences were those of degree, not of kind, and they were not in all cases even those of degree. Mining was carried on fundamentally as it had been carried on by the Pharaohs in the countries adjacent to the Red Sea.

The wares of the merchants of Boston, of Charleston, like the wares of the merchants of Nineveh and Sidon, if they went by water, were carried by boats propelled by sails or oars; if they went by land, were carried in wagons drawn by beasts of draught or in packs on the backs of beasts of burden. The ships that crossed the high seas were better than the ships that had once crossed the Ægean, but they were of the same type, after all — they were wooden ships propelled by sails; and on land, the roads were not as good as the roads of the Roman empire, while the service of the posts was probably inferior.

In Washington's time anthracite coal was known only as a useless black stone; and the great fields of bituminous coal were undiscovered. As steam was unknown, the use of coal for power production was undreamed of. Water was practically the only source of power, save the labor of men and animals; and this power was used only in the most primitive fashion. But a few small iron deposits had been found in this country, and the use of iron by our countrymen was very small. Wood was practically the only fuel, and what lumber was sawed was consumed locally, while the forests were regarded chiefly as obstructions to settlement and cultivation.

Such was the degree of progress to which civilized mankind had attained when this nation began its career. It is almost impossible for us in this day to realize how little our revolutionary ancestors knew of the great store of natural resources whose discovery and use have been such vital factors in the growth and greatness of this nation, and how little they required to take from this store in order to satisfy their needs.

RESOURCES AND GROWTH OF THE UNITED STATES

Since then our knowledge and use of the resources of the present territory of the United States have increased a hundredfold. Indeed, the growth of this nation by leaps and bounds makes one of the most striking and important chapters in the history of the world. Its growth has been due to the rapid development, and alas! that it should be said, to the rapid destruction, of our natural resources. Nature has supplied to us in the United States, and still supplies to us, more kinds of resources in a more lavish degree than has ever been the case at any other time or with any other people. Our position in the world has been attained by the extent and thoroughness of the control we have achieved over nature; but we are more, and not less, dependent upon what she furnishes than at any previous time of history since the days of primitive man.

Yet our fathers, though they knew so little of the resources of the country, exercised a wise forethought in reference thereto. Washington clearly saw that the perpetuity of the States could only be secured by union, and that the only feasible basis of union was an economic one; in other words, that it must be based on the development and use of their natural resources. Accordingly, he helped to outline a scheme of commercial development, and by his influence on Interstate Waterways Commission was appointed by Virginia and Maryland.

It met near where we are now meeting, in Alexandria, adjourned to Mount Vernon, and took up the consideration of interstate commerce by the only means then available, that of water. Further conferences were arranged, first at Annapolis and then at Philadelphia. It was in Philadelphia that the representatives of all the States met for what was in its original conception merely a waterways conference; but when they had closed their deliberations the outcome was the Constitution which made the States into a nation.

The Constitution of the United States thus grew in large part out of the necessity for united action in the wise use of one of our natural resources. The wise use of all of our natural resources, which are our national resources as well, is the great material question of to-day. I have asked you to come together now because the enormous consumption of these resources, and the threat of imminent exhaustion of some of them, due to reckless and wasteful use, once more calls for common effort, common action.

Since the days when the Constitution was adopted, steam and electricity have revolutionized the industrial world. Nowhere has the revolution been so great as in our own country. The discovery and utilization of mineral fuels and alloys have given us the lead over all other nations in the production of steel. The discovery and utilization of coal and iron have given us our railways, and have led to such industrial development as has never before been seen. The vast wealth of lumber in our forests, the riches of our soils and mines, the discovery of gold mineral oils, combined with the efficiency of our transportation, have made the conditions of our life unparalleled in comfort and convenience.

PRESENT DRAIN ON OUR RESOURCES

The steadily increasing drain on these natural resources has promoted to an extraordinary degree the complexity of our industrial and social life. Moreover, this unexampled development has had a determining effect upon the character and opinions of our people. The demand for efficiency in the great task has given us vigor, effectiveness, decision, and power, and a capacity for achievement which in its own lines has never yet been matched. So great and so rapid has been our material growth that there has been a tendency to lag behind in spiritual and moral growth; but that is not the subject upon which I speak to you to-day.

Disregarding for the moment the question of moral purpose, it is safe to say that the prosperity of our people depends directly on the energy and intelligence with which our natural resources are used. It is equally clear that these resources are the final basis of national power and perpetuity. Finally, it is ominously evident that these resources are in the course of rapid exhaustion.

This nation began with the belief that its landed possessions were illimitable and capable of supporting all the people who might care to make our country their home; but already the limit of unsettled land is in sight and, indeed, but little land fitted for agriculture now remains unoccupied, save what can be reclaimed by irrigation and drainage. We began with an unapproached heritage of forests; more than half of the timber is gone. We began with coal fields more extensive than those of any other nation, and with iron ores regarded as inexhaustible, and many experts now declare that the end of both iron and coal is in sight.

The mere increase in our consumption of coal during 1907 over 1906 exceeded the total consumption in 1876, the centennial year. The enormous stores of mineral, oil, and gas are largely gone. Our natural waterways are not gone, but they have been so injured by neglect, and by the division of responsibility and utter lack of system in dealing with them, that there is less navigation on them now than there was fifty years ago. Finally, we began with soils of unexampled fertility, and we have so impoverished them by injudicious use and by failing to check erosion that their crop-producing power is diminishing instead of increasing. In a word, we have thoughtlessly, and to a large degree unnecessarily, diminished the resources upon which not only our prosperity but the prosperity of our children must always depend.

We have become great because of the lavish use of our resources, and we have just reason to be proud of our growth. But the time has come to inquire seriously what will happen when our forests are gone, when the coal, the iron, the oil, and the gas are exhausted, when the soils shall have been still further impoverished and washed into the streams, polluting the rivers, denuding the fields, and obstructing navigation. These questions do not relate only to the next century or to the next generation. It is time for us now as a nation to exercise the same reasonable foresight in dealing with our great natural resources that would be shown by any prudent man in conserving and widely using the property which contains the assurance of well-being for himself and his children.

Two Classes of Resources

The natural resources I have enumerated can be divided into two sharply distinguished classes accordingly as they are or are not capable of renewal. Mines, if used, must necessarily be exhausted. The minerals do not and can not renew themselves. Therefore, in dealing with the coal, the oil, the gas, the iron, the metals generally, all that we can do is to try to see that they are wisely used. The exhaustion is certain to come in time.

The second class of resources consists of those which can not only be used in such manner as to leave them undiminished for our children, but can actually be improved by wise use. The soil, the forests, the waterways come in this category. In dealing with mineral resources, man is able to improve on nature only by putting the resources to a beneficial use which in the end exhausts them; but in dealing with the soil and its products man can improve on nature by compelling the resources to renew and even reconstruct themselves in such manner as to serve increasingly beneficial uses — while the living waters can be so controlled as to multiply their benefits.

Neither the primitive man nor the pioneer was aware of any duty to posterity in dealing with the renewable resources. When the American settler felled the forests, he felt that there was plenty of forest left for the sons who came after him. When he exhausted the soil of his farm he felt that his son could go West, and take up another. So it was with his immediate successors. When the soil-wash from the farmer's fields choked the neighboring river he thought only of using the railway rather than boats for moving his produce and supplies.

Now all this is changed. On the average the son of the farmer of to-day must make his living on his father's farm. There is no difficulty in doing this if the father will exercise wisdom. No wise use of a farm exhausts its fertility. So with the forests. We are over the verge of a timber famine in this country, and it is unpardonable for the nation or the States to permit any further cutting of our timber, save in accordance with a system which will provide that the next generation shall see the timber increased instead of diminished. Moreover, we can add enormous tracts of the most valuable possible agricultural land to the national domain by irrigation in the arid and semi-arid regions and by drainage of great tracts of swamp land in the humid regions. We can enormously increase our transportation facilities by the canalization of our rivers so as to complete a great system of waterways on the Pacific, Atlantic, and Gulf coasts, and in the Mississippi valley, from the Great Plains to the Alleghenies, and from the northern lakes to the mouth of the mighty Father of Waters. But all these various uses of our natural resources are so clearly connected that they should be coördinated, and should be treated as part of one coherent plan and not in haphazard and piecemeal fashion.

It is largely because of this that I appointed the Waterways Commission last year, and that I have sought to perpetuate its work. I wish to take this opportunity to express in heartiest fashion my acknowledgment to all the members of the Commission. At great personal sacrifice of time and effort they have rendered a service to the public for which we cannot be too grateful. Especial credit is due to the initiative, the energy, the devotion to duty, and the far-sightedness of Gifford Pinchot, to whom we owe so much of the progress we have already made in handling this matter of the coördination and conservation of natural resources. If it had not been for him this convention neither would nor could have been called.

Duty of the Nation

We are coming to recognize as never before the right of the nation to guard its own future in the essential matter of natural resources. In the past we have admitted the right of the individual to injure the future of the republic for his own present profit. The time has come for a change. As a people, we have the right and the duty, second to none other but the right and duty of obeying the moral law, of requiring and doing justice, to protect ourselves and our children against the wasteful development of our natural resources, whether that waste is caused by the actual destruction of such resources or by making them impossible of development hereafter.

Any right-thinking father earnestly desires and strives to leave his son both an untarnished name and a reasonable equipment for the struggle of life. So this nation, as a whole, should earnestly desire and strive to leave to the next generation the national honor unstained and the national resources unexhausted. There are signs that both the nation and the States are waking to a realization of this great truth. On March 10, 1908, the Supreme Court of Maine rendered an exceedingly important judicial decision. This opinion was rendered in response to questions as to the right of the Legislature to restrict the cutting of trees on private land for the prevention of droughts and floods, the preservation of the natural water supply, and the prevention of the erosion of such lands, and the consequent filling up of rivers, ponds, and lakes. The forests and water power of Maine constitute the larger part of her wealth and form the basis of her industrial life, and the question submitted by the Maine Senate to the Supreme Court and the answer of the Supreme Court alike bear testimony to the wisdom of the people of Maine, and clearly define a policy of conservation of natural resources, the adoption of which is of vital importance, not merely to Maine, but to the whole country.

Policy of Preservation

Such a policy will preserve soil, forests, water power as a heritage for the children and the children's children of the men and women of this generation; for any enactment that provides for the wise utilization of the forest, whether in public or private ownership, and for the conservation of the water resources of the country, must necessarily be legislation that will promote both private and public welfare; for flood prevention, water-power development, preservation of the soil, and improvement of navigable rivers are all promoted by such a policy of forest conservation.

The opinion of the Maine supreme bench sets forth unequivocally the principle that the property rights of the individual are subordinate to the rights of the community, and especially that the waste of wild timber land derived originally from the State, involving as it would the impoverishment of the State and its people, and thereby defeating one great purpose of government, may properly be prevented by State restrictions.

The court says there are two reasons why the right of the public to control and limit the use of private property is peculiarly applicable to property in land: "First, such property is not the result of productive labor, but is derived solely from the State itself, the original owner; second, the amount of land being incapable of increase, if the owners of large tracts can waste them at will without State restriction, the State and its people may be helplessly impoverished, and one great purpose of government defeated. . . . We do not think the proposed legislation would operate to 'take' private property within the inhibition of the Constitution. While it might restrict the owner of wild and uncultivated lands in his use of them, might delay his taking some of the product, might delay his anticipated profits and even thereby might cause him some loss of profit, it would nevertheless leave him his lands their product and increase, untouched, and without diminution of title, estate, or quantity. He would still have large measure of control and large opportunity to realize values. He might suffer delay but not privation. . . . The proposed legislation . . . would be within the legislative power and would not operate as a taking of private property for which compensation must be made."

The Court of Errors and Appeals of New Jersey has adopted a similar view, which has recently been sustained by the Supreme Court of the United States. In delivering the opinion of the court on April 6, 1908, Mr. Justice *Holmes* said:

"The State as quasi-sovereign and representative of the interests of the public has a standing in court to protect the atmosphere, the water, and the forests within its territory, irrespective of the assent or dissent of the private owners of the land most immediately concerned. . . . It appears to us that few public interests are more obvious, indisputable, and independent of particular theory than the interest of the public of a State to maintain the rivers that are wholly within it substantially undiminished, except by such drafts upon them as the guardian of the public welfare may permit for the purpose of turning them to a more perfect use. This public interest is omnipresent wherever there is a State, and grows more pressing as population grows . . . . We are of opinion, further, that the constitutional power of the State to insist that its natural advantages shall remain unimpaired by its citizens is not dependent upon any nice estimate of the extent of present use or speculation as to future needs. The legal conception of the necessary is apt to be confined to somewhat rudimentary wants, and there are benefits from a great river that might escape a lawyer's view. But the State is not required to submit even to an æsthetic analysis. Any analysis may be inadequate. It finds itself in possession of what all admit to be a great public good, and what it has it may keep and give no one a reason for its will."

These decisions reach the root of the idea of conservation of our resources in the interests of our people.

FROM THE MESSAGE OF PRESIDENT ROOSEVELT, DECEMBER 3, 1907

Inland Waterways. The conservation of our natural resources and their proper use constitute the fundamental problem which underlies almost every other problem of our National life. We must maintain for our civilization the adequate material basis without which that civilization cannot exist. We must show foresight, we must look ahead. As a nation we not only enjoy a wonderful measure of present prosperity but if this prosperity is used aright it is an earnest of future success such as no other nation will have. The reward of foresight for this Nation is great and easily foretold. But there must be the look ahead, there must be a realization of the fact that to waste, to destroy, our natural resources, to skin and exhaust the land instead of using it so as to increase its usefulness, will result in undermining in the days of our children the very prosperity which we ought by right to hand down to them amplified and developed. For the last few years, through several agencies, the Government has been endeavoring to get our people to look ahead and to substitute a planned and orderly development of our resources in place of a haphazard striving for immediate profit. Our great river systems should be developed as national water highways; the Mississippi, with its tributaries, standing first in importance, and the Columbia second, although there are many others of importance on the Pacific, the Atlantic, and the Gulf slopes. The National Government should undertake this work, and I hope a beginning will be made in the present Congress; and the greatest of all our rivers, the Mississippi, should receive especial attention. From the Great Lakes to the mouth of the Mississippi there should be a deep waterway, with deep waterways leading from it to the East and the West. Such a waterway would practically mean the extension of our coast line into the very heart of our country. It would be of incalculable benefit to our people. If begun at once it can be carried through in time appreciably to relieve the congestion of our great freight-carrying lines of railroads. The work should be systematically and continuously carried forward in accordance with some well-conceived plan. The main streams should be improved to the highest point of efficiency before the improvement of the branches is attempted; and the work should be kept free from every taint of recklessness or jobbery. The inland waterways which lie just back of the whole eastern and southern coasts should likewise be developed. Moreover, the development of our waterways involves many other important water problems, all of which should be considered as part of the same general scheme. The Government dams should be used to produce hundreds of thousands of horsepower as an incident to improving navigation; for the annual value of the unused water power of the United States perhaps exceeds the annual value of the products of all our mines. As an incident to creating the deep waterway down the Mississippi, the Government should build along its whole lower length levees which taken together with the control of the headwaters, will at once and forever put a complete stop to all threat of floods in the immensely fertile Delta region. The territory lying adjacent to the Mississippi along its lower course will thereby become one of the most prosperous and populous, as it already is one of the most fertile, farming regions in all the world. I have appointed an Inland Waterways Commission to study and outline a comprehensive scheme of development along all the lines indicated. Later I shall lay its report before the Congress.

Reclamation Work. Irrigation should be far more extensively developed than at present, not only in the States of the Great Plains and the Rocky Mountains, but in many others, as, for instance, in large portions of the South Atlantic and Gulf States, where it should go hand in hand with the reclamation of swamp land. The Federal Government should seriously devote itself to this task, realizing that utilization of waterways and water-power, forestry, irrigation, and the reclamation of lands threatened with overflow, are all interdependent parts of the same problem. The work of the Reclamation Service in developing the larger opportunities of the western half of our country for irrigation is more important than almost any other movement. The constant purpose of the Government in connection with the Reclamation Service has been to use the water resources of the public lands for the ultimate greatest good of the greatest number; in other words, to put upon the land permanent home-makers, to use and develop it for themselves and for their children and children's children. There has been, of course, opposition to this work; opposition from some interested men who desire to exhaust the land for their own immediate profit without regard to the welfare of the next generation, and opposition from honest and well-meaning men who did not fully understand the subject or who did not look far enough ahead. This opposition is, I think, dying away, and our people are understanding that it would be utterly wrong to allow a few individuals to exhaust for their own temporary personal profit the resources which ought to be developed through use so as to be conserved for the permanent common advantage of the people as a whole.

Public Lands. The effort of the Government to deal with the public land has been based upon the same principle as that of the Reclamation Service. The land law system which was designed to meet the needs of the fertile and well-watered regions of the Middle West has largely broken down when applied to the dryer regions of the Great Plains, the mountains and much of the Pacific slope, where a farm of 160 acres is inadequate for self-support. In these regions the system lent itself to fraud, and much land passed out of the hands of the Government without passing into the hands of the home-maker. The Department of the Interior and the Department of Justice joined in prosecuting the offenders against the law; and they have accomplished much, while where the administration of the law has been defective it has been changed. But the laws themselves are defective. Three years ago a public lands commission was appointed to scrutinize the law, and defects, and recommended a remedy. Their examination specifically showed the existence of great fraud upon the public domain, and their recommendations for changes in the law were made with the design of conserving the natural resources of every part of the public lands by putting it to its best use. Especial attention was called to the prevention of settlement by the passage of great areas of public land into the hands of a few men, and to the enormous waste caused by unrestricted grazing upon the open range. The recommendations of the Public Lands Commission are sound, for they are especially in the interest of the actual home-maker; and where the small home-maker can not at present utilize the land they provide that the Government shall keep control of it so that it may not be monopolized by a few men. The Congress has not yet acted upon these recommendations; but they are so just and proper, so essential to our National welfare, that I feel confident, if the Congress will take time to consider them, that they will ultimately be adopted.

Some such legislation as that proposed is essential in order to preserve the great stretches of public grazing land which are unfit for cultivation under present methods and are valuable only for the forage which they supply. These stretches amount in all to some 300,000,000 acres, and are open to the free grazing of cattle, sheep, horses and goats, without restriction. Such a system, or rather such lack of system, means that the range is not so much used as wasted by abuse. As the West settles the range becomes more and more over-grazed. Much of it can not be used to advantage unless it is fenced, for fencing is the only way by which to keep in check the owners of nomad flocks which roam hither and thither, utterly destroying the pastures and leaving a waste behind, so that their presence is incompatible with the presence of home-makers. The existing fences are all illegal. Some of them represent the improper exclusion of actual settlers, actual home-makers, from territory which is usurped by great cattle companies. Some of them represent what is in itself a proper effort to use the range for those upon the land, and to prevent its use by nomadic outsiders. All these fences, those that are hurtful and those that are beneficial, are alike illegal and must come down. But it is an outrage that the law should necessitate such action on the part of the Administration. The unlawful fencing of public lands for private grazing must be stopped, but the necessity which occasioned it must be provided for. The Federal Government should have control of the range, whether by permit or lease, as local necessities may determine. Such control could secure the great benefit of legitimate fencing, while at the same time securing and promoting the settlement of the country. In some places it may be that the tracts of range adjacent to the homesteads of actual settlers should be allotted to them severally or in common for the summer grazing of their stock. Elsewhere it may be that a lease system would serve the purpose; the leases to be temporary and subject to the rights of settlement, and the amount charged being large enough merely to permit of the efficient and beneficial control of the range by the Government, and of the payment to the county of the equivalent of what it would otherwise receive in taxes. The destruction of the public range will continue until some laws such as these are enacted. Fully to prevent the fraud in the public lands which, through the joint action of the Interior Department and the Department of Justice, we have been endeavoring to prevent, there must be further legislation, and especially a sufficient appropriation to permit the Department of the Interior to examine certain classes of entries on the ground before they pass into private ownership. The Government should part with its title only to the actual home-maker, not to the profit-maker who does not care to make a home. Our prime object is to secure the rights and guard the interests of the small ranchman, the man who plows and pitches hay for himself. It is this small ranchman, this actual settler and home-maker, who in the long run is most hurt by permitting thefts of the public land in whatever form.

Forests. Optimism is a good characteristic, but if carried to an excess it becomes foolishness. We are prone to speak of the resources of this country as inexhaustible; this is not so. The mineral wealth of the country, the coal, iron, oil, gas, and the like, does not reproduce itself, and therefore is certain to be exhausted ultimately; and wastefulness in dealing with it to-day means that our descendants will feel the exhaustion a generation or two before they otherwise would. But there are certain other forms of waste which could be entirely stopped — the waste of soil by washing, for instance, which is among the most dangerous

of all wastes now in progress in the United States, is easily prevent-
able, so that this present enormous loss of fertility is entirely unnecessary. The preservation or replacement of the forests is one of the most
important means of preventing this loss. We have made a beginning
in forest preservation, but it is only a beginning. At present lumbering
is the fourth greatest industry in the United States; and yet, so rapid
has been the rate of exhaustion of timber in the United States in the
past, and so rapidly is the remainder being exhausted, that the country is unquestionably on the verge of a timber famine which will be felt
in every household in the land. There has already been a rise in the
price of lumber, but there is certain to be a more rapid and heavier rise
in the future. The present annual consumption of lumber is certainly
three times as great as the annual growth; and if the consumption and
growth continue unchanged, practically all our lumber will be exhausted
in another generation, while long before the limit to complete exhaustion is reached the growing scarcity will make itself felt in many blight-
ing ways upon our National welfare. About 20 per cent of our forested
territory is now reserved in National forests; but these do not include
the most valuable timber lands, and in any event the proportion is too
small to expect that the reserves can accomplish more than a mitigation
of the trouble which is ahead for the nation. Far more drastic action is
needed. Forests can he lumbered so as to give to the public the full
use of their mercantile timber without the slightest detriment to the
forest, any more than it is a detriment to a farm to furnish a harvest;
so that there is no parallel between forests and mines, which can only
be completely used by exhaustion. But forests, if used as all our forests have been used in the past and as most of them are still used, will
be either wholly destroyed, or so damaged that many decades have to
pass before effective use can be made of them again. All these facts
are so obvious that it is extraordinary that it should be necessary to
repeat them. Every business man in the land, every writer in the
newspapers, every man or woman of an ordinary education, ought to
be able to see that immense quantities of timber are used in the country,
that the forests which supply this timber are rapidly being exhausted,
and that, if no change takes place, exhaustion will come comparatively
soon, and that the effects of it will be felt severely in the every-day life
of our people. Surely, when these facts are so obvious, there should be
no delay in taking preventive measures. Yet we seem as a nation to be
willing to proceed in this matter with happy-go-lucky indifference even
to the immediate future. It is this attitude which permits the self-
interest of a very few persons to weigh for more than the ultimate interest
of all our people. There are persons who find it to their immense pecuniary benefit to destroy the forests by lumbering. They are to be blamed
for thus sacrificing the future of the Nation as a whole to their own
self-interest of the moment; but heavier blame attaches to the people

at large for permitting such action, whether in the White Mountains, in the southern Alleghenies, or in the Rockies and Sierras. A big lumbering company, impatient for immediate returns and not caring to look far enough ahead, will often deliberately destroy all the good timber in a region, hoping afterwards to move on to some new country. The shiftless man of small means, who does not care to become an actual home-maker but would like immediate profit, will find it to his advantage to take up timber land simply to turn it over to such a big company, and leave it valueless for future settlers. A big mine owner anxious only to develop his mine at the moment, will care only to cut all the timber that he wishes without regard to the future — probably not looking ahead to the condition of the country when the forests are exhausted, any more than he does to the condition when the mine is worked out. I do not blame these men nearly as much as I blame the supine public opinion, the indifferent public opinion, which permits their action to go unchecked. Of course to check the waste of timber means that there must be on the part of the public the acceptance of a temporary restriction in the lavish use of the timber, in order to prevent the total loss of this use in the future. There are plenty of men in public and private life who actually advocate the continuance of the present system of unchecked and wasteful extravagance, using as an argument the fact that to check it will of course mean interference with the ease and comfort of certain people who now get lumber at less cost than they ought to pay, at the expense of the future generations. Some of these persons actually demand that the present forest reserves be thrown open to destruction, because, forsooth, they think that thereby the price of lumber could be put down again for two or three or more years. Their attitude is precisely like that of an agitator protesting against the outlay of money by farmers on manure and in taking care of their farms generally. Undoubtedly, if the average farmer were content absolutely to ruin his farm, he could for two or three years avoid spending any money on it, and yet make a good deal of money out of it. But only a savage would, in his private affairs, show such reckless disregard of the future; yet it is precisely this reckless disregard of the future which the opponents of the forestry system are now endeavoring to get the people of the United States to show. The only trouble with the movement for the reservation of our forests is that it has not gone nearly far enough, and was not begun soon enough. It is a most fortunate thing, however, that we began it when we did. We should acquire in the Appalachian and White Mountain regions all the forest lands that it is possible to acquire for the use of the Nation. These lands, because they form a National asset, are as emphatically national as the rivers which they feed, and which flow through so many States before they reach the ocean.

There should be no tariff on any forest product grown in this country; and, in especial, there should be no tariff on wood pulp; due notice of the change being of course given to those engaged in the business so as to enable them to adjust themselves to the new conditions. The repeal of the duty on wood pulp should, if possible, be accompanied by an agreement with Canada that there shall be no export duty on Canadian pulp wood.

Mineral Lands. In the eastern United States the mineral fuels have already passed into the hands of large private owners, and those of the West are rapidly following. It is obvious that these fuels should be conserved and not wasted, and it would be well to protect the people against unjust and extortionate prices, so far as that can still be done. What has been accomplished in the great oil fields of the Indian Territory by the action of the Administration, offers a striking example of the good results of such a policy. In my judgment the Government should have the right to keep the fee of the coal, oil, and gas fields in its own possession and to lease the rights to develop them under proper regulations; or else, if the Congress will not adopt this method, the coal deposits should be sold under limitations, to conserve them as public utilities, the right to mine coal being separated from the title to the soil. The regulations should permit coal lands to be worked in sufficient quantity by the several corporations. The present limitations have been absurd, excessive, and serve no useful purpose, and often render it necessary that there should be either fraud or else abandonment of the work of getting out the coal.

SENATE DEBATE ON FOREST RESERVATIONS [1]

Mr. Spooner. Now, all I started out to say was that the policy of the Government has been, so far as the forestry laws are concerned, exercising the option which it possesses to hold its timber lands in order to conserve the timber supply of the States and of the country rather than to open it, except in a qualified way, to homestead settlement. It would be opening it, as I said a few moments ago, to corporations cutting, manufacturing, and selling lumber, enabling them to save their own timber supply and obtain that for present uses from homesteaders. The average homesteader can not carry on to any large extent lumbering operations. They clear a little piece for agricultural purposes, for the erection of a cabin. They fence a little space, but for many, many years they do not go beyond that. It is a work of years, and many years ordinarily, to clear a forest farm, and, as the Senator from Utah [Mr. Smoot] says to me, half of it is lost.

Mr. President, that is not all. The Congress had another thing in view in establishing the forest reserves, and that is of the utmost con-

[1] *Congr. Record*, Feb. 19–23, 1907.

sequence to the people of the West, of some consequence to those States whose forests have been denuded or destroyed, and that was to conserve the water supply. That is of peculiar consequence to all the people living in the semiarid region of the country. That plays an important part in carrying to successful consummation the splendid irrigation scheme which is upon the statute book and is now being wrought out. The water supply in the far West and its conservation is of the utmost consequence. Congress had a wise purpose expressed in the act for the establishment of these reserves. The act of June 1, 1897, provides —

No public forest reservation shall be established, except to improve and protect the forest within the reservation, or for the purpose of securing favorable conditions of water flows, and to furnish a *continuous* supply of timber for the use and necessities of citizens of the United States.

Without this forest-reserve policy, leaving the land open to settlement, except upon the mountain tops, where no man could live, it would not be twenty years until the State of Idaho would have supplied the East and the Middle States with her timber, and her own forests would, in the main, be gone.

Mr. HEYBURN. Will the Senator permit me to suggest something?

Mr. SPOONER. Certainly.

Mr. HEYBURN. I looked at the question from that standpoint four years ago and three years ago. It so happened at the last session of Congress that I was ill and unable to be present. I had therefore kept in the law an exception in the interest of Idaho, providing that lumber should not be shipped by the Government out of the State of Idaho, but during my absence last winter that provision was stricken out. I am going to ask that it be inserted this year.

Mr. SPOONER. Why should it not be shipped out of the State of Idaho?

Mr. HEYBURN. Why should the Government ship it out of Idaho if the forests are being conserved for the future uses of the people of Idaho?

Mr. SPOONER. The conservation of the forests requires that some timber shall be cut.

Mr. HEYBURN. But let it be sold in Idaho.

Mr. SPOONER. Dead and down timber must be removed. A hurricane sweeps through the forest. The timber affected should be cut away, and for two reasons. It will otherwise be destroyed by worms, and worse than that, it invites a fire which may devastate the whole region. That is what conservation of the timber supply means. It means to take out those trees which ought to be taken out in the interest of the timber conservation, and it means that all cutting in the forest reserves shall be done in a manner which will not invite fires, and, second, which will not prevent reforesting.

I am not speaking without some personal knowledge of this particular phase of it. I am not speaking of the details. You may have some things to complain of, and no one would be more prompt to aid in correcting them than I. I am speaking — for there has been generalization here without limit on this subject — in support of this great national policy for the benefit of all the people, both as to the conservation of the forests and the conservation of the water supply; and if I am not very, very, very much mistaken no people anywhere have as acute interest in it as the people who occupy these States and those who are yet to occupy these States.

I once spent six weeks in a city in the West, and during all that time I could not see a vast mountain not far away, because it was obscured by the smoke of forest fires which destroyed millions, untold millions, of property and which worked a lasting harm to people who yet are to go into these sections. So it will not do to say the Government has no right to hold its lands, if it chooses, nor will it do to say that the Government is not far-sighted and kindly in the policy which it has adopted to hold its lands and to protect its lands, and so to utilize them as to benefit the people of the localities and benefit the people of the country.

When Senators balk about the Government becoming a lumber merchant, that is incidental. The forests would be swept away by fire, spoliation, and otherwise but for these timber reservations. You would have the same experience we had, and we had forests which, I have been told, could not be exceeded anywhere in beauty — white pine — except in a part of Idaho. I met one man who had years ago ridden through the Bitter Root Mountains and down along the stream for miles and for days, and he told me that he never had seen such a forest in his life; and he had seen forests. Ten days' fire would have ruined it for miles and miles; and there is no one on earth who hungers more for such trees and who have more money with which to buy them than a great many lumber corporations. It is a legitimate business. I am not reprobating them, but there is no reason, founded in public policy, why the Government of the United States should open to homestead entry every 160-acre tract of timber land which it owns, provided that land when denuded of its trees would be arable. And that doctrine, I repeat, would simply destroy the forests and turn over — not to be too carefully exercised, either, in the public interest as to the manner of cutting and clearing — to corporations and wealthy firms the timber supply of the West.

Thousands of men who have been driven out by the destruction of our forests in Wisconsin have gone to Idaho and to other Western States to purchase timber. They are good men.

Mr. HEYBURN. May I make a suggestion to the Senator from Wisconsin?

Mr. SPOONER. If it pertains to this subject.

Mr. HEYBURN. I should like to suggest that those who got the most of the forests of Wisconsin and realized the benefit of them are now in Idaho. I admit that.

Mr. SPOONER. I do not know anything about that.

Mr. HEYBURN. I do.

Mr. SPOONER. That makes no difference. The lumberman of Wisconsin is, I think, as good as the lumberman from Idaho or anywhere else in the world. There is no distinction to be drawn between people of different States on that basis.

The question is, Shall the Government dispose of these lands, take no care for the future either as to the water supply or the timber supply, or shall it go along in a wise, not extravagant, but liberal prosecution of the work of forest reservations? For myself, I have no doubt about it. I know it has its hardships to the people of Idaho, to the people of Montana, and to the people of other Western States. I know in a way it deters settlement. I know perfectly well the truth of what the Senator from Oregon and the Senator from Idaho say, that a man with a family is loath to settle upon a piece of land to live for years without neighbors, unable to establish schools, and all that.

But, Mr. President, this law, notwithstanding, is a wise and generous law. I have traveled for days in beautiful valleys along the Snake River and other streams in Wyoming, fertile, susceptible of cultivation, which could be entered under this law. The mountains are full of valleys, some of them extensive, other less so, susceptible of cultivation and all open to settlement under existing law.

There has been no conflict, and is none between the Government and the States as to the enforcement of the game laws. I am told that the officials of the Forest-Reserve Service are under instructions to coöperate in the enforcement of the State laws in respect to game, and that they are doing it.

As to coal, we have a bill pending here which without impeding the development from the agricultural standpoint of the State in which there are deposits of coal owned by the Government, the coal can be conserved by disposing of the surface for agricultural purposes and reserving to Government the coal and under reasonable conditions to permit its being taken out.

There is a wise public policy in that, Mr. President. So taking it by and large I have no doubt that this forest-reserve policy as a policy is of the greatest benefit to the people of this country, and especially to the people of the far West.

Now, take the lumber business. I want to read a few words, better used than I could use them, from a statement which I asked from Mr. Pinchot. The Senator from Colorado spoke of him as a person of miraculous excellence. I am sure he claims no perfection. I am sure he would not ask any man to put him above his fellows. But he is remarkable for his knowledge in a practical and a theoretical way of forestry, of conserving the existing forests and of planting and rearing trees for future forests. He is remarkable for another thing, that being a young man, a man of brains, a man of wealth, a man of education, to whom larger possibilities in politics or business open themselves, but has chosen to devote himself, sacrificially in some respects, to this great work of forest conservation, of perpetuating for the people yet to come, who will inhabit the valleys and the arable lands and the semiarid lands of the West, a water supply without which it is an irreclaimable desert. He does it for the love of it, not for your little pitiful salary. There are not many men within my knowledge who have been willing to do that.

Instead of being criticised he deserves the highest commendation, Mr. President, in my judgment. Of course he may have made mistakes. This policy began not many years ago. It has made great progress, not simply in the increase in acreage of the forest reserves, but in the system, in the methods adopted, and in the results. It has gone far enough under his supervision to vindicate the policy as one of great public value.

He sent me this statement at my request, and I will read a part of it. It is a statement in which I have the utmost confidence.

In the creation of reserves agricultural land is carefully excluded so far as possible, but since the nature of the country makes it impossible to avoid including occasional small isolated areas, such areas, when shown to be in fact agricultural are opened to bona fide settlers under the act of June 11, 1906.

All the resources of the reserves — wood, water, and grass — are open to the fullest use and development, the only restriction being that they shall be so used as to be *permanently* usable.

That is the object and the value of the policy. It looks not simply to to-day, but to long years to come; not simply to the people who are living in the section now, but to the people who are yet to come and who will come.

I ask leave to incorporate this statement in my remarks, Mr. President, and I have nearly finished.

The VICE-PRESIDENT. Without objection, permission is granted.

The matter referred to is as follows:

The forest reserves cover mountainous land in the West more valuable for forestry than for any other purposes. The act of June 4, 1897, specifically provides that no forest reserves shall be established except to improve and protect the forest or to secure favorable conditions of water flow, and to furnish a continuous supply of timber for the use of citizens.

In the creation of reserves agricultural land is carefully excluded so far as possible, but since the nature of the country makes it impossible to avoid including occasional small isolated areas, such areas, when shown to be in fact agricultural, are opened to bona fide settlers under the act of June 11, 1906.

All the resources of the reserves — wood, water, and grass — are open to the fullest use and development, the only restriction being that they shall be so used as to be permanently usable.

The mineral laws apply in forest reserves exactly as they do outside, as provided in the act of June 4, 1897.

Timber on the forest reserves which can be cut safely and for which there is actual need is for sale. Applications to purchase are invited. Green timber is for sale except where its removal makes a second crop doubtful or reduces the timber supply below the point of safety for local needs or injures the streams. All dead timber is for sale.

So far as the requirements of law for sale after advertisement to the highest bidder will permit, sales are made to small men, so as to prevent monopoly by disposing of timber to large corporations.

Timber valued at $500,945.76 was sold during the last fiscal year. The time allowed for cutting was from one to five years, and amount actually received for timber cut and removed amounted to $242,668.23.

Settlers and residents are given free use of timber in establishing and maintaining their homes. During the last calendar year 13,575 free-use permits were issued, to the value of $68,547.41.

Living trees to be cut are carefully selected and marked. Careful and effective provision is made for the reproduction and safety of the forests.

The grazing industry of the West depends on the forest reserves, because the summer range, without which the winter range is useless, lies almost wholly in the mountains. Grazing animals are excluded from cut-over areas to safeguard the reproduction.

It would be impossible to exclude all grazing from the western reserves without ruining the live-stock business of the country and raising the price of meat. Under proper regulation the grazing does little or no harm.

Since the transfer of the Forest Service to the Department of Agriculture two years ago the area of the reserves has increased from 58,000,000 to 127,000,000 acres; the personnel has more than doubled; the use of the reserves by the western people has increased many fold, and yet under the estimates the total cost to the Government of forest work during the coming fiscal year will have increased only from $800,000 to $900,000.

During the last fiscal year of the administration of the reserves in the Land Office the total expenses of the Government forest work in the Interior and Agricultural Departments were $800,000 and the receipts were $60,000, a net charge of $407,000. During the first full fiscal year of administration by the Forest Service the expenses were $1,195,000, the receipts $767,000 — a net cost to the Government of $430,000.

The policy thus inaugurated, if allowed to continue, would have made the Forest Service self-sustaining in five years from the transfer, or three years more, and while vastly increasing the use of the reserves by the western people and the efficiency of their administration over an area more than double.

Protection against fire is very successful, fires having almost disappeared. The last fiscal year they burned over less than one-tenth of 1 per cent of the total area.

Trespass is practically at an end.

The best supporters of forest reserves are the people who live in them or immediately about their borders. The great associations of stockmen, lumbermen, miners, and others support the policy.

The following instructions from the Secretary of Agriculture to the Forrester outline the policy:

"In the administration of the forest reserves it must be clearly borne in mind that all land is to be devoted to its most productive use for the permanent good of the whole people and not for the temporary benefit of individuals or companies. All the resources of forest reserves are for use, and this must be brought about in a thoroughly prompt and businesslike manner, under such restrictions only as will insure the permanence of these resources. The vital importance of forest reserves to the great industries of the Western States will be largely increased in the near future by the continued steady advance in settlement and development. The permanence of the resources of the reserves is therefore indispensable to continued prosperity, and the policy of this Department for their protection and use will invariably be guided by this fact, always bearing in mind that the conservative use of these resources in no way conflicts with their permanent value.

"You will see to it that the water, wood, and forage of the reserves are conserved and wisely used for the benefit of the home builder first of all, upon whom depends the best permanent use of lands and resources alike. The continued prosperity of the agricultural lumbering, mining, and live-stock interests is directly dependent upon a permanent and accessible supply of water, wood, and forage, as well as upon the present and future use of these resources under businesslike regulations, enforced with promptness, effectiveness, and common sense. In the management of each reserve local questions will be decided upon local grounds. The dominant industry will be considered first, but with as little restriction to minor industries as may be possible; sudden changes in industrial conditions will be avoided by gradual adjustment after due notice, and where conflicting interests must be reconciled the question will always be decided from the standpoint of the greatest good to the greatest number in the long run."

In a word, the object of the Forest Service, as the President has declared, is to create and maintain prosperous homes and conserve the natural resources upon which those homes depend.

Just what does it mean when unreserved public lands are proclaimed public forest reserves? Let us get down to simple facts and see what kind of a change really takes place.

We have, to start with, throughout the Rocky Mountains and Pacific coast regions vast areas of high and rocky land, sometimes densely, sometimes sparsely timbered, frequently covered with brush, and usually producing good crops of grass and other herbage; vast areas which contain the sources of innumerable streams, the waters of which are used for irrigation, power, and transportation. These lands are worthless for settlement. If unreserved, they will not be taken up for homes or cultivated for the support of families. Their altitude, their generally poor soil, their very nature makes agriculture impossible or unprofitable. That they are in no sense of the word homestead lands has been determined beyond all doubt through careful examinations on the ground by western men familiar with western conditions; by men who know from practical experience what lands can be cultivated and what lands can not be cultivated with success.

What are these vast areas good for?

The production of timber and wood, for one thing. The production of summer range for cattle and sheep for another thing. And last, but not least, they are the all-important conservers of the water supply for the farms and manufactures of the lowlands. They are the great reservoirs upon which the solid prosperity of the valleys depends. '

How are these resources used when the lands are still unreserved?

The timber is rapidly taken up by individuals under several of the land laws. From individuals it passes to companies and corporations, by whom the most valuable portion of it is cut and marketed. That which remains is burned up, and nine times out of ten the land becomes a nonproductive waste, utterly valueless to the county, State, and nation. The large timber owner profits, but only by what he makes on the timber cut. The county and State profit, but only temporarily, while taxes come in and before the land becomes a waste. The wage-earner profits, but also only temporarily. When the timber is gone beyond repair his occupation goes with it. The Government receives at the most but $2.50 an acre for timber which has an actual market value of from $5 to $100 an acre or more.

When this unreserved public land is made into a forest reserve the timber is still available. It is not locked up or withdrawn from market. It is not left to rot from age and be wiped out by fire. It is still ready to assist in the general development of the region concerned. Anybody can buy it — a thousand feet or ten million feet. It is there to be used by the settler, or, if the settler does not need it, by the big corporation; neither is excluded. But with this very important difference — the land must be *wisely* used — so used that it will continue to produce timber, the greatest possible quantity of it, and forever. The timber is so harvested that future crops are assured, just as with cotton, wheat, or corn. The lands are protected against fire, and millions of dollars' worth of timber are saved to the Government each year which on the unreserved public domain goes up in smoke. The timber resources are made permanent. The lands are kept productive, and the county, State, and nation reap the benefit. The prosperity which use brings is lasting prosperity, not a transitory boom. Present greed is forced to yield to the requirements of future development. Moreover, the nation receives a fair price for its own. If private or corporate timber in the same locality sells for $50 an acre, the United States can sell its own timber for $50 an acre — for what it is worth. Is there any reason why it should be given away for $2.50 an acre, as it must be if the land is unreserved?

So far, then, as timber is concerned, throwing the public lands into forest reserves means simply that their timber resources are better and more wisely used, for the general benefit, now and in the long run. That is all. There is no other difference.

How is the range used when the lands are still unreserved?

STOCKMEN

It is open to all, without restriction or regulation. As a consequence, there is continual warfare between the big stockmen and the little stockmen, between sheep and cattle men, and the range deteriorates constantly from overgrazing. Take almost any part of the West and ask the old settlers how the grass compares with that of former years. In many localities the range is almost totally destroyed.

If a forest reserve is made out of this public land, the range is not locked up. It does not cease to benefit the general welfare. It is grazed by cattle and

36

sheep. It is used by the small man and the big man. But with this important difference — its use is so regulated that the big man and the small man are both assured of the share which rightfully belongs to them through prior use and settlement; and the grazing is so regulated that the range will support the total number of stock allowed without deterioration. It is kept at its highest productive capacity. It is precisely the same with the range as with the timber. A forest reserve makes sure of a better and wiser use and a permanent prosperity. The stockman wants it.

What happens to these vast areas from the standpoint of water supply when they are still a part of the unreserved public domain?

They are left to the ravages of fire, to destructive lumbering, and destructive grazing. Their cover of forest, brush, and grass is slowly, but surely destroyed. They gradually lose their sponge-like properties as great reservoirs for holding and regulating the waterflow. The rains rush quickly down the slopes, causing floods in the wet season and droughts in the dry seasons.

In forest reserves these lands are systematically protected. The most important protection is from fire. There is an organized force on the ground whose business it is to prevent this destruction. It is not a perfect force at present, but it is all the time becoming more efficient. If anyone doubts the effectiveness of this systematic protection, let him compare the chaotic conditions on the unreserved public domain with those on the forest reserve. The results are there to speak for themselves.

Let us look at this whole matter from the standpoint of what it really means. In many of the Western States there are very considerable areas of public lands brought together into forest reserves. Maps which show these areas colored in green seem to conjure up grave fears in the minds of the opponents of the Government's policy, and these green areas are pointed to as if they were huge tracts surrounded by stone walls dropped upon the mountains as a blanket to all future development. The cry goes up that so and so many million acres have been closed to settlement. The truth is that settlement is impossible from the nature of the case. If there were a chance of settlement, these areas would not be in forest reserves. Nobody wants to make forest reserves out of agricultural lands.

Then the cry is raised that the resources are locked up and that the present and future development of the region is crushed beyond hope. This objection is absolutely without foundation for the simple reason that all the resources on each and every forest reserve are *now being used*.

They are being used by those who have the best right to their use. They are being used for the greatest good of the greatest number in the long-run. And their use will continue in just this way.

Forest *reserve* is an unfortunate term. As a matter of fact, the resources of these mountain areas are not reserved, they are conserved. In other words, they are wisely used. The name misleads.

Mr. Spooner. It is a question which is the wisest and best, to do away with this policy, except up on the mountains where the land never can be utilized for farming purposes, or keep it for the people's use.

Mr. Heyburn. What people?

Mr. Spooner. The people who live out there now and the people who are to live out there after the Senator — which I hope will be a great many years — shall have passed to his last sleep. It is not for to-day, and that is where the mistake is. It is in looking upon Idaho purely from the standpoint of to-day. You can pay too much for the too rapid development of a new State. You can pay too much for rapid increase in population in such States. You can lay now a foundation deep and broad and strong for future wealth for all the people of Idaho and the West generally. I think this policy does it. I think Congress ought not to be penurious in carrying it on. I think this notion that no money shall be expended in a work of this kind without estimates is fatal to the work. It is full of vicissitudes. More men may be required to-morrow by a thousand than are required to-day. It depends upon fire; it depends upon whether a whirlwind shall sweep over the timber, as to what will be required to take it out and preserve it. There are many things, Mr. President.

*   *   *   *   *   *   *   *

Mr. PATTERSON. When you say my proposition is a subtle plan to destroy the forest reservation, that is pretty near to charging a motive.

Mr. SPOONER. I did not intend to impugn any improper motive to the Senator.

Mr. PATTERSON. I do not take offense at it, but I want to make a statement in that connection. Then I will give way to the Senator.

The VICE-PRESIDENT. Does the Senator from Wisconsin yield to the Senator from Colorado?

Mr. SPOONER. Certainly.

Mr. PATTERSON. Mr. President, the Senator from Wisconsin utterly mistakes my attitude and the attitude of the people of my State upon the question of forest reserves. I want to say to him that I am heartily in favor of forest reserves, and if there were a proposition to abolish absolutely those which have been made, as far as I am able I would be. in the front rank to oppose their abolition, for I want to tell you that we in the mountains realize far more keenly than you gentlemen of the plains the benefit to us of forest reserves in the way of restraining the melting snows in the spring and early summer.

We are at the source of the water supply of nearly all of our great streams, in whatever direction they flow and to whatever ocean, and as a rule our waters flow through our State with tremendous speed and velocity and power. Now and then, when the snows melt under a suddenly heated atmosphere, we have great calamities in the mountains by reason of the unusual and unrestrained volume of water. Therefore we want the forest reserves held intact. We desire to cherish them, to help to maintain them, to support them, to regulate them, and to do whatever is necessary to preserve them from fire and to extinguish fires when they occur.

Let me suggest another thought with which those who do not live in the mountains, perhaps, are not familiar, and that is that we do not

have homesteads made by clearing forests. In my thirty-odd years'
experience in Colorado — and I have traveled from one end of the
State to the other, in all forms of conveyances and upon all sorts of
animals — I want to say to the Senator from Wisconsin I have not
known of a single farm or homestead made by clearing the land of
timber. The general rule is that our timber lands are not good agricultural lands, and therefore we do not desire to denude the lands of
timber for the purpose of opening them up to settlement, for we have
had no settlements upon such lands and no desire to make settlements
on timber lands. As a rule spruce and pine timber lands do not make
good agricultural land, especially in the mountain section of the country.

Then, what motive can we have? Certainly those of us who live
there do not wish to see the timber of the country go into the hands of
great speculators. We want so much timber as may be needed for
domestic uses or even for outside commerce cut and disposed of under
wise rules and regulations, and we want the Government to get the
benefit of the value of every stick of timber that is cut from the public
domain. That is the attitude of the Senators and Representatives from
the mountain States upon the subject of forest reserves.

And why should we have a subtle or any other plan to destroy forest
reserves when forest reserves were first championed by western Senators,
and when those of us who are making this struggle upon the floor of the
Senate to-day are the real friends of forest reserves and may be required
to interpose our influence to preserve them, if this method of their administration is continued? It is a serious matter, Mr. President, to take
from a great State two-thirds or a fourth or a fifth of its agricultural area
and turn it over to live stock and to silence when men and women and
children are hungry for land; and the desire for land ownership is
the dominating desire of the real patriotic American citizen. We do
not want this system to break down. So indignant are the people of
the western portion of the State I represent about the administration
of forest reserves that they are to-day in a state of rebellion, and
meeting after meeting has been called where resolutions have been
passed resolving to interpose all obstacles to the continuation of such
an administration and refusing to pay the license fees demanded of
them before they can put a head of stock of any kind within a forest
reserve.

The truth of it is that within forest reserves in my State there are
millions upon millions of acres which are not forest lands at all, but
they are agricultural and grazing lands, which are taken from the portion
that is open to the people of the country for settlement, and we shut
them up to meet the hobby of the gentleman who is at the head of this
Bureau. Like the Senator from Idaho, whoever represents Colorado
and whoever continues to represent the mountain States and the States
affected by this new-fangled system of taking care of the public lands

within them will fight, and they must fight all such institutions as this. If they do not they will be rejected by their constituencies, for to hold an office of this kind from the West a man must represent the sentiment of his people.

Mr. SPOONER. Mr. President, I do not yield my assent to the proposition made by the Senators from the Western States that they are the only members of this body who have to do with this question, or the imputation, if I may call it such, or criticism, which is suggested as to those of us who do not live in the far West, for having the temerity to entertain or to express views upon this subject. We are all Senators of the United States. The Senator from Idaho is a Senator from Idaho, but he is not a Senator of Idaho. He is a Senator of the United States from Idaho. I am a Senator of the United States from a State. My first duty, and the first duty of every Senator, as I understand it, is to represent the general public interest, and subordinate to the general public interest the local interest of his State. The Senator from a State in which there happens to be fifteen, twenty, twenty-five, or fifty million acres of Government land can not ask that he and his colleague shall be permitted to say, all others by courtesy following them, what disposition shall be made of that property belonging to the Government within his State.

This is property of the United States, 127,000,000 acres, in forest reserves; and it is not only the right, but it is the duty of every Senator of the United States to give the matter thought, and to determine, if it be possible to do it, upon that line of policy with reference to its disposition which will best conserve the general public interest of the United States and the interest as well of the State in which that land happens to be located.

I do not live in a mountainous State, but I live in a State the northern portion of which was covered within my memory with magnificent forests. It is gone, and within a very few years vast quantities have been wasted, affecting detrimentally the water supply and affecting in economic ways injuriously the people of that State. Taking account of my observation in a lumber region in which I live, reasoning from the past to the future, knowing or having reason to believe that, if unrestricted, what happened in Wisconsin forests will happen in Idaho, and will happen in other States having virgin forests of timber. I believe with all my heart that in the interest of those States on general principles, as well as in the interest of all the people, it is important that the forest reservation policy be not essentially crippled.

If land in large bodies has been included within forest reservations that ought to be without them, that is one thing. I would not ask nor would I vote to exclude, because of a forest reservation, settlers from occupying the land in any State of the West; and if lands ought to be taken out of the reservation, if the lines of the reservation should be changed in order to throw open to homestead, to settlement, to occupation, and cultivation lands in Idaho or anywhere else I would not for one moment oppose it. But, Mr. President, to take valleys within a reservation, not along its border, but in its heart or near it, fit for agriculture, out of the reservation would be to destroy the reservation. To my mind it is impossible to go further than the law now goes in the direction of throwing open such land within the reservation to settlement without destroying the reservation.

I am in favor of the Appalachian reservation when the facts in regard to it can be ascertained. I believe it will be a wonderful boon to the South and as well of vast advantage in many ways to some of the Northern States, and a matter of great wealth in the long run to the country at large. I am in favor of the policy. If lands are devoted under improper regulations to sheep raising or grazing, let those regulations be changed. No one can object to that change. If it be improper from a governmental standpoint to charge stock owners and sheep owners for grazing privileges on the Government lands let that practice be abolished. That and all of those matters might very well be urged by way of amendment to the forest reservation act instead of being projected or attempted to be projected into this bill, the object of which is to maintain and support the general policy. There is not an item of either of these amendments proposed to be offered to this bill which is in order. They all propose to change the existing law and they are general legislation.

I hope when my friend from Idaho reads some of his observations uttered this morning he will feel, as I feel, that he allowed himself to indulge in suggestions, as to some of those who support this general proposition and have advocated a larger appropriation, far away from any foundation in justice. I would not be willing that the Senator from Idaho should consciously and deliberately impute to me or to my action upon a public measure here personal friendship for an official or social fondness for an official. Senators who deal with the public interest, under oath, can not be supposed to do that. I have met but few times the Chief Forester. What I have said of him is of his ability and knowledge of the subject as it impresses me. Except for my belief in the policy and my belief in the present administration, subject, perhaps, to some remodeling in matters complained of which can be easily disposed of, I would not support this nor any other bill or appropriation on personal ground, nor do I know any Senator here who would.

That is all I want to say, Mr. President.

SPEECH OF SENATOR ALBERT J. BEVERIDGE ON THE FOREST SERVICE [1]

The Senate having under consideration the bill (H. R. 24815) making appropriations for the Department of Agriculture of the fiscal year ending June 30, 1908 —

Mr. BEVERIDGE said:

Mr. President: The question immediately before the Senate is whether or not the appropriation for the Forest Service, which the other day, perhaps without full information, was reduced, is to be restored. After the very long attack upon the Government's policy, I may be permitted some time to explain and defend it. No debate which has occurred this session has been so useful as this in informing both the Senate and the country on a policy of such high importance.

There are those of us who were deeply interested in this question and yet who were not informed about what this Service meant and about the priceless work for the whole country which it was doing. There have been in the course of this debate some points made, charges made, and various statements made which require some attention; and it is to do this that I rise to address the Senate before we take any vote, if a vote, indeed, shall be necessary upon this amendment.

SIGNIFICANCE OF RESERVE POLICY

The Senator from Wyoming [Mr. Clark] the other day began his remarks by asking the question, "What does this great forest-reserve system," which he said included some 200,000 square miles, "mean?" Since then, Mr. President, the question has been pretty fully answered. It means, perhaps, a wiser piece of public policy, so far as the present and future prosperity of this people is concerned, than any one single other piece of public policy affecting our lands. It means, Mr. President, at the bottom the conservation and the distribution of the waters, upon which agriculture depends, and upon which the population of the Senator's State and of other States similarly situated depend for its growth more than upon any one other single element that can be named.

RESERVES THE MAINSTAY OF IRRIGATION

Mr. President, we are spending now, or arranging to spend, some $50,000,000 for the irrigation of what was once thought was the "arid West." I remember very well the great fight which was made for the irrigation law. It was finally put through the Senate and the House

[1] *Congr. Record*, Reported March 1, 1907.

against the counsel of some of the most conservative members of each body, but I think its wisdom now is universally recognized by men of all parties and men of all sections.

But, Mr. President, you can not irrigate with a word — you have to irrigate with water. You can not irrigate merely by digging a hole in the desert; not enough water is supplied. In the last analysis it must come from rainfall in the mountains. The Senator knows better, no doubt, than I do that unless the forests on those mountains are conserved irrigation is impossible. Because if the forests are felled the rain which falls in equal abundance sweeps down in torrential floods and either takes away the reservoirs or fills them up with silt. So the basis of the whole irrigation system, which means so much to the western country, and therefore to the whole country, rests upon the foundation of the forest-reserve system.

Mr. F. H. Newell, Chief of the Reclamation Service, has repeatedly emphasized the very great importance of forest reserves in connection with the Government's irrigation work. In the second annual report of the Reclamation Service (1902–03) Mr. Newell stated: "One of the most important matters in connection with the permanent development of the water resources of the country is the protection of the catchment basins from destructive influences. It is essential to preserve in such locations a certain amount of forest cover, and to prevent the destruction of these by fire or by overgrazing. The headwaters of many of the important streams are already included within forest reserves, and some of the important reservoir sites are thus guarded from injury. In other localities the forest reserve boundaries should be extended to include the country from which comes the greatest part of the run-off. This land usually has no value for cultivation, is rugged, and suitable only for the production of trees. Grazing to a limited extent is practicable and will not interfere with the best use of the waters, but if unrestricted, the number of cattle and sheep may be increased to such an extent that the grass is destroyed and the bare soil is washed by storms."

Again, at the hearing before the Committee on the Public Lands of the House of Representatives (January 11 to 30, 1901), Mr. Newell explained himself as follows:

"As Mr. Walcott has outlined, the great undertaking of national importance is first to hold the timber-clad mountains of arid country from which the water comes in forest reserves, not keeping the timber from use, but letting it be cut under such restrictions as will enable the matured timber to be taken and keep the forest itself as a perpetual crop. This has already been entered upon by the National Government."

All Reserves Conserve Timber or Water

Forest reserves are created for these main objects: To conserve and regulate stream overflow, and to maintain a permanent supply of timber.

Some forest reserves are valuable for both these purposes; others are valuable mainly for their effect upon stream flow. In southern California, for example, forest reserves have been created in the San Gabriel Mountains, not with the chief purpose of the production of timber, because these mountains are largely covered with brush known as chaparral and have few trees growing upon them. But these southern California reserves serve a most valuable purpose in maintaining the flow of streams rising in them, which supply important cities, such as Los Angeles, and are essential for the development of water power, and, above all, in the conservation of streams used in the irrigation of arid lands. Again, large areas in these reserves are capable of growing trees, although no trees are growing upon them at present. As rapidly as its funds permit, and conditions warrant, the Forest Service is planting up these areas.

To make the boundaries of forest reserves conform exactly to the boundaries of existing forests would be to leave out of these reserves large areas which are of immense value as a protection to the water flow, and which have grown trees and will grow trees again under proper methods. Obviously the boundaries of forest reserves must be drawn not to conform to the boundaries of existing forests, but based on the actual character of the country in its relation to the objects for which reserves are created. Brush and grass covered areas of natural forest land in the mountains, even if they do not now produce trees, ought to be given exactly the same protection as existing forests receive, because they often exercise a not less important effect in conserving and regulating stream flow.

The Forest Service has never recommended the creation of a single reserve the land inclosed in which can not serve its main purpose either by the regulation of stream flow or by the production of timber. No considerable bodies of open range are included in forest reserves. So far as open range is included, it has been included not as range land, but because it is necessary to the protection of stream flow or because it is suitable for forest planting.

Reserves Based on Thorough Examination of Lands

Mr. President, the Senator from Wyoming [Mr. Clark] said further — and it was a most important charge, one that we should carefully consider, one that the country should know the truth about — that the reserves had been created without knowledge of actual conditions upon the ground. So far from that being accurate (and I am satisfied that neither the Senator nor any other Senator who spoke meant to make an inaccurate statement) perhaps as much as in the case of any other scientific department of the Government the most careful, detailed, painstaking, and scientifically accurate examinations were made.

These reserves, I say, are created after the most painstaking, comprehensive, and scientific examination of conditions on the ground. If it were earlier in the day, I should stop here first to read to the Senate the details of the plan upon which information is gathered for determining whether or not a forest reserve shall be made. None of us could have more valuable information upon that subject, which is quite as important as any other subject we now have before us, than the method by which this vast reserved forest system, which is the heart and source of all the water for the great irrigation system, is made.

I hold in my hand, and I shall ask to have entirely inserted in the *Record* in my remarks, the instructions to the field men who make the examinations.

The VICE-PRESIDENT. In the absence of objection, it will be so ordered.

The matter referred to is as follows:

The following outline must be considered in the examination and used in writing the full report, or it will be returned for correction:

1. Location and area.
2. Description and topography.
3. Climate, showing any difference between the reserve and adjacent agricultural regions. Precipitation, prevailing rain-laden winds, etc.
4. The forest.

(a) A map on a scale of 2 miles to the inch, showing the distribution and character of the cover (to be compiled by the drafting division from data furnished by the examiner). The following classes of cover should be distinguished and mapped:

1. Commercial forest. — Actual saw, stull, or tie timber, irrespective of its accessibility. A merchantable forest.
2. Timber land. — Land-bearing commercial species, either reproduction under 20 feet high or too scattering to be a merchantable forest. Potential forest land capable of producing merchantable timber.
3. Woodland. — Juniper, piñon, oak, aspen, etc., without mixture of commercial species. It may be a cord-wood forest.
4. Cut-over land. — Wherever logging has been carried on, whether stripped or merely culled.
5. Burns. — Where the cover has been totally destroyed.
6. Chaparral.
7. Open grass land. — Parks or open range.
8. Sagebrush.
9. Cultivated land.
10. Cultivable land.
11. Barren land. — Above timber line, slide rock, cliffs, etc.

(b) A brief description of the various silvicultural types of forest cover; reproduction.

(c) A rough estimate of the amount of merchantable timber, according to watersheds or logging units; its accessibility, and means of logging that must be used, and prevailing stumpage price. Definite recommendations as to stumpage prices and method of sale to be pursued in the event of creation of the reserve.

5. The forest as a protection cover: Its effect on the regulation of the water flow. Use of water for irrigation and power at present and possible acreage and value of irrigated and irrigable lands dependent on the reserve for water supply. Location of reservoir sites and possibility of ditch applications. Any areas or slopes from which timber should not be sold.

6. Industries: Nature, relative importance, dependence on water and timber in proposed reserve and adjacent affected regions. Extent and value of most important interests.

7. Settlements: Location, size, importance, and industry. Table of alienated lands, showing area in acres of each class and per cent of recommended reserve.

8. Roads, trails, and railroads.

9. Lumbering: Extent of lumbering in the past and at present. Its effect upon the forest. The condition of cut-overlands. Effect which creation of reserve would have upon lumbering. Need for reserve timber. Means of supplying it from elsewhere. Standing and retail prices of different species in the local market.

10. Grazing: To what extent the prosperity of the local residents depends upon live stock, and to what extent is the stock dependent on this range. How many stock now using reserve and how distributed. Where owned. Whether stockmen own ranches or reside in reserve.

To what extent as a summer range proposed reserve limits use outside range. Whether it includes lambing grounds. Conflicting interests, such as between sheep and cattle, local and outside stock, etc. Merits of the controversy.

Description of pasture lands, their nature, brush, grass, etc. Extent of open parks and pasture in timber. To what extent grazing has injured the range or forest. Manner of handling. Size of herds.

Areas, if any, from which stock should be excluded. Division of pasture lands. Give plan, number to be allowed, length of season, any special regulation necessary. Practicability of a division of range into individual ranges. Necessity for counting wings, drift fences, dipping vats, windmills, etc. Cost and location.

11. Fire: Damage from fire; usual causes. Threatened points. Season. History of burns. Prevention. Area burned. Outline a definite plan of protection and patrol. Are fire lines feasible?

12. Situation. A brief description of the political and economic situation of the locality (settlements, county, or State) in its bearing on the reserve question. From whom will opposition come and why? Attitude and motives of influential men or corporations. Any illegal settlements or operations. Any concessions that the Forest Service should make. Labor prices and cost of living in the surrounding communities.

13. Local sentiment in regard to the creation of a forest reserve: A special effort should be made to obtain all arguments possible both for and against the creation of a reserve.

14. Conclusion and recommendations: A clear recommendation for or against the creation of a reserve.

15. If recommended, boundaries to be shown on maps in red pencil. If not,

write "not recommended" in red pencil on the map and on the title page of the report.

16. Administration. Number of men needed to handle current business. Ranks and rates of pay. Length of service. How many men in summer? In winter? Indicate ranger districts on map where ranger should be stationed in each district.

In what town should the officer in charge make his headquarters. What are office, mail, railroad, telegraph, and telephone facilities there. Regions where patrol is most needed. Where sales, free use, trespass, and privilege cases will be numerous. Improvement work, such as cabins, phones, pastures, roads, or trails necessary at once and cost of each. Special regulations desirable, not in present rules. Revision of present rules or practice.

The administrative feature is a very important one, and complete plan of administration for the proposed reserve should be outlined.

Names and addresses of men who would make good forest officers.

The importance of photographs can not be overestimated. They should be taken to illustrate particular points in the reports. Also views over considerable areas, showing the general character of the country should be taken.

Mr. BEVERIDGE. Furthermore, I have here, and will exhibit that the Senate may see it, a map of the Shoshone or Coeur d'Alene Reserve in Idaho. The Senate will notice the various colors. This deep green here [indicating] in the southwest portion is the heavily forested portion of this reservation. These brown patches [indicating] throughout that reservation are the burnt-over districts, where millions of dollars, the property of the United States, has been destroyed by forest fires. The lighter portions here [indicating] are the young timber. There are other portions that represent sagebrush.

With reference to this green portion here [indicating], within these lines, heavily wooded, *it is nearly all taken up by the State or by settlers.* That is the "ruthless" and "infamous" way in which the Government of the United States has destroyed the resources of the State, as Senators have charged.

TIMBER FREE TO SMALL USERS FOR HOME BUILDING AND OTHER NEEDS '

Mr. President, having located a reserve, what occurs? In the first place, it is again carefully mapped, classified, and examined. The Department knows just exactly what kind of timber is in every part of the reserve. What is done with that timber? Two things are done with it. It is given away by the Government to the small users without charge — to the settler, to the homesteader, to those men that we have been led to believe were so badly treated by this "tryannical" Government — and who with this timber build their homes. Lumber and timber are given free of charge. Not only is the place to build their homes given them, but all the timber they need.

In order to show how fairly and with what careful detail the law providing for the free use of timber and stone is applied, I will quote the regulation in this respect:

' "Regulation 10. The free-use privilege may be granted to settlers, farmers, prospectors, or similar persons who may not reasonably be required to purchase, and who have not on their own lands or claims, or on lands controlled by them, a sufficient or practically accessible supply of timber or stone for the purposes named in the law. It may also be granted to school and road districts, churches, or coöperative organizations of settlers desiring to construct roads, ditches, reservoirs, or similar improvements, for mutual or public benefit. Free use of material to be used in any business will be refused, as, for example, to sawmill proprietors, owners of large establishments or commercial enterprises, and companies or corporations. The free-use privilege will not be given to any trespasser."

Timber Sold so that Forest is Conserved

Next certain timber is sold, and to whom? To those who wish it, whether in small or in large quantities; not for their own use, but for commercial purposes. Ought the Government give it to *them?* Heretofore men have made millions sawing into lumber the timber that belonged to the people of this Nation. Shall we return to that policy?

Now, then, what timber is sold?

I will come in a moment to the question of policy that was raised as to "the Government being a merchant."

Not only is what is known as "down" timber, to which the Senator from Wisconsin [Mr. Spooner] referred yesterday, sold, but what is called "ripe" timber is sold.

Mr. Spooner. I said that.

Mr. Beveridge. I did not hear the Senator when he said it. Perhaps I had been called out of the Chamber. Then the Senator did cover that. The truth about it is that these forest reserves are merely great natural wood factories, and unless reserves are so treated, and trees cut that should be cut and *when* they should be cut the result is *bad* to the forest itself. It is blown down, it rots, and is itself a source of decay. What shall the Government do? Let it fall and let it rot? It is the Government's property, just as much as the chairs in this Chamber; just as much as the money we seem to be so afraid to appropriate is Government property.

The prime object of the forest reserves is use. While the forest and its dependent interests must be made permanent and safe in preventing overcutting or injuring the young growth, every reasonable effort is made to satisfy legitimate demands. Timber cut from forest reserves may be handled and shipped like any other timber, except that it is not sold for shipment in regions where local construction requires the entire supply, or is certain to do so in the future. Anyone may purchase timber except trespassers. Forest rangers are authorized to sell timber in amounts not exceeding $20 in value; forest supervisors not more than $100 worth, and the Forester larger sales.

We talk about "economy." Economy of what? Of the Government's *resources*, and those resources consist in cash, in land, in trees, in ships, in anything else that the Government *owns*. So, if we are conserving these trees, and derive revenue from them, we are practicing the highest economy just as much as if we are careful — and we should be careful — of the actual dollars appropriated.

So that, Mr. President, is what is done with that wood, and that is not only bringing a revenue into the Treasury, but it is creating a continuous revenue from the same source for the future. I ask any Senator who objects to the Government being a "merchant," as we have heard, whether or not any Administration could be justified in not saving to the people of the United States the revenue that comes from the sale of this timber. What else would you do with it?

Would you give to one man to receive freely and sell for his own profit the timber for which another man stands ready to pay two or three or five dollars a thousand feet — millions upon millions of feet of it? For there is no other choice than this — either some favored individual or the people of the United States must receive the benefit. Under sales already made the Government will receive hundreds of thousands of dollars. The timber sold cannot be removed except in large quantities; expensive plants must be provided to make it possible to utilize the timber at all. Should the Government abstain from receiving this revenue that some private individual may gratuitously reap a fortune? If so, on what principle shall selection of the person to receive this princely favor be made?

Technical Investigations Add to Country's Wealth

But this is not all, Mr. President, nor is it perhaps the most important thing. We are developing this country, developing its resources. I very greatly doubt whether we have had any source of tangible wealth to the people so great as the aid that has been given the people in information, scientific direction, and help by the department of Agriculture. An entire day might be most usefully spent, both so far as the people and the Senate are concerned, in reviewing the actual practical help to the people by the information that is gathered and given to the farmers of the country by the Department of Agriculture.

So the next thing the Forest Service does is to constantly test the trees and the various kinds of wood for new uses. It is found that some woods which formerly were supposed to be worthless are most valuable;

so that, as one kind of timber is cut off and the lumber disappears another kind of timber is found.

I cite as examples of that two trees with which some Senators here will be especially familiar. One is the western hemlock and the other the southern gum. The southern gum was a tree which afforded excellent lumber, but which immediately warped, so that the stock expression of a lumberman was that if you were to go to sleep on one side of a southern gum board you would wake up next morning on the other side of it, because it would warp so. But the Department has found a method of cutting and treating it so that it has become one of the considerable resources of the States where it grows. It has taken the place of wood which heretofore was used almost exclusively, but which now has become practically exhausted, just because we did not have such forest preservation as is now proposed.

Another is the western hemlock. Up to a few years ago the western hemlock was supposed to be like the eastern hemlock, unfit for lumber. This Department has developed the fact that it makes an admirable lumber; and now it constitutes a source of real revenue to the States where it grows.

The Forest Service is active in finding new uses for sawmill waste; testing new woods to be used for paper in place of those which are becoming exhausted or too expensive; testing new woods for mine props, railroad ties, box boards, vehicle woods, wooden pavements, cooperage, and many other uses. It is studying methods of preserving woods against decay, and is thus increasing enormously the service that can be got out of wood in some of its commonest uses. In this one field its work is equivalent to increasing the timber resources of the country by creating out of nothing thousands and hundreds of thousands of acres of standing forest. Both by promoting economy in the use of wood and by preventing waste in harvesting the forest crop it has added millions of dollars' worth of material to the national wealth in private ownership.

Mr. President, that is not only creating wealth for the Government as such, but it is creating wealth for the people, because, of course, most everybody knows that most of the forest land of the United States is held by private owners. I think perhaps less than one-fifth — the Senator from Wyoming may know about that, and I want to be corrected if the statement is wrong, and that it is too high, if anything — is held in Government reserves.

Mr. CLARK of Wyoming. It is very much too low.

Mr. BEVERIDGE. You mean that much more than the amount I named is held by private owners?

Mr. CLARK of Wyoming. Yes.

Mr. BEVERIDGE. I think that very much more than I have stated is held by private individuals, but the private owners do not and can not, unless they operate upon a scale almost as great as the Government itself, make these scientific examinations which discover the unknown properties of their wood. So in this one way the Department is creating enormous wealth for the American people.

Mr. CLARK of Wyoming. Right on that point, will the Senator allow me a question as to the scientific work of the Bureau?

The VICE-PRESIDENT. Does the Senator from Indiana yield to the Senator from Wyoming?

Mr. BEVERIDGE. Certainly.

Mr. CLARK of Wyoming. Is it not a fact that nearly all of the seientific experiments of the kind to which the Senator is referring are conducted by the private owners, and that nearly all these experiments are made upon private timber lands? I ask him if that is not the general fact.

Mr. BEVERIDGE. No; not all of them by any manner of means. I understand the fact to be ——.

Mr. CLARK of Wyoming. I did not say all of them; I said pretty generally the experiment was not a united experiment between the private owner of the timber and the Government.

COÖPERATION WITH PRIVATE OWNERS AND INDUSTRIES

Mr. BEVERIDGE. I understand the fact to be — and I desire to get it right and I will put it in the *Record* right if I do not get it correct now, because we are trying to get information and we have no pride of opinion, and if any of us find that we have made a mistake we are all equally willing to admit it — I understand the fact to be about these experiments that they are conducted to ascertain the best uses of timber on the Government's forest lands, and also the best uses of timber on the lands of private owners. Where any private owner of forest land desires to test his wood, the Government coöperates very cheerfully, and even invites such coöperation. I am sure that every Senator here, no matter what may be his opinion upon any other subject, would approve that plan as a wise and common-sense thing.

In addition to coöperative work in timber tests, the Forest Service gives advice and assistance to private owners of timber lands all over the country. Unless these forests also are preserved, a timber famine not less dangerous than a coal famine is in sight. Applications for help of this kind come from both owners of small wood lots and holders of large timber tracts. What are called "working plans" are made; that is, certain rules are recommended for the proper protection, management, and utilization of the timber, to the end that the owner may be assured of a continuous supply of wood, at the same time cutting what is necessary for present needs.

The object of the wood-lot work is to give, free of cost to farmers and other small owners, advice and assistance in the improvement and use of their woodlands. The coöperative work on large timber tracts embraces the whole country, and in many cases the plans recommended by the Forest Service are now actually being carried out very successfully.

Coöperative work is also undertaken with the various States, and this branch of the work has been taken up with the greatest detail in California.

So, Mr. President, we see what the Department is doing. I am trying to forward the work as much as possible. Of course there is a tremendous and far-reaching and deeply founded policy beneath it which I stated in the beginning, and that is the prevention of that portion of this country — and, if we could, of every portion of this country — from continuing a desert or being made into one if it is not one already. We are in a great work — and how characteristically American it is — the work of reclaiming, of saving, of developing, of making two blades of grass grow where none grew before. We have passed the period of destruction. We have abandoned that ruinous exploitation which was called "development," but was the reverse. We are replacing as fast as we can those gigantic resources which, in the strength and in consequence of our national youth, we so ruthlessly and thoughtlessly destroyed. It is a great constructive policy designed to create conditions that will supply homes for hundreds of thousands and millions in the near future and even a denser population in the more distant future.

RESERVES ·NATURAL FOREST LAND

I come now to a statement made — and it was an illustrative statement — yesterday afternoon by the Senator from Colorado [Mr. Patterson] — and I am sorry that he is not in his seat. But the Senate has heard him — and I think possibly one or two other statements were made like it. The Senator from Colorado yesterday described, with that vigorous eloquence which so characterizes him and charms us all, the establishment in Colorado of a great reserve, larger, he said, than some States, without a single tree upon it or any tree ever having grown upon it. I took pains to look up the *facts* as to that statement; and what are the facts?

It is true, in part, Mr. President, that such a reserve has been taken up so far as the existing trees are concerned. But it was originally land every foot of which was covered with magnificent woods which have long since been burned away until parts of the mountains — and it is a mountain region — where that reserve is are as bare of trees as three mountains I saw in the States of Colorado and California — though they were bare from a different cause — as the surface of this desk. But it is natural forest land. It is ideal for reforesting; it is being reforested. But the reforesting is impossible if all the herds and all the flocks of Colorado belonging to her great cattle and sheep kings and princes — and I have no objection to them; I should like to be a king of that kind myself — are allowed to pasture over that reserve at will and without control as well as without charge.

Mr. President, it was held out by intimation, if not by direct statement, that this land was fit for agricultural purposes and that the policy of the Department, therefore, had been to despotically take a principality in size, where no trees grew, and keep off the "sweeping tide of immigrants " from "founding homes." The fact is that it is above the agricultural line where homes are not "founded,"'and "immigrants " do not "pour in tides " or "pour " in any other way. Most of it is over 8,000 feet above the sea level, where farms are not practicable, except, I believe, a certain kind of farming, which is not worth taking into account. It is one of nature's natural forest reservoirs of water for the purpose of distributing that water for the uses of the people where the land farther down is agricultural.

What exists with reference to that land now is this: It is grown over with grasses; those grasses are good for grazing, and over that great extent, which belongs to the Government of the United States, the stockmen and the sheep men of Colorado have been fattening their herds. And they ask to do it still more — and that, too, without paying the Government a dollar.

Reserves not Unpeopled Solitudes

Let us bear in mind the actual conditions. A forest reserve contains lands "chiefly valuable for timber." Yet if the farmer finds up and down some valley that creeps back into these mountains a site for settlement, it is open to him as much as any other part of the public domain, if he enters in good faith. The reserves have been pictured as vast stretches of unbroken wilderness, empty solitudes trod only by the forester. In point of fact, they contain thousands of ranches; they contain hamlets, villages, and towns, to say nothing of lumber camps and railroad construction camps and mining camps. Wherever signs of mineral can be found the prospector stakes out his claim. In summer they are alive with those who resort thither for health and recreation — 50,000 of them in one season in southern California alone — and with the cowboys and sheep herders, who guard and care for the 7,000,000 head of animals that last year grazed in the forest reserves.

Benefits of Regulated Grazing

These forests of. the West are unlike those of the East. They are often open and park like, with forage plants growing beneath the trees. These grasses, like the trees themselves, will be wasted if they are not used. For this reason the Forest Service permits grazing in the reserves, but in every case is careful to exclude grazing from areas in which it has been found harmful. For example, grazing is not permitted in forests "under reproduction," as the Forester speaks of it — that is, forests in which cuttings are in progress to invite young growth. Forest reserves have never been created out of lands which are merely grazing lands. Yet this resource is like the forest in that it may be greatly impaired and even destroyed by unwise use. Unrestricted admittance of all stock would bring, and in many cases has brought, a decline in the number which the range would support. By licensing only so many head as the range can well support the Forest Service has proved to the satisfaction of the stockmen themselves that the carrying power of the range season after season is actually increased.

It was said that this was the crowning "infamy" of the Department, that the Department actually charged a "license fee" before any of these men were permitted to graze their cattle. I ask the Senate what else could the Government do? Ought the Government to give that privilege to the cattle and the sheep men, and if the Government ought not to give it to them can anybody imagine a safer or more practicable system of charging than the permit system?

Responsibility for Lieu Land Abuses

Now I come to the question of lieu land. I thought when I heard the Senator from Oregon make his charge the other day that he made a very serious charge, and when it was renewed by the Senator from Montana it appeared to me even grave. I knew that neither one of those Senators would make such a charge as that thoughtlessly. I have looked it up, and, in my opinion, that charge is entirely true.

I think it is entirely well founded, and after my investigation I think the language of the Senator from Montana, which I thought at the time was severe, is entirely justified, when he said that the relations of the Department at one·time with the land-grant railroads would bear looking into.

I find that it is true, as the Senator from Oregon described, that large tracts of land in Washington which were worthless had been released and lieu lands taken up in valuable portions of Oregon. But what has this Bureau to do with that? What are the facts? Let us be just to everybody. Nobody intends to accuse any man falsely nor condemn any man unjustly. The truth is that was done under a construction of the law by the *Land Office* some years ago, *and one of the first objections to it that was made within the Government itself was made by the Bureau of Forestry and personally by Gifford Pinchot, the Chief Forester.*

The Senator from Minnesota, who was most active in repealing that law to which a false meaning had been given by this construction of the Land Office will bear me out in that.

Mr. CARTER. Will the Senator permit an interruption?

Mr. BEVERIDGE. I will.

Mr. CARTER. The situation of which complaint is made presented this aspect, to wit: This Government owned large areas of very valuable timber land. The ownership of the Government over the land was undisputed. The superb character of the timber growing upon the land no one questioned and everybody knew. That character of land was not included in forest reservations until a lot of destitute, barren land in Arizona and elsewhere had been included in forest reserves — land which at the time of such inclusion was largely in the ownership of railroad companies, and that private ownership of these barren lands gave to the railroad companies the right to exchange the barren lands for the superb timber lands to which I referred.

Now permit me to ask why these great, superb, and valuable timber lands were not first withdrawn as forest reservation, so as to be protected from the rapacious grasp of the land-grant railroad, seeking lieu land for its trifling land in Arizona and elsewhere?

Mr. BEVERIDGE. The original fault was in Congress, which made the law capable of the construction the Land Department put upon it.

Mr. CARTER. Mr. President ——

Mr. BEVERIDGE. Let me answer your question. The secondary fault was in the Land Department for putting that construction upon it *and the remedy for which* — and let us spend no more time on that point, because the Senator ought generously to admit it — was suggested by the present Chief of the Bureau. So the fault, whatever there is, lies with us.

Mr. CARTER. Will the Senator inform us now why it was, when this great body of splendid timber land was in peril, the power of the Government was not exercised to protect it by withdrawing it and putting it in a forest reserve, and thus beyond the grasp of the lieu-land speculator?

Mr. BEVERIDGE. That has been a long time ago, and was because of the law which we ourselves had passed ——

Mr. CARTER. Mr. President ——

Mr. BEVERIDGE. Now pardon me. I have gone over this two or three times — and which this Bureau, and the head of this Bureau as one of this Commission, *was the first to suggest the correction* of.

Mr. CARTER. But the law which allowed poor land to be withdrawn certainly allowed good timber land to be likewise withdrawn. Why was not the good land withdrawn first?

Mr. FLINT. Mr. President ——

The VICE-PRESIDENT. Does the Senator from Indiana yield to the Senator from California?

Mr. BEVERIDGE. Certainly.

Mr. FLINT. I would like to ask a question of the Senator from

Montana. How long was it after the Secretary of the Interior had made the ruling he has mentioned before Congress acted and repealed the statute permitting the selection of good lands for the bad lands surrendered?

Mr. CARTER. From the very beginning it was within the power of the Interior Department to protect all the valuable timber land in the United States by including it in a forest reserve before any barren land at all was put in a forest reserve. The policy pursued was to put the barren land in forest reservations first and leave the superb timber land open, to be taken in exchange for the base lands in the forest reserves.

Mr. BEVERIDGE. If that was the policy, it never has been the policy under the present administration of the office.

Mr. CARTER. I refer to things done and not to policy. I refer to accomplished facts and public records and not to chimerical policies or uncertain data.

Mr. BEVERIDGE. That is rhetoric, but as a matter of fact the Senator must be as fair to me as I was to him and admit, and not only admit, but gladly assert, and I know the Senator will, that none of the things of which the Senator complains had its source in the present administration of the Forestry Bureau.

Mr. CARTER. I admit that Mr. Pinchot complained early and earnestly of the law.

Mr. BEVERIDGE. Yes.

Mr. CARTER. I place the responsibility where I think it belongs ——

Mr. BEVERIDGE. That is right.

Mr. CARTER. On the shoulders of those who so connived with the construction of this law as to pass to the land-grant railroads the splendid timber lands of Washington, Idaho, and western Montana in exchange for chaparral land in Arizona.

Mr. BEVERIDGE. I heartily agree with the Senator.

EFFECTIVE ADMINISTRATION OF THE NATIONAL FORESTS

Mr. President, I have examined briefly the policy, the three grounds of public good upon which this whole forest-reserve system rests. Now as to the question of administration, by which we mean the management of the reserves, it includes several things. After the reserves have been located in the painstaking way they are, as I have shown here by these maps and by the instructions to the locators of reserves, they are remapped. They are classified as to trees. There is now under the actual practical administration of this Bureau 128,000,000 acres, I believe. The Senator from Montana will correct me if I am wrong.

Mr. CARTER. One hundred and twenty-seven million acres.

Mr. BEVERIDGE. One hunderd and twenty-seven million acres. Now, through that runs a great system of forest patrol. It is policed by a network of forest rangers. One Senator yesterday referred to the fact that the examination of the land could not have been thorough, because one man had gone over 4,000,000 acres in two weeks. Was it not that? It was something like that, in any event, Mr. President. What does that mean? Merely that instead of cutting down the appropriation for the proper care of the reserves it ought to be increased. As a matter of fact, the forest policing is very careful, thorough, systematic. They police the forests, and I will tell in a minute what that means. If any man thinks that a forest police is not valuable, I shall show in a moment that there is no individual service in this Government that is more valuable or more delicate.

This policing is done by the rangers — 900 of them employed last year to patrol 100,000,000 acres of land — one ranger to 110,000 acres, or 172 square miles. In the highly profitable forests of Prussia there is one forest guard on the average to every 1.7 square miles. Small wonder that the cost of administration in the United States in spite of the higher scale of wages has been kept below that of any other European country except Russia.

The Forest Service is now expending annually, in administering the reserves, 1.6 cents per acre. Doubtless it should spend more, and must spend more as use of the reserves increases, for wise use means supervision and supervision means expense. Every live tree that is cut on the reserves is first marked by the forest ranger's axe; every log that is used is scaled; and this is but one of their many duties, which include guarding the range against trespass and the forests against fire. And all this with one ranger to 172 square miles! It needs no further evidence to show that these are not invalids, or Eastern tenderfeet, or college-bred, impractical theorists. They are men of the West, woodsmen, cowboys, lumberjacks — men who can ride the mountain trails and live a frontiersman's life. As to their efficiency, the record of forest fires throws some illumination on that point. I shall have something to say on that subject presently.

The next thing that the Forest Service does in the actual administration, after the test of the trees, after the marking of the "ripe" or mature timber, after arranging for the sale of that and the "down" timber, is to make trails and build roads, so that it is possible to communicate with one part of the reservation from another, and, further, so that if any agricultural lands are taken up by homesteaders there is a system of communication.

Then along this road there are built telephone lines, so that if in one portion of the forest a fire starts a ranger who finds himself unable to put it out may instantly telephone for help, so that men may be sent there and extinguish the fire while it is still young. Also, they build bridges, so that instead of a wild, ruinous, and rotting tangle of forest land you have a forest land which is woven together by trails, by a network of roads, and by telephones. You have the "'ripe" timber cut and taken off so as to increase the growth of that which is left. You have the "down" timber disposed of by selling it instead of permitting it to rot. You create a natural and healthy and perpetual forest, and therefore a profitable forest.

SUCCESS OF PROTECTION AGAINST FOREST FIRES

Mr. President, about the question of fires. In conversation yesterday I said that one of the most valuable services the Forest Service does was to preserve the forests from fires. I myself have had a little experience with forest fires and considerable observation about them, and there are Senators here from the West who have had a great deal more. It was suggested to me that the men who put out the fires are not the foresters, but really farmers. But that shows that there is still not as much knowledge in the Senate or the country as there ought to be as to what this Bureau is doing in the way of practical administration; because nearly all the fires that are now started in these mighty western forests are extinguished before they are old fires.

When a forest fire gets under way hardly all the farmers in a State could stop it; and I, in common with other Senators, have seen great areas of forest land, where millions — and I might also be accurate in saying tens of millions — of dollars' worth of Government property has been destroyed in less than two weeks' time. Then this is another part of its administration, and so excellent has it been — and I call the attention of the Senator from Montana to this, because he will know better than I — so excellent has this fire protection been that *the entire West has been practically clear of smoke during the summer time for the last two years.*

Mr. President, that last circumstance is something which, to those who live near great forest districts, is of absolutely incalculable consequence. I myself have seen in the forests of the Northeast mighty conflagrations raging which swept away villages and towns; and in one such fire, I remember, more than a hundred human beings lost their lives. I have seen, and the Senator from Montana has seen much more that I, the whole atmosphere clouded for weeks with smoke from these criminal acts of negligence — because that is what they are. When the Forest Service of the United States stops *one* of these fires they have saved more money to the Government than ten appropriations like this. We speak of economy, but we mean economy of resources, and trees are resources and soil is a resource as much as actual dollars.

The Forest Service keeps careful records of all fires on the reserves. These include even the smallest fires, which are put out before they have covered more than a few square rods — fires which, but for the vigilance of the forest officers, might become great conflagrations, but which are extinguished without cost beyond the salary of the rangers who patrol these forests as a part of their regular duties. During the year 1906, out of a total of 97,000,000 acres under administration, one-eighth of 1 per cent was burned over, and three one-hundredths of 1 per cent of the estimated standing timber was destroyed. But of over 1,100 fires reported, 450 were extinguished without one cent of extra cost to the Government. Nearly 700 large fires were fought, at a total cost of less than $9,000 for extra labor and supplies. That is pretty good evidence of the efficiency of the protection which the Forest Service gives, at a lower cost per acre, as I have already shown, than any European country except Russia — and Russia's figure is so low because the greater part of her forests are not under administration at all.

Increase in the Flow of Streams

The next thing is the exactly opposite thing, and yet closely connected with it — I am now talking about the actual tangible administration of this Service. The next thing which shows how completely the Service is practical and results in a definite and tangible benefit to the people is whether or not, as a matter of fact, it increases the waterflow in the streams. If we can show that it has kept the West, that mighty area of imperial forests, clear of smoke for two summers, we have vindicated it. But now if we can show, as a matter of fact, it has kept the streams' banks full, we have done more than that.

As a matter of fact, actual stream measurements made in southern California show an increase of 25 per cent in the flow of water since the reserves were created. No wonder the two Senators from California are hearty supporters of this policy. That means life to the people of California. That means prosperity to the people of that region. That means happy homes for hundreds and thousands of people. And so the Senators from California, speaking from actual experience, can testify, as they have so repeatedly testified, to the practical excellence of the tangible administration of these reserves. The same is true elsewhere.

So we see that in all the details of actual administration the Bureau is well-nigh perfect. I do not use that adjective unwittingly or lightly. I do not use it without having something of an official nature to support it. It is my purpose in the Senate to make no statement that I can not substantiate by something recognized as authoritative. I myself have never been greatly impressed by statements, however powerful they may seem, which could not be sustained by authorities.

The Department's conduct of these reserves has been criticised, even as to its administration here in Washington. This Department and all of the Executive Departments were examined by a commission called "the Keep Commission." I do not know whether that Commission is very popular or not, and the question is not whether it is. The question is whether what that Commission found of this Department is true. I wish to state in the beginning that a member of that Commission was Mr. Pinchot. But the man who testified before the House Committee on the Expenditures of the Agricultural Department was not Mr. Pinchot. It was Mr. Garfield, who is about to be the Secretary of the Interior. They went through all the Departments and one model department was found as to its actual administration, and particularly as to its system of auditing accounts, particularly as to the extreme care it took of the people's money. And so admirable was this Bureau found to be that it has been taken as an example upon which to recast and remodel other Departments and bureaus of the Government.

* * * * * * * *

Mr. President, I think that we have gone pretty thoroughly into this thing. I have tried to do it briefly, and still I have tried not to forget anything. I have here some other data which I shall ask the permission of the Senate to insert in my remarks without reading.

The VICE-PRESIDENT. Without objection, permission to do so is granted.

The matter referred to is as follows:

The administrative policy under which the forest reserves are managed was laid down by the Secretary of Agriculture in his letter to the Forester dated February 1, 1905:

In the administration of the forest reserves it must be clearly borne in mind that all land is to be devoted to its most productive use for the permanent good of the whole people, and not for the temporary benefit of individuals or companies. All the resources of forest reserves are for *use*, and this use must be brought about in a thoroughly prompt and businesslike manner, under such restrictions only as will insure the permanence of these resources. The vital importance of forest reserves to the great industries of the Western States will be largely increased in the near future by the continued steady advance in settlement and development. The permanence of the resources of the reserves is therefore indispensable to continued prosperity, and the policy of this Department for their protection and use will invariably be guided by this fact, always bearing in mind that the *conservative use* of these resources in no way conflicts with their permanent value.

You will see to it that the water, wood, and forage of the reserves are conserved and wisely used for the benefit of the home builder first of all, upon whom depends the best permanent use of lands and resources alike. The continued prosperity of the agricultural, lumbering, mining, and live-stock interests is directly dependent upon a permanent and accessible supply of water, wood, and forage, as well as upon the present and future use of these resources under businesslike regulations, enforced with promptness, effectiveness, and common sense. In the management of each reserve local questions will be decided upon local grounds; the dominant industry will be considered first, but with as little restriction to minor industries as may be possible; sudden changes in industrial conditions will be avoided by gradual adjustment after due notice, and where conflicting interests must be reconciled the question will always be decided from the standpoint of the greatest good of the greatest number in the long run.

Mr. BEVERIDGE. Mr. President, I do not know that I should have gone so much into the discussion — but I am glad I have gone into it — if it had not been for the original question of the character of the services rendered by that remarkable public servant, the Chief Forester of the United States, whom I have known intimately since I' was chairman of the Forestry Committee of the Senate years ago, and whose work I have observed with increasing wonder and admiration — a man who never spares himself mental or physical fatigue. Mr. President, when that man shall have completed his work on earth his monument will be no shaft of stone or image of brass. No! it will be the great and splendid forest reserves reclothed with nature's garment. It will be mighty mountain peaks now bare, then covered with the woods nature once put there and which he has restored. It will be the streams now dry, running bank full for the welfare of the people. It will be human welfare and human happiness.

THE NATIONAL FOREST POLICY[1]

SINCE Mr. Roosevelt has been President and Gifford Pinchot chief of the forest service, forest reserves in the West have been increasing with such rapidity as to provoke a great deal of criticism from Western Senators and lumber interests. The forest service, beginning as an unimportant bureau in the Department of Agriculture, has now come to have an entity of its own and broad powers over selected portions of the public lands. In the closing days of Congress Easterners, who give but little attention to matters in the far Western States, were considerably surprised at the concerted attack made by several Western Senators on the forest policy of the Administration.

This opposition to the forest service is declared by those in a position to know best, to have sprung from two sources — opposition to the general public lands policy urged by the President, and misconception of the actual purpose and probable results of the forest service policy. For reasons not unremotely allied to this wave of criticism, and because the name was a misnomer, the designation National Forest has been substituted for forest reserves.

The discussion by the President, in his successive messages to Congress, of public land questions seems to have aroused a very general feeling of alarm among Western men. Naturally, the interests which have found their profit in fraudulent operations under the present laws — land-grabbers, timber-grabbers, and range-fencers — were not likely

[1] *New York Evening Post*, March 20, 1907.

to favor the changes intended to put a stop to their operations. It would be a mistake, however, to suppose that desire for illicit gain is the motive which actuates the majority of the Western people not willing to follow the President's lead.

The whole tendency of things in the West tends to promote recklessness in the use of national resources, and to cause many Western people to look with leniency on questionable methods of acquiring title to property from the public domain. The people are too new to the region, too unattached, too hustling, to give great thought to the distant future. Boom development is far too much the ideal for which most people are working. The distinction between exploitation and real upbuilding is that between the man who develops the country and the man who skins the land. This is the Administration argument:

' THE ADMINISTRATION ARGUMENT

The national forests are undeveloped properties. They contain resources basic to the industrial life of the several Western States, so that their wise conservation is essential to the permanent welfare of these States. But, to make them useful, large capital expenditures are necessary. Even to protect them properly calls for a far greater sum than Congress would be likely to vote. Nor would it be just for Congress to take from the national Treasury this money, which would be expended for local benefits, when the money can be raised perfectly well by a moderate charge upon the users of the national forests for valuable privileges or materials. The only way to find the means for developing the national forests at the present time as they should be developed lies in securing a revenue from them.

State	Number of reserves	Acres
Arizona	13	9,450,825
California	19	19,882,487
Colorado	16	12,698,825
Idaho	16	19,048,806
Kansas	1	97,280
Montana	20	17,344,883
Nebraska	3	556,072
Nevada	4	766,959
New Mexico	12	7,024,504
Oklahoma	1	60,800
Oregon	12	12,500,728
South Dakota	4	1,263,720
Utah	16	6,731,300
Washington	5	7,785,606
Wyoming	8	8,637,366

The area of the national forests in 1891 was 2,437,120 acres. This has increased steadily except during the period from 1893 to 1896 inclusive, until to-day the acreage of the national forests is 148,281,230. On February 1, 1907, there were 136 forest reserves in the United States with a total acreage of 123,850,161. How these were located and their acreage are shown in the above table.

THE PRESIDENT'S RECENT PROCLAMATION

One of the last acts of Congress before adjournment this month was to pass a law forbidding the creation of forest reserves, except by Congress in the six States of Washington, Oregon, Montana, Idaho, Wyoming, and Colorado. The effect of this act would have been to delay the extension of national forests in these States had not the President, as soon as he became aware of the purpose of Congress, rendered the legislative will practically void by adding 17,000,000 acres to the national forest area in those States by executive order. This great acreage is divided into thirty-two separate reserves of forests.

It is impossible to say how much remaining public land — though probably but a very small proportion — is adapted for national forest purposes, because no satisfactory examinations have been made of this land to determine its best use. Instead of answering this question, the following statement, comparing the stumpage of the national forest with the stumpage of the Western States as a whole, may prove interesting:

The estimated stumpage of the national forests is 330 billion feet. An estimate of the Western States, which includes only some of the States for certain species, and omits several species, gives 800 billion feet as the total stumpage of the region. Probably only 25 per cent of the timber of the States in which they are located is included in the national forests.

The only lands among the national forests which have been thrown open to settlement are those which were restored to the public domain March 16 last. This was not forested land, but a part of it was intended to be used for experiments in forest planting. It was restored because agriculture on part of the area had become possible by means of the Campbell system of dry farming.

Lands temporarily withdrawn from entry, comprising 550,000 acres in Colorado and 370,000 in Washington, were released this month. No other areas of importance have recently been released, though it is the active policy of the Forest Service to withhold no land more important for other purposes than for forest growth.

Under the Administration of President Harrison 13,416,710 acres were added to the forest reserve; under President Cleveland the total became 25,686,320, and under President Roosevelt the total is 56,876,934. The following table shows the growth in area of the national forests from 1891 to the present time:

GROWTH IN AREA OF THE NATIONAL FORESTS

1891 2,437,120	1900 46,571,359
1892 5,752,840	1901 46,082,719
1893 17,928,070	1902 59,966,090
1894 17,928,070	1903 62,962,849
1895 17,928,070	1904 63,093,164
1896 17,928,070	1905 97,716,860
1897 39,103,030	1906 127,154,371
1898 43,744,424	1907, March 15 148,281,230
1899 46,726,879	

'In area the reserves were increased during the fiscal year 1905 to 1906 from 85,693,422 to 106,999,138 acres. In revenue they brought in $767,219.96, as against $60,142.62 for the previous year. In timber sales there were disposed of for immediate or early removal nearly 300,000,000 board feet of lumber at stumpage prices ranging up to $4 per .thousand (besides other material to a large value), as against 96,060,258 board feet, with a maximum price of $2.50 per thousand in 1904–5 and 69,257,710 board feet in 1903–4. The number of free-use permits granted in the same years also showed progressive increase. In the year 1904–5 the reserves were under forest service control only after February 1.

Local sentiment has sometimes been unfavorable to the creation of reserves before their effect upon the public welfare was understood; but opposition has always dissolved under the test of actual experience. The reserves do not withhold land from agricultural use. Though they were made from the most rugged and mountainous parts of the West and were intended to include only land unsuited for agriculture, by the act of June 11, 1906, the right is given settlers to homestead within the reserves wherever strips and patches of tillable land can be found. At the same time, through their water-conserving power, these forests fix in regions of scanty rainfall the amount of land which can be brought under the plough, since at best much otherwise fertile land must go uncultivated for want of water. Without forest preservation much of the land now under irrigation would have to be abandoned again to the desert.

NOT A MONEY-MAKING SCHEME

It is not the policy of the forest service to make money out of the reserves of the Government. They are administered on the same principle that a private estate is administered by an executor; to make it pay the greatest returns to the beneficiaries — in this case the people of the United States. By an act of Congress, 10 per cent of the gross receipts from the national forests are made over to the several States in which the reserves are situated, for the benefit of the counties which would otherwise receive no revenue from a part of their area. This redressed a real grievance. Eventually, it is hoped, the counties affected will find themselves far better off than they would have been without the reserves, for, it is argued, private ownership followed by exploitation would have destroyed the sources of revenue by leaving little or nothing of permanent taxable value.

On the floor of the Senate opponents of Mr. Pinchot's forest policy conceded that he had won over the stockmen to his way of thinking. On this point Secretary Wilson said:

I wish to commend the heartiness and good spirit with which the associations of Western stockmen have coöperated in our efforts to enforce fair and just measures for the regulation of grazing in the interest of all users of the forests, and in the interest of the public, to whom these forests belong. The charge of a grazing fee, made for the first time during the last year, though reasonable in view of the advantages of grazing regulation to the stockmen and the cost of reserve administration to the Government, and justly due to the interest of the public, might have been expected to cause dissatisfaction and friction. On the contrary, as soon as the reasons for the charge and the method in which it would be applied had been explained, it was generally approved and paid willingly and promptly. It was followed by no falling off in the number of stock grazed in the reserves. In some cases the associations of stockmen have voluntarily aided the service in settling local difficulties. Their whole conduct has shown remarkable moderation, far-sightedness, and readiness to recognize and accept what is in the permanent interest of their industry, even though it involves the sacrifice of immediate personal advantage.

SPEECH OF SENATOR FRANCIS G. NEWLANDS ON INLAND WATERWAYS [1]

Mr. Newlands said:

Mr. President, the agitation for a deep waterway from St. Louis to the Gulf and from the Lakes to the Gulf has reached such proportions as to create a general demand from every section of the country that a broad and comprehensive plan should be inaugurated for the improvement of all the navigable waterways of the country, and that legislation should be adopted creating a fund for continuous and uninterrupted work, securing a fair apportionment of the work between the different sections of the country, and providing for a businesslike administration with reference both to examination and construction.

The President, realizing this demand, determined to investigate the matter with a view to recommending to Congress such a broad and comprehensive plan; and, as a step in that direction, appointed the Inland Waterway Commission to look into the various questions relating to the inland waterways and their full economic development, and to

[1] *Congr. Record*, reported Jan. 6, 1908.

report to him, with the expectation that, if their recommendation was approved by him, it would be submitted to Congress for its action. The Commission has been in frequent sessions since April last. It has visited nearly every section of the country. Several members of the Commission visited the Pacific coast and inspected the Sacramento, the San Joaquin, and the Columbia rivers. The entire Commission took a tour of the Great Lakes, and also made a trip from St. Paul to the Gulf upon the Mississippi River. Subsequently a majority of the Commission made an examination of the Missouri River.

WATERWAY CONVENTIONS

In addition to this the Commission has been represented at various conferences and conventions which have been held throughout the country from the Pacific to the Atlantic and from the Lakes to the Gulf upon this important question.

The general interest which the country is showing in the improvement of waterways is manifest in the organization of various river-improvement associations in all parts of the country and in meetings of these and other associations, the principal object of which is to consider waterway improvement. I shall enumerate some of these.

The Inland Waterways Commission is now engaged in framing a preliminary report to the President, but it has not yet reached a final conclusion. I wish to say, as a member of that commission, that I simply express here my individual views and that I have introduced in the Senate a bill (S. 500) providing for the appointment of an inland waterway commission for the development of the inland waterways of the country, purely in a tentative way. I invite suggestion, criticism, and amendment, so that the commission may have the advantage of the consideration of this question by Members of both bodies of Congress and by the country at large before it reaches a final conclusion.

GOVERNMENT WORKS

In the past, Mr. President, it has been the general view of the country that the Government was unable to do constructive work; that it was unable to do such work efficiently; that it was unable to do it economically; that it was unable to do it quickly. The experience of the country within the past few years with two great systems of constructive work has proved the contrary and has proved that the Government is able to do its own work.

Mr. BEVERIDGE. I will ask the Senator what are the two examples to which he refers?

Mr. NEWLANDS. Those two exceptions are the construction of the Panama Canal and the work of the Reclamation Service. For the work of the Panama Canal service $75,000,000 has already been appropriated, of which about $39,000,000, I believe, has already been spent. The Reclamation Service has a fund of about $39,000,000, a very large proportion of which has already been spent on about twenty-three different projects in fourteen or fifteen different States and Territories. I will not enlarge upon the work of either one of these services. It is sufficient to say that the country is satisfied with the work of both. So far as the region which I represent is concerned — the arid and semiarid region — there is a feeling of universal satisfaction with the energetic and efficient work and the thoroughly organized work that has been done by the Reclamation Service.

Now, Mr. President, in shaping this bill I have endeavored to unite the best features of both those bills.

Mr. BEVERIDGE. Mr. President ——

The VICE-PRESIDENT. Does the Senator from Nevada yield to the Senator from Indiana?

Mr. NEWLANDS. If the Senator will permit me a moment further ——

Mr. BEVERIDGE. I am profoundly interested in what the Senator is saying on this whole great plan, and I think the Senator might enlarge there upon the fact that the Reclamation Service and the Panama Canal, as enterprises, are conducted also by officers of the Government, and in the case of the Panama Canal it finally came down to the most efficient work by the officers of the Regular Army. Those two instances I call to the Senator's attention, so that he might put them into his speech.. They, however, are not the only ones. There is the telegraph service in Alaska, covering 8,000 miles or more, and other things of that kind.

I ventured to interrupt the Senator for the purpose of directing his attention more particularly to those facts.

Mr. NEWLANDS. I am very glad to receive the suggestion of the Senator from Indiana. It is true, as he says, that both of these services are being conducted by officers of the Government.

My individual view is that within the next ten years the United States should expend at least $500,000,000 in the improvement of its inland waterways; that we ought to enter upon this work contemporaneously in every section of the country; that we should enter upon the work of the rivers of the Pacific coast, upon the rivers of the Atlantic coast, upon the Gulf coast, and upon the Mississippi River and its tributaries, and upon the coastal canals or sheltered waterways which will connect the rivers of the Gulf and Atlantic coast from Texas to Maine. All these works should be commenced and prosecuted contemporaneously. I wish to say further that that is the sentiment of the people of the United States, and Congress will, I have no doubt, accommodate itself to that view of the great public.

A Broad and Comprehensive Treatment

Now, I ask, what is a broad and comprehensive treatment of a river that is to be used in interstate or foreign commerce for navigation? Take the Mississippi, so far as its western tributaries are concerned; the Missouri, and its tributaries; the Yellowstone; the Madison; the Gallatin; and the Jefferson rivers; farther down, the Platte and the Kaw; farther down, the Arkansas River. All these rivers have their source in the region to which the Senator and I belong — in the snows of the mountains.

Prevention of Floods

Now, what does a rational treatment of that river, so far as concerns its utilization for navigation, involve? It involves for one thing the prevention of floods, for these waters rush down in torrential streams in the spring months and destroy property, and then during the summer and fall months, the waters having rushed down to the ocean and having been wasted, the river itself is reduced to an attenuated stream upon which boats can not float. What does a rational treatment of that river involve? Obviously storage, all along the line, wherever it can be done practicably and economically and with a view to the reasonable cost of the entire enterprise. What does storage upon those upper rivers mean? It means the construction of artificial reservoirs in which these waters are impounded during the period of flood, and from these reservoirs waters are led over the great plains, the arid and the semiarid plains, and used for purposes of cultivation. These plains absorb the water like a sponge and gradually give it out by the process of seepage to the tributary streams of the great river. Give it out when? Give it out when it is most needed for navigation, during the months of July, August, and September. So irrigation is a proper method of treating the river for navigation, for it is one method of impounding the flood waters of these tributary streams, preventing those flood waters from creating destruction below in the spring and preserving them for a beneficent purpose later on in the summer and fall months. In the more humid regions, in which irrigation is not required and in which evaporation is less rapid than in the arid and semiarid districts, the reservoir may be used for the storage of storm and thaw waters, which may be kept impounded, as is now done, for example, in the upper Mississippi and in some foreign countries, until the time of low water, when the contents may be let out in such manner as to maintain navigation throughout the summer.

Now, the Senator's view doubtless would be that the Government has no power to enter upon the reclamation per se of arid lands not in its own ownership. There is no power expressly granted in the Constitution for that purpose, and I believe with the Senator from Colorado that this is a Government of granted powers, and that we can only exercise the granted powers. I shall simply contend for the full exercise of these powers. No one will deny the full power of the Government over the question of interstate and foreign commerce. No one will deny the power of the Government to make a river navigable. If you do not deny that, then the Government can adopt any practicable means to make it navigable, and it need not confine itself to digging a channel when it can by this process of the storage of waters at the heads of these streams and by this process of spreading those waters over the vast arid and semiarid plains suspend the flow of that water until by the process of seepage it gradually goes back to the streams at the time when it is most needed for the maintenance of a full, safe, and sure channel for the purposes of navigation.

FORESTRY

So it is with forestry. The forests are the conservators of moisture. In a state of nature the streams gathering in forests run clear and in fairly uniform volume throughout the year. The soil is protected from the beating of the storm by the branches and foliage, which break the drops into spray, and this trickles gently down the trunks and along the roots, so that the soil remains open and pervious. This soft, spongy soil is further protected by a mulch of partly decayed leaves, twigs, and shreds of bark and wood; and in the mulch and friable mold the waters of rains and thaws are absorbed as in a sponge, and do not flow off quickly in rills and freshets, but seep slowly through the soil into the permanent springs by which the streams are fed. Denude large areas of their forests, and the rains falling from the heavens rush off the lands in torrential streams and increase the volume of the floods that are so destructive below. We all know that one of the causes of these great and destructive floods has been the destruction of our forests. If, then, the forests are conservators of moisture, if they are natural storage reservoirs of moisture, and if the impounding of these waters in artificial reservoirs for the purpose of holding them until they can swell the volume of the stream below for the purpose of navigation is constitutional, can we not make use of the reservoirs that nature has created and develop them; and if we can do that, can we not take control over large areas of land and replace the forests that have been destroyed?

Of course the Constitution grants no power to the National Government to enter into the timber business or the lumber business as such, but it has the power to make a sure, stable, equal stream for purposes of navigation; and if it can accomplish this by developing the forests, the natural reservoirs of the country, so as to hold these waters in suspense until the time when they are most needed, it has the power to preserve and protect the existing forests, it has the power to replace the forests; and certainly in that connection it has the power to plant trees; and if it has the power to plant trees, it has the power to sell the timber which is planted when it becomes unnecessary to the main purpose of the enterprise — the conservation of moisture.

If the forest becomes too crowded, is there any objection to the removal of useless trees, and can you say that because the Constitution has not granted to the Government the power to enter into the lumber business it therefore can not sell that timber as a part of the compensation of the enterprise itself? Would you say with reference to these great reclamation enterprises, which constitute a rational method of treating the river for the purpose of navigation, that the Government can not compensate this fund and diminish the cost of the entire enterprise by selling irrigation rights, thus getting back proportionately from all the lands benefited the cost of the reclamation work and diminishing the cost of the main enterprise — the promotion and development of a navigable stream?

RECLAMATION OF SWAMP LANDS

But the comprehensive plan for the development of these waterways not only involves reclamation by irrigation and the protection and replacement of forests, but it also involves the drainage of swamp lands below. The reclamation of swamp lands is the antithesis of the irrigation of arid lands. There is too little water on the land above and there is too much below. Why is there too much below? Because the river breaks through its banks, divides itself into numerous channels, creates bayous and sloughs, and thus dedicates vast areas of cultivable land, the richest in the world, to proverty and death.

Mr. BEVERIDGE. Will the Senator from Nevada permit an interruption?

Mr. NEWLANDS. Certainly.

Mr. BEVERIDGE. As I said, and as the Senator from New Hampshire said, I think this is one of the very greatest subjects before the American people, and one, perhaps, in which they are as much interested as any other just at the present time. I wish the Senator would follow, till he establishes it more closely, the analogy between the Government's power over the conservation of waters and their control as navigable waters and the power of the Government over forests. For example, one of the most fundamental rules in statutory and constitutional interpretation is that if the power is conceded it carries with it any incidental power necessary to make it complete. So if it be conceded — and that has been thrashed out — that we have the right as a Government to control certain forest reserves, it follows as an incident of that that it is not only our right and our power, but our duty to dispose of what is called "down timber" and "express timber"; and therefore the Government not only has the right, but it becomes its duty, to become a lumber merchant to that extent.

Again, our power to build the Panama Canal is conceded, let us say. That carries with it the power to do what the Government is now doing; that is, to operate a line of steamships and also to operate a railroad across the Isthmus of Panama. So it can be carried out in numberless instances.

I would be glad if the Senator would spend a little more time in establishing the analogy between the Government's power over the conservation of waters and their control as navigable waters and these other things which the Senator has referred to.

If the Senator from Nevada will permit me for just a moment further. In reference to what was said by the Senator from Colorado, of course it has been held, since *Gibbons* v. *Ogden* until now, that the power of the National Government over navigable waters, even wholly within a State, goes to the point that signals and lights may be maintained by the National Government, and it may do everything else that is necessary. The State has no right to establish lights, or signals, even in its own waters, because they might interfere with the navigation of commerce that passes beyond the State lines.

So again, the National Government, in improving waterways, for which we now expend scores of millions every year in the river and harbor bill, has the right to prevent the State from in any way obstructing that waterway. If that was not conceded, of course, it would be destructive of the power to improve it. Therefore, if the establishment by the State of an electric-light plant upon the waters running through the State, which were navigable, interfered with that purpose, the National Government would have the right to prevent the erection of such an electric-light plant. But per contra, if the erection of such an electric-light plant became necessary as an aid to the navigability of the waters, it would necessarily follow, would it not, that we would have the right to construct it?

The Senator will pardon me, but I think it is a vital point in his argument, and if he will follow that analogy a little more closely, it will be agreeable to many of the friends of his measure.

Mr. NEWLANDS. I have already gone further into the argument of these questions than I intended when I rose. My purpose was simply to present a statement of the bill and an explanation of its provisions, but I have been drawn out somewhat by the challenge of the Senator from Colorado. It was not my intention to go into all these refinements. However, I will pursue the argument that I was pursuing regarding the various uses of the waters of a stream which tend to the promotion of its navigability, and I will take up in its turn the suggestion that the Senator from Indiana makes with reference to electric power.

I was upon the question of the reclamation of swamp lands, which I stated was the antithesis of the reclamation of arid lands, the swamp lands being at the lower reaches of the streams, the arid lands at the sources of the streams. We all know that a great river in making its way through these lowlands during periods of flood divides itself into numerous channels, which make bayous and sloughs, and create these vast areas of swamp lands, incomparably rich, for they are composed of alluvial soil, and yet are incapable of cultivation because of an excess of moisture. Now, the reclamation of swamp lands as such, unless the Government is the owner of those lands, would not be one of the functions of Government under the granted powers of the Constitution. But the control of the river for purposes of navigation is; and if the control of that river involves the construction of levees along its banks so as to keep the river in its channel, so that the large volume of water can scour the bottom and create a channel fit for navigation, then that is clearly within the powers of the Government. In like manner, when the needs of navigation demand, it is competent for the Government to maintain the volume and regimen of rivers required for commerce by laying drains in such manner as to maintain a flow at low-water stages. The reclamation in both cases is simply incidental and collateral.

COMPENSATORY PROJECTS

Would you say that when the Government goes to this great expenditure, which involves an incidental benefit to the lands of private owners, it can not seek in some way compensation to the fund for this beneficial work, and thus diminish the cost of the primary enterprise? Can not the Government by cooperation with States, by cooperation with districts, so organize this work as to divide the cost between the States or the localities affected and the National Government? The project might not be feasible at all unless the Government could diminish the cost by putting a certain amount of the cost upon incidental and collateral works of this kind. And so this great plan of developing a river for navigation may involve, and in most cases does involve, the actual reclamation of large areas of swamp land.

WATER POWER

Now we come to the question of water power. The Government will be compelled not only to construct dams on the tributary streams for irrigation, but sometimes on the great river itself — for the purpose of constructing locks through which vessels can pass, and thus avoid dangerous rapids. If the Government does construct such a dam for the purpose primarily of promoting navigation, will the Senator from Colorado contend that the Government can not diminish the cost of the enterprise by selling the water power created by that dam?

Mr. TELLER. Does the Senator want me to answer his question now?

Mr. NEWLANDS. Yes.

Mr. TELLER. That is the very point I wanted to bring to the Senator's attention. That is exactly what I wish to deny. The Government has not any power under the Constitution, for any purpose whatever, to go into business of that character. It has not any right to create a water power and sell the power. If the State did not interfere, the Government would have no such authority under the Constitution. But the State, if it had a proper conception of its rights, would not allow that to be done. The State would say it would do it if it was to be done; and if the Senator will pardon me, some day I will present him a brief on this subject which I think will convince him that my suggestions are fully supported by the decisions of the Supreme Court of the United States.

I am not afraid that the Senate will go into anything of that kind. But I do not want to have this initial step, as it were, in this waterway business complicated by what will appear to those who study the law on the subject as an utter impossibility.

Mr. NEWLANDS. I take issue with the Senator upon that question. I shall be very glad to read the brief to which he has referred me, but I can not question the power of the Government to build a dam in a river for the purpose of constructing locks which will be serviceable to navigation.

Mr. TELLER. The Senator has no business to put me in that category. I have never suggested that the Government could not do that.

Mr. NEWLANDS. I was going one step further.

Mr. TELLER. I say most emphatically the Government may do that, but the Government has no right, then, to establish an electric-light plant on it and sell the light. That is what I assert.

Mr. NEWLANDS. If the Senator had heard my sentence through, I think he would not have taken exception to it. I will repeat part of what I did say and add to it what I intended to say.

I do not doubt for a moment the power of the Government to construct a dam for the purpose of establishing a lock which will be serviceable to navigation.

Mr. TELLER. Neither do I.

Mr. NEWLANDS. Thus far the Senator agrees with me. Now, I was going to add, nor do I doubt the power of the Government to diminish the cost of that enterprise to the Government by availing itself of the sale of the power created by that dam.

Now, another thing. If the Senator insists that the Government can not do that without the consent of the State, then I say we should take steps in this bill for obtaining the consent of the State.

Mr. TELLER. I deny the right of the Government to do it even with the consent of the State. This Government can not go into any commercial business of that kind.

Mr. NEWLANDS. I would not expect the Government to go into the commercial business of peddling out light ——

Mr. TELLER. Or water.

Mr. NEWLANDS. Of constructing poles and stringing wires and distributing light throughout an entire community, or distributing power throughout an entire community, but I do contend that it would be entirely within the governmental function to diminish the cost of the great work; and if it can accomplish that result by some method of leasing the power, at the same time so controlling the lease that it will not result in monopoly and oppression, I should say it had that power as a means of diminishing the cost of the enterprise.[1]

But if there is anything in our dual government that prevents the nation from acting without the consent of the State, then I see no reason why the two sovereigns affected should not confer together about the matter — the Union of States, the one sovereign, the individual State where the dam is located, the other. Can we doubt that they would come to some rational conclusion? Would the lesser sovereign deny to the greater sovereign the right to get a value out of that which it itself had created that would be in a measure compensatory of its own expenditures? The two sovereigns can do business with each other just as individuals can; and there is no reason why the Union of States should not enter into an arrangement with an individual State that will present a just solution of the question. If the State has the property rights, for which the Senator contends, it can share with the nation the burden of cost of a work necessary or useful for both navigation and power. If the Government spends millions of dollars in the construction of a dam, it should certainly have compensation for the power which it itself has created. Common honesty would dictate that.

I did not intend at this time to discuss the question of governmental functions at all; it is a matter of business, and that is what I hope to see established as the basis of this enterprise. I hope to see this great work put upon a business basis. I believe the Government can do work in a businesslike way in carrying out the granted powers, and I believe in giving its agents a pretty free hand to enable them to do business effectively.

[1] In fact, that is just what the Government is doing now, and has done for several years, under statutory authority. The legislation has so often been repeated and has so long remained unquestioned that the governmental policy with respect to water power may be regarded as established. Under this policy the Federal Government reserves the right, when authority is given to private corporations to dam actually or possibly navigable streams for the development of power, to use without charge so much of that power as may be required for specific uses by the Government, this reservation being in the nature of a consideration. When the works are constructed coöperatively between the Federal Government and prospective powers users, then the Government reserves rights of administration and specific uses, and also limits the lease or authority to the private party to use the power to a specified period; while, if the work is constructed at the cost of the Federal Government, then the statutes authorize the leasing of the power developed thereby under customary governmental restrictions as to advertising, etc.

The reason why I present this bill now is because I fear that in the future should we enter upon this work Congress may without considering these related questions of use and compensation and coöperation put the administrative agents of the Government in a strait-jacket and thus prevent them from conducting the work in a businesslike way.

I do not intend, Mr. President, to be drawn off into nice refinements as to constitutional power. I do not propose to balance the power of the National Government with the power of the State in an individual matter. Here is an enterprise which is of the greatest importance to the entire country. We propose in aid of the development of commerce between the States, and commerce with foreign nations, exclusively within the jurisdiction of the National Government, to enter upon this great work of utilizing our rivers in a businesslike way for every beneficial purpose to which they can be put.

We must realize that it is not wise to take up simply one use of the river, for navigability, and lose sight of all the other uses, when the adoption of the other uses and the development of the other uses will diminish the cost of the enterprise and make it more efficient for the public good. The cost might be entirely prohibitory if it were not for the correlated uses and the contribution or compensation secured through them, for this is a work which can be accomplished either by the National Government itself or by the coöperation of the National Government with States, with corporations, with municipalities, and with individuals.

CLARIFICATION OF STREAMS

We can not only take up this question of the utilization of water power beneficial to the entire people, and with a view to economy in the enterprise itself, but we can take up with it the question of the clarification of the streams. That is a matter, you say, of sanitation, affecting the people of the towns and cities along the borders of the streams. But you must recollect that these great rivers are full of sediment and sand, every particle of which is a destructive tool when directed against the banks of the river. Clear waters are not nearly so destructive or obstructive as muddy waters, as water filled with sand or soil. It is well demonstrated that every particle of soil, every particle of sand in the water, is a destructive agent. When deposited in the shoals and bars it obstructs the channel. When suspended in the water and driven by the force of the current against the banks of the river it breaks them down, and the broken bank carried down in the current sinks within a few miles and makes the shoal or bar.

What do we find in the great rivers that pass through alluvial bottoms? The banks dissolve like sugar when the force of the water is directed against them. A capricious stream like the Missouri River makes its way through a bottom of this kind from Kansas City to St. Louis, a distance of about 300 miles, a valley from 4 to 10 miles in width, bounded by bluffs on either side; and that river, during the period of flood, its banks dissolving like sugar before the force of the water, can make its way anywhere in the alluvial bottom between the bluffs, so that the farm of to-day becomes the swamp to-morrow, and the river bed of to-day becomes the cultivated farm to-morrow.

We can clarify that turgid water, swollen with sediment and sand. How? By the prevention of soil waste and by the protection of the banks by willow and stone revetment. There washes down the Mississippi River every year pretty nearly a continent of the best soil. At New Orleans to-day the alluvial soil is twelve hundred feet deep.

The great problem we have had in the lower reaches of the Mississippi has been the control of the passes, the river making its way to the Gulf through three passes, building up on either side, by the deposit of sand and sediment, a continent. So it is hardly an exaggeration to say that in time the great Gulf itself will become a continent.

Now, is the Government simply to dredge out that sand and sediment when it settles down in the bed of the stream and deposit it somewhere else, whence it will make its way gradually back to the stream, or can it take measures to prevent that sediment and sand from coming into the stream? Can it not take measures to prevent this soil waste and this bank destruction? It is fair to say that in time the prevention of soil waste can be brought about by proper methods of cultivation enjoined by the National Government, perhaps as a matter of persuasion at first, though it might well become a matter of compulsion. The conservation and development of the natural resources of the country — the forest, the land, the water — for every purpose require the scientific treatment of a stream and the full consideration of every related use.

How is this to be done? In the first place, this fund is created to which I have referred, a fund for uninterrupted and continuous work, the dedication of $50,000,000 immediately to this work. The Senator from Idaho says it may lie idle for a time. There is $250,000,000 or $300,000,000 in the Treasury now that is lying idle. The Treasury deposits a large portion of it in banks of the country and receives no compensation from it. It will be no more idle than it is now.

It is incumbent upon us to show our fixed and determined purpose that this work shall commence, and that it shall be prosecuted without interruption, and not in the elusive and disjointed way in which it has been prosecuted heretofore.

An Administrative Matter

Now, this bill gives the executive department great power, and I have no doubt that objection will be urged. I believe in giving the executive department full power in this matter, because it is an administrative matter. I believe in preserving the boundaries of the functions of the Government; and I insist upon it that Congress has attended too much to administrative matters, and the very reason of the inefficiency of our work upon our rivers and harbors has been that Congress has sought to do administrative work and has done it badly, as it always will do it badly.

Ninety men in the Senate and four hundred or more in the House working on legislation for the country do not constitute efficient bodies for administrative work. Wherever administrative work is to be done I believe in intrusting it to the executive department and putting the responsibility upon the Executive. We did this with reference to the reclamation act. After having educated the entire country to the desirability of entering upon the great reclamation work, the Western men found that they were unable to move because they were divided among themselves as to what should be done. Each man wanted a project first undertaken in his own State and was unwilling to concede that another State had superiority or advantage as to priority. We were in confusion as to the methods of administration. Finally we got together, and what did we conclude to do? We passed a bill creating a fund derived from the sales of the public lands of the country and dedicated that fund forever to this work. Then we gave the power to the Secretary of the Interior to go ahead and investigate the projects and if he found them feasible, to do the work, and the only limitation put upon his power was that he should not let a contract unless the money for its payment was in the fund. That was the only limitation. We did not go into details regarding the organization. There can be no effective organization which is not the result of the process of evolution. Let Congress attempt to organize at the start a great working force of this kind, and it will always fail. They will have to come back to Congress for amendatory and supplementary legislation, all delaying the prosecution of the work. We did the simple thing and put the responsibility upon the Secretary of the Interior, and the Secretary of the Interior accepted the responsibility and held the responsibility. Congress of course reserved to itself all the powers of supervision, of criticism, of examination. Reports were required. The officers of the Service were compelled to come before the committees and give full expositions of their work. Committees visited the works themselves and made actual inspection, and then upon their return to Congress summoned the officials before them and examined them upon matters concerning which they desired information..

So the whole service, under the critical eye of Congress, but with full powers of administration, has advanced and accomplished a great work. It has in the short period of its existence removed, I believe, twice as many cubic yards of earth as have been removed in the Panama Canal. It has constructed works of great magnitude and has considered problems, many of which were as difficult as those involved in the Panama construe-tion. We have organized in the Reclamation Service a body of skilled engineers capable of undertaking any work of construction from the construction of a canal to the construction of a railroad and the development of the inland waterways themselves.

So it was with the Panama construction. Accidentally we blundered there into wise legislation. Congress was divided into contending forces as to whether we should have the canal at Panama or at Nicaragua. Different views prevailed as to whether it should be a lock canal or a sea-level canal. There would have been the widest divergence of views as to all the details of operation. But in the confusion a simple bill, I believe drawn by Senator Spooner of Wisconsin, appropriated $50,000,000 for the work and gave the President full power to go ahead and do it. We all know how that has worked out.

Suppose we had started in the first place and insisted upon it that all the plans should be submitted to committees of Congress with their differences of opinion, and to Congress itself with their differences of opinion, we would have been debating to-day over mere matters of detail. But out of the very necessity of the situation, inasmuch as Congress was unable to agree, a simple bill was prepared which gave the President full power. Does anyone contend that the President has abused that power? Is there any President whom we can elect who will be so dishonest or so inefficient as to abuse that power? He has gone about in a businesslike way to create an organization, each organization in itself tentative at the start. I believe the Panama Canal service has been reorganized three times. First we had the Walker Commission, and then we had the Shonts Commission, and then we had the Goethals Commission, a commission the same in number, authorized, I believe, by Congress, but maintained in organization at the will of the Executive. We were probably unwise in compelling the Executive to have a commission of nine men. He himself in a recent message or in a recent speech has indicated that perhaps a more efficient method of organization would be one commissioner, with subordinates, so that one person could be held responsible for the work.

The first two commissions held their sessions here. The last commission is located in Panama, and consists mainly of officers of the Government, an engineer officer of the Army, an engineer officer of the Navy, and a medical officer of the Army, who has done the sanitation work of that district. After various experiments the President has placed the control of the work in the Engineer Corps of the Army, noted for its efficiency, integrity, and high sense of honor — a corps which has been compelled thus far to adapt itself to the repressive policy of the nation as to rivers and harbors, but which, under a progressive policy and aided by the other scientific services of the Government in matters relating to their jurisdiction, will accomplish as brilliant a work in our inland waterways as it is now accomplishing at Panama. We have given the Executive a free hand, and we have been wise in giving him a free hand. Had we sought to impose upon him Congressional restraints and put him in a Congressional strait-jacket, the work would not have advanced as it has advanced.

So I contend that in this case we should give the President the power not only to enter upon the construction of the work, but to make the examinations and the surveys, and to do it without further authority from Congress, and to appoint such boards and commissions and agents and experts as in his judgment may seem proper, and to fix their salaries until Congress fixes them. The organization can best be worked out by an executive officer and not through the wisdom of Congress.

It will be observed that the Forest Service, the Reclamation Service and the Panama Canal Service are all engaged in a variety of works incidental to the main enterprises, and they are engaged not only in constructing them, but in operating them. Such works include water-works, electric-light plants, roads, railroads, electric roads, cement mills, and other works of similar character, all incidental and collateral to the main enterprises.

Can it be maintained that the Government should have less power when, in the interest of interstate and foreign commerce, it enters upon the artificialization of rivers and the construction of canals?

It will also be observed that the Panama Canal Service is to be made compensatory by the charging of tolls, the Forest Service by the sale of timber and by charges for grazing permits, and the Reclamation Service by the sale of water rights. So far as the Forest Service and the Reclamation Service are concerned, they will be absolutely self-compensatory. In the case of the Inland Waterways Service it is proposed that the artificialized rivers and canals shall be free to navigation and that no tolls shall be imposed. Is it not, therefore, of all the more importance that the collateral works undertaken by this service through other appropriate services of the Government for the purpose of fully developing every profitable and beneficial use of our rivers shall be made self-compensatory as far as practicable and that wherever the coöperation of States, municipalities, communities, corporations, or individuals is necessary to accomplish this purpose, such coöperation shall be secured? No one can measure the future value of the water power of the country in the development of electricity. It is probable that this new force has a future value equal to that of all the coal supplies of the country.

In organizing this great work, an ample fund should be immediately provided and as free a hand as possible given to the Executive. In the case of the Reclamation Service, the method of securing a revolving fund from the proceeds of the sales of public lands and of water rights has proven an incentive and an inspiration to the best efforts of these in charge of the work. The methods are those of a business house which knows its condition at all times. Under such a method the Government organization knows just what to depend upon. It can plan for the future and look ahead without uncertainty as to the size of appropriations. Furthermore, it is inspired to work for practical results, for early and considerable returns which, by the application of business methods, can be again applied to produce more returns. No questions of such magnitude, where a long look ahead is necessary and a comprehensive plan for the future imperative, should be hampered at its beginning by uncertainty of Congressional action. Those in charge should know at all times on what they can depend and what results are expected of them. It is therefore essential that an ample fund should be provided and that provision should be made for its replenishment by the sale of bonds whenever Congressional appropriation fails. As free a hand as possible in organization should be given, and particularly during the first few years. After the organization is perfected and its work reduced to a system, then Congress can, if it chooses, substitute the old plan of Congressional initiative as to investigation, as to projects, and as to construction in each particular case.

Breaking Down of the Railway System

Mr. Newlands. I wish to add that this question of waterway transportation is, of course, only a part of the general subject of transportation. The railway service of the country is much broken down. The railroads of the country, when there was less business than there is now, sought to increase their tonnage by carrying cheap and bulky products long distances at low prices, and they thus entered upon a carriage which has been mainly absorbed in other countries by waterways. This bulky carriage has absorbed so large a proportion of their facilities that suddenly, with the great increase in production and population, they found themselves unable to meet the demands of the country. At that time an agitation arose for the regulation of rates and for the better control of the railroads themselves. The railroads, on the one side, regarded their properties as private properties and resented legislative intrusion. The people, on the other hand, regarded them as public servants charged by the law with the performance of public duties, entitled only to a just compensation, that compensation to be fixed by the public either in the shape of tolls or the limitation of return upon capital in the shape of dividends. That contest has not yet reached the end.

The railroads have now reached the point where they admit in some degree the powers and the rights of the public. They now talk about coöperation; they will talk later on about obedience; and obedience is what the American people demand. The only limitation upon the power of the American people over the highways and over common carriers is that the legislation shall not be confiscatory in character. That contest is not yet ended. Meanwhile the finances of the railroads have been embarrassed; rates of interest have gone up; and the very agitation which has gone on has affected their negotiations in foreign countries for cheap money. They have been unable, even if they willed it, to keep up with the necessary construction in order to meet the demands of increasing population and of business. One eminent railway man declares that it will be necessary for these railroads to expend, I believe, within the next five years, five and one-half billions of money in order to meet the requirements of the country. We all realize that it is now impossible for them to get the money. We might enable them to get the money if we stopped this agitation; but the American people will not rest, whatever may be the consequences, until the true status of the common carrier is ascertained and determined as that of a public servant. So that we cannot hope for such conditions as will enable them to finance the construction that is necessary. It is therefore of great importance that we should develop these waterways and that we should develop them quickly.

COÖRDINATION OF RAIL AND WATER TRANSPORTATION

It would startle the country, perhaps, if we were to say that $100,000,000 annually for the next five years should be expended; but I believe it ought to be expended in order to meet the requirements of transportation, and the public mind must become accustomed to it. After it is all expended the business of the railroads will not be injured. They will have more than they can then carry, and their carriage will be of products more compensatory than the cheap and bulky products that will be carried by water transportation.

We have had a most marvelous railroad development in this country, which has surpassed that of any other part of the world. But our development has not been as rational, as comprehensive, and as scientific in the matter of transportation as has that of Germany. Her railway transportation, her river and canal transportation, and her ocean transportation have been dovetailed together in such a fashion as to make her carriers the most efficient servants of production and of commerce in the world.

This movement is not one of hostility to the railroads. It is one that supplements the railroad system of the country. If we can add to our ocean service so that that ocean service and the river and canal service and the railroad service of the country will act in coöperation as the handmaidens of production and commerce, we shall have marvelous results.

After we get these waterways developed the question then will be, How shall we administer them? Are the railroads to be allowed to put down their rates during the navigation season to the destruction of their river competitors and to put them up during the winter season when that competition ceases? Shall we permit one public servant to destroy another public servant necessary to the public good? We might crowd these rivers with boats, but capital, regardful of the bitter experience of the past, will hesitate to enter upon the enterprise. As we passed down the Mississippi River we hardly saw a boat. On both sides of the river we saw long trains of cars carrying the products to the country. If the railroads refuse to act in coöperation with the rivers in the future, as they have in the past, they may paralyze the very instrumentalities which we create for interstate and foreign commerce.

We must ourselves — the nation must — create the corporations that are to act as waterway carriers. We should not submit the incorporation of these great public servants engaged in interstate carriage to the shifting legislation of 46 different States. There is no river boat that on its course will not in going from bank to bank move from one State to another in interstate commerce. The nation should create its own public corporate servants, and we should protect them.

We may find it necessary in creating these instrumentalities of interstate commerce to exempt them from taxation, State and national, for a limited period. The power is, in my judgment, clear. The nation can certainly exempt them from its own taxation, and can refuse to permit a sovereign State, without the nation's consent, to place a burden that might be destructive upon a national instrumentality. We may have to protect them against unfair and unjust competition. We may have to compel the coördination of the railroads with them. The railroads to-day have all the terminal facilities upon the rivers. They have the depots and the stations and the tracks. They have all the spaces that will be required for river commerce. The nation cannot permit these national instrumentalities to be subject to the caprice of selfish interests.

All this can be adjusted if we only go further and provide that as to the great national system of railways, eight or ten in number, each one of them having from ten to twenty thousand miles of track and traversing between fifteen and twenty States — these mergers shall come under a national charter. We shall then ourselves have created the public agents of the nation the servants of the nation for the adequate development of interstate and foreign transportation.

THE NATIONAL POWERS

It may be said that we have not the power to compel the merger of such corporations under a national charter. I admit that we can not forcibly go into a State and compel a State to force a State corporation to come within the national merger, but the nation can authorize public carriers, common carriers, incorporated under its laws, to construct new interstate lines, and it can, by the process of persuasion, induce the States, driven by the demands of their own people, to permit these parts of great interstate systems to get together under one national control and charter.

The change will not mean an invasion of the powers and rights of the States. At present we have State corporations engaging also in interstate transportation. Is it not just as logical to have national interstate corporations engage in State transportation? The same public agent, whether State or national, can now engage in both State and interstate transportation. As to the former it would be subject to the State regulation; as to the latter it would be subject to national regulation, whether the corporate agent were incorporated under State or national charter. Nor would the police powers of the States or the jurisdiction of the State courts be affected by national charter. The National-bank Act, under which the jurisdiction of State courts is maintained, is an illustration of that. If we can nationally incorporate these great railway carriers, and if we can nationally incorporate river carriers, and if we can nationally incorporate ocean carriers, the entire people will then have these public servants under their control, and by the unity and simplicity of the operation the service can be made profitable to the carriers, just to the public, and efficient in the promotion of interstate and foreign commerce.

I am aware that some of my friends call this a centralization of power. Some of my friends on this side of the House are accustomed to apply that term to any power which is exercised by the National Government.

The National Government has not, in my judgment, commenced to exercise its powers under the interstate commerce clause of the Constitution. It has been prevented from exercising the powers which the people granted to the nation for a beneficent purpose. The main purpose of the formation of the Union was to unite all the States in matters relating to the national defense and to the protection of interstate and foreign commerce. The development of interstate and foreign commerce was the primary cause of the Constitution and of the Union. The growth of transportation has been an accidental growth from a point in one State to another point in the same State. Gradually this accidental growth has advanced until, either under the laws of the States, or outside of the law, or against the law, or in evasion of the law, great systems of railways have been in fact, though not in law, nationalized, unionized, running almost from the Atlantic to the Pacific and from the Lakes to the Gulf. Will any one deny that the combination has been beneficial, whatever we may say about the methods employed, about the capitalization issued, about the power in politics exercised by these great political masters that ought to be public servants?

Would you to-day enter upon a process of decentralization? Would you attempt to divide these systems up into the units of which they were once composed, each unit comprised within State lines? You would not?

Then legalize them under proper restraints as to capitalization, under proper restraints as to profits, and legalize them by the action of the only sovereign capable of dealing with the question.

Not Centralization, but Unionization

Centralization! Is that the right term? I should say "unionization." The exercise of the granted powers of the Constitution does not involve the centralization of power. It involves simply the unionizing of the forces of the entire people of the country in matters clearly intrusted to the Union of States. This union is composed of forty-six States. We are all parts of this Union. This nation is not a separate entity afar off, exercising jurisdiction and control and dominion without our participation in it. The States constitute this Union; and they entered into this Union for certain beneficial purposes, one of which was the advancement of interstate and foreign commerce. That involves the creation of the instrumentalities for interstate and foreign commerce, the creation of the public servants that are to engage in interstate and foreign commerce by the nation and not by a single State of the least public virtue, absolutely controlled by the corporate carriers, who ought to be the servants of the nation. There is no centralization about it. We unionize the forces of the nation under the powers granted to the nation, of which each State forms a component part. If the States were all separate, then would they not have to get together by treaty and settle many matters? We have the best kind of treaty making under our system, the treaty making of this legislative body and the other legislative body — the Congress of the United States — a permanent treaty-making Congress, imposing its will upon each one of the forty-six sovereign States in matters intrusted to it for final determination.

39

XI

ARMY AND NAVY

FROM PRESIDENT ROOSEVELT'S MESSAGE, DECEMBER 3
1907

The Army. Not only there is not now, but there never has been, any other nation in the world so wholly free from the evils of militarism as is ours. There never has been any other large nation, not even China, which for so long a period has had relatively to its numbers so small a regular army as has ours. Never at any time in our history has this nation suffered from militarism or been in the remotest danger of suffering from militarism. Never at any time of our history has the Regular Army been of a size which caused the slightest appreciable tax upon the tax-paying citizens of the Nation. Almost always it has been too small in size and underpaid. Never in our entire history has the Nation suffered in the least particular because too much care has been given to the Army, too much prominence given it, too much money spent upon it, or because it has been too large. But again and again we have suffered because enough care has not been given to it, because it has been too small, because there has not been sufficient preparation in advance for possible war. Every foreign war in which we have engaged has cost us many times the amount which, if wisely expended during the preceding years of peace on the Regular Army, would have insured the war ending in but a fraction of the time and but for a fraction of the cost that was actually the case. As a Nation we have always been shortsighted in providing for the efficiency of the Army in time of peace. It is nobody's especial interest to make such provision and no one looks ahead to war at any period, no matter how remote, as being a serious possibility; while an improper economy, or rather niggardliness, can be practiced at the expense of the Army with the certainty that those practicing it will not be called to account therefor, but that the price will be paid by the unfortunate persons who happen to be in office when a war does actually come.

I think it is only lack of foresight that troubles us, not any hostility to the Army. There are, of course, foolish people who denounce any care of the Army or Navy as "militarism," but I do not think that these people are numerous. This country has to contend now, and has had to contend in the past, with many evils, and there is ample scope for all who would work for reform. But there is not one evil that now exists, or that ever has existed in this country, which is, or ever has been, owing in the smallest part to militarism. Declamation against militarism has no more serious place in an earnest and intelligent movement for righteousness in this country than declamation against the worship of Baal or Astaroth. It is declamation against a non-existent evil, one which never has existed in this country, and which has not the slightest chance of appearing here. We are glad to help in any movement for international peace, but this is because we sincerely believe that it is our duty to help all such movements provided they are sane and rational, and not because there is any tendency toward militarism on our part which needs to be cured. The evils we have to fight are those in connection with industrialism, not militarism. Industry is always necessary, just as war is sometimes necessary. Each has its price, and industry in the United States now exacts, and has always exacted, a far heavier toll of death than all our wars put together. The statistics of the railroads of this country for the year ended June 30, 1906, the last contained in the annual statistical report of the Interstate Commerce Commission, show in that one year a total of 108,324 casualties to persons, of which 10,618 represent the number of persons killed. In that wonderful hive of human activity, Pittsburg, the deaths due to industrial accidents in 1906 were 919, all the result of accidents in mills, mines, or on railroads. For the entire country, therefore, it is safe to say that the deaths due to industrial accidents aggregate in the neighborhood of twenty thousand a year. Such a record makes the death rate in all our foreign wars utterly trivial by comparison. The number of deaths in battle in all the foreign wars put together, for the last century and a quarter, aggregate considerably less than one year's death record for our industries. A mere glance at these figures is sufficient to show the absurdity of the outcry against militarism.

But again and again in the past our little Regular Army has rendered service literally vital to the country, and it may at any time have to do so in the future. Its standard of efficiency and instruction is higher now than ever in the past. But it is too small. There are not enough officers; and it is impossible to secure enough enlisted men. We should maintain in peace a fairly complete skeleton of a large army. A great and long-continued war would have to be fought by volunteers. But months would pass before any large body of efficient volunteers could be put in the field, and our Regular Army should be large enough to meet any immediate need. In particular it is essential that we should possess a number of extra officers trained in peace to perform efficiently the duties urgently required upon the breaking out of war.

The Medical Corps should be much larger than the needs of our

Regular Army in war. Yet at present it is smaller than the needs of the service demand even in peace. The Spanish war occurred less than ten years ago. The chief loss we suffered in it was by disease among the regiments which never left the country. At the moment the Nation seemed deeply impressed by this fact; yet seemingly it has already forgotten, for not the slightest effort has been made to prepare a medical corps of a sufficient size to prevent the repetition of the same disaster on a much larger scale if we should ever be engaged in a serious conflict. The trouble in the Spanish war was not with the then existing officials of the War Department; it was with the representatives of the people as a whole, who for the preceding thirty years, had declined to make the necessary provision for the Army. Unless ample provision is now made by Congress to put the Medical Corps where it should be put disaster in the next war is inevitable, and the responsibility will not lie with those then in charge of the War Department, but with those who now decline to make the necessary provision. A well organized medical corps, thoroughly trained before the advent of war in all the important administrative duties of a military sanitary corps, is essential to the efficiency of any large army, and especially of a large volunteer army. Such knowledge of medicine and surgery as is possessed by the medical profession generally will not alone suffice to make an efficient military surgeon. He must have, in addition, knowledge of the administration and sanitation of large field hospitals and camps, in order to safeguard the health and lives of men intrusted in great numbers to his care. A bill has long been pending before Congress for the reorganization of the Medical Corps; its passage is urgently needed.

But the Medical Department is not the only department for which increased provision should be made. The rate of pay for the officers should be greatly increased; there is no higher type of citizen than the American regular officer, and he should have a fair reward for his admirable work. There should be a relatively even greater increase in the pay for the enlisted men. In especial provision should be made for establishing grades equivalent to those of warrant officers in the Navy which should be open to the enlisted men who serve sufficiently long and who do their work well. Inducements should be offered sufficient to encourage really good men to make the Army a life occupation. The prime needs of our present Army is to secure and retain competent noncommissioned officers. This difficulty rests fundamentally on the question of pay. The noncommissioned officer does not correspond with an unskilled laborer; he corresponds to the best type of skilled workman or to the subordinate official in civil institutions. Wages have greatly increased in outside occupations in the last forty years, and the pay of the soldier, like the pay of the officers, should be proportionately increased. The first sergeant of a company, if a good man, must be one of such executive and administrative ability, and such knowledge of his trade, as to be worth far more than we at present pay him. The same is true of the regimental sergeant major. These men should be men who had fully resolved to make the Army a life occupation and they should be able to look forward to ample reward; while only men properly qualified should be given a chance to secure these final rewards. The increase over the present pay need not be great in the lower grades for the first one or two enlistments, but the increase should be marked for the noncommissioned officers of the upper grades who serve long enough to make it evident that they intend to stay permanently in the Army, while additional pay should be given for high qualifications in target practice. The position of warrant officer should be established and there should be not only an increase of pay, but an increase of privileges and allowances and dignity, so as to make the grade open to noncommissioned officers capable of filling them desirably from every standpoint. The rate of desertion in our Army now in time of peace is alarming. The deserter should be treated by public opinion as a man guilty of the greatest crime; while on the other hand the man who serves steadily in the Army should be treated as what he is, that is, as preëminently one of the best citizens of this Republic. After twelve years' service in the Army my own belief is that the man should be given a preference according to his ability for certain types of office over all civilian applicants without examination. This should also apply, of course, to the men who have served twelve years in the Navy. A special corps should be provided to do the manual labor now necessarily demanded of the privates themselves.

Among the officers there should be severe examinations to weed out the unfit up to the grade of major. From that position on appointments should be solely by selection and it should be understood that a man of merely average capacity could never get beyond the position of major, while every man who serves in any grade a certain length of time prior to promotion to the next grade without getting the promotion to the next grade should be forthwith retired. The practice marches and field maneuvers of the last two or three years have been invaluable to the Army. They should be continued and extended. A rigid and not a perfunctory examination of physical capacity has been provided for the higher grade officers. This will work well. Unless an officer has a good physique, unless he can stand hardship, ride well, and walk fairly, he is not fit for any position, even after he has become a colonel. Before he has become a colonel the need for physical fitness in the officer is almost as great as in the enlisted man. I hope speedily to see introduced into the Army a far more rigid and thoroughgoing test of horsemanship for all field officers than at present. There should be a Chief of Cavalry just as there is a Chief of Artillery.

Perhaps the most important of all legislation needed for the benefit of the Army is a law to equalize and increase the pay of officers and enlisted men of the Army, Navy, Marine Corps, and Revenue-Cutter Service. Such a bill has been prepared, which it is hoped will meet with your favorable consideration. The next most essential measure is to authorize a number of extra officers as mentioned above. To make the Army more attractive to enlisted men, it is absolutely essential to create a service corps, such as exists in nearly every modern army in the world, to do the skilled and unskilled. labor, inseparably connected with military administration, which is now exacted, without just compensation, of enlisted men who voluntarily entered the Army to do service of an altogether different kind. There are a number of other laws necessary to so organize the Army as to promote its efficiency and facilitate its rapid expansion in time of war; but the above are the most important.

The Navy. It was hoped The Hague Conference might deal with the question of the limitation of armaments. But even before it had assembled informal inquiries had developed that as regards naval armaments the only ones in which this country had any interest, it was hopeless to try to devise any plan for which there was the slightest possibility of securing the assent of the nations gathered at The Hague. No plan was even proposed which would have had the assent of more than one first class Power outside of the United States. The only plan that seemed at all feasible, that of limiting the size of battleships, met with no favor at all. It is evident, therefore, that it is folly for this Nation to base any hope of securing peace on any international agreement as to the limitation of armaments. Such being the fact it would be most unwise for us to stop the upbuilding of our Navy. To build one battleship of the best and most advanced type a year would barely keep our fleet up to its present force. This is not enough. In my judgment, we should this year provide for four battleships. But it is idle to build battleships unless in addition to providing the men, and the means for thorough training, we provide the auxiliaries for them, unless we provide docks, the coaling stations, the colliers and supply ships that they need. We are extremely deficient in coaling stations and docks on the Pacific, and this deficiency should not longer be permitted to exist. Plenty of torpedo boats and destroyers should be built. Both on the Atlantic and Pacific coasts, fortifications of the best type should be provided for all our greatest harbors.

We need always to remember that in time of war the Navy is not to be used to defend harbors and sea-coast cities; we should perfect our system of coast fortifications. The only efficient use for the Navy is for offense. The only way in which it can efficiently protect our own coast against the possible action of a foreign navy is by destroying that foreign navy. For defense against a hostile fleet which actually attacks them, the coast cities must depend upon their forts, mines, torpedoes, submarines, and torpedo boats and destroyers. All of these together are efficient for defensive purposes, but they in no way supply the place of a thoroughly efficient navy capable of acting on the offensive; for parrying never yet won a fight. It can only be won by hard hitting, and an aggressive sea-going navy alone can do this hard hitting of the offensive type. But the forts and the like are necessary so that the Navy may be footloose. In time of war there is sure to be demand, under pressure of fright, for the ships to be scattered so as to defend all kind of ports. Under penalty of terrible disaster, this demand must be refused. The ships must be kept together, and their objective made the enemies' fleet. If the fortifications are sufficiently strong, no modern navy will venture to attack them, so long as the foe has in existence a hostile navy of anything like the same size or efficiency. But unless there exists such a navy then the fortifications are powerless by themselves to secure the victory. For of course the mere deficiency means that any resolute enemy can at his leisure combine all his forces upon one point with the certainty that he can take it.

Until our battle fleet is much larger than at present it should never be split into detachments so far apart that they could not in event of emergency be speedily united. Our coast line is on the Pacific just as much as on the Atlantic. The interests of California, Oregon, and Washington are as emphatically the interests of the whole Union as those of Maine and New York, of Louisiana and Texas. The battle fleet should now and then be moved to the Pacific, just as at other times it should be kept in the Atlantic. When the Isthmian Canal is built the transit of the battle fleet from one ocean to the other will be comparatively easy. Until it is built I earnestly hope that the battle fleet will be thus shifted between the two oceans every year or two. The marksmanship on all our ships has improved phenomenally during the last five years. Until within the last two or three years it was not possible to train a battle fleet in squadron maneuvers under service conditions, and it is only during these last two or three years that the training under these conditions has become really effective. Another and most necessary stride in advance is now being taken. The battle fleet is about starting by the Straits of Magellan to visit the Pacific coast. Sixteen battleships are going under the command of Rear-Admiral Evans, while eight armored cruisers and two other battleships will meet him at San Francisco, whither certain torpedo destroyers are also going. No fleet of such size has ever made such a voyage, and it will be of very great educational use to all engaged in it. The only way by which to teach officers and men how to handle the fleet so as to meet every possible strain and emergency in time of war is to have them practice under similar conditions in time of peace. Moreover, the only way to find out our actual needs is to perform in time of peace whatever maneuvers might be necessary in time of war. After war is declared it is too late to find out the needs; that means to invite disaster. This trip to the Pacific will show what some of our needs are and will enable us to provide for them. The proper place for an officer to learn his duty is at sea, and the only way in which a navy can ever be made efficient is by practice at sea, under all the conditions which would have to be met with if war existed.

I bespeak the most liberal treatment for the officers and enlisted men of the Navy. It is true of them, as likewise of the officers and enlisted men of the Army, that they form a body whose interests should be close to the heart of every good American. In return the most rigid perform-ance of duty should be exacted from them. The reward should be ample when they do their best; and nothing less than their best should be tolerated. It is idle to hope for the best results when the men in the senior grades come to those grades late in life and serve too short a time in them. Up to the rank of lieutenant-commander promotion in the Navy should be as now, by seniority, subject, however, to such rigid tests as would eliminate the unfit. After the grade of lieutenant-com-mander, that is, when we come to the grade of command rank, the unfit should be eliminated in such a manner that only the conspicuously fit would remain, and sea service should be a principal test of fitness. Those who are passed by should, after a certain length of service in their respective grades, be retired. Of a given number of men it may well be that almost all would make good lieutenants and most of them good lieutenant-commanders, while only a minority will be fit to be captains, and but three or four to be admirals. Those who object to promotion otherwise than by mere seniority should reflect upon the elementary fact that no business in private life could be successfully managed if those who enter at the lowest rungs of the ladder should each in turn, if he lived, become the head of the firm, its active director, and retire after he had beld the position a few months. On its face such a scheme is an absurdity. Chances for improper favoritism can be minimized by a properly formed board; such as the board of last June, which did such conscientious and excellent work in elimination.

If all that ought to be done can not now be done, at least let a begin-ning be made. In my last three annual Messages, and in a special Message to the last Congress, the necessity for legislation that will cause officers of the line of the Navy to reach the grades of captain and rear-admiral at less advanced ages and which will cause them to have more sea training and experience in the highly responsible duties of those grades, so that they may become thoroughly skillful in handling battleships, divisions, squadrons, and fleets in action, has been fully explained and urgently recommended. Upon this subject the Secretary of the Navy has submitted detailed and definite recommendations which have received my approval, and which, if enacted into law, will accomplish what is immediately necessary, and will, as compared with existing law, make a saving of more than five millions of dollars during the next seven years. The navy personnel act of 1899 has accomplished all that was expected of it in providing satisfactory periods of service in the several subordinate grades, from the grade of ensign to the grade of lieutenant-commander, but the law is inadequate in the upper grades and will continue to be inadequate on account of the expansion of the personnel since its enactment. Your attention is invited to the following quotations from the report of the personnel board of 1906, of which the Assistant Secretary of the Navy was president:

"Congress has authorized a considerable increase in the number of midshipmen at the Naval Academy, and these midshipmen upon graduation are promoted to ensign and lieutenant (junior-grade). But no provision has been made for a corresponding increase in the upper grades, the result being that the lower grades will become so congested that a midshipman now in one of the lowest classes at Annapolis may possibly not be promoted to lieutenant until he is between 45 and 50 years of age. So it will continue under the present law, congesting at the top and congesting at the bottom. The country fails to get from the officers of the service the best that is in them by not providing opportunity for their normal development and training. The board believes that this works a serious detriment to the efficiency of the Navy and is a real menace to the public safety."

As I stated in my special Message to the last Congress: "I am firmly of the opinion that unless the present conditions of the higher commissioned personnel is rectified by judicious legislation the future of our Navy will be gravely compromised." It is also urgently necessary to increase the efficiency of the Medical Corps of the Navy. Special legislation to this end has already been proposed; and I trust it may be enacted without delay.

It must be remembered that everything done in the Navy to fit it to do well in time of war must be done in time of peace. Modern wars are short; they do not last the length of time requisite to build a battle-ship; and it takes longer to train the officers and men to do well on a battleship than it takes to build it. Nothing effective can be done for the Navy once war has begun, and the result of the war, if the combatants are otherwise equally matched, will depend upon which power has prepared best in time of peace. The United States Navy is the best guaranty the Nation has that its honor and interest will not be neglected; and in addition it offers by far the best insurance for peace that can by human ingenuity be devised.

I call attention to the report of the official Board of Visitors to the Naval Academy at Annapolis which has been forwarded to the Congress. The report contains this paragraph:

"Such revision should be made of the courses of study and methods of conducting and marking examinations as will develop and bring out the average all-round ability of the midshipman rather than to give him prominence in any one particular study. The fact should be kept in mind that the Naval

Academy is not a university but a school, the primary object of which is to educate boys to be efficient naval officers. Changes in curriculum, therefore, should be in the direction of making the course of instruction less theoretical and more practical. No portion of any future class should be graduated in advance of the full four years' course, and under no circumstances should the standard of instruction be lowered. The Academy in almost all of its depart- ments is now magnificently equipped, and it would be very unwise to make the course of instruction less exacting than it is to-day."

THE WAR DEPARTMENT—MILITARY ADMINISTRATION [1]

By Brigadier-General William H. Carter, U. S. A.[1]

When the great Civil War Secretary, Edwin M. Stanton, took up the work of the Department, which for four years laid such a mental and physical strain upon him as few men could bear, he found a condition calculated to bring discouragement to the stoutest heart. The relations between the Secretary of War and the Commanding General of the Army had long been of such a character that the latter officer had removed his headquarters to New York City. He was now brought back to the seat of government with the expectation that his staunch loyalty, knowl- edge of the army and professional ability would render him useful in the hour of peril. Advancing years, however, soon compelled his retirement from active service.

Immediate measures were taken to insure the safety of the Capital and to bring into service armies sufficient in size and number to cope with the grave question of preserving the Union. It became necessary to reorganize the business methods of the various bureaus to meet the exceptional tasks confronting them in the organization, equipping and supplying of an army suddenly increased from about ten thousand to ultimately more than one million men in actual service.

The general system of administration was similar to that pursued during the Mexican War, and much reliance was placed on the veterans of that conflict. It did not take long to make it evident, to thoughtful and alert friends of the Union, that the magnitude of the conflict then raging was little understood by the general public, and that preparation, in the shape of money, material, and men, for a prolonged and bloody war was the immediate duty of the War Department. The history of the great struggle is still fresh in the minds of the American people, but it may be safely stated that only a very limited number have a proper appreciation of the great administrative work performed by the War Department during the days and nights of the whole four years of war. There were periods of marching, of battle, and of monotonous camp life

[1] Part of an article in *Scribner's Magazine*, June, 1903. Reprinted by permission. Copyright.

for the average regiment; but for the Secretary of War and his coadjutors there was one unending round of high tension work.

Armies are useless without food, clothes, ammunition and transportation, and to obtain and distribute these essential requisites in the quantities demanded during the Civil War required administrative and executive ability of a high order. The absence of a directing and co-ordinating professional authority in the scheme of army organization threw an immense strain upon the Secretary of War and President. No student of the art of war can read the war orders and instructions of President Lincoln without noting the rapid and wonderful growth of his mind during the early years of the war, especially as to the military policy and grand strategy. It was his knowledge of the value of co-ordinated and united action that led him to a constant effort to have all the various armies operate under a general policy, and prevent the Confederates from continually availing themselves of interior lines of communication to reënforce threatened points. It took a long time and untold millions to bring all the separate armies to a condition of readiness, but when this agressive, hammer-and-tongs policy was instituted all along the line the Department was able to see the end of the enormous burden the country was patiently bearing, in the drain upon its resources.

Nothing in all military history equals the business administration of the War Department as exemplified in the muster-out and transportation of the great volunteer armies to their homes at the close of the Civil War. The great burden of current expense was quickly reduced, a matter of vital importance at the time.

After so much experience in handling large numbers of men during four years of war, the preparation of General Sheridan's army, for a descent upon the French troops in Mexico, was attended with no special difficulties. Fortunately wise counsels prevailed in the French nation, and this, together with some rather active pressure on the part of the Mexican people, caused the withdrawal of Bazaine's army from our neighboring republic, and enabled the War Department to dispense with the volunteers assembled in Texas.

Following close upon the muster-out of the volunteers a reorganization of the regular army, involving an increase of the various staff departments and a considerable augmentation of the line, took place. A portion of the new army was destined for service in the Southern States during the reconstruction period. The duties required of the army during the long and disastrous efforts at sustaining "carpet-bag" governments were intensely distasteful to both officers and men, as well as to the better element amongst the Southern people. To be sure the Civil War had just closed, and it was necessary to reëstablish law and order throughout a vast territory inhabited by a negro population, which regarded the army as the embodiment of that power which had struck off the shackles of slavery. The use of the army at the polls and in civil matters generally has ever been repugnant to American ideas, and at this period it only succeeded in embittering the Southern people to such an extent that one of their first and most insistent policies, after the reconstruction, was to demand a reduction of the regular army. Under this pressure the strength of the army was fixed and remained at 25,000 men until the outbreak of the war with Spain.

During the quarter of a century following the close of the Civil War the army was constantly overworked in the Far West, where advancing civilization was resisted by the warriors of nearly all the Indian tribes in their fruitless effort to stem the tide, which was steadily circumscribing and overflowing their hunting grounds. The wasteful slaughter of millions of buffaloes within the brief period of half a dozen years completely changed the history of the nomadic Plains Indians. The many stories of wagon trains, and even railroad trains, being stopped to wait the passing of countless thousands in some of the great migrating buffalo herds now read like visionary tales of disordered minds.

The War Department had continued in charge of the Indians until the close of the Mexican War, after which period their affairs were managed by Indian agents, with minimum salaries and maximum temptations. Many times the army was compelled to stand idly by and witness the perpetration of wrongs, and when the Indians, in desperation, "broke out," the War Department was called upon to produce another era of peace. Year after year regiments were summoned to the field, sometimes under tropical suns, and again in the land of blizzards, where the icy winds made campaigning miserable alike to pursuer and pursued. With each recurring surrender the Indians were restored to the tender mercies of the agent and his harpies, only to find their grievances multiplied.

As years wore on the settlers, with their wire fences, closed in slowly but surely around the reservations, and the fact dawned upon the Indians that the wild, free life of the Golden West had gone. The march of civilization had swept away the old life and left but mere remnants of once proud tribes stranded as drift-wood along the shores of progress. Encountering only the worst elements amongst the whites, too often the mere outcasts of society, the poor warriors, shorn of the power wielded by their ancestors, turned restlessly for some light to those with whom they had battled and at whose hands they had often suffered defeat. Army officers were again installed as Indian agents and gradually laid the foundations of lasting peace by showing the Indians the utter futility of contending against inevitable fate.

The Indian question having been practically settled for all time, a plan was adopted by the War Department of bringing together the scattered fragments of the regular army, which in its entirety did not equal in numbers a single army corps. The necessity for guarding isolated and exposed points had for years presented proper instruction of officers and men in the administration and maneuvers of battalions, regiments, and brigades, but in minor warfare they were not outclassed by any soldiers the world over. To accomplish the best results numerous small posts were abandoned and regimental posts established. Coincident with the inception of this plan, work of construction proceeded along the seacoast under the general scheme adopted under authority of Congress. During actual Indian hostilities the urgent need for men in the cavalry and infantry had caused a reduction in the strength of artillery organizations, which rendered them incapable of fulfilling their proper functions in seacoast defense. To meet this emergency in a mediocre way, two troops of each cavalry regiment and two companies of each infantry regiment were "skeletonized." This scheme left the cavalry regiments with two squadrons and a half, but gave the infantry regiments two complete battalions, that branch having at the time only ten companies to each regiment. One of the results of recent experience has been to fix by statute a minimum limit for each troop of cavalry and company of infantry, so that in future it will not be legal to skeletonize any portion of the army.

The unwillingness of Congress to recognize the urgent need of men to garrison the growing coast defenses, while continuing to spend millions upon fortifications and guns, caused the Department grave concern. After years of pleading for proper legislation, a piteous appeal was finally made for two additional regiments of artillery, and action was slowly maturing in this regard when other events occurred which rapidly roused the country to action.

For more than half a century Cuba had been a source of incessant anxiety and trouble to every administration. Forty years back — December, 1858 — President James Buchanan, in complaining in a message to Congress of past conditions, said: "Spanish officials under the direct control of the Captain General of Cuba have insulted our national flag, and in repeated instances have from time to time inflicted injuries on the persons and property of our citizens. . . . All our attempts to obtain redress have been baffled and defeated. . . . The truth is that Cuba, in its existing colonial condition, is a constant source of injury and annoyance to the American people. . . . It has been made known to the world by my predecessors that the United States have on several occasions endeavored to acquire Cuba from Spain by honorable negotiation. . . . We would not, if we could, acquire Cuba in any other manner. This is due to our national character. . . . Our relations with Spain, which ought to be of the most friendly character, must always be placed in jeopardy whilst the existing Colonial government over the island shall remain in its present condition."

There was a widespread sentiment throughout the United States in behalf of the Cubans in their insurrection against Spanish domination.

Many well-informed newspapers protested against the circulation of unreliable stories calculated to create false sympathy, but the tide was flowing full, and the minority in Congress constantly twitted the majority because of the failure to intervene in the Cuban struggle. Captain General Weyler was held up to universal scorn because he had turned back the methods of war to the days of the Spanish Inquisition. The establishment of reconcentrado camps, done to prevent Spanish soldiers from being murdered in a war in which there were no battles in the open, brought down upon Spain the antagonism of all Cuban sympathizers.

The Secretary of War and his co-workers were advised of the unprepared state of the army and of the defenses for immediate war. Everything which could be legitimately done at the time was hastened forward to make up for past neglect, but guns, ammunition and armies do not appear by magic. When the battleship Maine met destruction in Havana harbor on the fateful night of February 15, 1898, the nation was so horrified that it required all the wisdom and statesmanship of President McKinley to delay the inevitable conflict while preparations were hurried forward. On March 8th Congress unanimously voted $50,000,000 for the national defense, but as the new Spanish Minister, Señor Palo y Bernabe, entered upon his duties at Washington a few days later, the appropriation was not regarded as a war measure. The brief period· intervening before the passage of the resolutions authorizing intervention in the Island of Cuba was used to advance preparation for war, but the Secretary of War was greatly embarrassed by the failure of Congress to pass any measure for raising an army until after war was actually declared. The nation was unprepared, yet when war was declared every shoulder was put manfully to the wheel, and Europe saw with amazement the capacity of the young giant whose whole energies had long been turned to the upbuilding of new States and the extension of an industrial development hitherto unknown to any like period of the world's history.

The country had not engaged in war since the close of the gigantic struggle of 1861 to 1865; no progress in legislation had been made in a hundred years so far as utilization of organized militia was concerned, and there was no law extant under which the President could take any of those preliminary steps so essential to success in war. During April all of the little regular army which could be spared was assembled in Southern camps and organized in brigades and divisions. This was a measure of extreme precaution; the results at Santiago prove it to have been one of those fortunate strokes upon which the fate of nations often hang.

Within a few hours after the passage of the Act authorizing a volunteer army a call for 125,000 men was made; this was followed by another for 75,000, which, with the increase of the regular army, made a total of nearly 250,000 men. The volunteers under the first call were put in the field in thirty days, and the entire work of organization — the mighty task of putting a quarter of a million men under arms and equipping them for service, in face of all obstacles — was completed in ninety days. There was no lack of volunteers; on the contrary the War Department was embarrassed with offers of service.

Notwithstanding all this, well-informed officials recognized that the country had not advanced in military methods one iota in half a century, for every effort of the War Department to profit by the lessons of the past met with opposition. There was a determination in many States to cast aside the one pronounced lesson of the Mexican and Civil Wars, and it was only through President McKinley's acceptance of the views of experienced officers that a complete breakdown of the system was avoided. To be more explicit on this important point; in our military system, organization and recruitment pertain to the adjutant general's bureau of the War Department; that bureau insisted that the scheme which allowed volunteer regiments to be mustered in with all their officers, but with only half a quota of men, to be soon reduced below a basis of efficiency, should not prevail. The anxiety to get mustered into service caused many excellent officers of the National Guard to join in a movement, which was calculated to break down the whole militia system, and did cause it to lose the respect of well-informed veterans of the Civil War. The pressure brought by Pennsylvania was so great that it secured a modification of the rule which Grant, Sherman, and all the great leaders of the Civil War, had contended for as of vital importance in maintaining the efficiency of volunteer armies. As soon as the first call was completed, President McKinley came to the rescue by making another call for 75,000 men, and giving an order that no new organization should be accepted from any State until the ranks of all existing volunteer organizations from that State should be recruited to the maximum. This is a military principle indispensable to economical success with volunteer armies.

Coincident with this work, the selection and appointment of general officers of the line and officers of the various staff and supply departments went on apace. In anticipation of war the Department had for some years been preparing lists of graduates of the officers' service or post-graduate schools in the regular army, with a view to the assignment of specially qualified officers to staff duty with the brigades, divisions and corps of volunteers. The first promotions and assignments were made from experienced regulars; then followed a rush of applicants urged by congressional delegations and those with official and social influence. The test of efficiency and experience was necessarily abandoned under this pressure, and appointments followed the usual lines of patronage and expediency. In these modern days, wars are of too short duration to justify appointment of inexperienced men to important military offices; it is a matter within the control of the President, and if he gives way to the fierce pressure, the army and country must suffer during the period while the new men are learning the trade of arms. Notwithstanding the many years of threatening clouds, there was no well-defined plan for organizing the army when called into active service. Brigades, divisions and corps gradually came into being through the expediency of the moment. A heterogeneous mass of staff officers was distributed to the general officers, and in many instances, instead of being useful, they proved to be encumbrances. In numerous cases the generals in command detailed subordinate regular officers to perform the duties while the volunteer officers held the higher staff rank and drew the pay of offices requiring technical knowledge, which is not immediately supplied through patriotism and willingness to serve. The humiliating experience of some of the great volunteer camps should be enough to prevent a repetition of such mistakes, but there is no assurance that like methods will not obtain in the next war unless some change in our military system is brought about.

. Having in view the advantage to be derived by not overcrowding railway terminals and docks, provision was made for distributing the forces destined for service over sea at New Orleans, Mobile and Tampa. Influences of various kinds prevailed against this scheme with the result that Tampa will always be to the army and the people a synonym of blunder and reproach. Taking advantage of the sharp criticisms brought upon the department because of conditions at Tampa, certain railroad and hotel interests urged the pretended advantages of Miami, and in face of adverse reports on the site by military experts, an order was given to move a division of troops to that point, with no good results.

The need for ships was urgent, and the navy was seeking them at the same time as the army. Our officers had had no previous personal experience with transports, and the history of the Vera Cruz expedition of the Mexican War appeared to have been forgotten; so General Shafter's magnificent corps was sent to Santiago, inadequately equipped, and had the navy not come to the rescue, the whole campaign must of necessity have been a failure through the impossibility of, or long delay in, effecting a landing. Once in contact with the enemy, the American army, as usual, added laurels to its already long list of successful campaigns. In face of all theory and academic teaching victory was wrested from brave and well-armed adversaries, but the general and honest opinion of army men well qualified to judge is, that an extremely lucky star hovered over America during the war with Spain.

The expedition to Porto Rico, and that across the wide Pacific to Manila were sent with less haste, and therefore better equipped. But experience was being obtained, and now, after having become possessed of a magnificent fleet of transports, the quartermaster department is enabled to point with just pride to four years of such successful endeavor that its record is not exceeded by that of any of the great steamship lines. This service ultimately reached such a degree of efficiency that thousands of troops have been transported seven thousand miles across the Pacific in sufficient comfort to have them ready for immediate field service on arrival.

With the signing of the protocol, it became necessary to reduce the forces, but as the Spanish army in Cuba was still intact, it was decided to proceed at once with the muster out of only 100,000 volunteers. The occupation of posts in Cuba to be evacuated by Spanish garrisons employed 50,000 troops. The question of withdrawing the volunteers from the Philippine Archipelago caused the War Department much concern. Peace once an accomplished official act, all volunteers would become entitled to discharge. The department concluded, therefore, to ask outright for a regular army of 100,000 men, and the House of Representatives passed a bill to that effect, but the minority in the Senate took up a line of speechmaking concerning the administration's Philippine policy and stifled the bill. To avoid an extra session, the minority was allowed to dictate a compromise of a temporary regular army and another force of volunteers. The muster out of the volunteers for the war with Spain was completed as rapidly as possible, having in mind the economy of the moment as well as protection from fraudulent claims for pensions in the future.

In the Philippines the army was confronted with many serious problems, the solution of which demanded a showing of well-organized force. The enlistment and transportation of volunteers to a scene of action ten thousand miles from their homes for a comparatively brief service, involved such an appalling expenditure of public funds that the President withheld his consent to the organization of the new regiments until conditions became so critical that the reënforcement could no longer be delayed. The excess of cost of this force of volunteers over what the cost would have been had regulars been employed, with the usual three years' enlistments, has been estimated by the various staff bureaus to be $16,374,009.04, quite an item even in these days of abounding prosperity. The new volunteer regiments were raised and commanded by regular officers, and were splendid organizations, but they were of necessity brought home and mustered out with an average of fifteen to eighteen months' service over sea, altogether a very expensive proceeding.

The exchange of troops in the Philippines to enable the volunteers who went out in the first expedition to come home, was effected during active insurrection which continued until a force of nearly 70,000 men was assembled in the Islands. The War Department has been subjected to much criticism concerning the conduct of the army while quelling the insurrection. While the Department has not come unscathed from the wordy conflict, the fact remains, if recent political events are correctly interpreted, that the army has never stood higher in the confidence and esteem of the people than now. Whatever motives may have actuated the detractors of the army, it can only be regretted that the conduct of the Philippine campaigns has been made a matter of political controversy. In the years to come the names of the heroes of the swamp and jungle campaigns of the recent past will be found upon the pages of history with those of Yorktown, Molino del Rey, and the Wilderness.

It became evident that makeshift devices would no longer serve the purpose, and the Secretary of War presented the needs of the service in carefully prepared legislation, which, while not accomplishing everything desired, gave the Department a sufficient force to meet the urgent demands upon the army in Cuba, Porto Rico, the Philippines, Alaska, and at home. In addition to an increase of strength, the Department secured the long-contested-for three battalion organization for the infantry branch. The artillery was largely increased and merged into a corps which enabled the department to concentrate the defense of each harbor or district, including submarine adjuncts, under the control of the senior artillery officer.

The Secretary of War, after a careful study of the situation, with particular reference to the difficulties encountered at the outbreak of the war with Spain, urged and secured a change in the laws which had hitherto perpetuated the staff departments as close corporations by virtue of life appointments. A detail system was introduced which will gradually supersede the old method of permanent appointments.

The variegated character of the militia system in the past caused the entire force which volunteered in bodies at the outbreak of the war with Spain to be judged by the weakest and most inefficient organizations. This was unjust to many excellent regiments, but the penalty paid by them for the association may be considered very light if the knowledge gained by the country at large eventuates in the honest reformation of the whole system and the placing of the organized militia upon a basis of self-respecting efficiency. Even under the favorable legislation recently enacted, it will require a long time to perfect the details of the system which is intended to secure immediate and efficient service from the militia at the outbreak of war. Our forefathers dreamed of the militia as the bulwark of a nation, yet the system failed utterly in the War of 1812. The "Continentals" left an indelible impression on the pages of Revolutionary history. The Mexican war proved the value of United States Volunteers in contradistinction to militia, and the world never saw better armies than those composed of the volunteers of 1861 to 1865. The National Guard organizations were recognized in 1898, but no effort was made to call into service the "militia," as contemplated by the Constitution. In all proposed legislation for improving the militia many varying opinions are advanced as to interpretations of the Constitution. This does not obtain in regard to United States Volunteers, who, once mustered into the service, are on the same footing exactly as regulars, except as to length of enlistment. At the outbreak of the war with Spain, Congress enacted that hereafter, in war, the army shall consist of the regular army and the volunteer army; in the former, enlistments are for three years, and in the latter for two years. This departure from the teachings of the Civil War was not called for by any emergency; an enlistment for "three years or the war" should be required of all volunteers, for, if this is not done, it makes it difficult to fill the ranks of old and valuable regular regiments where the three years' enlistment prevails.

Ever since the spring of 1898 the officials of the War Department have discussed the confusion which arose at Tampa and elsewhere, and have constantly sought the best means of preventing a repetition of conditions which might lead to humiliation and temporary defeat in a war with an enterprising and audacious enemy. After mature consideration, the Secretary of War settled upon a plan for the establishment of a General Staff Corps, with a chief at its head who will be Chief of Staff for the whole army. Under this plan the misnamed office of Commanding General will disappear. It has ever been a delusion and a disappointment for the distinguished soldiers who have occupied it, with constant but fruitless efforts to invest the office with something more than a name. This is the final army reform of a general nature, to the accomplishment of which Secretary Root has devoted himself. It will be a fitting capstone to the long series of definite and comprehensive improvements secured in the War Department and army methods by the Secretary. The new scheme once in successful operation, all the business of the army will be brought under the advisory control of a selected and highly trained body of experts, who, working in harmony with all the bureau chiefs, should accomplish coöperation and achievement of the most satisfactory character.

And now, with the advent of the third year of the new century, the great wave of prosperity which followed the close of the war with Spain, a not uncommon result of·wars, has reached dimensions far beyond the expectations of the most optimistic of our public men. The extension of American commerce is following in the trail of war, and all our people are participating in its practical results. The conduct of our troops, and the frankness and honesty of our policies, in Cuba, the Philippines and China, has challenged the attention of the civilized world. American diplomacy, backed by our highly civilized and intelligent troops, has become a synonym for fair dealing and unswerving honesty. There is abundant cause for pride in the respect now entertained for the United States throughout the world, as evidenced by the treatment of our representatives. Resting under the ægis of the Constitution and an honest interpretation of the Monroe doctrine, there is no possibility of the military arm ever becoming a tool to subvert our own or the liberties of other people. Sophistry and concealment find no place in our treatment of other nations, and this country will fulfil its duties as a newly discovered world power with only such an army and navy as will prevent a decadence of the military art, and yet strong enough not to offer an invitation to attack.

SPEECH OF HON. ALBERT F. DAWSON ON NAVAL ADMINISTRATION [1]

THE House being in Committee of the Whole House on the state of the Union, and having under consideration the bill (H. R. 20471) making appropriations for the naval service for the fiscal year ending June 30, 1909, and for other purposes —

Mr. Dawson said:

Mr. Chairman: We have heard the naval subject discussed here this afternoon from a scientific standpoint, a sentimental standpoint, and, I am almost tempted to add, from a hysterical standpoint. I would like to ask the committee at this hour to consider it from the business standpoint, and to direct attention to one of the most important questions in the whole naval service — the question of naval administration.

Mr. Chairman, this is not a sentimental proposition; this is a great business proposition, involving as it does the expenditure of the $100,000,000 which we appropriate annually for this great arm of the national defense. Upon this problem of administration rests the question of whether these millions are expended economically and wisely or whether they shall be expended wastefully and extravagantly. But this question of naval administration, Mr. Chairman, is even more than a business proposition. It is a question which goes to the very root of the efficiency of the naval service itself; it has a most important bearing upon the efficiency of the material of the Navy; it is vital to whether or not we will have good guns, good ammunition and good ships; it is vital likewise to the personnel of the Navy, because on the question of administration depends the esprit de corps of the officers and men of the entire Navy.

It may be a matter of surprise to some Members of the House to know that the present administrative organization of the Navy Department is almost seventy years old. Is it any wonder, Mr. Chairman, with the tremendous advances that have been made, both in naval and in commercial matters, during these seventy years that the present administrative system in the Navy Department does not measure up to present-day business standards? I say, is it any wonder that this system of administration is outworn, out of date, and obsolete?

The present plan of administration in the Navy Department was

---

[1] *Congr. Record*, Reported April 15, 1908.

adopted in 1842, and the law has been only slightly amended since. At that time, upon the recommendation of Secretary Upshur, Congress passed a law creating five bureaus in the Navy Department. Since that time three other bureaus have been added, with some rearrangement and readjustment of duties, and now we have in the Navy Department eight separate bureaus, as follows:

Navigation, having charge of the personnel and the movements of the fleet, under the direction of the Secretary of the Navy.

Yards and Docks: The construction and maintenance of public works in navy yards and at naval stations.

Supplies and Accounts: Provisions, clothing, small stores, accounts, and pay of the Navy.

Medicine and Surgery: Its name explains its duties.

Construction and Repair: The ships' hulls, turrets, ammunition hoists, etc.

Steam Engineering: Steam-propelling machinery of the ships.

Ordnance: Guns, ammunition, and parts of the electrical machinery on the ships.

Equipment: Equipment of ships, and supplying most of their electrical apparatus.

It should be remembered, Mr. Chairman, as we go along, that the Bureau of Construction and Repair, the Bureau of Steam Engineering, the Bureau of Ordnance, and the Bureau of Equipment are the ones principally concerned in the construction and the repair of ships.

Under the law as it stands now it is provided that the orders of these chiefs of bureaus, pertaining to their respective duties, shall be considered as emanating from the Secretary of the Navy, and "shall have full force and effect as such." Mark that. The orders of each chief of bureau shall have the full force and effect as though the orders had been issued by the Secretary of the Navy himself. In other words, instead of one head of Department we have under this old organization nine heads operating within one Department.

There is nothing in existing law which provides for any coöperation or any coördination among those several bureaus. Each is entirely independent, subject only to the Secretary himself. They all stand on an equal footing. Under the law each bureau may proceed in its own way according to the chief's idea of what is for the best interest of that bureau. The system is lacking in that one feature that is most essential for good administration and best results—there is no single controlling influence below the Secretary to correlate the work of the different bureaus. Thus responsibility is divided among eight different heads, which has the effect of there being practically no responsibility at all for the work as a whole. Secretary Moody, when he was at the head of that great Department, recognized and set forth in his annual report some of the defects of the system as he found them. What did he say?

The distribution of business among bureaus independent of and correlated to each other (except through the action of the Secretary) unquestionably creates the condition out of which grow conflicts of jurisdiction between the bureaus, sometimes injurious, and a tendency to consider the interests of the bureaus rather than the interests of the Navy. The division of business in the bureaus extends to the navy yards and even to some extent to ships in commission. This leads sometimes to excessive and cumbersome organization, and lack of harmony of effort resulting from the fact that there is no coördination except by the voluntary action of the bureau chiefs.

That is testimony of one who was in the Department long enough to familiarize himself with conditions there. But, Mr. Chairman, how does this system operate, both in the Department and in the navy yards throughout the country? Perhaps we can best determine the character of its operation by examining its work in the repair of ships, which is conducted at these navy yards. Last summer the Committee on Naval Affairs made a tour of inspection of all the navy yards on the Atlantic coast from Norfolk north to Portsmouth, and we went in and examined carefully the condition at each of these yards. This examination disclosed a wasteful duplication and multiplication of plants, buildings, and equipment which can not be otherwise than extravagant in the expenditure of the public money, and it emphasized the necessity for some consolidation of bureaus. Each of the four bureaus which have to do with the repair or the construction of ships had at the different navy yards a separate and independent plant. Each had sought to build up its own bureau there, that it might be entirely independent of all the others. Thus, at every one of these navy yards, instead of finding one complete, fully organized, well-trained enterprise, we found what was virtually four separate plants at each yard.

Each of the bureaus has its own force of workmen, each has its own machinery, its own buildings, and its own peculiar method of doing business. For instance, at the navy yard at New York we found that the Bureau of Construction and Repair had a paint shop, and so did the Bureau of Yards and Docks, the Bureau of Equipment, and the Bureau of Steam Engineering — Equipment maintaining a shop with three painters, while the Steam Engineering had another shop in which was employed one lone painter. The same was true of the carpenter shops, except the Ordnance Bureau had one in addition to these other four, making five carpenter shops in a single yard. Of those five shops, three were employing less than ten men each. And so it went. What was true of paint shops and carpenter shops was equally true of pattern shops, blacksmith shops, coppersmith shops, and foundries.

Will anyone contend that this is anything except a most wasteful and extravagant method of carrying on a purely industrial business, because the repair of ships is not military in its character, it is purely the industrial side of the Navy? Such a plan of course requires a useless duplication of machinery, of buildings, and of supervising force. But this condition is only the natural result of a system which makes each bureau independent of the other, and where at every navy yard each bureau is watching every other bureau with jealous eye. With Congress making separate appropriations for each of these bureaus, it becomes, as one naval officer tersely stated it, simply a game of "grab." If a given bureau has secured an appropriation for a new building at a certain yard, the following year each of the other bureaus are supplicating Congress to treat it with like liberality.

This whole bureau system, as exemplified at the navy yards, is unbusinesslike; it is cumbersome and extravagant and, as Secretary Long so well said in one of his official reports while he was Secretary of the Navy, "No private business in the world would be run on such a wasteful and inharmonious plan."

But how does the present bureau system operate in the Navy Department itself? The public has had many striking instances within the last year of the friction and contentions that arise in that Department by reason of the fact that there are eight separate and independent bureaus, each practically supreme in the duties which are assigned to it by the Secretary of the Navy. The heads of these bureaus are but human, and it is too much to expect that they will not take advantage of every opportunity which occurs that will increase the magnitude or the importance of their respective duties. As Secretary Moody says, the operation of the system has a tendency to cause the bureau chiefs to consider "the interests of the bureaus rather than the interests of the Navy."

I hope gentlemen will understand that I am not criticising individuals. I am simply offering these suggestions regarding a system which prevails, in the hope that we can accord to the Navy Department in due course better and more modern machinery with which to conduct the work of that great Department.

I need not relate in detail the incidents which have arisen from time to time, and some of which have been alluded to in this debate, showing the clashing of interests and authority under this system of independent bureaus, each, mind you, with the power to issue independent orders of the same authority as those issued by the Secretary of the Navy himself.

If we are in any doubt as to the workings of this system in the Department, let us summon a witness here who is eminently qualified to speak with authority, one who by experience, by knowledge, and by courage is entitled to the consideration of this House. I allude to the Hon. John D. Long, who for five years was Secretary of that great Department, and it might be added parenthetically, that he was in charge of that Department for a longer period than any other man who has held that portfolio in the last decade. He was there long enough to understand the workings of that Department and to master its defects. He recognized the faults of the existing bureau system, and in his annual report for 1899 he recommended that three of these bureaus, these three bureaus that have to deal with the construction and fitting out of vessels, should be merged into a single bureau. That recommendation was as follows:

Consolidation of Bureaus

In the opinion of the Department it would be in the interest of good business organization and economy to consolidate the three Bureaus of Construction and Repair, Steam Engineering, and Equipment under one head — the Bureau of Ships. These Bureaus have to do with the construction and fitting out of vessels; in one word, the material of the ship. It is an integral work. When a contract is made for the construction of a ship, it is made with one builder. It is not given part to a constructor of hulls, part to a steam-engine manufacturer, and part to an outfitting firm. Whatever various trades enter into the work are all under one head. This is the method of private shipyards which build the largest ships and which are not left to the administration of three heads between whom delicate questions of respective authority and responsibility are liable to arise, resulting in delays and too often in friction and lack of harmony of coöperation.

Each of the above Bureaus has now, during the construction of naval vessels, its separate inspectors at each yard. A consolidated bureau could, of course, be run much cheaper than three bureaus, and a great saving made by a reduction of the now three separate working forces, both clerical and mechanical, especially in our navy yards. Fewer naval officers would be needed, as there would be but one staff instead of three, so that more officers would be available for other duty. Under the present system one Bureau brings its work to the point of readiness for the work of another, which is not always ready for it. There is necessarily a lack of that adaptation and harmony of movement which one head would secure.

If this consolidation were effected, the matter of furnishing coal and other current supplies, which is now under the direction of the Bureau of Equipment, could be easily transferred to the Bureau of Supplies and Accounts, and such other incidental changes made as became necessary.

The foregoing suggestion is made solely with a view to an improvement in departmental organization, and with the highest appreciation of the ability and dutifulness with which these Bureaus have been administered under their present heads. Efficient as they have been, however, their consolidation is recommended, because it is believed that if consolidated under the direction of any one of their present heads, or of any competent officer, that efficiency would be still greater, less expense incurred, and a better business organization would succeed.

The terms of office of the chiefs of the three Bureaus will all expire in a little more than a year, one of those officers then going upon the retired list, and it is due to them all, as an assurance that the change is recommended on systematic and not personal grounds, to suggest that if made, it shall not go into effect until the beginning of the fiscal year after the expiration of their said terms.

It is most interesting, in the consideration of the workings of the present system, to note what he has to say in his annual report for the year 1900 when he renewed that recommendation. Here is what he said:

Consolidation of Bureaus

The recommendation heretofore made that the organization of the Navy Department be simplified by the consolidation of the three Bureaus of Construction and Repair, Steam Engineering, and Equipment is renewed. Under the present system, from the inception of its design until completed and placed in commission, the plans and specifications of a naval vessel are in the hands of three bureaus, each with a distinct organization, each having exclusive jurisdiction within certain lines, and all charged with the duty of carrying on work within, but not beyond, their respective provinces, as nearly as may be at the same time.

Such a system is, in practical administration, cumbrous and expensive, and from its very nature tends to develop controversies respecting the scope of each bureau's duties and to occasion friction, delay, and want of harmony in doing whatever approaches border lines of jurisdiction. It is to the credit of the officers in charge of the bureaus concerned that work upon ships now under construction has been carried on without more friction; but the system itself is none the less objectionable, and is a source of inconvenience, delay, largely increased cost, and occasional confusion.

The present divided organization is the outgrowth of conditions which no longer exist. The hull, the propelling machinery, and the articles of equipment of a modern steamship no longer constitute simple, distinct, and separable elements in construction, but, on the contrary, in their multiplicity of details are so interwoven as to render embarrassing their supervision by three sets of independent administrative officials.

The union of these three bureaus, the chief function of which is to deal with the material of the ship, into one bureau, which might appropriately be called the " Bureau of Ships;" the consolidation of their several corps of assistants and inspectors, and the conduct of the really integral work of building and equipping vessels, under the management of one responsible chief instead of three chiefs, would promote the efficient and economical administration of this important part of the business of the Navy Department.

A chief of bureau is practically an assistant secretary. The proposed consolidation would not only reduce three of these assistants to one, but in like manner reduce the supervising, mechanical, and clerical forces in every navy yard, and thus save great and unnecessary expense. At present each of these bureaus in question has at each yard its separate shops, inspectors, foremen, and workmen, all often doing the same kind of work. No private business is run on such a wasteful and inharmonious plan. I renew the recommendation in this respect of my last annual report.

Let me cite to the House one or two instances to show the complications arising out of the present divided organization in the Navy Department to which Secretary Long alluded. In the installation of the fire-control apparatus on a battle ship — and you all understand what the fire-control apparatus is; it is, in comparison with the other elements of the ship, a very simple matter — it would naturally be supposed that one bureau would be sufficient to install the fire-control apparatus, and yet under the existing system three separate and distinct bureaus have cognizance of the installation of this apparatus on a battle ship. Again, we find that the Bureau of Steam Engineering owns the steam pipes on the pumps and the engines which are under the jurisdiction of the Bureau of Construction and Repair. The Bureau of Steam Engineering likewise controls the deck hatches and gratings leading to the boiler and engine rooms, and also that part of the hull-drainage pipes that drain these compartments. Countless other instances might be cited to show that the lines of authority between the different bureaus within a single battle ship are mixed in bewildering confusion. These are not faults of the bureau method, but they are faults of the bureau system which, in its present form, can not be adjusted to suit the natural divisions in shipbuilding which have come about by reason of the change from wooden sailing vessels to steel steamships.

I am not one of those Members of this House who believe that he has done his duty in any matter when he has pointed out the defects. It is easy enough to criticise; anybody can find fault. I believe it is equally a part of his duty to come forward with some remedy to correct existing defects as he may find them. In my judgment, Mr. Chairman, the remedy for the present situation which exists in the administration of the Navy Department rests in reorganization and in the consolidation of certain bureaus in that Department.

NAVAL ADMINISTRATION [1]

By T. G. Roberts, Naval Constructor, U. S. N.

It is necessary to recognize, in the first place, that three separate and distinct methods of administration are found within the operations of the Navy Department, comprising what we understand as naval administration. These three divisions may be classified under the heads (1) Political, (2) Military, and (3) Industrial.

The political system is represented by the head of the Navy Department, who is, and ever will be, a civilian, because the spirit and essence of our Government is based on a subjection of the military to the civil institution.

The political administration, as above classified, is frequently referred to as civil administration, which it is; but so also is industrial administration, and to avoid confusion, the foregoing classification will be adhered to throughout.

Military administration refers to that under the line officers, who alone are eligible to the supreme command of a ship, a squadron, or a

[1] Part of a paper read before the United States Naval Institute in 1905, and reprinted in the *Congr. Record*, April 15, 1908.

fleet. Line officer means a naval officer in the line of promotion to such command. The functions are purely military, and the purely military field of operations finds its most correct example on board a ship or in a fleet. Shipboard administration will be considered the exact expression of military administration in the Navy. The strategy and directing power of a fleet are included in the same definition.

By industrial administration is meant that portion engaged in the production and manufacture of a ship and its accessories, which may be more closely defined as those departments engaged in procuring materials and operating civilian mechanics in producing the ship. Navy-yard administration is industrial in all that applies to workshop and civil employees as found to exist in the analogous institution of a private shipyard, being military only by virtue of the supreme authority vested in a commandant.

(1) POLITICAL ADMINISTRATION

The Secretary of the Navy represents the political administrator. Politics is our method of securing government of the people, by the people, for the people. The politically successful man is one selected by the majority as their representative, because of personal attributes most acceptable to the people, whose actions the people believe will be most agreeable to themselves concerned. He is, presumably, the embodiment of our form of government, and to his authority the military and industrial considerations must bow.

The political feature finds its expression in various ways in naval administration, over and above all other considerations contemplated in the military establishment as laid down in the Navy regulations. If a ship must be overhauled and repaired and two navy yards desire to get the work, the workmen's representatives that clamor loudest usually get it, that being the will of the majority that care anything about it. Within the service the opinion always holds that such matters, as all others, should be determined by the absolute merits of the case, regardless of clamors. The military administrator must determine his actions by merit, that being the root and foundation of his education and training, and he cares little about the will of the people where his position is not influenced by such a regard. A naval officer is not in the best position to be a political administrator — he can read from the mercurial barometer an approach of a storm at sea, but he is handicapped where it comes to feeling the pulse of the people from the touch of the political barometer.

Political administration finds its way into the service in shifting ships and work from one station to another, in shifting personnel in like manner, in the location of navy yards and naval stations, in appropriations for new buildings and new expenditures of all kinds at the various stations; it determines whether vessels shall be built or repaired at navy yards. In time of war political considerations divert naval vessels from the fleet to patrol the coasts in the vicinity of frightened political communities. It has given high position to political favorites and has determined the command of ships and squadrons. Sometimes it goes even farther and influences the actions of naval boards in their duties under the regulations. Boards have been known to have their recommendations returned for revision until they meet the political desires, or another board may be called to reverse their actions, and so on until the desired results are attained. This operates to promote personnel in some cases, or discharge or retire it in others. It operates sometimes to increase the pay of the navy-yard mechanic. Its existence has been alleged in political contests against nonpartisan shipbuilders in the trials of vessels, and it shows itself in various forms in the distribution of contracts for new ships, and is constantly at work in the purchase and acceptance of all sorts of materials for Government use. The head of a Government Department is sensitive to the representations of the people; if he is not, someone soon takes his place who is. Of course there have been abuses, as in every other department of life, but a good administrator knows enough not to try to reform the people or the political system of which he is a part; he does his part best if he recognizes facts as they exist; and he concedes to political demands, if they are logical, where it makes no material difference otherwise, and where it does not interfere with the object for which his institution was created.

I am not attempting to lay down rules, but merely to place an estimate on what appears to have been the guiding features of political administration from the evidences that have come to notice in the past.

Is such a political government an abuse? Should the people rule the people? If the public's wishes be disregarded, the Government becomes autocratic by definition, and how else can their wishes be made known except through their representatives? If reform, who will attempt it, and how? Would the creation of a general staff, or any other sort of a mechanism inside the Navy Department destroy, limit, or influence in any way the politics of the head of the Department as it applies to the military and industrial establishments? It may as well be conceded, in the light of history, that the political administration, whatever its good or evil, will remain untrammeled as long as our form of government exists.

(2) Military Administration

Only on board a naval vessel does military discipline hold complete sway. The order of the captain is the law and must be obeyed without question, argument, or appeal to a higher power. The captain must confine his actions to the limits prescribed by law, but inside those limits he can cover almost any sort of overbearing conduct toward those beneath him, officers and men alike. He can not strike them, or punish them physically beyond the lawful limit; but he can harangue them and institute such a personal bearing toward them as to punish them mentally beyond degree. There is no appeal from an order, which must be obeyed with alacrity whether right or wrong, and he who refuses classifies his actions with the mutineers, the limit of which, in grave cases, is death. He who answers back goes to prison, but he can not resign or be discharged. I am merely specifying the limits in order to distinguish more clearly between military and industrial administration and to show that a trained military administrator is as different from an industrial as from a political administrator.

Our bureau system is represented in miniature on the ship. The captain represents the Bureau of Navigation, which directs his own actions and the movements of the ship. Although the other bureaus are represented, not one of them has any right or power of appeal that would modify in the least the perfect and absolute control of the directing administrative bureau and its captain in the wielding of the ship as a fighting machine. In this point it differs from navy-yard administration, as we shall see presently. The executive officer represents the Bureau of Construction and Repair, and the ordnance, equipment, medical, pay, and marine officers represent the corresponding bureaus. In the operation of the bureau system in the use of tools, stores, etc., there are no conflictions; they are used where needed indiscriminately by shipboard authority or without. If one bureau's machine breaks down another bureau's force repairs it, if more handy. The bureau representatives themselves are not expert in the lines of demarcation and coguizance of the bureaus, a line officer representing a staff bureau, and there is no provision for appeal beyond the ship if one should so desire. In other words, the captain has complete control of the ship and all her accessories, and the bureau system divides the duties of officers into a convenient distribution of the work. Military efficiency is attained by drilling, innate intelligence, alacrity in obedience to orders, and the good example and rigid discipline that must be maintained by the officers at all hazards. Admiral Farragut laid down a military rule for all time when he said to his officers: "Whatever is to be done must be done quickly." Shipboard efficiency consists in preparedness and alacrity. It has little to do with dollars and cents. Military economy is exercised in taking care of the materials and avoiding waste, in about the same way as one would take care of a new suit of clothes, or would eat sparingly of his provisions during a long journey. It has nothing to do with saving money by a judicial distribution of the laboring forces, to obtain the best returns for the money expended, which forms the essence of industrial administration.

On the contrary, shipboard administration contemplates expending

the maximum amount of labor in order to fill up the time. Those who have been to sea know the monotony of having nothing to do, which tends to generate the spirit of unhappiness. Hence, the sailor's proverb that the best commander keeps his crew happy by keeping them busy. Happiness is healthy for the mind, labor is healthy for the body, and these essentials permit of the attainment of military preparedness, alertness, and efficiency. Industrial economy is a different profession. It is a law of humanity that a man is most proficient in the line of his ambitions. The highest ambition of a line officer is to command at sea. In that position the eyes of the whole world may be turned on him in war, and his name may be in every mouth. He may bring honor or disgrace to his country. He must be a specialist in the strictest sense, but not a general practitioner. Besides familiarity with the methods of wielding the men and the tools at his disposal, he must be familiar with strategy, international law, naval history, navigation, and tactics. None can afford to be an indifferent expert in these branches, for a single blunder in one might lose all. No profession in civil life forms any sort of analogy or comparison to that of a line officer, and it is a matter of current belief that the easy habits and disciplinary notions of naval training unfit an officer for civil pursuits; and it is likewise apparent that civilians never have been, and can not be, eligible to the position of a line officer without the necessary course of training. It requires no analytical mind to discern the irreconcilable differences between industrial and military administration.

(3) INDUSTRIAL ADMINISTRATION

The peaceful arts of the shipbuilding mechanics comprise the industrial features of naval administration, as is represented by a navy yard. The business of such an institution is to manufacture, repair, or assemble the vessel and her outfit. The production of the vessel belongs purely to civil industry, being the product of the shipbuilding trades under the cognizance of labor unions. The pay of a sailor is merely nominal in comparison with that of the mechanical tradesman, which furnishes an opening for a considerable loss of funds unless the quality of administration secures the best combination in outlay of plant, in the purchase and handling of materials, and, most important of all, in the distribution and handling of the difficult and very expensive labor that fills up the navy yards. The workmen may not be tongue-lashed, nor put in the brig, but they may be discharged if the administrator has a good case.

Now, let us examine the operations of the bureau system as it applies to the industry of a navy yard. The local representatives of bureaus comprise the corresponding departments of Construction and Repair, Steam Engineering, Equipment, Yards and Docks, Ordnance, Supplies and Accounts, and Medicine and Surgery. The Bureau of Navigation is represented by the commandant.

The division of work assigned to each bureau or department is a development of the natural and convenient divisions that existed in shipbuilding when the bureaus were first formed in 1842. The original Bureau of Construction, Equipment, and Repair controlled practically all the industry that was required to build a ship. It included all that is now represented by the three bureaus Construction and Repair, Equipment, and Steam Engineering, the latter subdivisions having been made in 1862 during the stress of war. Had the Construction Bureau not been thus subdivided there would be a different tale to tell about the cost of navy-yard administration to-day. But no one could have foreseen the effect at that date. The subdivisions were natural ones, inasmuch as the Chief Constructor before that time had an engineer as assistant to look after the steam machinery of the new motive power.

The wood shipbuilder viewed with suspicion the advent of steam, and the motive power of the future passed out of his hands to those who were willing to master it. A ship was then a simple affair, and there was no question as to where the propelling machinery left off and where the ship began. The Equipment Bureau undertook to relieve the Construction Bureau of assembling movable articles not strictly a part of a ship, but corresponding more nearly to the furnishings, such as sails, rigging, anchors and chains, the electrical outfit, and the like. With the changes that have come about in modern shipbuilding, the steel ships of to-day, with their complex machinery, have merged all professions into one. The wood shipbuilder, as represented in the modern shipwright, has been driven almost out of business. His cognizance included the whole vessel in 1842, while now he is limited to the decks and the outside sheathing, if any. The steam engineer finds himself replacing his own auxiliary machinery with equipment motors, and he has to tolerate rival steam engines that form essential portions of the equipment and construction machinery. Likewise the Equipment Bureau finds rivals with electrical machinery in the Bureaus of Steam Engineering and Construction.

The original natural divisions of these three bureaus have become unnatural and very complex and illogical. All three operate both steam and electrical machinery, and generally throughout are trying to do similar work that now falls under one profession. I shall not endeavor to relate all the unreasonable subdivisions or the work in these bureaus, but will cite only a few samples. As new methods have been adopted, each bureau has claimed as much of the work as possible, and each head of department, disagreeing, has written out his case, and all the papers have gone to the Secretary of the Navy for decision. In the meantime, in many instances the work has waited several months until the matter was settled. The decisions have not followed any rule, but the bureau in most favor at the time has generally won. If the question was referred to a board composed mostly of line officers, the decision was given very frequently to the line officer contestant, if there was the slightest possible justification for it. I would remark here that with a general staff of pure line officers to pass on such questions, the bulk of industrial administration would pass from the staff bureaus into the hands of the military administrators, in case human nature should not unexpectedly reform. To-day the department of Steam Engineering owns the steam pipes of Construction pipes and engines, the deck hatches and gratings and their fastenings leading to the boiler and engine rooms, and also that portion of the hull drainage pipes that drain these compartments; Equipment owns the dynamos, and the dynamo foundations if there are any, and the railing around them if attached to these foundations. Shall I go any further? Suffice it to say, that the lines of cognizance between these bureaus are more mixed up than the present Navy pay table. The fault is not in the bureau method, but in the fact that the bureau system has not been readjusted to suit the natural divisions of shipbuilding as they exist since the steel ship has created a revolution in shipbuilding methods.

Shipbuilding was originally made up of several professions, but to-day it has merged into a single profession, and it not only includes the production of the whole ship, but it operates the shipbuilding plant, by which it controls the profit which forms the measure of efficiency in industrial administration. The remedy is the simplest business proposition in the country — consolidation. There is no economy in shifting cognizance from one bureau to another, as now organized; each department has developed according to its needs, by virtue of experience, and to shift its power, plant, or shop to some other department only acts to deprive the one that needs it and prevents the responsible party from controlling its own profits. There is a great deal of talk about consolidating the power plants of a navy yard. The idea seems to be that only the power plants are duplicated. That is a .very great error. Everything is duplicated and multiplied. In the navy yard with which the writer has been associated for the past five years there are in the several departments the following shops, viz.:

Six power plants, eight machine shops, five joiner shops, five paint shops, five laborers' lobbies, four blacksmith shops, four pattern shops, four tin shops, four fuel-oil plants, four testing laboratories, three electrical workshops, three copper shops, three riggers' gangs, three polishing shops, three fuel-gas plants, three foundries, two steel-plate shops, two electroplating shops, thirty-two storehouses under separate roofs, fifty material fields, or piles of materials not under cover, and thirteen coal sheds and bins under separate roofs.

The shops and forces of the departments being duplicated, it follows that the heads of departments, and hence the departments themselves, are pretty nearly duplicated, which is, actually, from a shipbuilder's point of view, a fact. Nothing short of industrial consolidation will be worth while, and the establishment should not only be consolidated, but it should be divorced from the military, so to speak; that is to say, the one shipbuilding department should be a unit under the one shipbuilding head, responsible for the economy of the work. Our navy yards would then be as in France. We are moving toward the French methods. We tried the British Admiralty Board from 1779 to 1781, but abolished it. It was tried again from 1815 to 1842 in the form of the Navy Commissioners, but it was again abolished as being unsuitable. Every young nation tries the British Admiralty method. It suits England for reasons purely English. The posts of honor and command are kept in the aristocracy for the benefit of the younger sons of the nobility. The line of the British navy is sought by them as a profession. The "Board of Commissioners for the Execution of the Office of Lord High Admiral of His Britannic Majesty's Navy," belongs to a privileged class. In this country we expect a man to be responsible only for what he knows; our lords of industry are the engineering nobility who have won their titles by actual achievement in their own particular line.

We have left the British Admiralty method far behind long ago and are approaching the French system. We hear of a general staff — that is what we sometimes erroneously translate the French état-major to mean. We hear that we need a "bureau of personnel" and a "bureau of matériel." That is all French in name and method, and all our own bureaus are adopted and named after the French. Then let us have the French "bureau of matériel" precisely as it exists, which consolidates all industrial shops and works under the one head of "naval construction"; its directing "personnel" is composed of "Ingenieurs des constructions navales." It includes also all ordnance workshops and fittings in navy yards. Unlike our ordnance, theirs is manufactured by civil industry and shipped to navy yards, where it is handled and installed by the department of naval constructions. French navy-yard industry is confined to the one department, which combines every shop and tradesman under a single head, and that not a military head, nor a number of mixed military and industrial heads, but rather an industrial head who is competent to take the responsibility for the things he knows, the things of his special education and training, the things of his pride and ambition, the only things by virtue of which eminent ability may permit him to rise to any sort of distinction. Not that he needs distinction and should be allowed to attain it, but that the human composition is such that the best efficiency can not be attained by any other inducements in a system where hope of reward must be the stimulus; where neither capital, salary, nor interest, from a personal investment, are at stake. "Individual responsibility reposing in the head who instructed in the things he is responsible for is at the root of efficiency." Our bureau method is preëminently such a method, and is the most perfect yet devised, but has become uneconomical for the plain reason that the system of the bureaus has not been readjusted to suit the natural subdivisions of the present times, until the supposedly "sharply defined duties and responsibilities of overspecialized bureaus," to adopt Captain Mahan's diction, have become interlaced, interwoven, and intertangled to such an extent as to exist only in theory and imagination, but have no semblance in reality.

The Bureaus of Construction and Repair, Steam Engineering, Equipment, and Yards and Docks should be combined under the heading of Bureau of Naval Construction; the Bureaus of Ordnance, Supplies and Accounts, and Medicine and Surgery to remain practically as at present; excepting that, as in France, the Bureau of Naval Construction should have cognizance of its own materials so as to control the economy in their purchase and handling.

The Bureau of Ordnance should remain as now, excepting that its duties should end with the manufacture and shipment of ordnance and armor; its plans should be limited to these items and should not include any portion of the vessel to which they are applied. This is in order to unify the manufacture of plans at the Navy Department and the plans and building work at shipyards as the nearest approximate measure of economy. Strictly speaking, ordnance and armor belong to the broad Division of Matériel, along with the rest of the ship, by definition, and by the example of the Navy furnishing us with the term, and hence, logically, should be combined with the other bureaus of matériel. In that event it would become advisable to detail line officers as inspectors, since in this country, unlike some other countries, naval ordnance has been developed and manufactured almost purely by line officers, and it would not be advantageous to take it out of their hands. This renders it less advisable to include the Bureau of Ordnance in the consolidation; but since the ordnance and armor factories are not situated so as to duplicate work of any kind, a result almost equal to consolidation will be obtained by consolidating the designs and building of ship and machinery, exclusive only of ordnance and armor, under the single industrial bureau. This arrangement need not exclude the inspector of ordnance when guns are being installed on shipboard, but should require his presence, as in France.

There is sufficient evidence to believe that the Bureau of Navigation has grown too large and that it should be separated into two bureaus, the new one to be called the "Bureau of Personnel." This bureau should take over the items suggested by its name, and other kindred duties that will leave only the items concerning strategy to the Bureau of Navigation. The latter bureau would retain, of course, the Intelligence Office, the War College, the direction of the fleet, war plans, and all those functions which go to make up the sum total of "the wielding of the Navy as a weapon"; and besides would inherit, from the defunct bureaus, the Naval Observatory, coaling stations, other naval stations, and in fact everything else except navy yards, stations, and docks engaged in the building or repair of vessels. I merely suggest, not advise, the latter subdivision. It can not, in any wise, affect industrial administration.

The present necessity is the unification of navy-yard industry, so that it can not duplicate itself, and so that naval industrial administration may operate in the full benefit of modern methods as developed with such eminent success in the private industries of this country. All power plants, shops, heads of departments, assistants, draftsmen, clerks, foremen, leading men, and mechanics may be combined into one set of each class or kind. The result would effect a reduction of the number of buildings in use, the working forces, and the total cost of the establishment by an amount that would be startling to predict. The military authority should remain supreme in a commandant, but the industrial establishment, being in subjection to the military, need not be subdivided into a number of mixed administrations interwoven as now, but combined and divorced as a pure industrial unit.

EVILS TO BE CURED

Of the present evils of greatest moment is the unsystematic method of laying out new yard plants and the distribution of shop buildings among the various departments. The sites for the plants themselves are selected, usually, by people having an eye only to the depth of water, facilities for military protection, and the nature of the soil. The most important economic industrial consideration contained in the contour of the site and water frontage and in the economic arrangement of shops have seemingly had no part whatever in the establishment of our navy-yard plants.

Economy in arrangement, whereby labor and material travel by the shortest route between shop and ship, is an asset which means a goodly percentage in profit as long as the plant endures. A steel plate that will travel 300 yards from plate rack to its place on the ship's side in a poorly arranged plant may travel only a hundred yards in its course from machine to machine in a well-arranged plant. The reduction in cost of handling is very appreciable; and if this be applied to all the multitude of articles that go to complete a modern ship, the difference in cost is considerable. The same condition obtains with labor, which is more important, because more expensive. The shipfitting and joiner shops belong nearest the building slips and fitting-out berths, so that the class of men that fit and refit from shop to ship will have to walk the shortest distance; for the similar reason that the engine and boiler shops would be at the rear, as near the fitting-out berths as possible, since the engines and boilers may be built complete in the shops, and when ready may be hauled any distance by rail to the fitting-out berths. Every shop has a logical location in a shipyard, yet no shop can have its proper place by our methods. Each department seeks the main business street as centrally located as possible. Sites and shops are let in a haphazard way, and, even if determined by a board, the most influential member gets the most central location. In the navy yard of my most intimate acquaintance the distance of the farthest buildings from the power house of one department is so great that the cost of the electric-power wires is something extraordinary; one department is widely separated into two large halves by another department lying between, and the joiner shop is farthest away from slips and berths, while the engine and boiler shops are nearest the slips and docks, just the reverse of where they ought to be. Yet the losses on first cost and circuitousness must appear in the figures of cost as long as the plant exists.

Another great source of loss lies in the lack of harmony that usually exists between the heads of departments. There are two sorts of inter-department administration; one where controversy is rife, another where obliging tact prevails. It may be observed here, incidentally, that the one who willfully enters into a squabble is a downright enemy to economy, for when at their best, heads of departments are far enough apart by the very nature of things. One department finishes its work to where another begins, and then endeavors to get the other department to supply the connecting link. The second department may have its men on a more pressing job, or may not even have obtained funds for the work in hand. The delay in connecting may be anywhere from an hour to a month. Worse than that has happened. These misconnections are very frequent, due to the simple fact that the various heads of departments have different trains of thought, and one can not divine what the other intends to do until the time arrives. The great effort of working ahead of time in all the mass of details is not to be expected from men whose capital or income does not bind them to it, and whose salary depends on the limits of the single duties of their own department as laid down in the Navy regulations. Unintentional misconnections between departments are the source of the greatest loss of time and money in the operation of the plants as they now stand. One department owns a crane, a second department is using it, while a third department waits for it. The time of making connections, getting permission, and waiting may keep a whole gang of men out of work for some time. One department builds a shop, the second department buys an elevator for it; the original plans made to fit are changed by one department without the knowledge of the other, and the elevator is found not to suit the shaft, so the floor just completed must be cut out again.

A load of steel plates arrives and must be immediately removed by one department from the receiving station. This causes one handling. Another department has the list of plates, what they are and who they are for, and retains it sometimes a week or two. When the list arrives the third department has to inspect them, one by one, to examine the inspector's mark on each. The first department does not find it convenient to handle them until the broken crane of the fourth department is mended, to avoid rehandling them twice again. At the end of some months the inspection is completed and the contractor has lost several months' interest on his money.

One department buys a lot of materials that it thinks the other department will need, and owing to a miscalculation of the other department's habits the goods lie in store for an indefinite time. Two departments disagree on a matter touching both. The first one begins the work and the other writes a letter to the commandant, who refers it to the first one for his arguments. If the work is important the commandant authorizes the one he thinks is right, and forwards the papers to the Assistant Secretary of the Navy for a decision to guide in future cases. If unimportant, the work may await the decision. Sometimes friction arises between two departments; they begin to make caustic remarks and indorsements to each other. The clerks, foremen, and workmen soon catch it, and there is a regular blockade of the interlying work between the two. When this happens, lords of old in feudal castles were not in more impregnable fortresses than are the two belligerent heads. The warfare is waged silently by mutual understanding; each puts the other out as much as possible, and there is no power on earth to stop them except by mutual consent. The commandant seldom has evidence of its existence. If anything comes up in correspondence he settles the point at issue; if one reports the other verbally or by letter, the other always has a plausible reason to offer. It is simply impossible for one to make the other come to time, and reports are liable to cut both ways, like a two-edged sword, and are out of fashion.

A dry dock belongs to one department, also its operating power plant. The operation of it belongs to the second department, and if the engines and boilers become old, dilapidated, and uneconomical, needing to be repaired or replaced, the first department must obtain the appropriations and make the repairs, if it approves the changes; its uninterested opinion governs, and in the meantime the second department bears on its books the unwilling losses from uneconomical operation, sometimes for a period of years.

The most unnatural scope of bureau cognizance is exemplified in the modern floating dry dock which falls under the bureau bearing a similar name, due undoubtedly to the circumstance of a name inherited from the graving dock. The design and building of a floating dock belongs purely to naval architecture (and not to civil engineering); yet the Government fails to utilize its own naval architects in such work, but pays the premiums, going to the naval architects of civil industry.

$$*\quad*\quad*\quad*\quad*\quad*\quad*\quad*$$

Each department is not complete in itself, but may require another department to do work it can not perform. One having no foundry may make requisition for the one with foundry to make its castings. The first department must furnish the materials, while the other department does the work and transfers back the charges so the labor may be paid from the appropriations of the department having cognizance of the work. Thus the cost appears against the first department, whereas it really had no hand in controlling the amount, which may be exorbitant. This occurs constantly, and it is evident the total expense account of a department includes a portion made outside of its control and for whose excess it can not be responsible. Another feature is illustrated in the effect of shifting cognizance from one department to another. Once the Government decided to economize by centralizing the lighting plants into a single department. The result was the department that needed light on ship work was supplied with inadequate lights, the ancient practice of using candles grew to an unnecessary extent, and hundreds of men have stood many hours in the dark, glad at the opportunity for a rest. The authority shifting the lighting from the department that controlled its cost and operation for its own work could not have understood how its details were going to work out. With all power plants shifted and consolidated under one department as the bureaus are now adjusted, the operation and cost of power would be beyond the control of the department using it, but the cost would be charged against that department, which would be held responsible for it notwithstanding, since this cost must have been included in the estimates and appears on the books against it. Such reform as that is truly "straining at a gnat and swallowing a camel."

Another illustration of interdepartmental methods may be shown by the following example: An appropriation is made to build a ship and is apportioned at Washington between the three bureaus producing the hull, machinery, and equipment. The department building the hull must be responsible for its cost. Incidentally, the building slip and launching ways must be prepared. A fourth department, having no allotment, must drive the piles by virtue of its cognizance as determined in the Navy regulations. The hull department must require the piles to be driven by the fourth department, and the latter determines all features included in the cost. The pile-driving department answers to nobody for expense, being the supreme judge of all matters touching its technical duties, while the cost is transferred back to the hull department, who must answer for it, though having no command over it. This requires the hull department to detail an inspector to watch the pile department to determine whether the men charged to the work have actually been present and properly engaged on the work as paid for. No regular inspectors having been provided for such work, this inspection is delegated to someone who is most handy; but only on large work of importance can inspection be employed, for there is so much small work going on of a similar character that it is impossible to anticipate it or to check it up after it is done; for in some cases where such charges have been transferred it has been found that men so charged for a whole day may have been engaged on the work only an hour, or perhaps a few of them may only have handled some of the material in the shops or may have done nothing at all on the work. This result may be quite unintentional and due to the methods of preparing accounts; but I shall not descend into those minutiæ. A day never passes but what every department transfers accounts of work done for the other departments, and they are of such varied and irregular character that practically no one can be held responsible for their correctness, much less for the economy exercised in producing them. The same is true of work within the cognizance of one department which has not the shops to do it with and must request another department to do it, with the same transferring of accounts and uncertainty of costs.

Is this evidence enough, or shall other instances be cited? How should it be remedied?

Shall the commandant be vested with authority to violate the Navy regulations defining bureau cognizance, or shall he be permitted to violate the appropriation act and charge the work to the most convenient appropriations, to avoid the paper and other evils? If so, will someone venture to explain in what features will navy-yard administration be benefited thereby?

If not that, then how will a General Staff, composed of military administrators, line officers only, interposed between the present bureaus and the Secretary of the Navy, ameliorate the situation?

There is no possible solution other than consolidation.

At the moment of this writing, out of a yard force of 1,426 workmen at the yard I have in mind, 761 of them belong to the construction and repair department and 665 to all other departments combined. At all navy yards in full operation the construction and repair department force is usually greater than all the others combined, and always has been. The reason is because navy yards exist principally for the construction and repair of ships. To consolidate the whole is not far to go.

Consolidation would cure also the spasmodic economy evil: One department has no money to do absolutely necessary work, while another department can not find enough work to expend all its funds; one can obtain all the material it needs, another has to take what it can get; one can supply motors for all its power on shipboard, another can not afford generators to give the crew electric lights; one can supply ma-

hogany furniture for every need, another can not replace an article of
furniture that falls to pieces from old age; one is worked to the limit
of mental and bodily strain to reduce the costs, another rocks along
easily, waiting for the quitting bell to ring. One wastes what the other
saves.

One of the most expensive luxuries indulged in by the Government
is a haphazard administrator — a merely accomplished officer, whose
only necessity is to know enough to keep out of trouble, and perhaps,
after some experience, to accumulate enough data to engage in a controversy. He is putty in the hands of his foremen. A ship arrives to
be overhauled. The foremen make his estimates for him, and in so
doing they determine the limits of the estimates. Shall this work be
repaired or renewed? The foreman says it must be made new, with
suitable gestures. The foreman's judgment usually governs the totals
of the estimates. One who is not in a position to know better than his
foremen must retreat when the latter present arguments which he knows
not how to refute. Likewise the foremen determine the actual limits
of the work undertaken, which may overrun the estimates. Foremen
are from among the workmen, who are their friends and companions,
and it is but natural to look out for new work and hold fast to that in
hand. Otherwise it means discharges for the tradesmen, which is not
a popular idea among them. Usually when an old ship gets safely moored
alongside a navy yard for a general overhauling she may bid farewell
to the world until there is other work in sight.

One must know more than his foremen and have the will power of
his convictions in order to be able to limit the work to its proper amount
and cost, and he must be very energetic and diplomatic in exemplifying
his superiority by a vigorous line of action. When several hundred expensive mechanics are engaged on a single ship, at a cost of several hundred dollars a day, more money can be sunk in shorter time than in
any other way at a navy yard, especially if the workmen are holding
on to the job like grim death, with no other work in sight, with a figurehead in charge of the department. If the electric lights go out and the
men stand idle for an hour, that is of little consequence where the work
of repairs may be drawn out for several months without half trying.

Recently the captain of a ship forwarded to Washington a letter accompanied by a sample copy of each of the different bureaus' blank
forms for survey, his contention being that all these forms should be
reduced to a single one, applying to all bureaus alike. The stores belonging to one bureau must be included on a separate form supplied by
that bureau, and the bureaus' forms differ on account of the differences
of the methods and usages of the bureaus themselves. The consolidation of the bureaus handling material would reduce these forms to unity,
and thus ameliorate a number of kindred inconveniences.

Another evil which combination would cure is to be found in the prevention of improvements to shipboard machinery where such improvement would transfer its cognizance to another bureau. Thus, steam auxiliaries have refused, at times, for such a reason to give way to motors, long after the auxiliary steam engine stands discredited everywhere else. The limit of bureau cognizance influences and injures the design of a ship in various details, and stands in the way of many improvements.

Likewise, no one may encompass, and be responsible for, the design of a ship as a whole. The art of shipbuilding is amply provided for in point of quality of workmanship, for where a poor job of work occurs the person who did it can always be definitely located; but the science of shipbuilding has no connecting link provided to unit the interdependent functions governing the mobility of a ship. The speed, vibrations, coal consumption, radius of action, economy of power, water consumption, and horsepower of a ship depend upon three separate and interrelated things, viz., the model, the propeller, and the engines. On the model depend the speed, vibrations, wake coefficient, bow and stern waves, and horsepower. The functions of the propeller influence and depend upon the model, wake coefficient, speed, revolutions, slip, vibrations, depth of water, coal and water consumption, radius of action, indicated horsepower, and economy of operation. On the engines depend the speed, vibrations, horsepower, coal and water consumption, revolutions, radius of action, and economy of operation. The bureau that designs the hull has no "say" with respect to the propeller and engines, and the bureau that designs the latter has no say about the hull; so that no competent person is provided for, or permitted, by the Government to design these three component parts, or to adjust them to secure the best results, or to locate the errors in the completed vessel.

If a new ship fails to attain the desired speed, it may be due to the insufficient horsepower or inefficient propeller of one bureau, or to the lines of hull, foul bottom, displacement, trim, or lack of depth of water at trial of another bureau's consideration. If there are excessive vibrations it may be due to an unbalanced engine, an improperly designed propeller, or a wrong location of the engines with respect to the hull's nodes of vibration of one bureau's cognizance. If the vessel is uneconomical and has a large coal and water consumption and a small radius of action, it may be due to a foul bottom, wrong propeller, excessive steam consumption of engines, or inefficient boilers. There is no one in a position to locate the fault and denote whether it belong to one bureau or the other, nor is anyone in a position to profit by the experience and correct future designs. There is greater reason to combine the design of the whole ship under one head than to combine the two departments building it. A ship is too small to separate its design or its building under any but one head. It may have been necessary forty-two years ago when the shipwright knew nothing of steam or electricity and the separate professions had to be employed to obtain the whole, but at this epoch when a war ship has merged into a machinery plant where hull, engines, boilers, dynamos, and all the other fittings are formed into shape by the same or similar machinery from iron, steel, brass, and copper by the same class of mechanics, there no longer remains an excuse for unnatural subdivisions descended from the olden times. The whole field of the shipbuilding profession to-day is not more than a specialized branch of mechanical engineering — steam engines, boilers, electricity, and naval architecture. Not even so diversified as the mechanical engineering of commerce, which encompasses the broad field covered by the great variety and differences in machinery, plants, and methods employed in the private industries of the country, but merely the comparatively narrow field of mechanical engineering applying to a shipyard plant only, and the architecture of naval vessels and machinery only; merely the same profession now covered by the curriculum of a single school and encompassed by a single diploma. There is no real barrier to the achievement of modern methods in our tape-ridden navy yards.

XII

THE AMERICAN FOREIGN SERVICE

[The growth of the national interest on the part of the United States in Foreign affairs has been accompanied with a desire to improve our foreign service especially by making the consular and diplomatic service a more satisfactory and continuous career. This policy is discussed by Mr. Huntington Wilson, now third assistant secretary of state, and in the discussions between Mr. Root and certain senators in a committee hearing. The article by Judge Francis C. Lowell upon American diplomacy brings out the advantage which the United States has derived through being represented in foreign affairs by men who, while they had not passed through a continuous diplomatic career, were representative of their country in the sense of being personages of national reputation and importance.]

THE AMERICAN FOREIGN SERVICE [1]

By Huntington Wilson [2]

THERE is evident a growing sentiment among Americans in favor of reorganizing and improving the foreign service, diplomatic and consular, and placing it upon a stable basis. Indeed, this feeling has become so general and so strong that but for our extreme conservatism something would have been done in that direction before the present time.

The diplomatic service is the machinery by which the relations of our Government with other Governments are carried on. It is the spokesman of our policies in the council of the nations; the channel through which flows peace or war. It is the eyes and ears of our Government in our foreign affairs; and it is the every-day means of attending to our rights and obligations towards other Governments and peoples. A hermit nation needs no diplomacy; but once a nation abandons isolation, the efficiency of its diplomacy is a matter of serious concern to every citizen.

The consular service is the machinery for carrying on, improving, and increasing foreign commerce. First, there is an enormous amount of routine business. For all goods imported into the United States invoices must be authenticated at our consulates at the ports of export or places of original shipment. Consulates are the custodians of the

---

[1] From the *Outlook*, March 3, 1906. Reprinted by permission.
[2] Secretary of Legation of the United States at Tokyo.

ship's papers of American vessels while at ports within their districts. They discharge sailors, assist destitute or sick seamen, adjust difficulties between ship's captains and their crews, and generally extend the control of the home Government over the merchant marine in foreign ports. Marriages of Americans in foreign countries must be witnessed by the Consul. Deceased Americans' estates in foreign lands are, to a degree varying in different countries, under consular protection. Deeds, powers of attorney, protests, affidavits, patent applications, and other instruments executed abroad to be effective in the United States, are attested at the consulates. Such are the ordinary administrative and notarial consular duties. In those countries where extraterritoriality is in force the consular officers exercise a much wider administrative function. There the American Consular Court is the only forum in which an American can be pursued by civil or criminal law.

After giving some idea of the variety and responsibility of the consular function, we come to what is to-day the all-important object of that service. That is, the extension and increase of American business by opening up, widening, and developing fields for our export trade. A consular district generally comprises all that part of the country in which a given consulate is situated which is nearer to it than to any other American consulate. It is the duty of the consul to make a deep and special study of the industrial and mercantile conditions existing in his district. He must know what the country needs or would take in raw materials, in commodities, and in manufactured articles. He should learn how these needs are being supplied, with particular attention to those of them which the American producer — farmer, miner, manufacturer, or merchant — might supply. He should investigate and report as to whether the American import could not, by a change in form or a variation in manufacture, by a different method of packing, by more convenient accommodation in payment, or in any other way, be brought into greater demand and American trade be thus increased.

Each consular district may reveal a peculiar phase of the general import possibilities of a country. Hence, general reports are made by an official who looks over the field as a whole. These reports are made at consulates-general, and sometimes also at embassies and legations. Of course the capital of a country affords the best facilities for obtaining from official sources information bearing on trade. Also, in some countries government contracts are an important item in the competition for import orders. Therefore it may be wise for us, as some European Governments have done, to appoint commercial attachés to some of our embassies and legations.   ·

Our consular service, then, exists to facilitate and promote the material and personal interests of the American people in foreign countries. Our diplomatic service adds a care for these same interests to its duty to protect and further America's political interests in the world.

The Department of State is charged with the duty of making the diplomatic and consular services of the greatest possible use to the Government and people. It is not generally realized how large a number of officers the State Department has under it in the service abroad, nor how vast and varied is the volume of its business. It has a personnel smaller and more poorly paid than that of the Foreign Office of Great Britain; but, besides being the American Foreign Office, it has a number of other duties superadded. The Secretary of State is keeper of the seal of the United States. He publishes the Federal laws of the land. Contentious matters between foreigners and the State sovereignties of the Union at times give rise to questions between those governments and the governments of foreign countries. All these have to be settled by elaborate domestic correspondence between the State Department and the Governors of our States, other departments, and various officials. So that functions corresponding in other countries to such offices as Keeper of the Seal, Chancellor of the Empire, etc., devolve upon the one Department. What with our new colonial possessions, it seems likely that the scope of the State Department's work may before long be still further extended. Yet the Department of State has a very small personnel and very small appropriations. The wonder is how its handful of officials acquit themselves so well in grappling with so enormous a volume of business. Certainly high praise is due them.

The fact is that all three components of the foreign service, that is, the Department of State and the diplomatic and consular services under it, were founded long ago on a small scale, just after our emergence from colonial days. They can never catch up with the country's present needs unless the will of the people express itself through Congress in the form of the required legislation, and Congress take a deeper interest in the work of the foreign service.

This brings me to one of the most distressing difficulties of our system. I refer to the lack of any constituted channel of communication for keeping Congress and the foreign service in sympathetic touch and effective coöperation. In other countries this undoubted need is supplied by a parliamentary secretary; or the Minister for Foreign Affairs speaks on the floor of the House. With us there are the President's occasional messages. Congress sometimes calls for correspondence when some question has become acute. Or, suppose a Senator or a Representative or an official of the State Department to be greatly interested in a piece of legislation touching foreign affairs, or in a treaty to be negotiated; he may by personal effort have a number of conversations which will greatly help both the Senate or Congress and the Department. But there is no sufficiently continuous keeping in touch between the Senate, the House, their committees, and the State Department; and the matter is too important not to be thoroughly provided for. Why should not an Assistant Secretary of State be charged with this duty?

Because of the heterogeneity of its business and the numerical inadequacy of its personnel, the State Department has been irreverently compared to the former Chinese Tsungli-Yamen. Our diplomatic and consular services have been, with less irreverence and more truth, called the "catch-as-catch-can system." There is enough truth in this pessimism to suggest that there is much room for improvement, and that the time is ripe and the way open for framing and putting into operation an ideal foreign service.

The Department needs a larger personnel to do its great intellectual work, and a more logical division of work. At present, in the Diplomatic Bureau the countries of the earth are apportioned for working purposes alphabetically. Yet it cannot be said that a knowledge of Cuba and Costa Rica is particularly useful to the men who must study the intricacies of Chinese policy. The Diplomatic Bureau should be divided into sections on some politico-geographical basis of reason. Several new bureaus and sections should be added. And, as said before, some official should be charged with keeping the Department in touch with the whole Congress on legislation respecting foreign affairs, and with the Senate on treaty matters.

The reform of first necessity is the extinction of the "spoils system" in filling offices in the foreign service. Here civil service is absolutely indispensable; but the application of it requires very careful working out.

Inefficiency in the foreign service may be divided, according to cause, into two classes. The first is inefficiency due to lack of natural qualifications, to inadequate professional education, and to want of experience. These are the vices of our unsystematized service. The zeal of a man trying to do a difficult thing quite new to him is sometimes its saving grace. The second is inefficiency arising from apathy and indifference. This is the vice of a thoroughgoing, closed civil service. Our problem is how to get the natural qualifications, the special education, and the experience, and at the same time to inspire zeal in the service.

Examinations will insure the special knowledge, a permanent service will supply the experience, promotion for meritorious work will secure the zeal. How are we to obtain the best men? Every college man knows that the men who pass the highest examinations are by no means always the ablest men in the class. Especially in diplomacy, a number of very intangible qualities are wanted. Tact, address, quick perception, an analytical mind, balance, and self-control are some of the natural qualities a good diplomatist has. These should therefore be sought in the young candidates for the service, and obviously they can not be detected by a written examination.

A famous Russian Minister for Foreign Affairs emphasized the indubitable importance of this personal element. It was his custom to have all the candidates who had successfully passed the diplomatic service examination call upon him next day. He then selected from among them the candidates to put into the service; and he is recorded as saying that his decision was based rather upon the impression each candidate personally made on him during the call than upon the relative merits of their examination papers.

Why should not the Secretary of State, perhaps assisted by a small board, select from among the successful candidates those to be put into the service after the examinations each year — the choice to be made after an informal and verbal examination of the men who had successfully passed the main written one?

Now that the days of the telegraph have made the envoy rather his Government's spokesman and advocate than its plenipotentiary statesman, some people too greatly minimize his duties. Surely it behooves us, as a practical people, to have for our Government the best possible spokesmen and advocates. In private life his personal abilities leave one advocate in the law to starve, while another's bring him a huge income. Success or failure in the Government's foreign affairs depends enormously — much more than people realize — upon the skill or the bungling of the Government's advocates abroad. And these are its diplomatic representatives.

For efficiency in a consular officer the personal factor presents somewhat fewer difficulties, yet it is questionable whether an examination should be the sole criterion for the admission of men eligible to all grades. Although the two services have a number of things in common, and what is true of the one is often to some extent true of the other, what next follows applies particularly to the diplomatic branch.

A charge which may be brought against an organized foreign service in which men spend their lives, except for occasional leaves of absence in going from post to post in foreign countries, is that they sometimes lose touch with the ideas of their own country. They are too long away from home. There is, however, a ready means of removing this danger.

The successful candidates for the service should first pass a year or more as clerks in the State Department, learning, from the big end, the practical work of their profession. These young men would be distributed in the bureaus and sections where the work would teach them most about their future duties, whether consular or diplomatic, and would be required to familiarize themselves with the general work of the Department.

Next, these clerks would be sent abroad to serve as attachés at embassies or legations, or as clerks in consulates, this depending upon which service they had been examined for and entered. Later, they would be transferred from one post to another, and, if they did good work, gradually promoted. In their respective services they would become third secretaries of embassy or legation, second secretaries, secretaries, and so on; and, in the consular service, higher grades of clerks, consular agents, vice and deputy consuls, consuls, consuls-general.

In connection with the regular diplomatic and consular service examinations there should be examinations for positions as student interpreters. A few years ago student interpreters were attached to our legation at Peking, and that was an admirable innovation. It should be extended, however, at least to our legation in Japan, and perhaps also to that in Turkey. The written language is practically the same in China, Japan, and Korea. These student interpreters, after an apprenticeship in the State Department, would be sent out and attached to the legations in the Far East. There they would spend several years in mastering the difficulties of the Oriental languages. After that they would be prepared to join the staffs of the consulates in China, Japan, and Korea as clerks, and so enter on a career in the Oriental consular service. The interpreters of our legations and their assistants would also be drawn from this body.

Now we come to the above-mentioned safeguard against a tendency to what may be loosely called expatriation. The plan which follows is most of all desirable because of the great benefits it carries with it.

It is difficult to gainsay that a man can do better work in the service abroad if he has first served in the Department at Washington. It also seems evident that it would be useful to have in the Department men who had made recent special studies of the political and trade conditions in various foreign countries. The suggestion, then, is that a mobility and interchange of posts be established, to a certain extent, between the Department of State and the diplomatic service, and perhaps also, in certain bureaus and sections, between the Department and the consular service. A parity of grade could be fixed between the posts in the Department and the posts abroad. For example, the different grades of clerks, the chiefs of section, the chiefs of bureau, and the assistant secretaries might correspond to attachés, to grades of secretaries of embassy or legation, to ministers resident, and to ministers plenipotentiary. A limited shifting between the two ends of the service could be ordered from time to time by the Secretary of State. Among other things, this system would give to the heads of the service a more intimate knowledge of the abilities of their personnel; and it is safe to say that in the long run it would be of great use to the Department and benefit to the diplomatic service.

Fairly frequent shifting between posts abroad is also desirable, and transfers should as far as possible invariably accompany promotions. For considerations which, if somewhat abstruse, are none the less cogent, it is best that a secretary should be transferred when promoted rather than be promoted to be minister at the same post. The two official characters of minister and secretary, and the subtle relations attaching to them, are different. Each position occupies a certain place in the mind of the local official circle; and these associations are not to be suddenly thrown off or assumed. An important reason why three or four years is generally long enough to leave a man at the same post is that he almost inevitably becomes somewhat "stale." His observation becomes less keen. Also, at difficult posts an energetic representative is not unlikely to wear out his welcome, and so lose much of his usefulness. Furthermore, frequent transfer gives wider experience and so increases efficiency. With this system each official would be commissioned by the President in a particular grade, and the Secretary of State would designate, from time to time, the post he should fill. From every point of view, a more mobile diplomatic service, including limited interchange to the State Department, has much to recommend it.

A closed service, in which a man has only to live in order to be steadily promoted and finally retired with a pension, tends to induce apathy. What we want is a service in which every man who gives his best years and energies to the work will be sure of a life career, and, at the end of his career, a pension. Only those who do signally fine work should expect to be rewarded with ultimate promotion to the highest grades. In this way justice is meted to faithful service and a reward is in store for brilliant service.

The best pension system would probably be to make retirement optional after, say, twenty-five years' service, with a pension computed on the salary of the grade from which the officer retired. The pension could be increased proportionally to the excess of the period of service rendered over twenty-five years. In private life it is deemed a hard lot when a man who has given the best twenty-five or thirty years of his life to a business or profession can not have accumulated enough to support him during his declining years. And if the foreign service is to have the good men it needs, their livelihood must not be made too precarious.

Nor would it be necessary to have an absolutely closed service. There is every reason why, with an organized service, the President should still have the power to appoint an ambassador or minister from outside the diplomatic service. The preëminent talents and conspicuous fitness of some countryman of ours, or the special nature of some mission to be carried out, may at times point unmistakably to such a selection.

Our ambassadors and ministers receive relatively small pay and no allowances worth mentioning, and are not provided with houses. Their colleagues representing other Powers receive generally better pay, besides funds for the costly and necessary outlays for "representation," and permanent buildings owned by their governments, in which to reside during their missions. Every truly democratic American should be shocked to realize that, because of our penury in this matter, only very rich men can possibly uphold the dignity of the United States at certain capitals. The very undemocratic result is that men of moderate fortune, however talented, can not be appointed to, nor could they afford to accept, those posts.

American travelers are constantly chagrined to find their legations and

In connection
nations there s
A few years a
Peking, and th
however, at lea
Turkey. The
and Korea. T
State Department
the Far East.
difficulties of t
pared to join t
as clerks, and
interpreters o
from this br

Now we
to what may
is most of all

It is difficult
abroad if he ha
seems evident th
who had made
in various fore
and interchang
Department of
certain bureaus
service. A part
partment and th
clerks, the chiefs
taries might corr
or legation,
limited shif
from time t
system wou
edge of the abilit
long run it woul
diplomatic servic
Fairly frequent
transfers should
For consideration
it is best that a s
than be promoted
characters of min
to them, are diffe
mind of the local
denly thrown off

HEARING ON THE REORG
ONSULAR SERVICE, 1906

reorganization which is
bill includes, first, the classification
the assignment of the members of the
accordance with their present positio

the salary, and the existing coditions of their present
ιuthority to the President to traɪfer these graded officers
.ion to another according to the ɪierests of the service.
ΛCON. The promotion then rɪuires a separate confir-

ↄooт. Yes; it provides for origɪal appointments only to
ιdes upon examination. An exɪination would be by a
sed of the Chief of the ◼◼◼ɪu, an officer of the
◼ ɪ chief examiner
ervice d by the Com-

ↄrsons as

ɪir

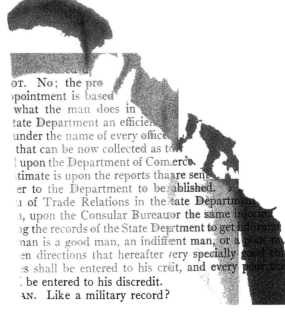

ↄт. No; the prↄ
ↄpointment is based
what the man does in
tate Department an efficiɪ
under the name of every offiɪ
that can be now collected as tↄ
l upon the Department of Comɪercↄ
ːtimate is upon the reports thaɪre senɪ
er to the Department to beɪblished.
ι of Trade Relations in theɪate Departmɪ
ι, upon the Consular Bureauↄr the same iɪ
ɪg the records of the State Deɪrtment to getɪ
nan is a good man, an indifɪent man, or a
en directions that hereafter ɪery speciallyɪ
ɪs shall be entered to his crɪit, and everyɪ
ɪ be entered to his discredit.
ΛN. Like a military record?

consulates abroad housed in a haphazard manner, comparing very unfavorably with those of other countries. Our Government owns legation
buildings only at Tokyo, Peking, Seoul, and Bangkok. The ownership of these was practically forced upon us by the peculiar conditions
existing in those countries. Similarly, we possess a few rather inferior
consular premises. Let us see what other countries do — countries
which place importance on foreign policy and its corollary, foreign commerce, as, for example, Germany and Great Britain. In every capital,
in every port or commercial center, they aim to have the eye met by an
embassy or legation or a consulate — substantial, permanent, and architecturally good — which stands in a foreign land as a reminder of the
dignity, the strength, and the enterprise of the country whose flag flies
over it. And then one finds (if, indeed, one can succeed in finding them)
the American embassy or legation, shabby or creditable, according to
the purse and generosity of the representative, and the consulate sometimes a dusty second floor in some back street. Is this what the American
people want?

I have outlined a number of points for a reorganization which I
believe would be entirely practical and feasible, and would vastly ameliorate the service. There are many minor reforms which can hardly be
taken up with any enthusiasm while the service is left in its present
unsettled condition.

A number of Senators and Representatives have done hard work and
have introduced bills which it was hoped would place the service on a
sound footing. But the ideal foreign service for which the way is now
open needs for its accomplishment the support of an active, not passive,
public opinion; and it needs the coöperation of the Senators and Representatives interested with the President and the Secretary of State,
and with some of those who have studied the service from within. The
foreign services of all countries must be studied and examined. What
is good must be adopted, or what is better must be devised. Then will a
bill be framed and passed which will give us the efficient foreign service
that a great commercial world power like the United States has the right
and the obligation to possess.

FROM A SENATE HEARING ON THE REORGANIZA-
TION OF CONSULAR SERVICE, 1906 [1]

SECRETARY ROOT. The scheme of reorganization which is embodied
in the first 11 sections of the bill includes, first, the classification of the
consular officers in grade, the assignment of the members of the present
force to those grades in accordance with their present positions, the

[1] Senate Report No. 112, 59th Congr., 1 Session.

importance, the salary, and the existing conditions of their present offices, and authority to the President to transfer these graded officers from one station to another according to the interests of the service.

Senator BACON. The promotion then requires a separate confirmation?

Secretary ROOT. Yes; it provides for original appointments only to the lower grades upon examination. An examination would be by a board composed of the Chief of the Consular Bureau, an officer of the State Department designated by the President, and the chief examiner of the Civil Service Commission or other person designated by the Commission — practically such examiner as they designate.

Senator LODGE. The examination is not competitive.

Secretary ROOT. No; the examination is to be of such persons as the President designates for examination.

Senator LODGE. Like the Marine Corps to-day?

Secretary ROOT. Yes, and the Army; the board to accompany their report of the list of those who pass the examination with a detailed statement of the reasons for their report and of the qualifications shown by the examination. The reorganization contemplates that the appointments made to the higher grades shall be by promotion — that is to say, the original appointments to be only to the lower grade, and the appointments to the higher grades to be by promotion from the lower grade.

Senator BACON. Pardon an inquiry right there, Mr. Secretary. In section 2 you speak of the number of consuls-general of the first class, then consuls-general of the second class, etc. Do I understand that there can be no original appointments to those positions?

Secretary ROOT. No; it is all by promotion.

Senator MORGAN. Based upon examination?

Secretary ROOT. No; the promotion is not based upon examination. The original appointment is based upon examination. The promotion is based upon what the man does in the service. We have already started in the State Department an efficiency record, under which there will be entered, under the name of every officer in the consular service, all the information that can be now collected as to what sort of an officer he is. I have called upon the Department of Commerce and Labor to inform me what their estimate is upon the reports that are sent in by the consuls and are sent over to the Department to be published. I have called upon the Bureau of Trade Relations in the State Department for the same information, upon the Consular Bureau for the same information, and I am searching the records of the State Department to get information as to whether a man is a good man, an indifferent man, or a poor man. Then I have given directions that hereafter every specially good thing that a consul does shall be entered to his credit, and every poor thing that he does shall be entered to his discredit.

Senator MORGAN. Like a military record?

Secretary ROOT. Yes. I am practically applying experience that I gained in the War Department in regard to the efficiency records of officers.

The two things to be gained by the classification and confining the appointments to a lower grade and filling the upper ones by promotion are, first, that it will enable the President to assign the officers to stations in accordance with the interests of the service. We have now a great many square pegs in round holes and round pegs in square holes. There are men in the service whose health is suffering and whose families' health is suffering, and they are holding on because there is no way to get out except to leave the service. There are men in places for which their peculiar faculties are not fitted, but they are holding on instead of being put in places where they could do far better work, because there is no way of remedying that situation except for them to get out of the service or turn somebody else out and reappoint them. I can not see any reason why they should not be assigned as the service requires, just as an army officer is assigned.

Senator MORGAN. Anywhere in the world?

Secretary ROOT. Anywhere. There is one man now, a gentleman Senator Cullom spoke to me about some time ago, who is consul in China, a most excellent man. I do not believe he is going to be able to stay at the place where he is. I think considerations of health will make it impossible. He has to go out of the service unless somebody else is turned out who perhaps ought not to be turned out, and this gentleman's name sent to the Senate upon an entirely new original appointment for another place. It is very difficult to find such a place, too, because you have either got to punish him because his health and his family's health will not stand the place where he is, by putting him in a place with a lower salary, or reward him for it, by putting him in a place with a higher salary, unless you can find one with just the same salary. There are many men who could do much better work in much better places, and we can not move them.

Senator BACON. The question as to the advisability of introducing this elastic feature into the service is somewhat different from the question which arises upon this classification in the matter of promotions.

Secretary ROOT. I was coming to that. That is the second advantage to be gained by classification, that it makes possible the filling of higher grades by promotion and confining the appointments to the lower grades. Now, it is not possible to have the best service from men who are hopeless of receiving any recognition of the best service. It is a fact that now it makes very little difference whether a consul does well or ill. He may be in a lower station, doing the highest kind of work, and a vacancy may occur in a better place in the very country where he is, and he expects nothing else but that somebody from home here will be shoved in over his head. He is away — "out of sight, out or mind." He is doing excellent service, but there is no recognition of it whatever, and there is no way of recognizing it unless we can have some established system under which the higher places shall be filled by promotion. That would give an incentive to good work. It would make it possible to recognize good work, and it would get us out of the rut that we are in, of having the consular service as an opportunity for retirement of gentlemen who have to be provided for because they have failed in life here.

Senator MONEY. I was going to ask a question along that line. There is nothing in the present system, is there, to prevent the recognition of a man who makes a splendid record? Why can he not be appointed, directly on your recommendation to the President, to this vacancy which occurs over him? There is no use of rushing anyone from here over there when he is on the ground and you know what he has done. You have his splendid record there before you.

Secretary ROOT. Senator, it is a long-established practice, and it is a practice which it will be exceedingly difficult to change without the consent of the Senate. The Senate is a part of the appointing power. The practice of making such appointments has continued ever since I have known anything about public life. It is embedded in the procedure of our Government, and I apprehend that if the President were to undertake now alone, by himself, to make an entire change in that matter, and were to say, "I will appoint no more citizens of the various States of consequence or importance whose interests are pressed by Senators and Representatives," without first having the approval of the Senate for the change, it would be regarded as revolutionary and would create ill feeling, and it would be an exceedingly difficult resolution to adhere to. I want you to say that that is the thing that ought to be done, and if it is the thing that ought to be done, it seems to me that, as a part of the appointing power, you ought to give it your approval; and if you approve this bill you do give that approval.

Senator BACON. Mr. Secretary, I recognize the force of what you say as to the value of the hope of promotion as an incentive to industry and good conduct, and possibly, within certain limitations, that principle could be advantageously applied. The thought in my mind, though, is as to the limitation of the appointment of these highest offices to those who are already in the service and having those offices filled by promotion. It is altogether possible that a man most eminently qualified for one of these highest consul-generalships may not have been in the consular service. Take, as an illustration, the case of Mr. Wynne, who is now consul-general at London. Under the proposed system he would not be eligible to that position. There is another case which is probably a little more marked in its application to this suggestion — the case of a man who was for a long time consul at Habana. I do not know whether he had the rank of consul-general or not.

Senator LODGE. Yes; he was consul-general.

Senator BACON. He was also highly esteemed by the commercial interests of the country. I assume he has gone out of the service and is possibly now beyond the age when he would be eligible; but, for illustration, suppose in the mutations of political fortune he had lost that place and an incoming Administration desired to reappoint him to a place where he had shown by his experience and his performances that he was eminently qualified for the place, his services could not be availed of. I recollect that I once went to see Mr. Cleveland, during his Administration, in the interest of a gentleman whom I thought would make a good consul-general at Habana. Williams had been appointed by a Republican President. Mr. Cleveland said to me that Williams was too valuable to be displaced, that a matter of politics could not be considered, and he must be retained because of the great interests of the country which were conserved by his retention.

I just gave that as an illustration, and what I say is more in the line of suggestion than argument. I do not wish you to understand me as taking issue with you upon that feature of the bill, but I think it is a matter of sufficient importance for consideration, whether this elastic feature might not of advantage be confined to some of the lower positions, or at least not extended to the higher positions.

I think it is frequently the case that men who make the most excellent subordinates makes very inefficient and poor principals. There have been a great many good colonels spoiled by being made generals.

Secretary ROOT. That is quite true, but it would be difficult to find a situation less open to that difficulty than this. That is very often the case in the Army and Navy. You will find that a good enlisted man often makes a poor lieutenant, and a good subaltern officer is very poor when he comes to be made a general officer; but here every consul has an independent command. The lowest-grade consul is an independent officer, and he is performing the same kind of duties that the highest consul-general is performing, and you have an opportunity to judge by the way he performs the duties of the lower-grade office how he would perform the duties of the high office.

Indeed, it is frequently the case that the lower-grade offices are the most difficult offices; but they are of the lower grade and lower salaries, because, while the duties may be much more difficult than those of the higher grade, they are less important. I do not know anything more difficult than the position of our consuls in some of the Central and South American countries, particularly consuls in countries where we have no resident minister. Some of them exhibit great ability, but they are low-grade consulates.

Senator LODGE. Your theory would be that by the time you got to the high grade of consul-general, you would have your men so thoroughly sifted out that you could not very well go wrong in getting a competent man?

Secretary ROOT. My idea is, that with the number we have of low-grade consuls — and the great bulk of these consuls are low-grade consuls — there is the best possible opportunity of determining whether a man is to hold one of the highest positions.

With regard to the Williams illustration, there would be no difficulty in framing this bill so that a reappointment could be made without going through the grades. It would be quite appropriate. That would cover the case like the one of Williams, going out and then being put back.

Senator LODGE. Going out from any cause?

Secretary ROOT. Yes; from any cause. If a man has once been in the service, I see no reason why he should not be treated, for the purpose of reappointment, just as a man who is in the service now for purposes of reassignment.

Senator CULLOM. His qualifications being already proven.

Secretary ROOT. Being already proven.

Senator MONEY. I do not recollect whether you said confirmations are necessary upon these promotions or not.

Secretary ROOT. Yes, sir.

Senator MONEY. Confirmations are necessary, just as in the case of an original appointment?

Secretary ROOT. Yes.

Then, as to the other illustration. Such an arrangement would have cut Mr. Wynne out, but I feel pretty confident on the general proposition that you would gain much more than you would lose. You would lose some good men, but you would gain by barring a great many men who are not good men. As a rule, I think it is safe to say that a man who has passed the age of the youngest of us at this table has become too old to learn new tricks.

Senator FRYE. He ought to be chloroformed?

Secretary ROOT. No; far from it. But he ought not to undertake an entirely new business and enter upon an entirely new field of action. There may be exceptional men who could, but the exceptions would be so few that, as a general proposition, in the interest of the service, men who have lived through the greater part of their lives ought not to be taken into the new field. The Government will have better service if it picks men comparatively young, who still have enthusiasm, energy, ambition, and the power of making a career, and lets them learn the consular business then, instead of taking men who have lived through the greater part of their lives and who have reached the time when they rather want rest.

Senator BACON. Mr. Secretary, what is the term of office proposed in this bill? Are they life appointments?

Secretary ROOT. There is no time fixed. It is left just as it is now.

Senator MORGAN. During good behavior.

Senator LODGE. It is not changed.

Senator BACON. I understand; but, then, the new system, if adopted, would raise some question on that subject. For instance, as it is now, when an administration changes it is perfectly competent and rather recognized as a rule that all of the consuls except such as those in the class to which Mr. Williams belonged should go out and the representatives of the other party come in.

Senator LODGE. That has been the great misfortune of the service.

Senator BACON. Under this you say there is no change. The right of the President to reappoint would be the same as now, but the original appointment could only be to the lowest grade. In other words, he could only displace the lowest grade.

Secretary ROOT. He could displace anybody he chose, filling his place by promotion and making vacancies in the lower grades.

Senator BACON. What I mean is this: He could not appoint a man to any position except the lowest grade.

Senator LODGE. Of course, constitutionally, he can disregard the law altogether.

Senator BACON. I am not so sure of that.

Senator LODGE. Consuls are specifically expressed in the Constitution, and we can not limit or restrict his right of appointment.

Senator BACON. You might say the same thing of an officer in the Army. I am not so sure about that.

Senator FORAKER. It would be better for the two Departments to work in harmony, especially when it comes to a matter of appropriations.

Senator BACON. Yes. I am asking that question simply for the purpose of seeing what the practical working of it will be. For instance, without any change of administration, the President could, of course, remove anyone from any grade; but then when he removes a man he can only fill the lowest place, and if there were a change in administration the same rule would hold good.

Senator LODGE. I would ask the Secretary if it is not the point of the law to give to the service greater stability, and whether that is not what it needs more than anything else.

Senator BACON. I think that, within bounds, is a very desirable thing.

Secretary ROOT. That does produce this effect, Senator. It takes away the opportunity to turn a given man out for the purpose of putting another given man in his place. I think that ought to be taken away. It leaves the opportunity to turn out a given man because he is not doing good work, thereby creating a vacancy in the lower grade which can be filled by somebody else. It leaves it still possible, in case of a change of administration, to effect a gradual substitution of men of one party for men of another party, but it makes it a little more difficult, which, I suppose, is about all that can be done. It takes the element of personal pressure out of it.

*   *   *   *   *   *   *   *

Secretary ROOT. I have written into the bill a few words which seem to me to accomplish the object that seemed to me to be the first impressions of the committee in regard to taking the consular service out of political limitations.

In section 8, on page 4 of the bill, insert, after the word "shall," in line 15, the words "without regard to their political affiliations."

Senator FORAKER. What precedes it?

Secretary ROOT. I will read the whole. Section 8 would then read:

That it shall be the duty of said board —

That is, the examination board —

to formulate rules for and hold examinations of applicants for admission to the consular service; and whenever a vacancy shall occur in the sixth or seventh class of consuls which the President deems it expedient to fill, the Secretary of State shall require the said board to examine such applicants as shall, without regard to their political affiliations, be designated therefor by the President.

Senator BACON. Mr. Secretary, is that sufficient? If you are going to take this out of politics, is it not necessary to do in that case as we do in some other instances where it is expressly provided that the offices shall be filled in certain proportions between the political parties?

Senator LODGE. That is where we fill boards. I do not think you could take an appointive service and do that.

Senator BACON. Pardon me a minute. In the civil service that is not necessary because it is competitive and any man is eligible to make the effort; but where the designation is exclusive, where no man can be eligible for examination unless he has the designation, it is quite different, and while it would possibly not be proper to say that they should be filled in the exact proportions that we provide for in the case of boards, it could be said that they shall be filled as nearly as practicable with an equal division between the parties, and I think also something ought to be said to desectionalize it.

Senator LODGE. That is going to be covered by the registered quota.

Secretary ROOT. I would say that it was desirable, with regard to that, to accomplish the object — it is only a suggestion; I am not bigoted about it — to employ a certain reserve in language in dealing with the exercise of the President's power to appoint consuls, which is specifically vested in him by the Constitution. I drafted it first with the statement "it shall be," and that grated a little in the treatment by Congress of the President's constitutional power, and it seemed to me that language a little more reserved, which really did establish a rule morally binding upon the President, was rather more to be desired.

Senator BACON. You could still regard that consideration and at the same time effect the purpose, which is to apply that moral obligation without a strict legal necessity to distribute them as nearly as possible equally between the opposing political parties; and this further is to be said, that while this might be construed or considered an attempt at limitation upon the constitutional authority of the President, it is not to be overlooked that this bill proposes to confer upon him very much enlarged powers, and to put, in the administration of the consular service, very much larger discretion and control in the hands of the President, really taking it out almost entirely from the legislative control.

So long as this statute remains upon the books, the only participation of Congress would be in the part of Congress which we represent in the confirmation or rejection of the nominees. Outside of that the service would be absolutely removed from all legislative control except the control which would still remain of the right and power to amend and change the law.

So that when we consider the question whether the suggestion would be an encroachment upon the executive constitutional power, there is to be taken into consideration the fact that it is a very great enlargement in other respects, and while you could not say it was a quid pro quo, the enlarged power which would be conferred by this would remove, I think, any possible suggestion that the effort was to limit the power of the President.

I can not entirely overlook in this consideration the fact that our system of government is very different from that of the English. The English put large powers in the hands of the executive. They are really putting them in the hands of the legislative department of the government, because the executive powers are exercised by the legislative branch.

Secretary ROOT. By a committee of the House of Commons.

Senator BACON. It is a very different thing here. The tendency here is exactly the other way, that the executive begins to control the legislative. People now, when they want legislation which will affect certain things, do not come to Senators and Representatives as formerly, but go to the White House and the Departments. I see they are even now going to the Bureau of Insular Affairs to get legislation about the Philippines. They are ignoring my friend on the other side of the table, the chairman of the Committee on the Philippines, and going to Edwards.

Senator McCREARY. I think Senator Bacon has raised the point that is of vital importance in this bill. I like the general provisions of the bill. I have felt and known for a long time that the consular service needed reorganizing. My experience with it was not encouraging at all. It needs reorganization very badly, and there are many things in this bill

I like very much; but the great obstacle, to me, has been that this bill of course seeks to put in for life certain men. If there is no provision in the bill such as is suggested by the Senator from Georgia, the probabilities are that pretty much all the people that would be put in would belong to one political party. The consular service is a great service. It seeks to accomplish great ends and good ends, and I think it ought to be just as nearly nonpolitical as possible.

Our Government, as the Senator stated, is different from the Government of Great Britain and from most of the other governments in Europe. Ours is a popular Government. While one party is in power to-day, another party may come into power by and by, and that party, if it should come into power, would of course find men in the service, unless we have something like that suggested by the Senator from Georgia, all differing, or most of them differing; and we ought to have in this bill some kind of provision which would necessitate, which would cause a division, so that each political party should have representation. I am not sure that I would contend for as much as Senator Bacon contends, that they should be equally divided, but there ought to be in the first place a distribution of the consuls among the States.

Secretary ROOT. In endeavoring to meet the suggestion on another point, I have drawn this clause in order to get something on paper for consideration:

So far as practicable, and except as the President shall otherwise determine in particular cases, the designation of candidates for examination shall be made in such manner as most effectively to distribute the appointments among the several States and Territories in proportion of their representation in Congress.

And such designation shall in all cases be made without regard to the political affiliations of the candidates.

I, naturally enough, had in mind the practice in army appointments, and I think it is worth your while to consider the experience which we have had in that regard. I do not think it is too much to say that we have taken the Army out of politics. I do not think, during the last years that I was in the War Department, that the Democratic Senators had any feeling that when there was a question of an appointment to the Army there was any difference between a Democrat and a Republican. I think I had the confidence of Senator Cockrell just as completely as I had the confidence of any Republican member of the Committee on Military Affairs, and that feature of it made no difference. The State of Virginia led in the number of appointments to the Army, and it led because it had the Virginia Military Institute, which has turned out a great number of very fine, able young fellows.

Senator BACON. I think there has always been a general feeling — I know I have had it — that there is a distinction between appointments in the military service and appointments in the civil service. I never asked for the appointment of anybody in the civil service. I have not hesitated to ask it in the military service. I thought they stood on different platforms altogether, and I think the Spanish war, which put so many of these young men in the line of appointment, had very much the effect that you have just stated, of breaking down anything like political distinctions in your appointments. Whether or not that could be accomplished in the consular service, which is more a matter of dollars and cents, is another question. Army appointments are not matters of revenue or income. They are on a different line altogether.

Secretary ROOT. It seems to me, Senator, that there is no branch of the service in which that rule ought to be applied more clearly than to the consular service. Under the present system I found the clerks in the State Department were keeping tab on appointments with reference to percentage of Republican vote. I think it is all wrong. It is a violation of the theory on which the Senate is expected to act in regard to appointments and in regard to foreign affairs generally. The President comes to the Senate for its advice without distinction of party. You vote on treaties, and you are not expected to vote in accordance with the distinction of party. That principle is intended by the Constitution to pervade the treatment of foreign affairs, because in foreign affairs every man who is sent abroad is representing the country, and the good name and credit of the country depend upon his being a creditable representative. It seems to me if there is any place where the distinction of party ought to be dropped it is when we pass beyond the confines of our country.

Senator BACON. Yet that is not so in practice.

Secretary ROOT. I know it is not so in practice, and I would like to see the practice changed.

Senator FRYE. Do you think you could put into a bill of this kind a provision that the appointments hereafter made in the consular service should be divided between the two political parties?

Secretary ROOT. I do not. I think that would be a bad provision.

Senator BACON. You say they should be designated without regard to political affiliations.

Secretary ROOT. Yes; I think that is right.

Senator BACON. And while the policy might make a difference, the principle is the same.

Secretary ROOT. One is excluding political considerations and the other is including political considerations. One is declaring what I believe to be the sound principle, that the question of party affiliations should not determine in the selection of a representative who is to represent us abroad, and the other is compelling the President to take into consideration party affiliations and compelling him to inquire whether a young man is a Democrat or a Republican before he determines in regard to the selection.

Senator BACON. He will always know that.

Secretary ROOT. No.

Senator MORGAN. That is just the difference between the two situations. I think the Secretary is right about it.

Secretary ROOT. I give you my word that in the four years and a half I was in the War Department there was never such a question asked — whether the young man was a Democrat or Republican.

Senator BACON. That is true in the military service.

Secretary ROOT. Well, it ought to be true of the consular service.

If you provide that the designations for examination in the consular service shall be made without regard to political affiliations, you have then established the same rule which is applied in the Army, and it seems to me the same result will follow, that it will stop inquiry, and necessarily that excludes the right of referees and chairmen of political committees to propose candidates and insist that they are entitled to have their recommendation taken for their section of the country. It causes the method of appointment to revert to the authorized representatives of the different States for advice, the men elected by the different States to represent them, no matter whether those representatives belong to one party or another party. It seems to me it is much better to put it in that shape.

Senator LODGE. The other way is forcing politics into it, it seems to me.

Senator McCREARY. I think when you use the words "without regard to party affiliations," that is a long step in the way of improvement over what we have had for so many years in both political parties. I am very glad you put that in. I know it would be a very great change to say now we should have half, and therefore I think the proposition made by the Secretary is a good step.

Senator BACON. I did not propose that such definite language as "one-half" should be used. The language I would suggest would be simply to the effect that they should be as nearly as may be equally divided; something of that sort.

Senator CLARK, of Montana. This relates to the examination, however, and not to the appointment.

Senator FORAKER. You could say that not more than one-half should be appointed from any one party.

Senator CLARK, of Montana. That would cover it.

Senator CLARK, of Wyoming. It seems to me, Senator Foraker, that would be unfortunate in view of the Secretary's statement, which I think is the proper one, that it should be taken out of politics instead of forced in.

Senator FRYE. I do not think anything of the kind ought to be in the bill at all.

Senator MORGAN. I agree with the chairman of the committee on that proposition. There never ought to be any active legislation by Congress. There should never be any reference to it at all. It is a matter about which the Executive has the right to determine for himself in making his selections for office, and I made the suggestion the other day with the view of trying to meet the difficulty in this committee, and with the hope that we would go before the Senate with a unanimous agreement that we could stand by on that very unsatisfactory and unfortunate proposition.

Secretary ROOT. I marked a month ago on a list of applicants an applicant from Georgia for appointment. I found that he had letters from Senator Clay, among others. I made a note, to send to Senator Clay when he got to Washington for further information about him. I do not want to inquire whether that young man is a Democrat or a Republican. I think the rule that he shall be considered without regard to his political affiliations is the true rule to apply to him, and I think Senator Clay, who has written a letter about him, is the proper person to apply to, and a statement that the appointment shall be made without regard to any political affiliations precludes any political committee or referee in the State of Georgia saying anything about him.

Senator FORAKER. I think that is a very good expression to use. If you were to undertake to describe the number beyond which any one party should not have representation, would not that raise a constitutional query as to whether or not we have power to restrict the President's selections to any particular class.

Senator BACON. You might say the same thing as to his appointment of an Interstate Commerce Commissioner.

Senator LODGE. No; the Interstate Commerce Commissioner is not provided for specifically in the Constitution.

Senator BACON. But he is a constitutional officer.

Senator LODGE. But in creating that office we can throw around it any conditions we choose.

Senator BACON. No; not so as to limit the power of the President where the Constitution says he shall have the power to nominate all officers.

Senator LODGE. He can not have it when we create it in that way.

Senator BACON. It is not simply those named in the Constitution. If you are correct, the numbers named in the Constitution are very few as compared with the vast number created by Congress, and if your theory is correct it would absolutely limit the power of the President to the appointment of few officers.

Secretary ROOT. Let me say that since the last meeting of the committee I have consulted the President specially on this subject, and he instructs me to say that he very heartily agrees with the idea of taking these appointments out of politics, of having them made without regard to political affiliations, and would be quite ready to accept such a provision.

There is only one further thing I want to say about this now, and that is that the agitation of this subject has been going on for many years. I have found ten favorable reports from committees of the Senate and House of bills to reorganize the consular service, and among them I have here a report made to this committee by Senator Morgan ten years ago, characterized by the thoroughness which is to be found in everything that Senator Morgan does, in which are laid down the main principles embodied in this bill, approved by this committee. In the meantime, the agitation has gone on in the country.

Now, there are many things agitated fictitiously. The mere fact that somebody comes here and is anxious to have some change of the law does not necessarily indicate that it ought to be made. Those agitations which are without substance die away. Those which have substance remain and grow. This has remained and it has grown, and we have communications from over three hundred commercial and business bodies scattered all over the country urging that something be done. It seems to me that the process has gone so far that Congress should, in due self-respect, take action, and that whatever conclusions you reach upon this subject should be conclusions not to be reported and lost in the shuffle, but to be put through and carried into effective legislation; that the due regard which the public ought to have for the efficiency of Congress as a practical legislating body calls for that attention to this particular business.

REGULATIONS GOVERNING APPOINTMENTS AND PRO-MOTIONS IN THE CONSULAR SERVICE OF THE UNITED STATES [1]

WHEREAS, The Congress, by Section 1753 of the Revised Statutes of the United States has provided as follows: —

"The President is authorized to prescribe such regulations for the admission of persons into the civil service of the United States as may best promote the efficiency thereof, and ascertain the fitness of each candidate in respect to age, health, character, knowledge, and ability for the branch of service into which he seeks to enter; and for this purpose he may employ suitable persons to conduct such inquiries, and may prescribe their duties, and establish regulations for the conduct of persons who may receive appointments in the civil service."

And, whereas, the Congress has classified and graded the consuls-general and consuls of the United States by the act entitled "An act to provide for the reorganization of the consular service of the United

[1] As amended by executive orders, etc., up to June, 1908.

that proposition. The never ought to b
Congress. There shod never be any retג
matter about which the Executive has theצ
self in making his selctions for office, atִ
other day with the viewf trying to meet
and with the hope that e would go before
agreement that we coul stand by on
fortunate proposition.

Secretary ROOT. I arked a m
applicant from Georgifor appointm
from Senator Clay, amng others.
Clay when he got to 'ashington
I do not want to inqu whether
Republican. I think th rule that
to his political affiliatics is the t
Senator Clay, who haswritten a
to apply to, and a statent that
regard to any politic filiation
referee in the State of Georgia

Senator FORAKER. Think
you were to undertakes dew
party should not have agree
tional query as to whether or
selections to any part ar

Senator BACON. Y ugh
of an Interstate Com ce

Senator LODGE. No th
provided for specifi llyn

Senator BACON. Bute

Senator LODGE. But
any conditions we choes

Senator BACON. Na
where the Constitu n
officers.

Senator LODGE. He

Senator BACON. It
If you are correct, th
few as compared wit
your theory is correct
to the appointment o

Secretary ROOT.
mittee I have consu
instructs me to sav
these appointments
political affiliations

ticable
ions of
Service
n him by
lent makes
general and
lways to the

ffice of consul
r grades
in t'

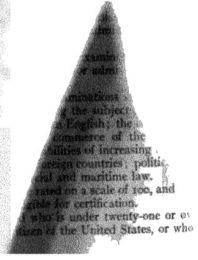

minations
the subject
English; the
commerce of the
ilities of increasing
reign countries; politi
al and maritime law.
ated on a scale of 100, and
ites for certification.
who is under twenty-one or ov
zen of the United States, or who

qualified for
)een specially
ısular service

r ninth class of
ill, the Secretary
ıall certify to him
ıccompanying the
ations, as revealed
be desired to fill a
nited States exercises
e sh

vice consul, deputy cons
upon passing such an ex
notion, as if appointed

intment subject o examination
n, due regard wl be had to the
equal merit, appintments should b
nal representation of all the States a
ervice; and neithe in the designation fo
or appointment will he political affiliations
red.

TEODORE ROOSEVELT.

1, 1906.

States," approved April 5, 1906, and has thereby made it practicable to extend to that branch of the civil service the aforesaid provisions of the Revised Statutes and the principles embodied in the Civil Service Act of January 16, 1883.

Now, therefore, in the exercise of the powers conferred upon him by the Constitution and laws of the United States, the President makes the following regulations to govern the selection of consuls general and consuls in the civil service of the United States, subject always to the advice and consent of the Senate: —

1. Vacancies in the office of consul-general and in the office of consul above class 8 shall be filled by promotion from the lower grades of the consular service, based upon ability and efficiency as shown in the service.

2. Vacancies in the office of consul of class 8 and of consul of class 9 shall be filled:

(a) By promotion on the basis of ability and efficiency as shown in the service, of consular assistants and of vice consuls, deputy consuls, consular agents, student interpreters and interpreters in the consular or diplomatic service, who shall have been appointed to such offices upon examination.

(b) By new appointments of candidates who have passed a satisfactory examination for appointment as consul as hereafter provided.

3. Persons in the service of the Department of State with salaries of two thousand dollars or upwards shall be eligible for promotion, on the basis of ability and efficiency as shown in the service, to any grade of the consular service above class 8 of consuls.

4. The Secretary of State, or such officer of the Department of State as the President shall designate, the Chief Clerk of the Department of State, and the Chief Examiner of the Civil Service Commission, or some person whom said Commission shall designate, shall constitute a Board of Examiners for admission to the consular service.

5. It shall be the duty of the Board of Examiners to formulate rules for and hold examinations of applicants for admission to the consular service.

6. The scope and method of the examinations shall be determined by the Board of Examiners, but among the subjects shall be included at least one modern language other than English; the natural, industrial and commercial resources and the commerce of the United States, especially with reference to the possibilities of increasing and extending the trade of the United States with foreign countries; political economy; elements of international, commercial and maritime law.

7. Examination papers shall be rated on a scale of 100, and no person rated at less than 80 shall be eligible for certification.

8. No one shall be examined who is under twenty-one or over fifty years of age, or who is not a citizen of the United States, or who is not

of good character and habits and physically and mentally qualified for the proper performance of consular work, or who has not been specially designated by the President for appointment to the consular service subject to examination.

9. Whenever a vacancy shall occur in the eighth or ninth class of consuls which the President may deem it expedient to fill, the Secretary of State shall inform the Board of Examiners, who shall certify to him the list of those persons eligible for appointment, accompanying the certificate with a detailed report showing the qualifications, as revealed by examination, of the persons so certified. If it be desired to fill a vacancy in a consulate in a country in which the United States exercises extraterritorial jurisdiction, the Secretary of State shall so inform the Board of Examiners, who shall include in the list of names certified by it only such persons as have passed the examination provided for in this order, and who also have passed an examination in the fundamental principles of the common law, the rules of evidence and the trial of civil and criminal cases. The list of names which the Board of Examiners shall certify shall be sent to the President for his information.

10. No promotion shall be made except for efficiency, as shown by the work that the officer has accomplished, the ability, promptness and diligence displayed by him in the performance of all his official duties, his conduct and his fitness for the consular service.

11. It shall be the duty of the Board of Examiners to formulate rules for and hold examinations of persons designated for appointment as consular assistant or as student interpreter, and of such persons designated for appointment as vice consul, deputy consul, and consular agent as shall desire to become eligible for promotion. The scope and method of such examination shall be determined by the Board of Examiners, but it shall include the same subjects hereinbefore prescribed for the examination of consuls. Any vice consul, deputy consul or consular agent now in the service, upon passing such an examination shall become eligible for promotion, as if appointed upon such examination.

12. In designations for appointment subject to examination and in appointments after examination, due regard will be had to the rule, that as between candidates of equal merit, appointments should be so made as to secure proportional representation of all the States and Territories in the consular service; and neither in the designation for examination or certification or appointment will the political affiliations of the candidate be considered.

THEODORE ROOSEVELT.

THE WHITE HOUSE,
June 27th, 1906.

REGULATIONS GOVERNING EXAMINATIONS

In pursuance of the Executive order of June 27, 1906, whereby the President promulgated regulations governing appointments and promotions in the consular service, the following rules have been adopted by the undersigned Board of Examiners, who, under that order, have been designated to formulate rules for and hold examinations of applicants for admission to the consular service whom the President shall have designated for examination to determine their eligibility for appointment therein:

1. The examinations will be the same for all grades and will be to determine a candidate's eligibility for appointment in the consular service, irrespective of the grade for which he may have been designated for examination and without regard to any particular office for which he may be selected.

2. The examinations will consist of an oral and a written one, the two counting equally. The object of the oral examination will be to determine the candidate's business ability, alertness, general contemporary information, and natural fitness for the service, including moral, mental, and physical qualifications, character, address, and general education and good command of English. In this part of the examination the applications previously filed will be given due weight by the Board of Examiners, especially as evidence of the applicant's business experience and ability. The written examination will include those subjects mentioned in the Executive order, to wit, French, German, or Spanish, or at least one modern language other than English; the natural, industrial, and commercial resources and the commerce of the United States, especially with reference to possibilities of increasing and extending the foreign trade of the United States; political economy, and the elements of international, commercial, and maritime law. It will likewise include American history, government, and institutions; political and commercial geography; arithmetic (as used in commercial statistics, tariff calculations, exchange, accounts, etc.); the modern history, since 1850, of Europe, Latin America, and the Far East, with particular attention to political, commercial, and economic tendencies. In the written examination, composition, grammar, punctuation, spelling, and writing will be given attention.

3. To become eligible for appointment, except as student interpreter, in a country where the United States exercises extraterritorial jurisdiction, the applicant must pass the examination outlined above, but supplemented by questions to determine his knowledge of the fundamental principles of common law, the rules of evidence, and the trial of civil and criminal cases.

4. The examinations to be given candidates for appointment as stu-

dent interpreters will follow the same course as in the case of other consular officers, provided, however, that no one will be examined for admission to the consular service as a student interpreter who is not between the ages of nineteen and twenty-six, inclusive, and unmarried; and, provided further, that upon appointment each student interpreter shall sign an agreement to continue in the service so long as his services may be required, within a period of five years.

5. Upon the conclusion of the examinations the names of the candidates who shall have attained upon the whole examination an average mark of at least eighty, as required by the Executive order, will be certified by the Board to the Secretary of State as eligible for appointment in the consular service, and the successful candidates will be informed that this has been done.

6. The names of candidates will remain on the eligible list for two years, except in the case of such candidates as shall within that period be appointed or shall withdraw their names. Names which have been on the eligible list for two years will be dropped therefrom and the candidates concerned will not again be eligible for appointment unless upon fresh application, designation anew for examination, and the successful passing of such second examination.

HUNTINGTON WILSON,
Third Assistant Secretary of State.

DEPARTMENT OF STATE,
Washington, December 13, 1906.

AMERICAN DIPLOMACY [1]

BY FRANCIS C. LOWELL

AT home and abroad there has been much criticism of American diplomatic representatives as compared with those of European countries. It is often said that our men are much inferior to their expert colleagues from Europe, and we are urged to adopt a system like the European, for their careful training and due promotion. That this criticism is valuable can not be denied. The extreme unfitness of some American envoys has discredited us, but there are advantages in our system, or want of it, which we ought not to overlook. In considering them here, we will pass over the consuls and limit ourselves to the regular diplomatic service.

Let us take a concrete case, and compare the American representatives in London with the English representatives in Washington. Since 1850 we have sent to England Joseph R. Ingersoll, James Buchanan, George M. Dallas, Charles Francis Adams, Reverdy Johnson, J. L.

[1] From the *Atlantic Monthly*, January, 1906. Reprinted by permission. Copyright.

REGULAIONS GOVI

IN pursuance othe Executive
President promulited regulatio
motions in the ccsular service, t
by the undersignl Board of Ex
been designated t formulate rule
cants for admissii to the consu
have designated r examination
pointment therein

1. The examittions will be t
determine a candate's eligibilit
vice, irrespective f the grade fo
for examination 1d without reg
he may be selectt.

2. The examittions will con.
two counting eqtily. The obje
determine the cadidate's busin
porary informatic, and natural
mental, and phycal qualificati
education and gtl command of
tion the applicatns previously
Board of Examirrs, especially
experience and 'ility. The w
subjects mentionl in the Execu
Spanish, or at list one moder
natural, industri and commerc
United States, esrcially with ref
extending the foign trade of t
and the elementsof internation:
will likewise inclle American
political and comercial geograp
statistics, tariff dculations, ex
history, since 18t, of Europe. I
particular attentii to political.
In the written examination, comp
and writing will e given attenti

3. To becomeligible for app
in a country whe the United .
tion, the applicat must pass th
plemented by qutions to dete-
principles of comon law, the .
and criminal cast.

4. The examittions to be gi

ll his colleagues
ally reaches the
whole, have
ss of an o
ierman A
-torical s
s are per
They r

ial |
anklii
onor fo
n. The
ore wrappe
distributing
ll about the
s never once
e Guildhall
relentlessly.
pathies, bid
refuse to be
a bust or a
ous English
he occasion.
should not
ms, Lowell,

Motley, R. C. Schenck, Edwards Pierrepont, John Welsh, J. R. Lowell, Edward J. Phelps, Robert T. Lincoln, Thomas F. Bayard, John Hay, Joseph H. Choate, and Whitelaw Reid. The English have sent to us Sir Henry Bulwer (Lord Dalling), J. F. T. Crampton, Lord Napier, Lord Lyons, Sir Frederick Bruce, Sir Edward Thornton, L. S. Sackville West, Lord Pauncefote, Sir Michael Herbert, and Sir Mortimer Durand.

Without dwelling on particular names, we see plainly that the Americans have been the more distinguished men. The English representatives have been well educated and trained, and have tried to do their diplomatic duty, with measurable success. No one of them at any time or in any place made considerable mark of any sort upon the history of his country or that of the world. No one held important office outside the diplomatic service. To establish an accurate standard of comparison is impossible. Distinction and importance can not be weighed. But of the Englishmen we may say that hardly one was of English cabinet rank, that is to say, had the importance which usually belongs in England to a cabinet minister. Among the sixteen Americans there are found one president, one vice-president, and an unsuccessful nominee of a great party for the latter office. Five served in our small cabinet: two secretaries of state, a secretary of war, and two attorneys-general; two others were lawyers at the head of their profession, one was a historian, and one a poet, both of high rank, and still we have not classified Mr. Adams, who did the greatest service of them all. The difference in the lists is striking.

*   *   *   *   *   *   *   *

Few of these Americans had long diplomatic experience; many of them served with little or none. Hence our range of choice has been much wider than that of those countries which have maintained a regular diplomatic service. Cabinet ministers, historians, poets, lawyers, teachers, are chosen to represent the United States. No country could keep permanently in its diplomatic employ so large a number of its leaders. There would not be enough left for other necessities. The American diplomat is a man of distinction, taken from public life, literature, or the bar, from a large business, or from a university, and set to a job for which he has had no special training. The typical European diplomat is a man of less ability and less general distinction, trained to a profession from his youth. What are the comparative advantages of the two systems?

The ordinary functions of a diplomat are matters of routine, the observation of proper formalities in public functions and in his official duties. Herein experience tells. Not only has the elaborate etiquette of courts and public offices become second nature to the ambassador who has practiced it since he was a boy, but, apart from the diplomatic career, the bringing up of a European gentleman, especially of a European nobleman, gives him the start of his American colleague, though the latter has grown up in the best society of New York or Washington. But important negotiations are now carried on by foreign secretaries, not by diplomats. The envoy who transmits messages between them is left little discretion. That he should have good manners is desirable, but want of ability and lack of initiative are not serious drawbacks. Thus far the European diplomat has the advantage. Yet emergencies may arise which call for ability in the diplomat himself as well as in his superior, the foreign secretary. There the European is at a disadvantage. His whole life has been given to the study of routine, until his initiative is gone. The American's ignorance of routine may be a positive help. He is accustomed to emergencies where something new and unexpected must be done. Business, politics, the law, literature, sometimes call for originality.

The success of American diplomacy in meeting these emergencies is illustrated by the career of Mr. Washburne as minister to France. He had been a member of the American House of Representatives and an experienced politician of Illinois, with little knowledge of Europe and almost none of the French language. His diplomatic rank in Paris was low. Nuncio, ambassadors, some ministers plenipotentiary, outranked him. The United States then had little reputation in Europe. But when the political revolution which followed the battle of Sedan perplexed European diplomats, Mr. Washburne made it his business to do the work which lay next his hand, and he found a good deal of it. Within a few weeks the envoy who had stood near the bottom of the list was become in effect the first diplomatic representative in France. How much credit for the gain was due to our Secretary of State, Mr. Fish, and how much to Mr. Washburne, is not known, but much was due to the latter. His protection of the Germans was efficient before and during the siege. When the French government moved to Versailles in consequence of the outbreak of the Commune, Mr. Washburne formally established his legation there, but spent most of his time in Paris. He was helped by his extraordinary courage, no doubt, but courage is not a rare virtue. His common sense, leading him to disregard diplomatic traditions, contributed more than his courage to his success. Thus he was able to save some proposed victims from the Commune, and to comfort in prison the Archbishop of Paris, though he could not save him. Much of his action was irregular, and his establishment in Paris was criticized. Thus he wrote: "This action, it must be admitted, was not entirely acceptable to the government at Versailles, and it was communicated to me, as coming unofficially from that government, that it would have been better for me to have joined all my diplomatic colleagues at Versailles, and not to have kept up any legation whatever in Paris. My answer to all this was that, while I desired to be as agreeable as possible to the government at Versailles, and not to be wanting in my loyalty to it, as minister of the United States, in any respect, yet that there were vast interests with which I was charged at Paris, and, however disagreeable it might be to remain there, I owed a greater duty to the interests with which I was charged than I did to the mere etiquette which would have required me to remain in Versailles."

That some disregard of diplomatic traditions on his part does not always discredit a diplomatic representative is proved by Mr. Washburne's experience. He had aided and protected the Germans. In this way he had obtained the gratitude of Germany; but the Germans were unpopular in France. He had dealt with the leaders of the Commune, some of them vile criminals as well as armed rebels. If his acts had strained our relations with France, his successes would have been dearly bought. But his tact and common sense conciliated France. Momentary irritation soon disappeared. The French ministers of foreign affairs were persons too considerable not to admire beneficent ability, even if its methods were unusual. Mr. Washburne's habit of dealing with men of all sorts as a man of business, not much troubled by the formalities of diplomatic etiquette, pleased every one. He earned the gratitude of the Germans, while keeping French good will. His conduct improved our position in Europe. At the other side of the world, nearly thirty years later, America was represented in China by Mr. Conger, an American politician of secondary importance, who had little knowledge of China and no diplomatic experience. An emergency arose, not provided for in the rules of diplomatic etiquette. While Mr. Conger's achievements in the Boxer troubles were not so great as Mr. Washburne's in France, yet it is understood that he was rather more than the equal of his trained brethren from England and the continent of Europe. We have just achieved diplomatic success in Russia, having disregarded diplomatic tradition so completely that our ignominious failure was generally predicted. This was the achievement of a president with neither diplomatic training nor a foreign secretary, speaking through an ambassador trained in business and politics.

Emergencies like these are infrequent, it is true, and the close observance of due formalities is called for every day. Granted that Mr. Washburne's success was brilliant, yet such instances are necessarily rare and have grown rarer. If our representatives in England, France, and Germany, can to-day do not more than observe diplomatic traditions, keep posted in the gossip of the capital, and avoid the little blunders upon which their colleagues, their colleagues' wives, and other persons of fashion like to dwell, then perhaps we may admit that emergencies may be left to take care of themselves, and that a trained diplomat may be most to our advantage. But some of our representatives, as it seems to me, have pointed out a new function for the diplomat which is of real benefit to his own country and to that which he visits.

An Englishman wrote at the time of Mr. Choate's departure: "In- ·

stinctively we separate the American Ambassador from all his colleagues in the Diplomatic Corps. He is the only one who really reaches the masses. He is the only one in whom the people, as a whole, have any interest. Of him alone it is expected that he will be less of an official and more of a man. One never hears of the Russian or German Ambassador being asked to lecture before a philosophical or historical society, or invited to a literary dinner. They and their colleagues are permitted to stand outside all but a fraction of the national life. They may entrench themselves behind the ramparts of society and officialdom, and none will seek to drag them forth. The public at large knows nothing of them, and does not care to know anything. They are what the American Ambassador never is, — they are foreigners, and treated as such. We surrender them cheerfully to Downing-Street, the Court, and the West End. . . . We never really give the poor man a moment's rest. We might almost be accused of trying to kill him with kindness. Even before he lands on English soil he is pounced upon by the Mayor and Corporation of Southampton, an address of welcome fired at him on shipboard, and a speech extorted from him in reply. And that is but a foretaste of what is to come. . . . But as it is, no sooner has he presented his credentials than the bombardment begins. I must admit at once it is most vigorously replied to. England and the American Ambassador set to forthwith to see which can spoil the other the most. Chambers of Commerce swoop down upon him and bear him off in triumph as their guest of honour. The Omar Khayyam Club points an invitation at this head, demanding unconditional surrender. The Dante Society insists on his escorting its members through the infernal regions. The Wordsworth Society, the Browning Society, the Boz Club, the Sir Walter Scott Club, — all press their claims. The Birmingham and Midland Institute insidiously elects him as its annual president, and exacts by way of tribute an address on Benjamin Franklin. The Edinburgh Philosophical Institution bestows the same honor for the price of a paper on Abraham Lincoln. And so it goes on. The big public schools, knowing that he is an American, and therefore wrapped up in education, play upon his weakness and lure him into distributing their prizes. Political leagues expect him to tell them all about the United States Supreme Court. The historic City companies never once let go of him. He is a standing feature on the toast-list of the Guildhall banquet. Charitable and philanthropic societies pursue him relentlessly. Working men's institutes, trading on his democratic sympathies, bid for an evening's loan of his presence and voice. Libraries refuse to be opened except by him. He is the obvious man to unveil a bust or a portrait. The organizers of a dinner in honor of a famous English cartoonist turn to the American Embassy for the orator of the occasion. After all, I suppose it is partly America's own fault. She should not send us such charming, cultivated, broad-gauged men. Adams, Lowell,

Edward J.
H

nsiderate fam
officialialary
me who
sar N
c
h
m

app
weal
lavish.
travaga
American
ought not
nation can
men have that
the small class
find in our foreign
aires would be in
are very large, whe
for his successor t prae
sador ought to sped in ou
should make the 1st guess.
intimate strongly nd officially
of living should corespond.

On the 4th
single member.
since then the C
inadequate force, ᴛ
me that a cordial sᴛ.
partial enforcement oꜰ
in aid of it.

Heretofore the book oꜰ
certifications were made uꜰ
This secrecy was the sourᴛ
di favoritism in the administᴛ
suspected; what is open can bᴛ
approval of all its members, haꜱ
public. The eligible lists for the cl..
are now publicly posted in the respeᴛ.
tions for appointments. The purpoꜱ.
absolutely to exclude any other consideratᴛᴛ
ments under it than that of merit as tested
business proceeds upon the theory that both tᴛ..
the appointing officers are absolutely ignorant aꜱ
and associations of all persons on the civil-servᴛᴛ
much to say, however, that some recent Congre
have somewhat shaken public confidence in the imp
tions for appointment.

The reform of the civil service will make no safe
vance until the present law and its equal administratio.
lished in the confidence of the people. It will be my ꜰ
my duty, to see that the law is executed with firmness aꜰ
If some of its provisions have been fraudulently evaded
officers, our resentment should not suggest the repeal ᴛ
reform in its administration. We should h ve one view

but a
·, and
h an
l by
m-
d

Phelps, Bayard, Hay, and Choate, — what other country has sent us representatives to compare with them? The capacity of a long line of American Ambassadors to warm both hands at the cheerful fire of English existence has been so palpable, their interests have been so manifestly stretched beyond the humdrum game of protocols and despatches, they touch life at so many more points than the ordinary professional diplomat, that we should hardly know what to do if the United States accredited to the Court of St. James anyone short of her best. A tongue-tied, unsociable, purely official American Ambassador has become unthinkable to this country. We calmly take it for granted that the representative of the United States, whoever he may be, will be a first-class after-dinner speaker, and able and willing at any time to deliver an address, preside at a meeting, or unveil a monument. And so he invariably is. Why, then, should we not use him for our profit and entertainment?"

The suggestion thus conveyed is valuable, now that our ambassadors are in hourly connection with Washington, and have become little more than messengers and clerks in their ordinary work. May they not be employed in acquainting people of one nation with the people of another? For this purpose miscellaneous ability is more effective than training. After he had become famous, Thackeray sought appointment as secretary of legation at Washington. The place was refused him because it had been promised to some one else, and also because some budding diplomat was deemed fairly entitled to it. We make ambassadors of men like Thackeray. To compare with him J. F. T. Crampton, Esq., at about that time British minister to Washington, seems to us absurd.

It is said that training is needed to avoid the blunders often committed by men who are unacquainted with the ways of courts. This is obvious, but how important are these blunders, after all? They give rise to the gossip common in the diplomatic circles of Pumpernickel and elsewhere, but, except in Pumpernickel, do the people of importance really care? Those who govern great states, be they sovereigns or ministers, are interested to find intelligence and capacity anywhere. They leave questions of precedence and clothes for the most part to their chamberlains and valets.

We have been successful in interesting the English people in our ambassadors, and their official position has not been much damaged by this interest. We have profited by the transaction, and this profit would have been impossible had we sent trained diplomats to London. In less degree we have profited elsewhere. We have certain advantages in supplying representatives of this sort, besides natural American adaptability. We draw from all the nations of Europe, and ought not to be strangers to any of them. Some of them are ripe for an ambassador who will talk to the people or to large classes of the people as our representatives have talked to the people of England for a generation. That one of our ambassadors appeals especially to men of letters, another to men of business, a third to men in public life, and still a fourth to teachers, but adds variety to the general interest aroused by the succession. In these latter days the people of one country are becoming curious about the people of another. International friendship and international tolerance, both important in their place, are advanced by international knowledge. The exchange of professors between our universities and those of continental Europe illustrates this growing interest of one people in another. Professor Wendell, lecturing last year in the provinces as well as in Paris, owed his welcome to his nationality as well as to his learning and literary skill. This year in Germany Professor Peabody has similar greeting from the Germans, and both will leave behind them sound knowledge and good feeling which the publication of their written lectures could not have effected. To expect our ambassador to open museums and to lecture on politics and literature seems, at first sight, to be asking him to go outside his vocation; but does not our English experience prove that the service he thus renders is in itself important, and that it does not interfere with duties more strictly diplomatic? Let us suppose, for example, that President Roosevelt, when he leaves his office, were sent to represent us for a while in some continental country. The people of that country would be immensely interested to see him and hear him. Seeing and hearing him, they would be interested in us, and would learn to know us better. With increased knowledge, they would lose some misconceptions and prejudices, and thus we should profit by our representative. That the President is not a trained diplomat is unimportant. It may well be that we can employ him more profitably than as an ambassador, but the suggestion explains my meaning.

Illustration may be found also in the diplomacy of other countries. In the Boxer troubles of 1900, China owed much to her envoy in this country. No doubt he discharged his diplomatic duty at Washington, but he did much more. In the face of the American people, he maintained the Chinese cause under extraordinary difficulties. We did not altogether believe what he said, but we were forced to hear him. He interested us, and, even against our will, made us feel human kinship with his people, while he showed such knowledge of ours.

A trained diplomat, indeed, can be of service to a lawyer, or poet, or college president, sent to represent us at a European court. If the secretary of legation will attend to the routine of the office and will coach the ambassador in the details of behavior and dress, the latter can attend to serious matters with more leisure and effect. But to carry out this plan, the promotion of our regularly trained diplomats must stop short of the highest places in our diplomatic service, and it is doubtful if reasonably intelligent young men will be attracted to a service in which they must remain subordinates. No professional training, however well directed, no experience, however extensive, will produce men to compare in general ability and distinction with our representatives in England, chosen almost at haphazard, during the last fifty years.

In the matter of payment, we touch upon one of our most serious difficulties. The salaries now paid are too low, especially for married men with considerable families. Private means are now needed to supplement the official salary, and so we are coming to appoint as ambassadors only those men whose private means are large. This may not be absolutely necessary. Mr. Roosevelt or Mr. Hay might live in London on $17,500 a year without loss of prestige, but it takes great distinction to make so little money go so far. We can not expect to get it in every case. As things go, the salary is not ordinarily large enough to enable our representative to live like his diplomatic colleagues. Therefore we appoint rich men ambassadors, to eke out the salary from their private wealth. Not only do they do this, but they outspend their colleagues so lavishly, that soon the merely rich man will be embarrassed by the extravagance of his predecessor. To curtail expense, especially for an American, is difficult. Yet the inability to live on his official salary ought not to lead an ambassador to spend ten times that amount. No nation can pay a salary like that. No nation ought to do so. But few men have that amount of money to spend, and not all the members of the small class of the very rich have the distinction which we ought to find in our foreign representatives. To limit our choice to multi-millionaires would be in every way unfortunate. If an ambassador's expenses are very large, whether he can afford them or not, he makes it harder for his successor to practice economy. To determine what an ambassador ought to spend in one place or another may not be easy, but we should make the best guess possible, fix the salary accordingly, and intimate strongly and officially to our representatives that their style of living should correspond.

XIII

CIVIL SERVICE

FROM THE FIRST ANNUAL MESSAGE OF PRESIDENT
HARRISON, 1889

ON the 4th of March last the Civil Service Commission had but a single member. The vacancies were filled on the 7th day of May, and since then the Commissioners have been industriously, though with an inadequate force, engaged in executing the law. They were assured by me that a cordial support would be given them in the faithful and impartial enforcement of the statute and of the rules and regulations adopted in aid of it.

Heretofore the book of eligibles has been closed to everyone, except as certifications were made upon the requisition of the appointing officers. This secrecy was the source of much suspicion and of many charges of favoritism in the administration of the law. What is secret is always suspected; what is open can be judged. The Commission, with the full approval of all its members, has now opened the list of eligibles to the public. The eligible lists for the classified post offices and custom-houses are now publicly posted in the respective offices, as are also the certifications for appointments. The purpose of the civil-service law was absolutely to exclude any other consideration in connection with appointments under it than that of merit as tested by the examinations. The business proceeds upon the theory that both the examining boards and the appointing officers are absolutely ignorant as to the political views and associations of all persons on the civil-service lists. It is not too much to say, however, that some recent Congressional investigations have somewhat shaken public confidence in the impartiality of the selections for appointment.

The reform of the civil service will make no safe or satisfactory advance until the present law and its equal administration are well established in the confidence of the people. It will be my pleasure, as it is my duty, to see that the law is executed with firmness and impartiality. If some of its provisions have been fraudulently evaded by appointing officers, our resentment should not suggest the repeal of the law, but reform in its administration. We should have one view of the matter,

683

affected by the consideration that time in power.

January, 1889, by an Executive the Railway Mail Service under

Provision was made that the state where   eligible list was

Mr. Lyman, then the only me in writing that it would not ly before May 1st, and requested of each class. They will be appropriately indated in the Official Register and in the report of the Department. Tlt a great stimulus would thus be given to the whole service I do not oubt, and such a record would be the best defense against inconsidera removals from office.

FROM THE FOURTH ANNUAL MESAGE OF PRESI DENT CLEVELAND,

~ss

ivil-service reform urnishes a cause for the
s survi the debts of its friends as well
t has gained permanent place among
politics at to improve, economize,

service pward of 84,000 places,
ruled from time to time since
it extension was made by
8o6, and if fourth-class
nt it may be said that
service law are now
e postmasterships,
d quiet of neigh-
n at present, I
ffice appropri-

and hold it with a sincerity that is not affected by the consideration that the party to which we belong is for the time in power.

My predecessor, on the 4th day of January, 1889, by an Executive order to take effect March 15, brought the Railway Mail Service under the operation of the civil-service law. Provision was made that the order should take effect sooner in any state where an eligible list was sooner obtained. On the 11th day of March Mr. Lyman, then the only member of the Commission, reported to me in writing that it would not be possible to have the list of eligibles ready before May 1st, and requested that the taking effect of the order be postponed until that time, which was done, subject to the same provision contained in the original order as to States in which an eligible list was sooner obtained.

As a result of the revision of the rules, of the new classification, and of the inclusion of the Railway Mail Service, the work of the Commission has been greatly increased, and the present clerical force is found to be inadequate. I recommend that the additional clerks asked by the Commission be appropriated for.

The duty of appointment is devolved by the Constitution or by the law and the appointing officers are properly held to a high responsibility in its exercise. The growth of the country and the consequent increase of the civil list have magnified this function of the Executive disproportionately. It can not be denied, however, that the labor connected with this necessary work is increased, often to the point of actual distress, by the sudden and excessive demands that are made upon an incoming Administration for removals and appointments. But, on the other hand, it is not true that incumbency is a conclusive argument for continuance in office. Impartiality, moderation, fidelity to public duty, and a good attainment in the discharge of it must be added before the argument is complete. When those holding administrative offices so conduct themselves as to convince just political opponents that no party consideration or bias affects in any way the discharge of their public duties, we can more easily stay the demand for removals.

I am satisfied that both in and out of the classified service great benefit would accrue from the adoption of some system by which the officer would receive the distinction and benefit that in all private employments comes from exceptional faithfulness and efficiency in the performance of duty.

I have suggested to the heads of the Executive Departments that they consider whether a record might not be kept in each bureau of all those elements that are covered by the terms "faithfulness" and "efficiency," and a rating made showing the relative merits of the clerks of each class, this rating to be regarded as a test of merit in making promotions.

I have also suggested to the Postmaster-General that he adopt some plan by which he can, upon the basis of the reports to the Department and of frequent inspections, indicate the relative merits of postmasters of each class. They will be appropriately indicated in the Official Register and in the report of the Department. That a great stimulus would thus be given to the whole service I do not doubt, and such a record would be the best defense against inconsiderate removals from office.

FROM THE FOURTH ANNUAL MESSAGE OF PRESIDENT CLEVELAND, 1896

THE progress made in civil-service reform furnishes a cause for the utmost congratulation. It has survived the doubts of its friends as well as the rancour of its enemies and has gained a permanent place among the agencies destined to cleanse our politics and to improve, economize, and elevate the public service.

There are now in the competitive service upward of 84,000 places, more than half of these having been included from time to time since March 4th, 1893. A most radical and sweeping extension was made by Executive order dated the 6th day of May, 1896, and if fourth-class postmasterships are not included in the statement it may be said that practically all positions contemplated by the civil-service law are now classified. Abundant reasons exist for including these postmasterships, based upon economy, improved service, and the peace and quiet of neighborhoods. If, however, obstacles prevent such action at present, I earnestly hope that Congress will, without increasing post-office appropriations, so adjust them as to admit in proper cases a consolidation of these post offices, to the end that through this process the result desired may to a limited extent be accomplished.

The civil-service rules as amended during the last year provide for a sensible and uniform method of promotion, basing eligibility to better positions upon demonstrated efficiency and faithfulness. The absence of fixed rules on this subject has been an infirmity in the system more and more apparent as its other benefits have been better appreciated.

The advantages of civil-service methods in their business aspects are too well understood to require argument. Their application has become a necessity to the executive work of the Government. But those who gain positions through the operation of these methods should be made to understand that the non-partisan scheme through which they receive their appointments demands from them by way of reciprocity non-partisan and faithful performance of duty under every Administration and cheerful fidelity to every chief. While they should be encouraged to decently exercise their rights of citizenship and to support through their suffrages the political beliefs they honestly profess, the noisy, pestilent and partisan employee, who loves political turmoil and contention or who renders lax and grudging service to an Administration not representing his political views, should be promptly and fearlessly dealt with in such a way as to furnish a warning to others who may be likewise disposed.

THE CIVIL SERVICE UNDER ROOSEVELT [1]

By WILLIAM B. SHAW

THE President of the United States, as every one knows who has read the Constitution of his country, is commander-in-chief of the army and navy. He is also the head of an organized body of civil servants, far outnumbering our standing military and naval forces, — a body unknown to the Constitution, since the very possibility of its existence was undreamed of by the fathers of the republic. There are about two hundred and eighty thousand of these men and women who toil daily in Uncle Sam's vineyard, and they are as truly the nation's servants as are the soldiers and sailors who fight its battles. Among them are some whose lives are by no means lacking in the heroic, — some whose devotion to duty is not less noble because their service has been rendered without trumpet-and-drum accompaniment.

A CIVIL-SERVICE PRESIDENT

It is no disparagement of the military arm to the Government to acknowledge that without the civil arm it would be powerless, and especially in a democracy like ours it would seem to be almost an axiom of successful administration that the executive civil service should be as thoroughly organized and trained to as high a degree of efficiency as the military or naval service. Yet it is only a short span of years since this truth began to be recognized by our government as a principle of conduct. Men who are hardly gray can recall the time when practically every salaried position on the Government's roster, from the department secretaryships down to the jobs of the messengers and charwomen in the corridors of the big Washington office buildings, was regarded as the legitimate loot of the place-hunter. In those days men were not esteemed for what they knew about the Government's work. It was not deemed necessary that a President should be familiar with the affairs of one or more of the executive departments. How many Presidents have entered office with any personal knowledge whatever of departmental business? For our Presidents we chose military heroes, Congressmen, or "favorite sons" of States, — never men experienced in the actual executive business at Washington. The fact is, that Theodore Roosevelt is the first occupant of the Presidential chair who has come to the office equipped with intimate knowledge, based on personal experience, of the practical work-

[1] *Review of Reviews*, March, 1905. Reprinted by permission.

ings of the great governmental machine. Some of the best years of his life had been given to the cause of civil-service reform, — not as an agitator on the outside, but as a practical administrator on the inside, holding the important post of president of the Civil Service Commission, facing grave problems of organization and method, of which the doctrinaire reformer had little conception, and gaining through it all an experience that has proved a valuable asset in the still broader responsibilities of the Presidency. That experience, supplemented as it was by his term of office as Assistant Secretary of the Navy, familiarized Mr. Roosevelt with the routine of executive business, so that now, as the head of the whole governmental system, his relation to the personnel may be likened to that sustained by an army's commander to the subordinate officers in successive gradations of rank through which he has himself risen.

It is only natural, then, that those who are working for the improvement of the national civil service should count on the Roosevelt administration as an active and vigilant ally. We have a President in office who knows as well as a man in his position can know what the system is and how it works, — its merits and its defects. Its problems and its difficulties he has made his own. He has had a hand in reforming its abuses, and more than once he has come to its defense when it was set upon by powerful enemies. Perhaps the inauguration of a "civil-service President" marks an appropriate time for a rapid survey of the conditions under which the government's work is performed by its army of civil servants. Changes more far-reaching, possibly, than the American public suspects, have within a few years so transformed those conditions that government employment in Washington and elsewhere now presents wholly new phases. Moreover, most of the discussion of the subject heretofore has been confined to the political or theoretical aspects of the situation, to the neglect of certain more concretely human aspects.

The Changes of Twenty Years

When Mr. James Bryce wrote "The American Commonwealth" he did not think it worth while to include a chapter on the public service, as he would almost certainly have done in writing a similar treatise on any of the European states; but it is not recalled that anybody noticed the omission. The truth is, that twenty years ago in this country, governmental employment, with a few exceptional instances, was anything but a dignified calling. It offered few attractions to the educated youth of the land. Its rewards were transitory at best. Every official's fortunes, however humble, depended on the coming and going of Presidents, Senators, and Representatives. To the great body of our citizenship, the whole business signified nothing more than a mad scramble, every four years, for place and pelt. The Government had not impressed the national imagination by its undertakings. Little was known of the official routine. Every job at Washington was believed to be a sinecure. Every office-holder was regarded as a spoilsman, who held his place only by the favor of some other spoilsman. Every office-holder was regularly and openly assessed a considerable part of his salary for campaign expenses at every election. Moreover, he was expected to neglect his official duties at election time and devote all his energies to electioneering for his party. What wonder that under such conditions the maxim that "public office is a public trust" seemed merely an empty platitude!

This state of affairs had developed gradually during the first century of the Republic's life, and it was not to be radically altered in a day. Some of the attendant evils are still with us. Yet it requires but a brief sojourn at the national capital to convince one that the general situation, as respects office-holding and all forms of public employment, is very different to-day from what it was, for example, when President Garfield took office and virtually sacrificed his life to the spoils demon. One now finds in the service of the Government hundreds of university-trained men who have entered on avenues of advancement in the public service that vie in attractiveness with academic careers. Furthermore, thousands of the purely clerical positions in the departments are filled by men and women who in training and equipment for their duties would do credit to the best-managed business houses in the land.

What the Law of 1883 Sought to Accomplish

An inquirer seeking a reason for this transformation (and it is nothing less) in the conditions affecting public employment in Washington and throughout the United States, will be told that the chief cause is to be found in the operation of the Civil Service Act of 1883, known for some years after its passage as the Pendleton Act, in recognition of the fact that it was fathered by the venerable Democratic Senator from Ohio. The passage of this law was the most effective blow ever dealt at the spoils system in this country. Yet its immediate results gave little promise of the increasing potency which has developed with each successive administration since that of President Arthur, when its machinery was set in motion. In brief, the law provided for the appointment of three commissioners, not more than two of whom should be adherents of the same political party, and made it the duty of the commission to aid the President in preparing suitable rules for the government of the civil service. It was required that these rules should provide, among other things, for open competitive examinations for testing the fitness of applicants for the classified service; that appointments should be made from among those passing these examinations with highest grades; that such appointments should be apportioned in the departments at Washington among the States and Territories; that there should be an appointment on probation before absolute appointment, and that the use of official authority to coerce the political action of any person or body should be absolutely prohibited. Provision was also made in the act for investigations touching the enforcement of the rules, and a penalty of fine or imprisonment, or both, was imposed for the solicitation by any person in the service of the United States of contributions to be used for political purposes of persons in such service, or the collection of such contributions by any person in any government building.

THE MEN WHO ENFORCED THE LAW

Now, as we look back to-day upon the immediate effects of the early enforcement of this law in the administrations of President Arthur and President Cleveland, it is hard to understand why such an outcry should have been made about it at the time, or why it should have been deemed so revolutionary in principle. Only fourteen thousand places were at first included in the classified service. This number was increased gradually during the first Cleveland administration, and more extensively in the Harrison administration, the second Cleveland administration, and the administrations of Presidents McKinley and Roosevelt, until at the present time more than one-half of the total federal civil service of the country, or, to be exact, 154,093 positions, are classified subject to competitive examination under the civil-service rules. In other words, there are eleven times as many persons who now owe their appointments in the civil service to the operation of competitive tests as were included within the scope of the rules when the commission first set them in operation. More than 133,000 persons were examined last year, of whom 103,718 passed, and 50,830 received appointments. It has been found necessary to divide the country into thirteen districts for the purpose of conducting examinations. Such an increase as this could not have been achieved had not the system itself, and its administration as well, commended themselves to Congress and to the heads of departments at Washington. An indifferent or lukewarm board of commissioners might at any time during the past twenty-two years have practically nullified the law and defeated its whole purpose, but the country has been fortunate in the character of the men who have served as Civil Service Commissioners. Beginning with George William Curtis, who declined the English mission in order to take the presidency of the first Civil Service Commission in Grant's administration, under an earlier law, the men who have served the Government's interests in this important office have set excellent examples of patriotism and devotion to public duty. The Commission has had Democratic presidents under Republican administrations and Republican presidents under Democratic administrations. Some of its members have been intense partisans,

44

and yet no charge of pernicious political activity has been laid at the Commission's door.

During President Harrison's administration, and in the first half·of President Cleveland's second administration, the president of the commission was Theodore Roosevelt. He was a Northern Republican, and he had as associates on the commission two Southern Democrats, — ex-Gov. Hugh S. Thompson, of South Carolina, and the late John R. Procter, the former State geologist of Kentucky. Mr. Roosevelt has himself said of his associates, both of whom had served in the Confederate army, that "it would be impossible for any one to desire as associates two men with higher ideals of duty, or more resolute in their adherence to those ideals." In the same connection, Mr. Roosevelt has declared that "in all the dealings of the commission in those years, there was no single instance wherein the politics of any person or the political significance of any action was so much as taken into account in any case that arose." Other commissioners of ability and eminence who succeeded Roosevelt were the Hon. William Dudley Foulke, of Indiana, and the Hon. James R. Garfield, of Ohio, now Commissioner of Corporations. The president of the commission at the present time is Gen. John C. Black, of Illinois, a lifelong Democrat, and with him are associated the Hon. Alford W. Cooley, of New York, and the Hon. Henry F. Greene, of Minnesota, both Republicans. The secretary of the commission, Mr. John T. Doyle, has held his present position throughout the commission's history, from the time when the entire effects and archives of the office were transported from one Washington building to another in an ordinary pushcart, until to-day, when an entire five-story building is inadequate for the work of the bureau. The present chief examiner of the commission, Mr. Frank M. Kiggings, served an apprenticeship at departmental duties before his connection with the commission, and is familiar with the examination problem in its most practical phases. The same thing is true of other members of the examining staff.

This matter of the commission's personnel is important in any consideration of the improvement and reform of the civil service. All the officials of the commission, from the beginning, seem to have been animated with a desire not merely to enforce the letter of the law, but to do everything possible to make it effective in the broadest sense. A continual campaign of popular education has been necessary in order to make the great outside public understand that its own interests were cared for and guarded by the commission, while, at the same time, no little persuasion was necessary in the early years in order to bring about the hearty coöperation of the heads of departments and the bureau chiefs. After more than a score of years of enforcement, it is the all but unanimous conclusion that the law has vindicated itself and·has amply justified its enactment. No head of a government department would to-day be willing to go back to the conditions of 1880, even if the law were to be repealed to-morrow. It is quite probable that in the event of such a repeal, the first action taken in most of the departments would be the establishment of a system of competitive tests based on the examinations now conducted by the Civil Service Commission. It should not, however, be inferred that the heads of all the executive departments and bureaus are unanimous in approval of examinations *per se*. As a bureau chief said to the writer a few days ago, "The examinations do not in every case form the best test. All that can be said of them is that for the purpose intended, applicable to the great mass of clerical positions in Washington, no better means has been devised for securing a fair competitive test."

EXAMINATIONS MADE PRACTICAL

Still, as the system has developed with the years, the practicality of the examinations has steadily gained, and the best proof of the general usefulness of the system is to be found in the fact that it brings to the various departments the types of candidates most desired. The heads of the scientific bureaus in Washington would be the first to resent any failure on the part of the commission to supply desirable material for positions in their specialties. The fact is, that under the workings of the examination system, specialists are continually coming to Washington and receiving appointments in one part or another of the service, who represent the best-trained intellects available in the country in those particular lines. Perhaps it is not fully understood outside of Washington to how great an extent the departments themselves now have in hand the framing of examination questions for these technical positions. Recognizing the fact that the department itself is the best judge of the qualifications required for appointees of this character, the Civil Service Commission has wisely sought the active coöperation of the departments in the framing of examination questions. It is decided, for example, that the Secretary of Agriculture desires to call to Washington for the government service a man trained in the study of noxious plant growths. The department itself knows better than any outsider possibly can what are the particular qualifications demanded in this position. At the same time, it is for the interest of the department that the spirit of the law should be fully observed, since better qualifications can in many cases be secured through competition than otherwise. The Civil Service Commission is notified by the department that it is desired to fill the vacancy in question, and the commission proceeds to request the department to suggest questions to be used in the competitive examination which is advertised to be held.

SIX HUNDRED DISTINCT EXAMINATIONS

The commission itself conducts at the present time more than six hundred different kinds of examinations, and it is not to be supposed that its examiners, unaided, can cover this entire field to the satisfaction of the departments. In the case which we are considering, the Agricultural Department frames its questions and submits them to the commission; the examination is held by the commission, and in due time the names of the successful candidates are sent to the department, which then makes its own selection of one name from three. If the department had the entire management of the matter in its own hands, it is difficult to see how it could make the test more practical or secure better results. In fact, the methods of the commission in the matter of examinations, from start to finish, all tend to the most practical results attainable. In the preparation of questions, the thing kept constantly in view is the nature of the duties to which the candidate will be assigned on appointment. The whole object of the test is to ascertain the candidate's qualifications for those particular duties. In the case of the special technical positions to which reference has been made, the difficulty experienced by an outside examiner in comprehending the nature of these specific duties is overcome by reference of the whole matter to the authorities directly concerned. Thus, the whole object of the law is secured, the department attains its end, the candidates are subjected to the fairest possible tests, and the general good of the service is promoted.

TESTS FOR MECHANICAL AND EXPERT POSITIONS

Turning from these positions, in which the highest form of technical ability is required, to the far more numerous places for which certain specific, practical tests are necessary, we find that the commission has steadily increased the efficiency of its examination system. The public has sometimes been led to suppose that persons applying for mechanical positions are subjected to purely literary tests. Nothing could be further from the truth. In examinations in mechanical trades, the subjects considered are not educational tests at all, but simply age, physical condition, and experience, the relative weights of which (on a scale of 100) are as follows: age, 20; physical condition, 20; experience, 60. Then, too, in classes of positions requiring expert knowledge of some particular trade or calling, the tests applied are of the most practical character. Take, for example, the examination of local and assistant inspectors of hulls, under the Steamboat Inspection Service. Here the relative weights of subjects, on a scale of 100, are: letter-writing, 10; arithmetic (comprising problems in common and decimal fractions, mensuration, and square root), 10; hull construction (comprising questions relative to the construction and strength of wood and iron hulls of vessels, and a description of the various parts and method of joining same), 30; pilot rules and inland navigation, 20; knowledge of lifeboats and life-rafts, 10; experience, 20. The criticisms of the examinations that were made in the early days of the commission have vanished before every thoroughgoing investigation into the scope and character of the questions themselves.

THE CASE OF THE RAILWAY MAIL SERVICE

The best answer to such criticisms, however, is to be found in the actual results produced by the system. As to these results, the men directly in charge of the departments and bureaus affected are, of course, best qualified to speak. Going back a few years, one of the most strik-ing instances of the effect of civil-service examinations on the standards of government employment is the notable improvement in the efficiency of the railway mail service as recorded from year to year in the official reports. It will be remembered that this important branch of the Post Office, after having been the football of both political parties for many years, was brought under the classified civil service during President Harrison's administration, in the year 1889. Prior to that time. Re-publican clerks had been turned out by a Democratic administration, and, in the early months of President Harrison's Republican administra-tion, a large number of Democratic clerks had in turn been dismissed. The whole service was utterly demoralized, and it probably reached at that time the lowest state of efficiency in its history. It was some months after the introduction of entrance examinations before the resulting change in the character of the appointees began to make itself felt in the general efficiency of the service. After a time, however, a marked im-provement was noted, and, in the opinion of those best qualified to judge, the advance was attributable mainly, if not wholly, to the application of the civil-service tests. For the fiscal year ended June 30, 1890, the errors in distribution committed by railway mail clerks amounted to the enor-mous total of 2,789,245. This meant that 2,834 pieces of mail matter were correctly handled to each error disclosed. Within the next twelve months, the number of errors had greatly decreased, and the number of pieces correctly handled to each error was found to be 4,261. There-after there was a steady decrease in the number of errors until the year 1898, when the number of errors had fallen below a million, and the number of "correct" pieces to each error was 11,960, the highest number ever reached by the service. Since that time the efficiency has been maintained at a relatively high level, the number of correct pieces to each error never falling below 10,000, and in 1904 exceeding 11,000. The sum of the whole matter is that in 1890, when the evils of the spoils system were still rife in the railway mail service, the clerks made an error to every 2,800 pieces of mail that they handled; while in recent years, the system, being manned by appointees chosen under the civil-service rules, the ratio of errors is one to every 11,000. This is a concrete case, in which every citizen is concerned, and it invites the attention of every business man who is interested in securing as high a state of efficiency in government work as has been attained by private enterprise.

General Gains in Economy and Efficiency

For obvious reasons, it has not been an easy matter to apply tests of this kind to the multifarious bureaus which make up the national civil service. The main difficulty is that many features of the arbitrary classification of clerkships, which was made more than fifty years ago, still survive. In most of the Government offices there is a failure to observe a logical division of duties. Thus, a $1,400 clerk will be found performing work of precisely the same character as that performed by a $1,200 clerk. Frequently a clerk promoted from $1,200 to $1,400 does exactly the same work after his promotion that he did before. All this confusion in the system makes it difficult to apply any general test showing how the efficiency of a bureau or department has been affected by the operation of the civil-service law. The officials of the Treasury Department will tell you, however, that in the customs service alone there has been an actual saving, in the matter of salaries, of at least 10 per cent. This would mean an annual saving to the Government of not less than two million dollars. Some years ago, it was estimated that altogether ten million dollars was saved to the Government in the various departments through the operation of the law, by the reduction in the required number of clerkships and the increased efficiency of the new employees. If this statement was justified when it was made, the saving to-day must be far greater, since many thousand offices have been added to the classified service within the last few years. That public opinion in the country at large has been favorably impressed by these object-lessons is shown by the agitations in various States and cities for local systems similar in principle and method to the federal civil-service establishment.

The Pay for Government Work

In regard to the compensation for government work, intelligent observation will probably confirm the epigrammatic statement in the newspaper witticism that has lately gone the rounds, to the effect that the pay is small for some public officials, but that some public officials are small for the pay. As a rule, the lower positions in the government service are paid more, and the higher positions less, than in private business. In most of the offices advancement is slower, but this is partly compensated for by the fact that the pay is higher on the whole in the earlier years. A man who has worked ten years for Uncle Sam will probably have had a gross income about equal to what a man of similar abilities, working the same length of time, would have received from a railroad company. At the start his salary would have been better than the railroad man's, but the latter in all likelihood would have caught up with him and outstripped him in the ten-year period. In the long run, one evens up with the other. This statement applies to the general departmental positions in Washington.

Young professional and scientific men of special qualifications are started on salaries corresponding pretty closely on the average with the salaries of "instructors" on college and university faculties. The government man has no long vacation in the year corresponding with that of the college professor. Furthermore, he is held more closely to the observation of office hours. Washington, however, has many attractions for this type of worker. He meets many men of his own degree of education and of similar aspirations, and in not a few cases scientific men, who have proved themselves capable investigators, have been put in responsible positions, where they virtually direct the work of many subordinates, and control the expenditure of considerable funds in the interest of scientific research. A few such men in Washington have undoubtedly attained such positions far more rapidly than would have been possible on any university faculty.

Washington offers further advantages to young men of promise who succeed in passing the examinations and obtain places in the departments. There are excellent law and medical schools in the city which accommodate their programmes of lectures to the department hours. It is quite the usual thing for young department clerks to pursue a three-year course of instruction, obtain degrees in law and medicine, and then resign their clerkships to embark upon professional careers. But this is by no means the whole purpose of such institutions as the George Washington University, which, under the vigorous administration of President Needham and Dean Tucker, of the Schools of Law, Jurisprudence, and Diplomacy, is making a serious and promising effort to provide courses of instruction that will actually qualify students to fill important posts, especially in the State Department, for which no other university makes systematic provision. There is an increasing number of positions in the departments, notably in the newly organized Department of Commerce and Labor, in which a sound knowledge of the law in one or more branches is a part of the qualifications required. A man entering on an ordinary clerkship may, by three or four years of study at the law school, qualify himself for one of these semi-technical legal positions. Such a man may reasonably expect quite as good an income in the form of a government salary as the average young lawyer gets in the early years of a private practice. As a life career, on the other hand, government work, it must be admitted, is less alluring to the young man of ambition. All the higher positions in the service are notoriously ill-paid. It is not at all unusual to find in Washington officials of long experience and the most thorough equipment, controlling the disbursement of many thousands of the Government's dollars, holding places of actual responsibility, and receiving a yearly stipend of $2,700, or even less. In some of the scientific bureaus there are compensating advantages, but in the general run of departmental positions, it is hard to discern any rewards at the top that are really worth striving for from the bottom. Most of the plums are on the lower branches of the tree.

FACTS ABOUT THE PERSONNEL

A great mass of information about the executive civil service, much of which it is impossible even to summarize in a magazine article, has recently been collected and published in Census Bulletin No. 12, by the Bureau of the Census. From the data thus compiled, it appears that of the 271,169 officers and employees in the service on June 30, 1903, 25,810 were employed within the District of Columbia, of which number 20,813 were included in the competitive class. The total number in the competitive class outside the District of Columbia at that time was 113,736. It also appears from these statistics that the ratio of men and women employed in Washington is 2.73 to 1, that outside of Washington it is 18.36 to 1, and that in the entire service it is 10.29 to 1. From the tabulation of salaries, excluding those classes of employees receiving less than $720 a year, and also those receiving more than $2,500 a year (most of whom are Presidential appointments), the approximate average annual salary of the Washington employee is $1,212, of those employed outside of Washington, $1,010, and of the entire service, $1,053. It is found that the average periods of service of employees were 10.55 years in Washington, 6.38 elsewhere, and 7.10 years in the entire service. In Washington, 5.54 per cent of the employees have served more than thirty years, while in the entire service the percentage is only 1.97. A comparison of the length of service of employees in the executive service with that of the employees of the New York Central & Hudson River Railroad, and the New York, New Haven & Hartford Railroad, revealed the fact that the government service contains a larger proportion of employees who have served over ten and less than twenty years; but, of those who served a longer period, the railroad companies can show a larger proportion.

As to the geographical distribution of government employees, the Eastern and central States of the Union are more fully represented than any other sections of the country among those who take examinations and receive appointments in the service. While Mr. Roosevelt was a Civil Service Commissioner, he made strenuous efforts to fill the quotas of the Southern States, which had long been far behind the North and

West in this regard. Much of the old prejudice against the administration of the law was overcome by Mr. Roosevelt's efforts, and it is believed that Southern young men and women are no longer deterred from entering the examinations by any feeling that they will fail to receive fair treatment. Nevertheless, the South is still backward in this respect, and the reason assigned by those who have given the matter special attention is that for the majority of Southern youth the opportunities for securing the kind of training necessary for a successful candidate in the examinations are relatively inferior to those possessed by young people in the North and West. Stenography and typewriting are almost invariably demanded at the present time as qualifications for a Washington clerkship. Throughout the Northern States, the facilities for qualifying in these branches have greatly multiplied within a few years, so that it is now possible for a young man or a young woman, even in the rural districts of Eastern or middle Western States, to secure a fair training in stenography and typewriting. This, however, is still impossible in large regions of the South.

The Moral Character of Appointees

A few months ago, the statement was carelessly made in an American magazine, that not five hundred of the Washington office-holders looked upon their offices as sacred trusts to the people. The author of the statement declared that public opinion among the civil-service employees regarded as clear gain anything that could be gotten out of the Government, whether an hour's time or a railroad pass for betraying the Government's interest under the care of the employees. Against such cheap and wholesale charges should be arrayed the undoubted consensus of opinion among those who have frequent business dealings with the departments, as well as among many disinterested observers in Washington who have had opportunities to study the facts that the average government employee is neither more nor less moral than the average man or woman employed in private business in any of our American cities. It will be recalled that in the post-office scandals of the past few years, the officials indicted have in every instance been political appointees; not one of the employees in the classified service has been found guilty of any form of corruption. The Government requires of all applicants for positions in its service just such indorsement of character as would be demanded by the head of any business house. It would be as reasonable to make wholesale charges of dishonesty against 98 per cent of the employees of the New York Central Railroad Company, as to make such charges against 98 per cent of Washington officialdom.

EXTENSION OF CIVIL-SERVICE RULES [1]

SIGNIFICANT of the present-day attitude has been the slight attention paid in any quarter to the orders amending the civil service rules, which the President signed just before his departure. The public merely notices that the screws have been turned a little tighter in the classified service, and there its interest ceases. This steady progress of the classified service is, however, having some notable results. Congressmen and friends of the Administration want a certain number of places, and the more fully the old ones are covered under the reform roof, the greater the enthusiasm for the creation of new positions, in order to have something to fill. This is one of the adverse effects of civil-service reform.

Privately, many congressmen are pleased to realize that there are now comparatively few spoils to be distributed. In public, especially when in the presence of constituents, they rail at the President and the Civil Service Commission. When Congress reconvenes, the House of Representatives will renew its old play of threatening to withhold all appropriations from the Commission. The President has gradually covered Government employees by the classified service until there are few places left with which the members of Congress may barter. Within the last three weeks, at least one hundred Republican members of the House of Representatives have searched every bureau of every department for some official crumbs that might be thrown to the hungry boys at home, and they all tell the same story — no crumbs are to be found.

In his first message to Congress President Roosevelt said that "the merit system of making appointments is, in its essentials, as democratic and American as the common school system itself. And wherever the conditions have permitted the application of the merit system in its fullest and widest sense, the gain to the Government has been immense."

A LIST OF THE EXTENSIONS

Within two months after he became President, Mr. Roosevelt turned his attention to those employees of the Government who were still outside the classified service. Here is a list of the extensions he has made since:

November 18, 1901 — Federal services, War Department, reincluded.

November 27, 1901 — Rural free delivery service, clerks, route inspectors, special agents, messengers, etc.

February 1, 1902 — Rural free delivery system carriers.

April 28, 1902 — At the President's suggestion temporary war emergency employees were transferred to the classified service by act of Congress.

July 1, 1902 — At the suggestion of the President Census Office employees were classified by act of Congress, March 6, 1902.

July 3, 1902 — Employees of the military government in Cuba appointed under special civil-service rules.

[1] *New York Evening Post*, April 7, 1905.

October 4, 1902 — Persons employed on construction of Government Printing Office building continued on War College and Washington Barracks under special civil-service rule.

February 11, 1903 — Temporary employees in insular naval stations transferred to the classified service.

February 11, 1903 — Employees at Post Office given free delivery between July 1, 1901, and June 30, 1903, covered by the classified service.

June 30, 1904 — By operation of the rules — employees in sixty-six post offices classified.

August 10, 1904 — The position of one clerk at each pension agency to act for the pension agent during his absence, transferred from the excepted to the competitive class.

March 26, 1904 — All positions under the War Department in the Philippines except those filled by persons employed as skilled laborers or persons appointed by the President, classified.

November 15, 1904 — Positions under the Isthmian Canal Commission, except those filled by persons employed as laborers, and persons whose appointment is confirmed by the Senate and engineers detailed from the army, classified.

November 23, 1904 — Positions of deputy collector, deputy surveyor, cashier, and naval officer in the customs service transferred from the excepted list to the classified service.

December 19, 1904 — Positions in the forestry service of the Department of the Interior made competitive.

June 22, 1904 — The positions of mail feeder and press feeder at the Philadelphia and New Orleans Mints included in the classified service at the request of the Treasury Department.

March 28, 1905 — Special agents of the Immigration Bureau on duty in foreign territory brought within the classified service.

April 3, 1905 — Positions of cashiers and finance clerks in post offices throughout the country, taken out of the excepted class, to be filled by promotion. Another order of the same date, relating to laborers in the departments at Washington, has been made familiar in recent despatches.

At the time Mr. Roosevelt became President there were, in round numbers, 83,000 persons in the classified service. The number is now 155,000. Within the last twelve months the service has shown a growth of about 14 per cent. Part of this is, of course, due to the natural growth of the system. In addition to these orders it has been provided that unclassified laborers at Washington and elsewhere should be selected by a system of competitive registration, taking account of age, physical condition, experience, and character. Thus 24,000 unclassified positions were made competitive.

RURAL FREE DELIVERY CLASSIFICATION

The order of the President that stands out most conspicuously is that placing the rural free delivery service in the classified list. At the time it was issued only 6,500 men were employed; now more than 25,000 are included.

One notable rule promulgated requires public officers in the Federal service to give testimony under oath before the Civil Service Commission when investigations are instituted. An honest effort has been made to cure abuses relating to transfers and reinstatements, and auditing and disbursing officers have been forbidden to pay salaries to persons holding positions in violation of the civil-service rules.

It is well understood that the President has further extensions of the classified service in mind. The rule that fourth-class postmasters are to be removed for cause may prove to be the forerunner of an executive order putting these public servants on a more secure basis. It is a reasonably safe guess that if the members of Congress do not accept without murmurings the rule that such postmasters shall be retained in office during good behavior and faithful service, the President will settle the whole controversy by classifying the 95,000 postmasters.

Back Door Closed

In their vain quest for places for constituents members of Congress have come to believe that the President has effectually closed the "back door" entrance to clerkships. From 1896 to 1901 it was an easy thing for a member of Congress with influence to find some back door through which he could push a constituent into a place without the trouble of consulting the Civil Service Commission. One of the favorite "back doors" led first to some remote country post office that was about to become a free delivery office. If the congressman had the proper amount of influence his constituent was put on the pay-roll of the remote post office, and as soon as it came into the classified service by reason of becoming a free delivery office the constituent was transferred to the place originally intended for him in one of the departments here. The post-office investigation revealed this crooked business, and in some instances persons who were found to be drawing salaries in post offices they had never seen, were made to give up their illegal salaries. The President soon put a stop to this by applying a rule that a transfer should not be made unless a person had actually served six months in the office from which he asked transfer, and also providing that the person in question must qualify for the new place by taking an examination.

Another "back door" which members of Congress found so convenient led to the laborers' rolls. Under the old régime, it was a common thing to appoint men as unclassified laborers and then, in due time, put them to work in the classified service. With the laborers covered by the classified service, this abuse no longer exists.

A Better Atmosphere

After all, it is the civil service "atmosphere" that is doing most to strengthen the merit system. The average departmental official, from the cabinet officer down, is about what the President of the United States wants him to be. The knowledge that Mr. Roosevelt believes in the merit system affects public sentiment mightily. A member of Congress from Indiana remarked, after he had failed to find places available for constituents, that officials said to him privately: "Of course, we might edge in a man notwithstanding the executive orders and the extensions of rules, but we do not dare do it."

Abuses of the system still exist. The late Senator Quay was not prosecuted for collecting campaign funds from the Federal appointees in Pennsylvania, while C. O. Self, a competent clerk in the internal revenue office at Terre Haute, was dismissed for the same offense. No one avers that the President did wrong in dismissing young Self, as that act settled the controverted question as to whether a person could be compelled to testify before the Commission, but to persons who watched the courses of the two cases it always seemed that the President ought to have insisted on a trial in the Quay case.

Undoubtedly the system needs corrective legislation, but Congress does not seem disposed to act. What to do with the men and women who have reached the age that unfits them for service is the great problem. Year by year the departments are becoming more topheavy. Cabinet officers have it within their power to discharge the aged and the infirm, but they will not do it, and perhaps they should not. Ten or twelve bills, offering remedies for this one defect, were before Congress last session, but none received consideration. The Civil Service Commission looks with favor on the plan to establish by law an annuity insurance system in the departments, and, generally speaking, the clerks favor this plan. Representative Gillett of Massachusetts, who was chairman of the Committee on the Reform of the Civil Service in the last Congress, and will probably be reassigned to that chairmanship, hopes for action of some kind at the coming session.

SENATOR HOAR ON APPOINTMENTS TO OFFICE [1]

[This extract deals briefly with the relations of the President to Congress in the matter of appointments.]

AMONG the great satisfactions in the life of public men is that of sometimes being instrumental in the advancement to places of public honor of worthy men, and of being able to have a great and salutary influence upon their lives. I have always held .to the doctrine of what is called Civil Service Reform, and have maintained to the best of my ability the doctrine of the absolute independence of the Executive in such matters, as his right to disregard the wishes or opinions of members of

[1] From Senator Hoar's *Autobiography*.

either House of Congress, and to make his appointments executive and judicial, without advice, or on such advice as he shall think best. But, at the same time, there can be no doubt that the Executive must depend upon some advice other than his own, to learn the quality of men in different parts of this vast Republic, and to learn what will be agreeable to public opinion and to the party which is administering the Government and is responsible for its administration. He will, ordinarily, find no better source of such information than in the men whom the people have shown their own confidence in by entrusting them with the important function of Senator or Representative. He will soon learn to know his men, and how far he can safely take such advice. He must be careful to see to it that he is not induced to build up a faction in his party, or to fill up the public offices with the partisans of ambitious but unscrupulous politicians. When I entered the House of Representatives, before the Civil Service Reform had made any progress, I addressed and had put on file with the Secretary of the Treasury a letter in which I said that I desired him to understand when I made a recommendation to him of any person for public office, it was to be taken merely as my opinion of the merit of the candidate, and not as an expression of a personal request; and that if he found any other person who would in his judgment be better for the public service, I hoped he would make the selection without regard to my recommendation.

I have never undertaken to use public office as personal patronage, or to claim the right to dictate to the President of the United States, or that the Executive was not entirely free, upon such advice as he saw fit, or without advice, if he thought fit, in making his selection for public office.

XIV

THE COURTS

FROM AN ADDRESS OF MR. JUSTICE FIELD DELIVERED
UPON THE OCCASION OF THE HUNDREDTH ANNI-
VERSARY OF THE COURT [1]

AND now, with its history in the century past, what is needed, that the Supreme Court of the United States should sustain its character and be as useful in the century to come? I answer, as a matter of the first consideration, — that it should not be overborne with work, and by that I mean it should have some relief from the immense burden now cast upon it. This can only be done by legislative action, and in determining what measures shall be adopted for that purpose Congress will undoubtedly receive with favor suggestions from the Bar Associations of the country. The Justices already do all in their power, for each one examines every case and passes his individual judgment upon it. No case in the Supreme Court is ever referred to any one Justice, or to several of the Justices, to decide and report to the others. Every suitor, however humble, is entitled to and receives the judgment of every Justice upon his case.

In considering this matter it must be borne in mind that, in addition to the great increase in the number of admiralty and maritime cases, from the enlarged commerce on the seas, and on the navigable waters of the United States, and in the number of patent cases from the multitude of inventions brought forth by the genius of our people, calling for judicial determination, even to the extent of occupying a large portion of the time of the court, many causes, which did not exist upon its organization or during the first quarter of the century, have added enormously to its business. Thus by the new agencies of steam and electricity in the movement of the machinery and transmission of intelligence, creating railways and steamboats, telegraphs and telephones, and adding almost without number to establishments for the manufacture of fabrics, transactions are carried on to an infinitely greater extent than before between different States, leading to innumerable

---

[1] Reprinted in Carson, History of the Supreme Court, I, 713.

controversies between their citizens which have found their way to that tribunal for decision. More than one-half of the business before it for years has arisen from such controversies.[1]

The facility with which corporations can now be formed has also increased its business far beyond what it was in the early part of the century. Nearly all enterprises requiring for their successful prosecution large investments of capital are conducted by corporations. They, in fact, embrace every branch of industry, and the wealth that they hold in the United States equals in value four-fifths of the entire property of the country. They carry on business with the citizens of every State as well as with foreign nations, and the litigation is enormous, giving rise to every possible question to which the jurisdiction of the Federal courts extend.

The numerous grants of the public domain, embracing hundreds of millions of acres, in aid of the construction of railways; also for common schools, for public buildings and institutions of much intricacy and difficulty. The discovery of mines of the precious metals, in our new possessions on the Pacific Coast, and the modes adopted for their development, have added many more. The legislation required by the exigencies of the civil war, and following it, and the constitutional amendments which were designed to give farther security to personal rights, have brought before the court questions of the greatest interest and importance, calling for the most earnest and laborious consideration. Indeed, the cases which have come before this court, springing from causes which did not exist during the first quarter of the century, exceed, in the magnitude of the property interests presented, all cases brought within the same period before any court of Christendom.

Whilst the constitutional amendments have not changed the structure of our dual form of government, but are additions to the previous amendments, and are to be considered in connection with them and the original Constitution as one instrument, they have removed from existence an institution which was felt by wise statesmen to be inconsistent with the great declarations of right upon which our government is founded; and they have vastly enlarged the subjects of Federal jurisdiction. The amendment declaring that neither slavery nor involuntary servitude, except as a punishment for crime, shall exist in the United States or any place subject to their jurisdiction, not only has done away with slavery of the black man, as it then existed, but interdicts forever the slavery of any man, and not only slavery, but involuntary servitude — that is, serfage, vassalage, villeinage, peonage, and all other forms of compulsory service for the mere benefit or pleasure of others. As has often been said, it was intended to make every one born in this country a free man

---

[1] [By the creation of Circuit Courts of Appeals in 1891, the volume of business in the Supreme Court was greatly diminished. These courts are final in matters such as are mentioned above, unless a question of constitutionality is involved.]

and to give him a right to pursue the ordinary vocations of life without other restraint than such as effects all others, and to enjoy equally with them the fruits of his labor. The right to labor as he may think proper without injury to others is an element of that freedom which is his birth-right.

The amendment, declaring that no State shall make or enforce any law which shall abridge the privileges or immunities of citizens of the United States, nor deprive any person of life, liberty, or property without due process of law, nor deny to any person within its jurisdiction the equal protection of the laws, has proclaimed that equality before the law shall forever be the governing rule of all the States of the Union, which every person however humble may invoke for his protection. In enforcing these provisions, or considering the laws adopted for their enforcement, or laws which are supposed to be in conflict with them, difficult and far-reaching questions are presented at every term for decision.

Up to the middle of the present century the calendar of the Court did not average 140 cases a term, and never amounted in any one term to 300 cases; the calendar of the present term exceeds 1,500. In view of the condition of the Court — its crowded docket — the multitude of questions constantly brought before it of the greatest and most extended influence — surely it has a right to call upon the country to give it assistance and relief. Something must be done in that direction and should be done speedily to prevent the delays to suitors now existing. To delay justice is as pernicious as to deny it. One of the most precious articles of Magna Charta was that in which the King declared that he would not deny nor delay to any man justice or right. And assuredly what the barons of England wrung from their monarch, the people of the United States will not refuse to any suitor for justice in their tribunals.

Furthermore, I hardly need say, that, to retain the respect and confidence conceded in the past, the Court, whilst cautiously abstaining from assuming powers granted by the Constitution to other departments of the government, must unhesitatingly and to the best of its ability enforce, as heretofore, not only all the limitations of the Constitution upon the Federal and State governments, but also all the guarantees it contains of the private rights of the citizen, both of person and of property. As population and wealth increase — as the inequalities in the conditions of men become more and more marked and disturbing — as the enormous aggregation of wealth possessed by some corporations excites uneasiness lest their power should become dominating in the legislation of the country, and thus encroach upon the rights or crush out the business of individuals of small means, — as population in some quarters presses upon the means of subsistence, and angry menaces against order find vent in loud denunciations — it becomes more and more the imperative duty of the Court to enforce with a firm hand every

45

guarantee of the Constitution. Every decision weakening their restraining power is a blow to the peace of society and to its progress and improvement. It should never be forgotten that protection to property and to persons can not be separated. Where property is insecure, the rights of persons are unsafe. Protection to the one goes with protection to the other; and there can be neither prosperity nor progress where either is uncertain.

That the Justices of the Supreme Court must possess the ability and learning required by the duties of their office, and a character for purity and integrity beyond reproach, need not be said. But it is not sufficient for the performance of his judicial duty that a judge should act honestly in all that he does. He must be ready to act in all cases presented for his judicial determination with absolute fearlessness. Timidity, hesitation, and cowardice in any public office, excite and deserve only contempt, but infinitely more in a judge than in any other, because he is appointed to discharge a public trust of the most sacred character. To decide against his conviction of the law of judgment as to the evidence, whether moved by prejudice or passion, or the clamor of the crowd, is to assent to a robbery as infamous in morals and as deserving of punishment as that of the highwaymen or the burglar; and to hesitate or refuse or act when duty calls is hardly less the subject of just reproach. If he is influenced by apprehensions that his character will be attacked, or his motives inpugned, or that his judgment will be attributed to the influence of particular classes, cliques, or associations, rather than to his own convictions of the law, he will fail lamentably in his high office.

THE SUPREME COURT OF THE UNITED STATES [1]

BY DAVID J. BREWER [2]

IT would be an easy and a pleasant task to point out how in many other ways the court has by its decisions affected the life of the republic, but the limits of my paper forbid. This must do for the past. As admitted by all careful students of history, the Supreme Court, whose organization and powers constitute the most striking and distinguishing feature of the Constitution, has been a most potent factor in shaping the course of national events. It stands to-day a quiet but confessedly mighty power, whose action all wait for, and whose decisions all abide. Turning to the future, every thoughtful man wonders what is coming to the republic, and many inquire what the Supreme Court will do in shaping that future, and how its decisions may affect the national life.

[1] Part of an article in *Scribner's Magazine*, March, 1903. Reprinted by permission. Copyright.
[2] Associate Justice.

The questions which now seem likely to arise and to be pressed upon judicial attention may be grouped in four classes: First, those growing out of the controversies between labor and capital; second, those that will spring from the manifest efforts to increase and concentrate the power of the nation and to lessen the powers of the States; third, those arising out of our new possessions, separate from us by so long distances and with so large a population, not merely of foreign tongue, but of a civilization essentially different from that of the Anglo-Saxon; and, fourth, those which will come because our relations to· all other nations have grown to be so close and will surely increase in intimacy.

Of these in their order. That the present relations of employer and employee differ from those which subsisted when the Constitution was framed is obvious. Three facts stand out in bold relief: First, the changes wrought by the countless inventions of the last half-century; second, the concentration of capital; and, third, the organization of labor. When all business was upon a small scale, when there were no large factories, and when the great volume of labor was hand labor, competition was regarded as a great solvent of all commercial troubles. Now competition has lost much of its force and as a result of the three facts that I have just noticed. I can not enlarge upon this subject, and yet a few words seem necessary. The industrial field was then occupied by the apprentice, the journeyman, and the employer. The apprentice was taught to do every part of the general work in which he was employed, and when so taught was recognized as a competent workman, a journeyman. The latter, master of his trade, could with a little economy soon establish a shop of his own, and himself become an employer. Take, for illustration, the manufacture of shoes. No one was considered a competent workman or anything more than an apprentice until he could do all the work in the making of a shoe, from cutting out the leather to polishing the uppers. The employer often worked with his employee, in the same shop, doing the same work. The number of his employees was few, and one by one the capable and industrious were opening shops of their own and starting in independent business. If the journeyman was dissatisfied with his employer or with the town in which he worked, there was little difficulty in finding another shop or another village. The avenues of employment were not crowded, and there was no blacklisting. The employer, if he found his business unprofitable, could easily move to another city and start a like business. If his prices were excessive some new man would start a rival establishment. Thus competition levelled prices and kept them reasonable. Not unnaturally there was a community of interest and at the same time an independence in both employer and employee. But to-day, through the inventive genius of the country, machines have superseded hand labor. The manufactory has taken the place of the shop, and labor finds its chief employment in the handling of machines, each employee doing only a special limited work. Some of the machines are costly and large amounts of capital are invested. For economy's sake the work is centered in large manufacturing establishments, where are gathered multitudes of machines and armies of laborers. The employer has become separated from his employees. They stand to him as meaning little more than the machines upon which they work. One significant and sad feature of not a few of our manufacturing establishments is the large boarding-house, where are gathered a multitude of laborers, like soldiers in barracks. Nor is there simply the large and separate manufacturing establishments; combinations have been formed by which all the factories of a single industry are brought under a single control. Difficult then is the position of the employee, who, familiar with only a particular and narrow work, finds, when discharged from one factory, the doors of all others closed against him. He feels that he must stay and accept the terms which the manufacturer has placed upon his service. So severe and stringent is the pressure upon him that not infrequently we hear his condition called the serfdom of labor. Nor is the pressure simply upon the employee. A combination of employers is often so rich and so powerful that one who would like to carry on an independent business is driven to the wall and has no other alternative than to go out of business or surrender to the combination. This which is true of manufacturing is also true of the mercantile business and of transportation; and combinations, some of them of immense wealth and far-reaching influence, have become the order of the day.

It is not strange, indeed it was the inevitable result of this subdivision of labor and such combinations of employers, that the laborers in the several departments should themselves organize. Labor organizations are as much the natural outgrowth of the economic conditions of the day as combinations of capital. We thus have, on the one hand, a few possessing or controlling immense amounts of capital and large industries, and, on the other hand, multitudes of laborers banded into organizations for self-protection. Self-interest (I will not call it selfishness) has operated to develop a great antagonism between these two factors in industry; each in seeking a greater control, a larger share of the profits resulting from the combined services of both. As organizations of laborers increase the influence and significance of a strike, which is one of their weapons in carrying on what is called the conflict between labor and capital, become greater. The summer of last year we stood face to face with one of immense magnitude, one affecting the business of the nation as none other has yet done. How shall these strikes be avoided? A man can scarcely count the suggestions which have been and are being made with a view of averting them in the future. The coal strike has precipitated more schemes of legislation, more suggestions of the extent of legislative and executive as well as judicial power than any which has preceded it. All legislative bodies, State and national, will be confronted with propositions to prevent or regulate struggles between labor and capital. Is it not reasonably certain that out of these conflicts and out of the legislation which may be enacted by Congress or the several State legislatures there will arise a multitude of questions, many of which will finally reach the Supreme Court of the United States?

Let me mention one or two which are frequently mentioned in the newspapers and discussed in private. Compulsory arbitration is thought by many to be necessary, and the only possible solution of these labor troubles. We are referred to New Zealand as furnishing an illustration of the possibility and wisdom of such an enactment. But what does such a scheme imply? On the one hand possibly the compulsion of the employer to pay more than he can afford or else quit business. On the other hand, of the laborer to work for an employer he does not like, and at less wage than he feels himself entitled to. How does such compulsion consist with that freedom of personal action which for more than a hundred years we have believed was the inalienable right of every individual? It is said in support of the proposed enactment that to prescribe the conditions under which an employer may carry on his business, leaving him free to abandon the business and pursue some other, and like compulsion of the laborer to work at a certain wage and place if he continues in a certain kind of employment, does not abridge any constitutional right of either when the larger interests of society demand such compulsion. But if compulsion may be introduced into one employment, why not into all? I can not spend the time to enlarge upon the arguments of either side, nor would it be proper to express any opinion as to the respective merits of such arguments. It is enough to say that if legislation be enacted looking toward compulsory arbitration it is obvious that there will be much to challenge the most careful consideration of the courts.

Again, we hear it said that the Nation or State should take the coal mines under condemnation proceedings and operate them for the public benefit. The power to do this is denied on the ground that private property can be taken only for public uses, and the furnishing of coal is said to be not a public service, that coal is no more a necessity of life than bread, meats, or clothing; that if the State can enter into the business of supplying coal it can into all these other matters, and for that purpose condemn all places in which such things are grown or manufactured. And it is contended by some that the State can under our constitutional limitations take to itself the control, ownership, and operation of all now known as private industries. On the other hand, and in reply to some of these arguments, it is said that the ordinary products of the soil can be grown or manufactured in many places, but that nature has created a monopoly in anthracite coal by locating it in only one or two portions of the United States; that by reason of the monopoly thus created by nature the power of the public to interfere and take possession is established.

I do not stop to notice the suggestions of government ownership of railroads, telegraph, telephones, electric lines, water and gas works, for as to them, or at least most of them, they are confessedly performing a public service, and the question of governmental possession and control is mainly one of expediency rather than of constitutionality, and the courts have nothing to do with questions of expediency.

Obviously in these and many kindred suggestions there is manifest a spirit of paternalism. The individual is not to be left to make his own contracts, determine his place and kind of work, or use his property in the way he sees fit. The government is to exercise the functions of a guardian, with the individual as its ward, to be in many respects protected, guided, and controlled. This is not wholly the idea that pervaded the old monarchical system, for there the king as a single ruler assumed the wisdom and the right to control the actions of all his subjects, while here the majority are the ruler, yet it is equally an assumption that the majority have the same right to control. It is true the belief is that such control is for the best interests of those controlled or of the general public. Yet it is unlike the thought which possessed the fathers at the foundation of the Republic. Their idea was expressed in the Declaration of Independence, "all men are created equal"; "inalienable rights of life, liberty, and the pursuit of happiness," and their purpose was to give the freest scope to individual action. The marvelous mystery which lies folded in the doctrine of the police powers of the government was to them unknown. I am not questioning either the necessity or the wisdom of the change. I only notice the fact that the thought of to-day is different from that which then existed, and that the tendency of legislation is in a different direction. Now the Constitution was framed by those who had large notions of individual liberty and a jealousy of governmental power, and the profound question is how far the language and guarantees of the Constitution are, if unchanged, consistent with legislation expressing these changed ideas. That it may be amended so as to be adjustable to any social order is provided by the Constitution itself. Without amendment how far is it adjustable? That many conditions and questions unknown to the fathers have been presented and found capable of solution without any change in the language of the Constitution the history of the past 115 years attests. In the judgment of not a few it is without amendment adjustable to any conditions, social and political, that may arise. Indeed, as one reads some of the propositions which are advanced, he is inclined to believe that the instrument possesses an elasticity which would make the manufacturers of india-rubber choke with envy. Fortunately and wisely, its grants, prohibitions, and guarantees were expressed tersely and yet in general terms, so that it has proved to be no cast-iron instrument applicable only to conditions then existing. But the question remains how far its general and comprehensive terms may be adjusted to the varying situations which the present and future days will present, and this matter of adjustability will bring before the court some of the profoundest and most important questions ever presented to any tribunal.

I pass now to notice some questions which may arise from the manifest effort to concentrate power in the United States and to lessen the powers of the respective States. Ever since the Civil War many have spelled nation with a big N, and there have been constant efforts to enlarge the activity, if not increase the powers, of Congress. The centralizing tendency has been marked. It is not unnatural. It harmonizes with the consolidating spirit of business, the unifying movement in all the activities of life. In matters over which it is manifest that Congress has no power under the Constitution, there is much clamor to so amend that instrument as to invest it with the desired control. Polygamy must be stamped out, and as only national action will reach everywhere in the Republic the Constitution must be amended so as to grant full control to the nation. Uniformity in the matter of marriage and divorce is desirable. The States do not agree in establishing such uniformity, therefore let by constitutional amendment Congress be given power to compel it. Commerce between the States is now subject to Congressional regulation, that within each State under its control, but those two branches of commerce are so interwoven as to produce much confusion and irritation. If all power in respect to commerce were taken away from the States and the entire control both of that between the States and that within the States vested in Congress, a desirable uniformity could be obtained, and in this direction is a clamor for a change in the organic law. The trusts are a dangerous factor in our commercial and political life. The States are not adequate to suppress them, hence the Constitution should be amended and full power over them vested in Congress. And so I might go on enumerating others. I simply mention these, not as suggesting matters for judicial decision, for under the power of amendment reserved in the Constitution the people may, if they see fit, engraft any of them upon the organic law and the courts have nothing to say. However wise or unwise any of these changes may be, if the people will it and amend the Constitution in the appointed way, that is the end of the matter.

But judicial questions may arise from efforts under the Constitution as it is to secure action by Congress in some one or other of these or kindred directions, and action which it is contended the Constitution withholds from the power of Congress and has reserved to the States or the people thereof. And because of the centralizing tendency of the day and the disposition to invoke the efficient action of the National Government there will doubtless be many such efforts. But as Chief Justice Chase said in *Texas* v. *White*, 7 Wall. 725: "The Constitution, in all its provisions, looks to an indestructible union, composed of indestructible States." And the Tenth Amendment to the Constitution provides that "the powers not delegated to the United States by the Constitution, nor prohibited by it to the States, are reserved to the States respectively, or to the people." It is the duty of the Supreme Court, as of all other courts, to enforce that provision of the Constitution as fairly and fully as any other. Any legislation of Congress, however desirable or beneficial it may appear, must, unless it comes within the powers given by the Constitution to that body, be declared invalid. Equally also must any action of a State in attempting to exercise dominion over matters the exclusive control of which is vested in Congress be adjudged unconstitutional. No one can predict the precise legislation coming either from Congress or the State legislatures which will challenge judicial inquiry upon the principles just stated. Both sides have strong adherents. The controversy between National authority and State's rights is as old as the Government. Hamilton and Jefferson have each to-day a large following. State's rights have always been and still are represented in Congress, and there have always been and still are in both Houses some of the ablest lawyers of the land, who will be careful that no legislation of that body trespasses on the powers of the States. Yet when public feeling is deeply aroused and the efficiency of national action is felt, popular pressure may be so great that Congress yields to it and enacts laws beyond its powers. At any rate, it is not only possible but probable that some of its legislation may be so near the boundary of power as to challenge judicial inquiry. Take, for instance, the Sherman Anti-Trust Act, which was framed with the view of exercising only those powers which are conferred upon Congress over interstate commerce, and yet its application was invoked in behalf of interference with manufactures wholly under State control. So also a difficult problem is to draw the dividing line between the exclusive control which Congress has over interstate commerce and the police powers which are reserved to the States. The reports of the court are full of cases on one side or the other of such line. In no class of cases has the court been more closely divided. *Leisy* v. *Hardin*, 135 U. S. 100, in which the power of a State to forbid the sale in the original package of imported liquor was denied is a well-known illustration. Two cases are now pending in which is challenged the power of Congress to restrain the transportation by express companies of lottery tickets from State to State. The great irrigation problem in respect to the arid lands in the West which is just now attracting legislative attention will very likely produce some sharp controversies in respect to the limits of State and National action. And so I might go on in enumeration. It is safe to say that the antagonism between National authority and State's rights which began with the Republic and which has become intensified by the vast interests affected by it, will bring into the Supreme Court an increasing number of important and difficult questions. Where millions are at stake the ingenuity of lawyers may be depended on to find some way of entrance to the court of last resort.

In the third place, questions will arise out of our insular possessions, and questions different from those which have attended previous acquisitions of territory, because unlike them these are densely populated with peoples speaking another tongue, of an essentially different civilization, alien in life and thought to Anglo-Saxon institutions. To what extent the provisions of the Constitution operate in those possessions is yet undetermined. It was held by the court in *DeLima* v. *Bidwell*, 182 U. S. 1, that by the treaty of peace between the United States and Spain the island of Porto Rico ceased to be a foreign country, within the meaning of the tariff laws. In *Downes* v. *Bidwell*, *id.* 244, the court, by five to four, held that Porto Rico was not a part of the United States, within the provision of the Constitution requiring uniformity in duties, imposts, and excises throughout the United States. From that conclusion four of the Justices dissented, and the majority did not agree in the reasoning by which that conclusion was reached. Justice White, one of the majority, speaking for Justices Shiras, McKenna, and himself, laid down these propositions: "Every function of the government being thus derived from the Constitution, it follows that that instrument is everywhere and at all times potential in so far as its provisions are applicable. . . . As Congress in governing the territories is subject to the Constitution, it results that all the limitations of the Constitution which are applicable to Congress in exercising this authority necessarily limit its power on this subject. It follows also that every provision of the Constitution which is applicable to the territories is also controlling therein. . . . In the case of the territories, as in every other instance, when a provision of the Constitution is invoked, the question which arises is, not whether the Constitution is operative, for that is self-evident but whether the provision relied on is applicable." In construing these declarations of three of the majority along with the views of the four dissenting Justices questions will naturally arise as to the force of the word "applicable." These are several provisions in the early amendments to the Constitution, designed to secure the liberty of the individual, such as that Congress shall make no law respecting the establishment of religion, or abridging the freedom of speech; forbidding that any person thall be held to answer for a crime except upon indictment of a grand jury; that he be twice put in jeopardy of life or limb, or compelled to be a witness against himself; granting him the right to a speedy public trial by an impartial jury of the district wherein the crime was committed; to be informed of the nature and cause of the accusation; to be confronted with the witnesses against him; to have compulsory process for obtaining witnesses and to have the assistance of counsel; and the further provision securing in suits at common law the right of trial by jury. Are any or all of these provisions applicable to these insular possessions? They have been applied in other territories having mainly a population as foreign to our language and institutions as that of these recent acquisitions. If some are and others are not, upon what principle is the distinction to be made? and if none are what provisions of the Constitutions are applicable? Obviously, as citizens of American birth move into these possessions, acquire property and engage in business, many questions of this nature will arise, and the court will be confronted with problems as difficult as any it has yet met and as important for the well-being of the Republic. An application was recently made for a *certiorari* to bring up a case involving as alleged the applicability in the Philippine Islands of the prohibition against being twice put in jeopardy of life or limb.

But I must not tarry. It is enough to say that the taking of these insular possessions is a new venture, and no one can anticipate all the novel questions which will arise therefrom and be presented to the Supreme Court for its decision. Do I in virtue of these possibilities and the responsibilities which will rest upon the court unduly magnify its office and function in the development of the history of the Republic?

The final class which I suggested is of cases growing out of our relations with other nations, which as all perceive are more intimate than in days gone by, and are surely to become much more so. I do not assume that this nation will forget Washington's farewell advice to avoid entangling alliances with foreign nations. But our rapidly extending commerce and our new possessions, especially those in the Orient, place us in close touch with the outer world. We can not, if we would, live to ourselves alone. We must sit in the council of the nations. The questions which will consequently arise are not all political; many are judicial. And our dealings with foreign nations must be had with a recognition of the fact that here, far more than anywhere else, those questions can not be finally determined for the nation save by the action of the judicial department. A pertinent illustration is found in the case of *Tucker* v. *Alexandroff*, recently decided and reported in 183 U. S. 424, 434. We had a treaty with Russia for the surrender of deserters from ships of war and merchant vessels. The Russian Government employed a Philadelphia firm to build a war ship, the Variag, and when near completion it sent a body of men over to serve as its crew. One deserted, was arrested at the instance of the Russian vice-consul at Philadelphia and committed for surrender to the Russian authorities. He sued out a *habeas corpus* for a discharge from that detention, and the case in due time came to the Supreme Court. The court was divided in opinion, but the majority held that the detention was justifiable and that the deserter should be surrendered to the Russian authorities. The interpretation of that treaty and the defining of the obligations of our Government to Russia were judicial questions, and the Supreme

Court prescribed the measure of this nation's duty. The recent Spanish War brought to the court many questions of prize in which the duties and obligations of neutrals were defined. Not merely in the construction of treaties, in matters of extradition and prize will the work of the court be seen, but in all the variety of questions which will grow out of the facts that our people are traveling through all countries of the world, our merchants trading in every city, our ships traversing every ocean and visiting every port. Further, we are contemplating such works outside our territorial limits as the Isthmian Canal for furthering the interests of the world's commerce, our own included, and who can predict all the questions that such enterprises will present to the courts?

Knowledge of international law has thus become a necessity, and the Supreme Court will be called upon to settle for this country what it is and what it requires. Our Federal system will also precipitate a class of questions not arising elsewhere. For instance, when some citizens of Italy were killed by a mob in New Orleans a demand was made by Italy upon this Government for the prosecution and punishment of the offenders, and the reply was in substance that the nation had no power in the matter; that prosecution for such crimes depended on the action of the State of Louisiana, and all that the nation could do was to call the attention of the authorities of that State to it and request action by them. A suggestion was made that Congress enact a law giving Federal courts jurisdiction in such cases, but the constitutionality of such an enactment was seriously challenged and nothing was done.

Time forbids any further illustrations of the variety of questions which are likely to come before the Supreme Court. Surely a tribunal called upon to decide such cases and questions must have great weight in shaping the destinies of the Republic. It will continue to be, as it has been, a most important factor in our national life. That its influence has been helpful few will doubt. That it should be shorn of none of its power is generally affirmed by disinterested observers. No specious plea against government by injunction should ever be permitted to take from it that wholesome restraining influence which has been so powerful for good.

May I add in closing that it is of the utmost importance that such a tribunal should be independent, free from partisan bias or political influence. Its members should, if not by constitutional amendment at least by the common action of all, be debarred from political office, so that no temptation of office or popular applause shall ever swerve from the simple path of justice, and the Constitution. In these days of newspaper reputation and ofttimes swiftly changing popularity it is well to have some tribunal of stability, one whose judgments do not vary with the varying opinions of the passing hours and do not, as Mr. Dooley says, simply "follow the election returns." The life tenure of its members does not make it an undemocratic factor in the life of the Republic. It does not govern the nation. The people are always the rulers. More than once have they reversed its judgments; but by reason of its stability and independence it has ever stood a check upon all hasty action; a brake on the swiftly moving wheels of popular passion, and holding ever the Republic close to the ways prescribed by the fathers in the Constitution. As it has been, so may it be. Each member of that tribunal should be animated by a noble ambition to be ever loyal to justice and the Constitution, no matter what may be temporary criticisms. He should appropriate in his life the spirit of the memorable words of Lord Mansfield, uttered in the presence of a mob demanding a particular decision: "I wish popularity, but it is that popularity which follows, not that which is run after. It is that popularity which sooner or later never fails to do justice to the pursuit of noble ends by noble means."

REMARKS OF MR. JUSTICE HARLAN ON THE METHODS OF THE SUPREME COURT [1]

THERE is one subject, Mr. Chairman, to which I am asked to reply and to which I deem it appropriate to refer. It is quite pertinent to the toast. I allude to the mode in which the business of the Supreme Court of the United States is conducted. In my intercourse with the members of the bar, I have found to my great surprise that the impression prevails with some that cases, after being submitted, are divided among the judges, and that the court bases its judgment in each one wholly upon the report made by some one judge to whom that case has been assigned for examination and report. I have met with lawyers who actually believed that the opinion was written before the case was decided in conference, and that the only member of the court who fully examined the record and briefs was the one who prepared the opinion.

It is my duty to say that the business in our court is not conducted in any such mode. Each justice is furnished with a printed copy of the record and with a copy of each brief filed, and each one examines the records and briefs at his chambers before the case is taken up for consideration. The cases are thoroughly discussed in conference — the discussion in some being necessarily more extended than in others. The discussion being concluded — and it is never concluded until each member of the court has said all that he desires to say — the roll is called and each justice present and participating in the decision votes to affirm, reverse or modify, as his examination and reflection suggests. The chief justice, after the conference, and without consulting his brethren, distributes the cases so decided for opinions. No justice knows, at the time he votes in a particular case, that he will be asked to become the organ of the court in that case; nor does any member of the court ask that a particular case be assigned to him.

[1] *American Law Review*, 30: 904.

The next step is the preparation of the opinion by the justice to whom it has been assigned. The opinion, when prepared, is privately printed, and a copy placed in the hands of each member of the court for examination and criticism. It is examined by each justice, and returned to the author, with such criticisms and objections as are deemed necessary. If these objections are of a serious kind, affecting the general trend of the opinion, the writer calls the attention of the justice to them, that they may be passed upon. The author adopts such suggestions of mere form as meet his views. If objections are made to which the writer does not agree, they are considered in conference, and are sustained or overruled as the majority may determine. The opinion is reprinted so as to express the final conclusions of the court, and is then filed.

Thus, you will observe, not only is the utmost care taken to make the opinion express the views of the court, but that the final judgment rests, in every case decided, upon the examination by each member of the court of the record and briefs. Let me say that, during my entire service in the Supreme Court, I have not known a single instance in which the court has determined a case merely upon the report of one or more justices as to what was contained in the record and as to what questions were properly presented by it. When you find an opinion of the court on file and published, the profession have the right to take it as expressing the deliberate views of the court, based upon a careful examination of the records and briefs by each justice participating in the judgment.

What I have said will give you some idea of the labor necessary to be performed by the members of the Supreme Court. How well it has been performed it is not for any member of the court to declare. Quite certain it is that the country believed that more was imposed upon the court than could be met with due regard to the interests of litigants, and to the prompt despatch of judicial business. Hence, the establishment of Circuit Courts of Appeals, whose decisions are final in large classes of cases of which the Supreme Court heretofore had jurisdiction upon appeal or writ of error. Time has vindicated, in the judgment of many, the scheme of the act of 1891, creating an intermediate Appellate Court in each Circuit. It is beyond question that that act will have the effect in a very short time to so reduce the number of cases which may, of right, be carried from the Circuit Courts directly to the Supreme Court of the United States, that that court will have no more cases upon its docket, at the beginning of each session, than can be disposed of during the term.

While at the beginning of the October term of 1890 the cases on the docket of the Supreme Court aggregated 1,406, the number on the docket at the beginning of the term to commence on the 12th day of the present month will not exceed 625. And it is safe to say that the entire number which will be on our docket at the beginning of the October term, 1898, will not exceed 350. Let this result speak for itself.

THE SUPREME COURT ON JUDICIAL POWER

[The following extract from the decision of the Supreme Court in the case of *Kansas v. Colorado*, 206 U. S. 46 (1907), announces a most important principle that the judicial power is subject only to express constitutional limitations. Mr. Gardiner in his essay on executive powers (see p. 12) had announced the same principle with regard to the executive. See also Senator Spooner's argument, *infra.*]

MR. Justice BREWER delivered the opinion of the court:

While we said in overruling the demurrer, that "this court, broadly speaking, has jurisdiction," we contemplated further consideration of both the fact and the extent of our jurisdiction, to be fully determined after the facts were presented. We therefore commence with this inquiry. And first, of our jurisdiction of the controversy between Kansas and Colorado.

This suit involves no question of boundary or of the limits of territorial jurisdiction. Other and incorporeal rights are claimed by the respective litigants. Controversies between the states are becoming frequent, and, in the rapidly changing conditions of life and business, are likely to become still more so. Involving, as they do, the rights of political communities which in many respects are sovereign and independent, they present not infrequently questions of far-reaching import and of exceeding difficulty.

It is well, therefore, to consider the foundations of our jurisdiction over controversies between states. It is no longer open to question that by the Constitution a nation was brought into being, and that that instrument was not merely operative to establish a closer union or league of states. Whatever powers of government were granted to the nation or reserved to the states (and for the description and limitation of these powers we must always accept the Constitution as alone and absolutely controlling), there was created a nation, to be known as the United States of America, and as such then assumed its place among the nations of the world.

The first resolution passed by the convention that framed the Constitution, sitting as a committee of the whole, was, "Resolved, that it is the opinion of this committee that a national government ought to be established, consisting of a supreme legislative, judiciary, and executive." 1 Eliot, Debates, p. 151.

In *M'Culloch v. Maryland*, 4 Wheaton, 316, 405, Chief Justice Marshall said:

"The government of the Union, then (whatever may be the influence of this fact on the case), is, emphatically and truly, a government of the people. In form and in substance it emanates from them. Its powers are granted by them, and are to be exercised directly on them, and for their benefit."

See also *Martin* v. *Hunter*, 1 Wheat. 304, 324, opinion by Mr. Justice Story.

In *Scott* v. *Sandford*, 19 How. 393, 441, Chief Justice Taney observed:

"The new government was not a mere change in a dynasty, or in a form of government, leaving the nation or sovereignty the same, and clothed with all the rights, and bound by all the obligations, of the preceding one. But, when the present United States came into existence under the new government, it was a new political body, a new nation then for the first time taking its place in the family of nations."

And in Miller on the Constitution of the United States, p. 83, referring to the adoption of the Constitution, that learned jurist said: "It was then that a nation was born."

In the Constitution are provisions in separate articles for the three great departments of government, — legislative, executive, and judicial. But there is this significant difference in the grants of powers to these departments: The first article treating of legislative powers does not make a general grant of legislative power. It reads: "Article 1, section 1. All legislative powers herein granted shall be vested in a Congress," etc.; and then in article 8, mentions and defines the legislative powers that are granted. By reason of the fact that there is no general grant of legislative power it has become an accepted constitutional rule that this is a government of enumerated powers.

In *M'Culloch* v. *Maryland*, 4 Wheat. 405, Chief Justice Marshall said:

"This government is acknowledged by all to be one of enumerated powers. The principle that it can exercise only the powers granted to it would seem too apparent to have required to be enforced by all those arguments which its enlightened friends, while it was depending before the people, found it necessary to urge. That principle is now universally admitted."

On the other hand, in article 3, which treats of the judicial department, — and this is important for our present consideration, — we find that section 1 reads that "the judicial power of the United States shall be vested in one Supreme Court, and in such inferior courts as Congress may from time to time ordain and establish." By this is granted the entire judicial power of the nation. Section 2 which provides that "the judicial power shall extend to all cases, in law and equity, arising under this Constitution, the laws of the United States," etc. is not a limitation or an enumeration. It is a definite declaration, — a provision that the judicial power shall extend to — that is, shall include, — the several matters particularly mentioned, leaving unrestricted the general grant of the entire judicial power. There may be, of course, limitations on that grant of power, but, if there are any, they must be expressed; for otherwise the general grant would vest in the courts all the judicial power which the new nation was capable of exercising. Construing this article in the early case of *Chisolm* v. *Georgia*, 2 Dall. 419, the court held that the judicial power of the Supreme Court extended to a suit brought against a state by a citizen of another state. In announcing his opinion in the case, Mr. Justice Wilson said (p. 453):

"This question, important in itself, will depend on others more important still; and may, perhaps, be ultimately resolved into one no less radical than this, — do the people of the United States form a nation?"

In reference to this question attention may, however, properly be called to *Hans* v. *Louisiana*, 124 U. S. 1.

The decision in *Chisolm* v. *Georgia* led to the adoption of the 11th Amendment to the Constitution, withdrawing from the judicial power of the United States every suit in law or equity commenced or prosecuted against one of the United States by citizens of another state or citizens or subjects of a foreign state. This amendment refers only to suits and actions by individuals, leaving undisturbed the jurisdiction over suits or actions by one state against another. As said by Chief Justice Marshall in *Cohen* v. *Virginia*, 6 Wheat. 264, 407; "The Amendment, therefore, extended to suits commenced or prosecuted by individuals, but not to those brought by states." See also *South Dakota* v. *North Carolina*, 192 U. S. 286.

Speaking generally, it may be observed that the judicial power of a nation extends to all controversies justiciable in their nature, and the parties to which or the property involved in which may be reached by judicial process, and, when the judicial power of the United States was vested in the Supreme and other courts, all the judicial power which the nation was capable of exercising was vested in those tribunals; and unless there be some limitations expressed in the Constitution it must be held to embrace all controversies of a justiciable nature arising within the territorial limits of the nation, no matter who may be the parties thereto. This general truth is not inconsistent with the decisions that no suit or action can be maintained against the nation in any of its courts without its consent, for they only recognize the obvious truth that a nation is not, without its consent, subject to the controlling action of any of its instrumentalities or agencies. The creature can not rule the creator. *Kawananakoa* v. *Polyblank*, 205 U. S. 349. Nor is it inconsistent with the ruling in *Wisconsin* v. *Pelican Ins. Co.*, 127 U. S. 265, that an original action can not be maintained in this court by one state to enforce its penal laws against a citizen of another state. That was no denial of the jurisdiction of the court, but a decision upon the merits of the claim of the state.

These considerations lead to the propositions that when a legislative power is claimed for the national government the question is whether that power is one of those granted by the Constitution, either in terms or by necessary implication; whereas, in respect to judicial functions, the question is whether there be any limitations expressed in the Constitution on the general grant of national power.

We may also notice a matter in respect thereto referred to at length in *Missouri* v. *Illinois*, 180 U. S. 208, 220. The 9th article of the Articles of Confederation provided that "the United States in Congress assembled shall also be the last resort on appeal in all disputes and differences now subsisting or that may hereafter arise between two or more states concerning boundary, jurisdiction, or any other cause whatever." In the early drafts of the Constitution provision was made giving to the Supreme Court "jurisdiction of controversies between two or more states, except such as shall regard territory or jurisdiction, "and also that the Senate should have exclusive power to regulate the manner of deciding the disputes and controversies between the states respecting jurisdiction or territory. As finally adopted, the Constitution omits all provision for the Senate taking cognizance of disputes between the states, and leaves out the exception referred to in the jurisdiction granted to the Supreme Court. That carries with it a very direct recognition of the fact that to the Supreme Court is granted jurisdiction of all controversies between the states which are justiciable in their nature. "All the states have transferred the decision of their controversies to this court; each had a right to demand of it the exercise of the power which they had made judicial by the Confederation of 1781 and 1788; that we should do that which neither states nor Congress could do — settle the controversies between them." *Rhode Island* v. *Massachusetts*, 12 Pet. 657, 743.

THE RIGHT OF THE GOVERNMENT TO APPEAL IN CRIMINAL CASES — INJUNCTIONS

FROM PRESIDENT ROOSEVELT'S MESSAGE OF DECEMBER, 1906

To the Senate and House of Representatives:

Appeal in Criminal Cases. Another bill which has just passed one House of the Congress and which it is urgently necessary should be enacted into law is that conferring upon the Government the right of appeal in criminal cases on questions of law. This right exists in many of the States; it exists in the District of Columbia by act of the Congress. It is of course not proposed that in any case a verdict for the defendant on the merits should be set aside. Recently in one district where the Government had indicted certain persons for conspiracy in connection with rebates, the court sustained the defendant's demurrer; while in another jurisdiction an indictment for conspiracy to obtain rebates has been sustained by the court, convictions obtained under it, and two defendants sentenced to imprisonment. The two cases referred to may not be in real conflict with each other, but it is unfortunate that there should even be an apparent conflict. At present there is no way by which the Government can cause such a conflict, when it occurs, to be solved by an appeal to a higher court; and the wheels of justice are blocked without any real decision of the question. I can not too strongly urge the passage of the bill in question. A failure to pass it will result in seriously hampering the Government in its effort to obtain justice, especially against wealthy individuals or corporations who do wrong; and may also prevent the Government from obtaining justice for wageworkers who are not themselves able effectively to contest a case where the judgment of an inferior court has been against them. I have specifically in view a recent decision by a district judge leaving railway employees without remedy for violation of a certain so-called labor statute. It seems an absurdity to permit a single district judge, against what may be the judgment of the immense majority of his colleagues on the bench, to declare a law solemnly enacted by the Congress to be "unconstitutional," and then to deny to the Government the right to have the Supreme Court definitely decide the question.

It is well to recollect that the real efficiency of the law often depends not upon the passage of acts as to which there is great public excitement, but upon the passage of acts of this nature as to which there is not much public excitement, because there is little public understanding of their importance, while the interested parties are keenly alive to the desirability of defeating them. The importance of enacting into law the particular bill in question is further increased by the fact that the Government has now definitely begun a policy of resorting to the criminal law in those trust and interstate commerce cases where such a course offers a reasonable chance of success. At first, as was proper, every effort was made to enforce these laws by civil proceedings; but it has become increasingly evident that the action of the Government in finally deciding, in certain cases, to undertake criminal proceedings was justifiable; and though there have been some conspicuous failures in these cases, we have had many successes, which have undoubtedly had a deterrent effect upon evil-doers, whether the penalty inflicted was in the shape of fine or imprisonment — and penalties of both kinds have already been inflicted by the courts. Of course, where the judge can see his way to inflict the penalty of imprisonment the deterrent effect of the punishment on other offenders is increased; but sufficiently heavy fines accomplish much. Judge Holt, of the New York district court, in a recent decision admirably stated the need for treating with just severity offenders of this kind. His opinion runs in part as follows:

"The Government's evidence to establish the defendant's guilt was clear, conclusive, and undisputed. The case was a flagrant one. The transactions which took place under this illegal contract were very large; the amount of rebates returned were considerable; and the amount of the rebate itself was large, amounting to more than one-fifth of the entire tariff charge for the transportation of merchandise from this city to Detroit. It is not too much to say, in my opinion, that if this business was carried on for a considerable time on that basis — that is, if this discrimination in favor of this particular shipper was made with an 18 instead of a 23 cent rate and the tariff rate was maintained as against their competitors — the result might be and not improbably would be that their competitors would be driven out of business. This crime is one which in its nature is deliberate and premeditated. I think over a fortnight elapsed between the date of Palmer's letter requesting the reduced rate and the answer of the railroad company deciding to grant it, and then for months afterwards this business was carried on and these claims for rebates submitted month after month and checks in payment of them drawn month after month. Such a violation of the law, in my opinion, in its essential nature, is a very much more heinous act than the ordinary common, vulgar crimes which come before criminal courts constantly for punishment and which arise from sudden passion or temptation. This crime in this case was committed by men of education and of large business experience, whose standing in the community was such that they might have been expected to set an example of obedience to law, upon the maintenance of which alone in this country the security of their property depends. It was committed on behalf of a great railroad corporation, which, like other railroad corporations, has received gratuitously from the State large and valuable privileges for the public's convenience and its own, which performs quasi public functions and which is charged with the highest obligation in the transaction of its business to treat the citizens of this country alike, and not to carry on its business with unjust discriminations between different citizens or different classes of citizens. This crime in its nature is one usually done with secrecy, and proof of which it is very difficult to obtain. The interstate commerce act was passed in 1887, nearly twenty years ago. Ever since that time complaints of the granting of rebates by railroads has been common, urgent, and insistent, and although the Congress has repeatedly passed legislation endeavoring to put a stop to this evil, the difficulty of obtaining proof upon which to bring prosecution in these cases is so great that this is the first case that has ever been brought in this court, and, as I am informed, this case and one recently brought in Philadelphia are the only cases that have ever been brought in the eastern part of this country. In fact, but few cases of this kind have ever been brought in this country, East or West. Now, under these circumstances, I am forced to the conclusion, in a case in which the proof is so clear and the facts are so flagrant, it is the duty of the court to fix a penalty which shall in some degree be commensurate with the gravity of the offense. As between the two defendants, in my opinion, the principal penalty should be imposed on the corporation. The traffic manager in this case, presumably, acted without any advantage to himself and without any interest in the transaction, either by the direct authority or in accordance with what he understood to be the policy or the wishes of his employer.

"The sentence of this court in this case is, that the defendant Pomeroy, for each of the six offenses upon which he has been convicted, be fined the sum of $1,000, making six fines, amounting in all to the sum of $6,000; and the defendant, The New York Central and Hudson River Railroad Company, for each of the six crimes of which it has been convicted, be fined the sum of $18,000, making six fines amounting in the aggregate to the sum of $108,000, and judgment to that effect will be entered in this case."

Granting of New Trials. In connection with this matter, I would like to call attention to the very unsatisfactory state of our criminal law, resulting in large part from the habit of setting aside the judgments of inferior courts on technicalities absolutely unconnected with the merits of the case, and where there is no attempt to show that there has been any failure of substantial justice. It would be well to enact a law providing something to the effect that:

No judgment shall be set aside or new trial granted in any cause, civil or criminal, on the ground of misdirection of the jury or the improper admission or rejection of evidence, or for error as to any matter of pleading or procedure unless, in the opinion of the court to which the application is made, after an examination of the entire cause, it shall affirmatively appear that the error complained of has resulted in a miscarriage of justice.

Injunctions. In my last message I suggested the enactment of a law in connection with the issuance of injunctions, attention having been sharply drawn to the matter by the demand that the right of applying injunctions in labor cases should be wholly abolished. It is at least doubtful whether a law abolishing altogether the use of injunctions in such cases would stand the test of the courts; in which case of course the legislation would be ineffective. Moreover, I believe it would be wrong altogether to prohibit the use of injunctions. It is criminal to permit sympathy for criminals to weaken our hands in upholding the law; and if men seek to destroy life or property by mob violence there should be no impairment of the power of the courts to deal with them in the most summary and effective way possible. But so far as possible the abuse of the power should be provided against by some such law as I advocated last year.

In this matter of injunctions there is lodged in the hands of the judiciary a necessary power which is nevertheless subject to the possibility of grave abuse. It is a power that should be exercised with extreme care and should be subject to the jealous scrutiny of all men, and condemnation should be meted out as much to the judge who fails to use it boldly when necessary as to the judge who uses it wantonly or oppressively. Of course a judge strong enough to be fit for his office will enjoin any resort to violence or intimidation, especially by conspiracy, no matter what his opinion may be of the rights of the original quarrel. There must be no hesitation in dealing with disorder. But there must likewise be no such abuse of the injunctive power as is implied in forbidding laboring men to strive for their own betterment in peaceful and lawful ways; nor must the injunction be used merely to aid some big corporation in carrying out schemes for its own aggrandizement. It must be remembered that a preliminary injunction in a labor case, if granted without adequate proof (even when authority can be found to support the conclusions of law on which it is founded), may often settle the dispute between the parties; and therefore if improperly granted may do irreparable wrong. Yet there are many judges who assume a matter-of-course granting of a preliminary injunction to be the ordinary and proper judicial disposition of such cases; and there have undoubtedly been flagrant wrongs committed by judges in connection with labor disputes even within the last few years, although I think much less often than in former years. Such judges by their unwise action immensely strengthen the hands of those who are striving entirely to do away with the power of injunction; and therefore such careless use of the injunctive process tends to threaten its very existence, for if the American people ever become convinced that this process is habitually abused, whether in matters affecting labor or in matters affecting corporations, it will be well-nigh impossible to prevent its abolition.

It may be the highest duty of a judge at any given moment to disregard, not merely the wishes of individuals of great political or financial power, but the overwhelming tide of public sentiment; and the judge who does thus disregard public sentiment when it is wrong, who brushes aside the plea of any special interest when the pleading is not founded on righteousness, performs the highest service to the country. Such a judge is deserving of all honor; and all honor can not be paid to this wise and fearless judge if we permit the growth of an absurd convention which would forbid any criticism of the judge of another type, who shows himself timid in the presence of arrogant disorder, or who on insufficient grounds grants an injunction that does grave injustice, or who, in his capacity as a construer, and therefore in part a maker, of the law, in flagrant fashion thwarts the cause of decent government. The judge has a power over which no review can be exercised; he himself sits in review upon the acts of both the executive and legislative branches of the Government; save in the most extraordinary cases he is amenable only at the bar of public opinion; and it is unwise to maintain that public opinion in reference to a man with such power shall neither be expressed nor led.

The best judges have ever been foremost to disclaim any immunity from criticism. This has been true since the days of the great English Lord Chancellor Parker, who said: "Let all people be at liberty to know what I found my judgment upon; that, so when I have given it in any cause, others may be at liberty to judge of *me*." The proprieties of the case were set forth with singular clearness and good temper by Judge W. H. Taft, when a United States circuit judge, eleven years ago, in 1895:

"The opportunity freely and publicly to criticize judicial action is of vastly more importance to the body politic than the immunity of courts and judges from unjust aspersions and attack. Nothing tends more to render judges careful in their decisions and anxiously solicitous to do exact justice than the consciousness that every act of theirs is to be subjected to the intelligent scrutiny and candid criticism of their fellow-men. Such criticism is beneficial in proportion as it is fair, dispassionate, discriminating, and based on a knowledge of sound legal principles. The comments made by learned text writers and by the acute editors of the various law reviews upon judicial decisions are therefore highly useful. Such critics constitute more or less impartial tribunals of professional opinion before which each judgment is made to stand or fall on its merits, and thus exert a strong influence to secure uniformity of decision. But non-professional criticism also is by no means without its uses, even if accompanied, as it often is, by a direct attack upon the judicial fairness and motives of the occupants of the bench; for if the law is but the essence of common sense, the protest of many average men may evidence a defect in a judicial conclusion, though based on the nicest legal reasoning and profoundest learning. The two important elements of moral character in a judge are an earnest desire to reach a just conclusion and courage to enforce it. In so far as fear of public comment does not affect the courage of a judge, but only spurs him on to search his conscience and to reach the result which approves itself to his inmost heart, such comment serves a useful purpose. There are few men, whether they are judges for life or for a shorter term, who do not prefer to earn and hold the respect of all, and who can not be reached and made to pause and deliberate by hostile public criticism. In the case of judges having a life tenure, indeed, their very independence makes the right freely to comment on their decisions of greater importance, because it is the only practical and available instrument in the hands of a free people to keep such judges alive to the reasonable demands of those they serve.

"On the other hand, the danger of destroying the proper influence of judicial decisions by creating unfounded prejudices against the courts justifies and requires that unjust attacks shall be met and answered. Courts must ultimately rest their defense upon the inherent strength of the opinions they deliver as the ground for their conclusions and must trust to the calm and deliberate judgment of all the people as their best vindication."

There is one consideration which should be taken into account by the good people who carry a sound proposition to an excess in objecting to any criticism of a judge's decision. The instinct of the American people as a whole is sound in this matter. They will not subscribe to the doctrine that any public servant is to be above all criticism. If the best citizens, those mose competent to express their judgment in such matters, and above all those belonging to the great and honorable profession of the bar, so profoundly influential in American life, take the position that there shall be no criticism of a judge under any circumstances, their view will not be accepted by the American people as a whole. In such event the people will turn to, and tend to accept as justifiable, the intemperate and improper criticism uttered by unworthy agitators. Surely it is a misfortune to leave to such critics a function, right in itself, which they are certain to abuse. Just and temperate criticism, when necessary, is a safeguard against the acceptance by the people as a whole of that intemperate antagonism towards the judiciary which must be combated by every right-thinking man, and which, if it became widespread among the people at large, would constitute a dire menace to the Republic.

Lynching. In connection with the delays of the law, I call your attention and the attention of the Nation to the prevalence of crime among us, and above all to the epidemic of lynching and mob violence that springs up, now in one part of our country, now in another. Each section, North, South, East, or West, has its own faults; no section can with wisdom spend its time jeering at the faults of another section; it should be busy trying to amend its own shortcomings. To deal with the crime of corruption it is necessary to have an awakened public conscience, and to supplement this by whatever legislation will add speed and certainty in the execution of the law. When we deal with lynching even more is necessary. A great many white men are lynched, but the crime is peculiarly frequent in respect to black men. The greatest existing cause of lynching is the perpetration, especially by black men, of the hideous crime of rape — the most abominable in all the category of crimes, even worse than murder. Mobs frequently avenge the commission of this crime by themselves torturing to death the man committing it; thus avenging in bestial fashion a bestial deed, and reducing themselves to a level with the criminal.

Lawlessness grows by what it feeds upon; and when mobs begin to lynch for rape they speedily extend the sphere of their operations and lynch for many other kinds of crimes, so that two-thirds of the lynchings are not for rape at all; while a considerable proportion of the individuals lynched are innocent of all crime. Governor Candler, of Georgia, stated on one occasion some years ago: "I can say of a verity that I have, within the last month, saved the lives of half a dozen innocent negroes who were pursued by the mob, and brought them to trial in a court of a law in which they were acquitted." As Bishop Galloway, of Mississippi, has finely said: "When the rule of a mob obtains, that which distinguishes a high civilization is surrendered. The mob which lynches a negro charged with rape will in a little while lynch a white man suspected of crime. Every Christian patriot in America needs to lift up his voice in loud and eternal protest against the mob spirit that is threatening the integrity of this Republic." Governor Jelks, of Alabama, has recently spoken as follows: "The lynching of any person for whatever crime is inexcusable anywhere — it is a defiance of orderly government; but the killing of innocent people under any provocation is infinitely more horrible; and yet innocent people are likely to die when a mob's terrible lust is once aroused. The lesson is this: No good citizen can afford to countenance a defiance of the statutes, no matter what the provocation. The innocent frequently suffer, and, it is my observation, more usually suffer than the guilty. The white people of the South indict the whole colored race on the ground that even the better elements lend no assistance whatever in ferreting out criminals of their own color. The respectable colored people must learn not to harbor their criminals, but to assist the officers in bringing them to justice. This is the larger crime, and it provokes such atrocious offenses as the one at Atlanta. The two races can never get on until there is an understanding on the part of both to make common cause with the law-abiding against criminals of any color."

Moreover, where any crime committed by a member of one race against a member of another race is avenged in such fashion that it seems as if not the individual criminal, but the whole race, is attacked, the result is to exasperate to the highest degree race feeling. There is but one safe rule in dealing with black men as with white men; it is the same rule that must be applied in dealing with rich men and poor men; that is, to treat each man, whatever his color, his creed, or his social position, with even-handed justice on his real worth as a man. White people owe it quite as much to themselves as to the colored race to treat well the colored man who shows by his life that he deserves such treatment; for it is surely the highest wisdom to encourage in the colored race all those individuals who are honest, industrious, law-abiding, and who therefore make good and safe neighbors and citizens. Reward or punish the individual on his merits as an individual. Evil will surely come in the end to both races if we substitute for this just rule the habit of treating all the members of the race, good and bad, alike. There is no question of "social equality" or "negro domination" involved; only the question of relentlessly punishing bad men, and of securing to the good man the right to his life, his liberty, and the pursuit of his happiness as his own qualities of heart, head, and hand enable him to achieve it.

Every colored man should realize that the worst enemy of his race is the negro criminal, and above all the negro criminal who commits the dreadful crime of rape; and it should be felt as in the highest degree an offense against the whole country, and against the colored race in particular, for a colored man to fail to help the officers of the law in hunting down with all possible earnestness and zeal every such infamous offender. Moreover, in my judgment, the crime of rape should always be punished with death, as is the case with murder; assault with intent to commit rape should be made a capital crime, at least in the discretion of the court; and provision should be made by which the punishment may follow immediately upon the heels of the offense; while the trial should be so conducted that the victim need not be wantonly shamed while giving testimony, and that the least possible publicity shall be given to the details.

The members of the white race on the other hand should understand that every lynching represents by just so much a loosening of the bands of civilization; that the spirit of lynching inevitably throws into prominence in the community all the foul and evil creatures who dwell therein. No man can take part in the torture of a human being without having his own moral nature permanently lowered. Every lynching means just so much moral deterioration in all the children who have any knowledge of it, and therefore just so much additional trouble for the next generation of Americans.

Let justice be both sure and swift; but let it be justice under the law, and not the wild and crooked savagery of a mob.

There is another matter which has a direct bearing upon this matter of lynching and of the brutal crime which sometimes calls it forth and at other times merely furnishes the excuse for its existence. It is out of the question for our people as a whole permanently to rise by treading down any of their own number. Even those who themselves for the moment profit by such maltreatment of their fellows will in the long run also suffer. No more shortsighted policy can be imagined than, in the fancied interest of one class, to prevent the education of another class. The free public school, the chance for each boy or girl to get a good elementary education, lies at the foundation of our whole political situation. In every community the poorest citizens, those who need the schools most, would be deprived of them if they only received school facilities proportioned to the taxes they paid. This is as true of one portion of our country as of another. It is as true for the negro as for the white man. The white man, if he is wise, will decline to allow the negroes in a mass to grow to manhood and womanhood without education. Unquestionably education such as is obtained in our public schools does not do everything towards making a man a good citizen; but it does much. The lowest and most brutal criminals, those for instance who commit the crime of rape, are in the great majority men who have had either no education or very little; just as they are almost invariably men who own no property; for the man who puts money by out of his earnings, like the man who acquires education, is usually lifted above mere brutal criminality. Of course the best type of education for the colored man, taken as a whole, is such education as is conferred in schools like Hampton and Tuskegee; where the boys and girls, the young men and young women, are trained industrially as well as in the ordinary public school branches. The graduates of these schools turn out well in the great majority of cases, and hardly any of them become criminals, while what little criminality there is never takes the form of that brutal violence which invites lynch law. Every graduate of these schools — and for the matter of that every other colored man or woman — who leads a life so useful and honorable as to win the good will and respect of those whites whose neighbor he or she is, thereby helps the whole colored race as it can be helped in no other way; for next to the negro himself, the man who can do most to help the negro is his white neighbor who lives near him; and our steady effort should be to better the relations between the two. Great though the benefit of these schools has been to their colored pupils and to the colored people, it may well be questioned whether the benefit has not been at least as great to the white people among whom these colored pupils live after they graduate.

Be it remembered, furthermore, that the individuals who, whether from folly, from evil temper, from greed for office, or in a spirit of mere base demagogy, indulge in the inflammatory and incendiary speeches and writings which tend to arouse mobs and to bring about lynching, not only thus excite the mob, but also tend by what criminologists call "suggestion," greatly to increase the likelihood of a repetition of the very crime against which they are inveighing. When the mob is composed of the people of one race and the man lynched is of another race, the men who in their speeches and writings either excite or justify the action tend, of course, to excite a bitter race feeling and to cause the people of the opposite race to lose sight of the abominable act of the criminal himself; and in addition, by the prominence they give to the hideous deed they undoubtedly tend to excite in other brutal and depraved natures thoughts of committing it. Swift, relentless, and orderly punishment under the law is the only way by which criminality of this type can permanently be suppressed.

XV

CENTRALIZATION AND CHANGES IN THE CONSTITUTION

[The expansion of the activities of the federal government has aroused much discussion. Those who believe in a strong national authority welcome the activity of the federal government as a symptom of strength in our national life. They see in it only the normal adaptation of instruments of government to social and economic needs of the nation. Others who believe strongly in local and state autonomy express the fear that the federal government may entirely supersede the states, and that there will result an over-concentration of political action. This matter has already been brought out in many of the extracts printed on preceding pages. The speeches of Senator Newlands and of Senator Beveridge, on national resources, express a strong belief in the justification of federal initiative. The same ideas are developed in the messages of President Roosevelt. The different points of view are very strongly presented in the following debates and addresses.]

HOW TO PRESERVE THE LOCAL SELF-GOVERNMENT OF THE STATES [1]

By Elihu Root

This gathering peculiarly represents two ancient Commonwealths, each looking back to a century and a half of colonial history before the formation of the American Union, each possessed of strong individuality, derived from the long practice of self-government, and both conspicuous among all the States for leadership in population and wealth, for commerce and manufacture, for art and science, and for the priceless traditions of great citizens in former generations. It seems appropriate to make here some observations upon a subject which is much in the minds of thoughtful Americans in these days.

What is to be the future of the States of the Union under our dual system of constitutional government?

The conditions under which the clauses of the Constitution distributing powers to the National and State governments are now and henceforth to be applied, are widely different from the conditions which were or could have been within the contemplation of the framers of the Constitution, and widely different from those which obtained during the

[1] A speech delivered by Secretary Root at the dinner of the Pennsylvania Society in New York, December 12, 1906.

early years of the Republic. When the authors of *The Federalist* argued
and expounded the reasons for union and the utility of the provisions
contained in the Constitution, each separate colony transformed into
a State was complete in itself and sufficient to itself except as to a few
exceedingly simple external relations of State to State and to foreign
nations; from the origin of production to the final consumption of the
product, from the birth of a citizen to his death, the business, the social,
and the political life in each separate community began and ended for
the most part within the limits of the State itself; the long time required
for travel and communication between the different centers of population, the difficulties and hardships of long and laborious journeys, the
slowness of the mails, and the enormous cost of transporting goods, kept
the people of each State tributary to their own separate colonial center
of trade and influence and kept their activities within the ample and
sufficient jurisdiction of the local laws of their State. The fear of the
fathers of the Republic was that these separate and self-sufficient communities would fall apart, that the Union would resolve into its constituent elements, or that, as it grew in population and area, it would split
up into a number of separate confederacies. Fo   he men of 178
would have deemed it possible that the Union   orming cou
be maintained among eighty-five millions of   ad over
vast expanse from the Atlantic to the Pacific   Lakes t
Gulf.

Three principal causes have made this p
One cause has been the growth of a N
at first almost imperceptible. The very   nt, wh
which our Nation was subjected in its c   nd hard
commerce, and the insults and indignitie   he injuri
of the contestants in the great Napol   n the p
Nation and National interests and N
the minds and in the feelings of the
swept westward, new states were fo:
to the older States as the homes of
and the origin of their laws and custo
and special separate political life of :
the supremacy of the Nation throug'
its sacrifices sanctified and made
Our country as a whole, the nobl
of every State, has become the ol
our people, North and South, with
Commonwealths, throughout that
of a separate empire culminating :
the far-distant shores of the Paci:
glowing loyalty to the Nation, s
become dim and faint in compari

The second great influence has been the knittig together in ties of common interest of the people forming the once separate communities through the working of free trade among the State. Never was a concession dictated by enlightened judgment for the common benefit more richly than that by which the States surrendered in the Federal Constitution the right to lay imposts or duties on imports or exports without the consent of Congress. To it we owe the domestic market for the products of our farms and forests and mines and factors without a parallel in history, and an internal trade which already exceeds the entire foreign trade of all the rest of the world; and to it we owe in a high degree the constant drawing together of all parts of our vast ad diversified country in the bands of common interest and in the improving good understanding and kindly feeling of frequent intercourse.

The third great cause of change is the marvous development of facilities for travel and communication produced by the inventions and discoveries of the past century. The swift trains that pass over our two hundred and twenty thousand miles of railroad, the seventy millions of messages that flash over the more than fourteen hundred thousand miles of telegraph wires, the conversations across vast spaces through our more than four million four hundred thousand telephone instruments,

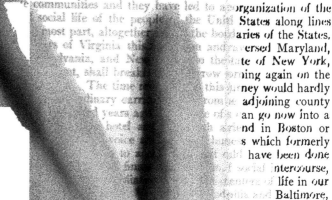

these have broken down the barriers between communities and they have led to a organization of the social life of the people of the United States along lines most part, altogether the boundaries of the States. of Virginia and traversed Maryland, vania, and to the state of New York, shall beginning again on the The time this journey would hardly nary can the adjoining county years can go now into a friend in Boston or s which formerly have been done social intercourse, life in our and Baltimore, early years of the Republic. When the authors of *The Federalist* argued and expounded the reasons for union and the utility of the provisions contained in the Constitution, each separate colony transformed into a State was complete in itself and sufficient to itself except as to a few exceedingly simple external relations of State to State and to foreign nations; from the origin of production to the final consumption of the product, from the birth of a citizen to his death, the business, the social, and the political life of each separate community began and ended for the most part within the limits of the State itself; the long time required for travel and communication between the different centers of population, the difficulties and hardships of long and laborious journeys, the slowness of the mails, and the enormous cost of transporting goods, kept the people of each State tributary to their own separate colonial center of trade and influence, and kept their activities within the ample and sufficient jurisdiction of the local laws of their State. The fear of the fathers of the Republic was that these separate and self-sufficient communities would fall apart, that the Union would resolve into its constituent elements, or that, as it grew in population and area, it would split up into a number of separate confederacies. Few of the men of 1787 would have deemed it possible that the Union they were forming could be maintained among eighty-five millions of people, spread over the vast expanse from the Atlantic to the Pacific and from the Lakes to the Gulf.

Three principal causes have made this possible.

One cause has been the growth of a National sentiment, which was at first almost imperceptible. The very difficulties and hardships to which our Nation was subjected in its early years, the injuries to our commerce, and the insults and indignities to our flag on the part of both of the contestants in the great Napoleonic wars, served to keep the Nation and National interests and National dignity constantly before the minds and in the feelings of the people. As the tide of emigration swept westward, new States were formed of citizens who looked back to the older States as the homes of their childhood and their affection and the origin of their laws and customs, and who never had the peculiar and special separate political life of the colonies. The Civil War settled the supremacy of the Nation throughout the territory of the Union, and its sacrifices sanctified and made enduring that National sentiment. Our country as a whole, the noble and beloved land of every citizen of every State, has become the object of pride and devotion among all our people, North and South, within the limits of the proud, old colonial Commonwealths, throughout that vast region where Burr once dreamed of a separate empire dominating the valley of the Mississippi, and upon the far-distant shores of the Pacific; and by the side of this strong and glowing loyalty to the Nation, sentiment for the separate States has become dim and faint in comparison.

The second great influence has been the knitting together in ties of common interest of the people forming the once separate communities through the working of free trade among the States. Never was a concession dictated by enlightened judgment for the common benefit more richly than that by which the States surrendered in the Federal Constitution the right to lay imposts or duties on imports or exports without the consent of Congress. To it we owe the domestic market for the products of our farms and forests and mines and factories without a parallel in history, and an internal trade which already exceeds the entire foreign trade of all the rest of the world; and to it we owe in a high degree the constant drawing together of all parts of our vast and diversified country in the bands of common interest and in the improving good understanding and kindly feeling of frequent intercourse.

The third great cause of change is the marvelous development of facilities for travel and communication produced by the inventions and discoveries of the past century. The swift trains that pass over our two hundred and twenty thousand miles of railroad, the seventy millions of messages that flash over the more than fourteen hundred thousand miles of telegraph wires, the conversations across vast spaces through our more than four million four hundred thousand telephone instruments, take no note of State lines; they have broken down the barriers between the separate communities and they have led to a reorganization of the business and social life of the people of the United States along lines which, for the most part, altogether ignore the boundaries of the States. I left the borders of Virginia this afternoon and traversed Maryland, Delaware, Pennsylvania, and New Jersey to the State of New York, and, barring accident, shall breakfast to-morrow morning again on the shore of the Potomac. The time required for this journey would hardly have sufficed for an ordinary carriage drive from the adjoining county of Westchester a hundred years ago. Any one of us can go now into a neighboring room in this hotel and talk with a friend in Boston or Chicago and recognize his voice and transact business which formerly would have required months to accomplish if it could have been done at all. The lines of trade, of financial operation, of social intercourse, of thought and opinion that radiate from the great centers of life in our country such as Boston and New York, and Philadelphia and Baltimore, and Chicago and St. Louis, and New Orleans and San Francisco, and many another great city, are perfectly regardless of State distinctions. Our whole life has swung away from the old State centers and is crystallizing about National centers; the farmer harvests his grain and fattens his cattle, not as formerly, with reference to the wants of his own home community, but for markets thousands of miles away; the manufacturer operates his mills and his factories to meet the needs of far-distant consumers; the merchant has his customers in many States; all — the farmer, the manufacturer, the merchant, the laborer — look for the supplies of their food and clothing, not to the resources of the home farm, or village, or town, but to the resources of the whole Continent. The people move in great throngs to and fro from State to State and across States; the important news of each community is read at every breakfast table throughout the country; the interchange of thought and sentiment and information is universal; in the wide range of daily life and activity and interest the old lines between the States and the old barriers which kept the States as separate communities are completely lost from sight. The growth of National habits in the daily life of a homogeneous people keeps pace with the growth of National sentiment.

Such changes in the life of the people can not fail to produce corresponding political changes. Some of those changes can be plainly seen now in progress. It is plainly to be seen that the people of the country are coming to the conclusion that in certain important respects the local laws of the separate States, which were adequate for the due and just regulation and control of the business which was transacted and the activity which began and ended within the limits of the several States, are inadequate for the due and just control of the business and activities which extend throughout all the States, and that such power of regulation and control is gradually passing into the hands of the National Government. Sometimes by an assertion of the interstate commerce power, sometimes by an assertion of the taxing power, the National Government is taking up the performance of duties which under the changed conditions the separate States are no longer capable of adequately performing. The Federal anti-trust law, the anti-rebate law, the railroad rate law, the meat-inspection law, the oleomargarine law, the pure-food law, are examples of the purpose of the people of the United States to do through the agency of the National Government the things which the separate State governments formerly did adequately but no longer do adequately. The end is not yet. The process that interweaves the life and action of the people in every section of our country with the people in every other section, continues and will continue with increasing force and effect; we are urging forward in a development of business and social life which tends more and more to the obliteration of State lines and the decrease of State power as compared with National power; the relations of the business over which the Federal Government is assuming control, of interstate transportation with State transportation, of interstate commerce with State commerce, are so intimate and the separation of the two is so impracticable, that the tendency is plainly toward the practical control of the National Government over both. New projects of National control are mooted; control of insurance, uniform divorce laws, child-labor laws and many others affecting matters formerly entirely within the cognizance of the State are proposed.

With these changes and tendencies in what way can the power of the States be preserved?

I submit to your judgment, and I desire to press upon you with all the earnestness I possess, that there is but one way in which the States of the Union can maintain their power and authority under the conditions which are now before us, and that way is by an awakening on the part of the States to a realization of their own duties to the country at large. Under the conditions which now exist, no State can live unto itself alone and regulate its affairs with sole reference to its own treasury, its own convenience, its own special interests. Every State is bound to frame its legislation and its administration with reference not only to its own special affairs, but with reference to the effect upon all its sister States, as every individual is bound to regulate his conduct with some reference to its effect upon his neighbors. The more populous the community and the closer individuals are brought together the more imperative becomes the necessity which constrains and limits individual conduct. If any State is maintaining laws which afford, opportunity and authority for practices condemned by the public sense of the whole country, or laws which, though the operation of our modern system of communications and business, are injurious to the interests of the whole country, that State is violating the conditions upon which alone can its power be preserved. If any State maintains laws which promote and foster the enormous overcapitalization of corporations condemned by the people of the country generally, if any State maintains laws designed to make easy the formation of trusts and the creation of monopolies, if any State maintains laws which permit conditions of child labor revolting to the sense of mankind, if any State maintains laws of marriage and divorce so far inconsistent with the general standard of the nation as to violently derange the domestic relations; which the majority of the States desire to preserve, that State is promoting the tendency of the people of the country to seek relief through the National Government and to press forward the movement for National control and the extinction of local control. The intervention of the National Government in many of the matters which it has recently undertaken would have been wholly unnecessary if the States themselves had been alive to their duty toward the general body of the country. It is useless for the advocates of State rights to inveigh against the supremacy of the constitutional laws of the United States or against the extension of National authority in the fields of necessary control where the States themselves fail in the performance of their duty. The instinct for self-government among the people of the United States is too strong to permit them long to respect any one's right to exercise a power which he fails to exercise. The Governmental control which they deem just and necessary they will have. It may be that such control would better be exercised in particular instances by the governments of the States, but the people will have the control they need either from the States or from the National Government; and if the States fail to furnish it in due measure, sooner or later constructions of the Constitution will be found to vest the power where it will be exercised — in the National Government. The true and only way to preserve State authority is to be found in the awakened conscience of the States, their broadened views and higher standard of responsibility to the general public; in effective legislation by the States, in conformity to the general moral sense of the country; and in the vigorous exercise for the general public good of that State authority which is to be preserved.

FROM PRESIDENT ROOSEVELT'S SPEECH AT ST. LOUIS, OCTOBER, 1907

Now that the questions of government are becoming so largely economic, the majority of our so-called constitutional cases really turn not upon the interpretation of the instrument itself but upon the construction, the right apprehension of the living conditions to which it is to be applied. The Constitution is now and must remain what it always has been; but it can only be interpreted as the interests of the whole people demand, if interpreted as a living organism, designed to meet the conditions of life and not of death; in other words, if interpreted as Marshall interpreted it, as Wilson declared it should be interpreted.

The Marshall theory, the theory of life and not of death, allows to the nation, that is, to the people as a whole, when once it finds a subject within the national cognizance, the widest and freest choice of methods for national control, and sustains every exercise of national power which has any reasonable relation to national objects. The negation of this theory means, for instance, that the nation — that we, the 90,000,000 people of this country — will be left helpless to control the huge corporations which now domineer in our industrial life, and that they will have the authority of the courts to work their desires unchecked, and such a decision would in the end be as disastrous for them as for us.

If the theory of the Marshall school prevails, then an immense field of national power, now unused, will be developed, which will be adequate for dealing with many, if not all, of the economic problems which vex us; and we shall be saved from the ominous threat of a constant oscillation between economic tyranny and economic chaos. Our industrial and therefore our social future as a nation depends upon settling aright this urgent question.

The constitution is unchanged and unchangeable save by amendment in due form. But the conditions to which it is to be applied have undergone a change which is almost a transformation, with the result that many subjects formerly under the control of the states have come under the control of the nation.

A hundred years ago there was, except the commerce which crawled along our seacoast or up and down our interior waterways, practically no interstate commerce. Now, by the railroad, the mails, the telegraph, and the telephone an immense part of our commerce is interstate. By the transformation it has escaped from the power of the state and come under the power of the nation. Therefore there has been a great practical change in the exercise of the national power, under the acts of Congress, over interstate commerce; while on the other hand there has been no noticeable change in the exercise of the national power " to regulate commerce with foreign nations and with the Indian tribes."

I believe that the nation has the whole governmental power over interstate commerce and the widest discretion in dealing with the subject; of course under the express limits prescribed in the constitution for the exercise of all powers, such for instance as the condition that "due process of law" shall not be denied. The nation has no direct power over purely intrastate commerce even where it is conducted by the same agencies which conduct interstate commerce.

The courts must determine what is national and what is state commerce. The same reasoning which sustained the power of congress to incorporate the United States bank tends to sustain the power to incorporate an interstate railroad or any other corporation conducting an interstate business.

There are difficulties arising from our dual form of government. If they prove to be insuperable, resort must be had to the power of amendment. Let us first try to meet them by an exercise of all the powers of the national government which in the Marshall spirit of broad interpretation can be found in the constitution as it is. They are of vast extent.

The chief economic question of the day in this country is to provide a sovereign for the great corporations engaged in interstate business; that is, for the railroads and the interstate industrial corporations.

At the moment our prime concern is with the railroads. When railroads were first built they were purely local in character. Their boundaries were not coextensive even with the boundaries of one state. They usually covered but two or three counties. All this has now changed. At present five great systems embody nearly four-fifths of the total mileage of the country. All the most important railroads are no longer state roads, but instruments of interstate commerce. Probably 85 per cent of their business is interstate business.

It is the nation alone which can with wisdom, justice, and effectiveness exercise over these interstate railroads the thorough and complete supervision which should be exercised. One of the chief, and probably the chief, of the domestic causes for the adoption of the constitution was the need to confer upon the nation exclusive control over interstate commerce.

But this grant of power is worthless unless it is held to confer thoroughgoing and complete control over practically the sole instrumentalities of interstate commerce — the interstate railroads.

47

The railroads themselves have been exceedingly shortsighted in the rancorous bitterness which they have shown against the resumption by the nation of this long neglected power. Great capitalists, who pride themselves upon their extreme conservatism, often believe they are acting in the interests of property when following a course so shortsighted as to be really an assault upon property. They have shown extreme unwisdom in their violent opposition to the assumption of complete control over the railroads by the federal government.

The American people will not tolerate the happy-go-lucky system of no control over the great interstate railroads, with the insolent and manifold abuses which have so generally accompanied it. The control must exist somewhere and unless it is by thoroughgoing and radical law placed upon the statute books of the nation it will be exercised in ever-increasing measure by the several states. The same considerations which made the founders of the constitution deem it imperative that the nation should have complete control of interstate commerce apply with peculiar force to the control of interstate railroads at the present day, and the arguments of Madison of Virginia, Pinckney of South Carolina, and Hamilton and Jay of New York in their essence apply now as they applied 120 years ago.

The national convention which framed the constitution, and in which almost all the most eminent of the first generation of American statesmen sat, embodied the theory of the instrument in a resolution to the effect that the national government should have power in cases where the separate states were incompetent to act with full efficiency, and where the harmony of the United States would be interrupted by the exercise of such individual legislation.

The interstate railroad situation is exactly a case in point. There will, of course, be local matters affecting railroads which can best be dealt with by local authority, but as national commercial agents the big interstate railroads ought to be completely subject to national authority. Only thus can we secure their complete subjection to and control by a single sovereign, representing the whole people and capable both of protecting the public and of seeing that the railroads neither inflict nor endure injustice.

Personally I firmly believe that there should be national legislation to control all industrial corporations doing an interstate business, including the control of the output of their securities, but as to these the necessity for federal control is less urgent and immediate than is the case with the railroads. Many of the abuses connected with these corporations will probably tend to disappear now that the government — the public — is gradually getting the upper hand as regards putting a stop to the rebates and special privileges which some of these corporations have enjoyed at the hands of the common carriers. But ultimately it will be found that the complete remedy for these abuses lies in direct and affirmative action by the national government.

I am not pleading for an extension of constitutional power. I am pleading that the constitutional power which already exists shall be applied to new conditions which did not exist when the constitution went into being. I ask that the national powers already conferred upon the national government by the constitution shall be so used as to bring national commerce and industry effectively under the authority of the federal government and thereby avert industrial chaos.

My plea is not to bring about a condition of centralization. It is that the government shall recognize a condition of centralization in a field where it already exists. When the national banking law was passed it represented in reality not centralization, but recognition of the fact that the country had so far advanced that the currency was already a matter of national concern and must be dealt with by the central authority at Washington. So it is with interstate industrialism, and especially with the matter of interstate railroad operation to-day.

Centralization has already taken place in the world of commerce and industry. All I ask is that the national government look this fact in the face, accept it as a fact, and fit itself accordingly for a policy of supervision and control over this centralized commerce and industry.

THE NATION AND THE CONSTITUTION

BY JUDGE CHARLES F. AMIDON [1]

OF late we have heard quoted again and again, from the Bench and from the platform, the language of Chief Justice Taney in the Dred Scott case, that the constitution "Speaks not only in the same words, but with the same meaning and intent with which it spoke when it came from the hands of its framers." The only objection to that fine phrase is that it is not true. The exact contrary would be nearer the truth, viz: That not a single distinctive word or phrase in the constitution has the same meaning to-day which it had when that instrument came from the hands of its framers. Such language is as reprehensible from that side of the controversy as on the other side are the words of the impassioned phrase-maker referred to by Senator Knox in his very able address at Yale. With a practical and rapidly progressive people like ours, the pharisaical doctrine that the nation exists for the constitution instead of the constitution for the nation, can never obtain permanent acceptance. The constitution performs its chief service when it holds the nation back from hasty and passionate action, and compels it to investigate, consider and weigh until it is made sure that the proposed action does not embody the passion of the hour, but the settled purpose of the years. A changeless constitution becomes the protector not only of vested rights but of

[1] An address before the American Bar Association, in 1907. Reprinted in part, by permission.

vested wrongs. As Bacon says, "He that will not apply new remedies must accept new evils, for time is the greatest innovator. . . . A forward retention of custom is as turbulent a thing as any innovation." A constitution which fixedly restrains a people from correcting their actual evils becomes associated in the popular mind with the evils themselves. When it performs that rôle, as ours once did, it becomes in the estimation of reformers a "compact with hell," and enlightened statesmen appeal from its provisions to a "higher law."

But it is now insisted with a zeal such as has not been heard since John Taylor of Caroline, that if the constitution is to be changed it must be done in the manner which the instrument itself provides for its amendment. To say that, however, is to say that it shall not be changed at all, for we are taught by a century of our history that the constitution can no longer be thus amended. Since 1804 more than two thousand amendments have been proposed. Many of them have been the subject of much public discussion, have found a place in party platform; some have received the requisite vote of one branch of Congress; but with the exception of the war amendments, all have failed of adoption.

The first twelve amendments may be regarded as merely formal, or as the result of the forces which produced the instrument itself. It required the fierce passions aroused by the civil war to bring about the only direct amendment of the constitution which has occurred apart from the period of its adoption. Even these amendments could not have secured the requisite number of states had it not been for the coercion of military power and political influence such as every lover of our country will hope can never be again employed for such a purpose. This, however, was not the worst feature of those amendments. The fierce passion necessary to secure their adoption was embodied in the amendments themselves. As a result they have been nullified in some of their most important provisions, and as to other features found in the Fourteenth Amendment, the Supreme Court in order to prevent their confounding our whole system of national and local government, was compelled in the Slaughter House Cases to resort to a construction which did violence to the language of the amendment, and defeated the avowed purpose of the men who employed that language. The most impressive lesson taught by the war amendments is that the constitution can not be amended in the manner which it provides except as the result of passions which wholly disqualify the nation for the work of constitutional amendment.

The vast enlargement of our country has made the method of amendment provided by the fathers far more difficult than they contemplated at the time. They also believed that they had forever foreclosed the possibility of government by party, and the inauguration of that system has made the plan which they devised unworkable; for any amendment which is proposed by one party encounters the opposition of the other.

If objection does not exist to the subject-matter, it is called forth by partisan considerations. No amendment, therefore, is possible except when one party controls the legislatures of three-fourths of the states, and a two-thirds majority in Congress. This condition has not existed since the early part of the last century, nor is it ever likely to occur again.

But probably the greatest force opposed to constitutional amendment is the fear of radicalism by the large business interests of the country. The wave of socialistic tendency, which is now sweeping over all western nations has greatly added to this alarm. Property knows that it is safe under the constitution as it is. There is a very general understanding that formal amendment is impossible. Every year that goes by without such a change strengthens that understanding; but if its power were once broken by an actual amendment, it is impossible to foresee the forces that might be set in operation. Hence with business interests it is the fact of amendment that controls, and not the subject-matter.

It is not only true that the constitution can not be amended in the method which it provides, but that such a change is neither needed nor best. Formal amendment is not suitable to bring about those slight but steady modifications of fundamental law which adapt it to the progressive life of the nation. It is far too violent a remedy for that purpose. The constitution has been and ought to be accommodated to the ever-changing conditions of society by a process as gradual as the changes themselves. Like the Kingdom of Heaven amendments such as these come not by observation. No political prophet can say of them, Lo, here! or Lo, there! As the result of more than a hundred years of experience the nation has become acquainted with this process of amendment and is satisfied with it. It must now be accepted as a part of our frame of government of equal validity with the constitution itself.

But if the constitution is changed by interpretation will it not be entirely swept away by the process? We hear much of this argument *in terrorem*. In the minds of its advocates the constitution is a kind of St. Rupert's drop, so fragile that if its elements be disturbed in the slightest degree, the entire combination will explode. Experience tells us that it is made of sterner stuff. After a century of such interpretation by which the instrument has been so altered that Mr. Ford tells us its authors would not know it, it is to-day performing its functions with far greater vigor than during the period following its adoption. Being a great instrument of government it can not be read in the library. As the late Justice Miller stated to a company of judges and lawyers at St. Paul a short time before his death: "The great questions of constitutional law are not to be finally settled by nine men, however wise, taking them off into a room and reading and studying about them. That is the way we start the process. We place the decision the best we can, according to that light, and then see how it works in its actual application to the national life. Very frequently that illumination shows us that we have gone far to one side of the true line. With this instruction of experience we place the next case on the other side and observe its application and so on, from time to time adding to our thought and study the results of experience and observation, we finally evolve the true solution by a process of exclusion and inclusion. The meaning of the constitution is to be sought as much in the national life as in the dictionary."

In our constitutional theory we habitually assume that the provisions of the constitution have but one meaning, and that plain and precise. But this is not its real character. As Marshall declares in *McCulloch* v. *Maryland*, "Its nature requires that only its great outlines should be marked, and its important objects designated. . . . It was intended to endure for ages to come, and to be adapted to the various *crises* in human affairs." An instrument of such a character must necessarily leave a wide latitude for construction. The fact that the Supreme Court in constitutional cases so frequently stand five to four, each division assigning weighty reasons for diametrically opposite views, shows plainly how much the constitution in actual application is a matter of interpretation. Now that questions of government are becoming so largely economic, the majority of our so-called constitutional cases turn not upon the interpretation of the instrument itself, but upon the construction of the living conditions to which it is to be applied. Let me illustrate: A statute of New York provided that women should not be employed in manufacturing establishments between the hours of nine o'clock at night and six o'clock in the morning. In a recent decision of the Court of Appeals of that state, this law is declared unconstitutional upon the ground that there is nothing in the nature and duties of woman which justify the legislature in discriminating as to her employment. The gist of this decision is not the meaning of the constitution, but the effect of labor in a manufacturing establishment upon the health of woman and her ability to perform the primary duties of home and motherhood; and while none of us would question the ability of the court to interpret the constitution wisely, some at least would feel that in that case it fell into grievous error in its interpretation of life. Constitutional cases are in the same manner frequently decided not upon the language of the constitution, but upon conflicting notions of life in which the courts assert doctrines at variance with both popular and legislative judgment. The danger of this practice is obvious. It gives us a government out of a law library, which, as Napoleon said, is the worst of all forms of government.

Courts are very fond of declaring that in the field of constitutional law they never exercise political power, but simply declare the private rights of parties. This is true as to the form but untrue as to the result. The ultimate effect of every constitutional decision is not only to declare the rights of the litigants, but to define the powers of government. If the constitution were precise, and capable of but one construction, then the courts in construing it would be simply declaring the rule and in no way making it. But in the case of the federal constitution in particular, its provisions are so general as to leave a wide latitude for judicial construction; and within the scope of that latitude the court in construing the constitution is exercising a political power second only to that of the convention that framed the instrument.

In the attempt to catch our constitution in a statement, we have been frequently told of late that "the powers of the federal government remain the same"; that the only change which has been wrought in our progressive history is the change of conditions to which those powers are applied. We would all agree, I think, that the powers of the federal government remain the same in number; but can any candid lawyer say they remain the same in extent? It is quite true that "no independent and unmentioned power" can rightfully be added to the federal government. But even such accurate statements can not settle constitutional questions. When the instrument comes to be applied to a given case the question will still be open, Is the power which has been attempted an independent power, or is it so related to one of the great powers of the constitution as to be an appropriate means for its execution? That question presents the old puzzle of the criterion of classification which Austin taught us was the most difficult problem of law, and which Madison pointed out in the Federalist to be as impossible of definite solution in the case of the constitution as it has been in natural history. What to Marshall was an appropriate means for collecting and disbursing the public revenue, was to Jefferson and his school the exercise of an independent power. It is because the constitution is thus general that it has been possible to adapt it to changing conditions, and make it the beneficent organ of a progressive nation.

What is needed to-day is not that the constitution shall be construed to mean precisely what it meant to Marshall or to Miller, Field, and Bradley, but that it shall be applied to present conditions by the same method and in the same spirit wherewith they applied it to the conditions of their times. In the performance of this, their highest duty, the federal courts are no part of the administration. They will not answer to its needs or its criticism. But they are a part of the nation, and in the past have responded, and ought always to respond to the deep, abiding organic changes in the national life.

There never was a time when the interpretation of the constitution required a more careful consideration of living conditions than to-day. Within the last fifty years economic forces have been introduced into our life that are as revolutionary of preëxisting conditions as the introduction of gun-powder was of the state of feudalism. Seward's statement in the debate of 1850 that "Commerce is the god of boundaries and no man now living can tell its ultimate decree" is far more true at present than when it was uttered. When the constitution was adopted the unit of our social and business life was the commonwealth. With the exception of the foreign and coasting trade, the commerce and industry of each state was confined to its own borders. The union was political instead of industrial or commercial. To-day our industry and our commerce are national. They are made aware of state lines only by conflicting and often narrowly selfish enactments. The units of commercial and industrial organization extend to many states, often to the entire nation. Instead of being required to obey one master, business is compelled to obey many. Coincident with this enlargement of business enterprise to embrace different states, has occurred a revolution in state activity. During the first half of the Nineteenth Century the doctrine of *laissez-faire* was the fundamental principle of government. The state left commerce and industry to private control. To-day that is all changed. Government is now present in all lines of business. When the state regulated but little, business was not much concerned who did the regulating. But now that all governments· are competing in their zeal for regulation, whether one government or many, the nation or the states, shall do the regulating, becomes a matter of paramount importance. These changed conditions in our actual life compel a reconsideration of our divided governmental authority to see what now belongs to the nation, and what to the states. The problem is not the same as it was; it can not be answered by reading history or studying precedents.

The new condition has manifested itself most conspicuously in two fields, the railroad and the interstate industrial corporation. At the beginning the railroads were local. There was a time when in making a shipment of freight from New York to Buffalo, at least three different bills of lading were required. Now five great systems embody more than three-fourths of the total mileage of the country, and the work of consolidation is still in progress. There are no longer state roads, but all are instruments of interstate commerce. Actual statistics are wanting, but persons in a position to know are of the opinion that the local business of the railroads does not exceed fifteen per cent of their entire traffic. In a case tried in one of our western states a few years ago, it was judicially found that the local business there involved amounted to less than three per cent. In the face of these conditions, it is impossible to maintain over common carriers the manifold control of the different states and the federal government.

There is no way in which local business can be separated from through business. The same roadbed serves both; both are carried in the same train and by the same crew. Back of every schedule of rates prescribed by government is the question, Are those rates reasonably compensatory? Under our present system that question as to state rates must be decided solely upon local business, and as to interstate rates solely upon interstate business. The court can not look to the entire traffic in judging of the reasonableness of either. While it is possible to ascertain what revenue is derived from each class, it is absolutely impossible thus to distribute the cost of operation and maintenance. The evidence upon that subject is wholly speculative and conjectural, consisting entirely of opinion testimony given by parties having a vital interest in the result of the litigation. In actual operation the railroads do not, and can not keep the two kinds of commerce separate. Why then should the law attempt to divide that which in actual life is a unit and indivisible?

Whenever a state prescribes a schedule of rates for local business, it thereby directly and necessarily regulates interstate business as well. There can be no sudden lifts and falls at state lines. They have no relation whatever to the cost of service, and can afford no justification for discrimination in rates. As the result of the schedule of rates prescribed by the State of Minnesota during the past winter, the rates on the western side of an invisible line were from twenty-five per cent higher than those on the eastern side. The railroads could not maintain both these rates without discriminating against North Dakota points in a manner which would constitute a gross violation of that portion of the interstate commerce act which forbids discrimination against any locality. The necessary result of the enforcement of the local rates was to compel a reduction of all through rates. This the Supreme Court has decided is such a direct interference with interstate commerce as to render the action of the state void. But further, if one state may prescribe a schedule of rates all states may, and the inevitable result of such a practice is to place the whole body of interstate commerce under the actual domination of state laws. In that way the authority which extends to only fifteen per cent of the business, regulates the entire business. The necessary consequence is that either the nation must take control of railroad transportation within the states or the states will take control of such transportation among the states. We deceive ourselves by a mere form of words when we speak of the separate regulation of local business by the state and through business by the nation. The state can not formulate and enforce any schedule of rates which will not necessarily and directly regulate interstate rates; neither can the nation formulate and enforce any schedule of interstate rates which will not necessarily and directly change local rates. The truth is that governmental regulation of rates is not a regulation of commerce, but of the railroads as an instrument of commerce, and when the nation and the state both prescribe to a railroad a schedule of rates, they are both regulating the same thing. This gives rise to a conflict of authority which Marshall declared in *Gibbons* v. *Ogden* ought never to be permitted to occur.

The chief domestic cause for the adoption of the constitution was to destroy the power of states over interstate commerce. But does not their control of railroads reëstablish that authority? To say that states shall not regulate commerce among the states, and at the same time

present than when it ws uttered. Wh
the unit of our social ad business life w
exception of the foreigiand coasting tr
of each state was confed to its own b
instead of industrial orommercial. T
merce are national. Tey are made awa
ing and often narrowl selfish enactme
and industrial organizion extend to
nation. Instead of beig required to o
pelled to obey many. Coincident wi
enterprise to embrace ferent states,
activity. During the fit half of the Ni
laissez-faire was the futamental princip
commerce and industrto private contr
Government is now psent in all line
regulated but little, buiness was not m
ulating. But now thaall governments
regulation, whether on government or
shall do the regulatin becomes a ma
These changed condins in our actua
of our divided govermental authority
nation, and what to thstates. The pro
it can not be answeredby reading histor

The new condition as manifested it
fields, the railroad ad the interstate i
beginning the railroadwere local. The
a shipment of freight fm New York to
bills of lading were riuired. Now fiv
than three-fourths of te total mileage o
consolidation is still iprogress. There
all are instruments of iterstate commer
ing, but persons in a psition to know a
business of the railroa does not exceed
traffic. In a case triedin one of our we
was judicially found tat the local busi
to less than three per nt. In the face
sible to maintain over ommon carriers t
ferent states and the feral government

There is no way in nich local business
business. The same rdbed serves both
train and by the same rew. Back of ev
by government is the qstion, Are those r
Under our present systn that question as
solely upon local busiss, and as to int
state business. The furt can not look

., to overleap
governments whose
·deral," "National,"
crican," these terms
are carrying on our
inding titles, but are
lucted. They have
al and international.
nployed three young
ze state laws passed
·ly upon the ground
·omparison between
tory statutes passed
tion. But the mass
great as to surpass
ition. The reports,
v in force are both
were those of the
ntined in the main
ose who had them
·equently manifold
recent govern-

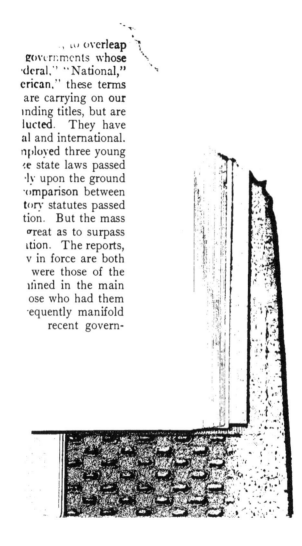

concede to them power to regulate the only instrumentalities by which that commerce is carried on, is to establish in practice what we deny in theory.˙ Hitherto state regulation has been inefficient and for that reason alone its localizing power has not become manifest. But now, through the investigations of economists and commissions, the general campaign of publicity, experience in rate litigation, the decreased influence of railroads over legislative bodies, there has come a new era in governmental regulation of carriers. State authority is becoming organized, energetic and effective. If continued it will work its inevitable results. In Commerce, as in politics, state governments will represent state interests. No rivalry can surpass that of our commercial centers, and the states in which they are located, let their power over carriers become effective, will exercise that power in support of their own cities. This is not theory. Only recently the commission of one of our most aggressive western states warned the railroads by a written communication that if they were not more considerate of the state as to interstate rates, the commission would retaliate by the exercise of its powers over local affairs. Other commissions, while not thus frank in their avowals, have been equally local in their practices. The severest critic of railroads can not deny that their policy has been splendidly national, and the most potent single factor in the creation of our vast domestic commerce. In thus maintaining the commercial supremacy of the nation, they have been compelled to withstand the importunities and fierce wrath of local interests. Now, however, the conflict is to be transferred from this field of economics to the field of government. Localism is to speak not by petition but by statute. Under this régime as governmental control increases in efficiency, the irrepressible conflict between local and national interests will increase in directness as well as in the frequency of its exhibition and the intensity of the passions aroused. It has already brought us to the verge of civil war in North Carolina, and been the occasion of the sharpest acrimony in other states. Such a ·conflict must in the end result in the complete supremacy of one authority or the other.

It is vain to appeal to states, as did Secretary Root in˙his New York address, to subordinate local advantage to the general welfare. Our whole history is a confirmation of the statement of Mr. Pinckney in the constitutional convention that "States pursue their interests with less scruple than individuals." They exhibit all that lack of conscience characteristic of those who exercise delegated power. As Justice Miller points out in his lectures on the constitution, had it not been for the dominant authority of the central government, the general welfare would have been as completely sacrificed to local selfishness under the constitution as it was under the articles of confederation. What states require is not exhortation but authority.

The situation in the field of industry presents the same general features. To abolish local control over matters extending outside of the state was

the origin not only of the article conferring power on the national government to regulate commerce among the states, but also of those provisions which forbid states to lay imposts or duties on exports or imports,
and which secure to the citizens of each state the privileges and immunities of citizens of the several states. These restrictions were placed in
the constitution not so much that men might be free, as that national
commerce and industry might be free. They have been largely nullified
in actual life by the fact that business is now carried on by corporations
instead of persons. When the constitution was adopted only twenty-
one corporations had been formed in the United States. These were
mainly for the construction of canals and turnpikes. There was but one
bank and two trading companies. As business agencies corporations
had no part either in life or thought, consequently they had no place in
the constitution. The Supreme Court has held that they are not citizens
within the meaning of the Fifth Amendment, and that each state may
either wholly exclude them, or impose as conditions of their entering or
remaining in the state such terms as local policy or interest may suggest. The result is that business which was intended to be free, has in
fact become subject to local authority. The abuses of corporate organization and management have heretofore commended this exercise of
local control. Ultimately, however, we shall become increasingly aware
of its injustice and folly. Business can not be conducted in this century
except through the agency of corporations; but the very enlargement
of that agency has caused industry, the same as commerce, to overleap
the bounds of states, and thus become subject to governments whose
only interest in them is that of the publican. "Federal," "National,"
"Union," "United States," "International," "American," these terms
find a place in the names of the corporations that are carrying on our
large business enterprises and are not mere high-sounding titles, but are
truly indicative of the scope of the business conducted. They have
taken national titles because their business is national and international.
While engaged in the preparation of this paper I employed three young
men in different libraries to examine and summarize state laws passed
since 1890, directed against foreign corporations solely upon the ground
of their alienage. My purpose was to institute a comparison between
laws of that character now in force, and discriminatory statutes passed
by the several states under the articles of confederation. But the mass
of material turned in by these investigators was so great as to surpass
any leisure at my command for its study and classification. The reports,
however, leave no room for doubt that the laws now in force are both
more vicious in character and varied in form than were those of the
earlier period. At that time discrimination was confined in the main
to taxation by states having ports of entry against those who had them
not. To-day they embrace not only double, and frequently manifold
taxation, but the thousand forms of regulation which recent govern-

mental activity in the field of business has developed. A condition which was then deemed sufficient to cause the framing and adoption of the constitution ought now to be adequate to compel the exercise of the power which the constitution vested in the federal government for the very purpose of controlling such conditions.

How far may the national government go in the control of those matters which have become in fact national? The situation fits exactly the terms of the resolution passed in the convention that framed the constitution, and which was the source of all the powers and restrictions embodied in that instrument. It presents a case "to which the separate states are incompetent and in which the harmony of the United States may he interrupted by the exercise of individual legislation." As to railroads there is no more reason why they should be subject to a divided authority than there is in the case of navigation. There will, of course, be in the one case as in the other, local matters that can be best dealt with by local authority. But as to all that affects them as commercial agencies, whether that commerce be local or interstate, the railroad is a unit; its activities are national, and it ought to be subject solely to national authority. Divided control is inefficient in protecting the public, and grossly unjust in the burdens which it places upon the carrier. During the last winter there were passed in the states west of the Mississippi River one hundred and seventy-eight statutes dealing directly with transportation and its instrumentalities. The number of such statutes now in force throughout the entire country extends well into the thousands. They are conflicting, oppressive, inefficient. They seldom represent intelligent investigation, but in the main have had their origin in agitation, often in popular frenzy. State legislatures have not yet learned that due process of legislation, like due process of law, proceeds upon inquiry, and legislates only after hearing. Protection to the public and justice to the carrier alike unite in the demand for a single governmental control. The power under the commerce clause of the constitution is plain. The decisions of the Supreme Court have placed that subject beyond the realm of controversy. If the railroad as an instrument of commerce can only be dealt with justly and efficiently by a single authority the federal government may assert and maintain its exclusive jurisdiction. Regulation is now inefficient because divided. If the federal government shall take exclusive control, it will then be responsible alone for such a control as shall be both efficient and just. Public opinion will have a single point for its direction, and will not be dissipated among many conflicting authorities. The subject does not demand separate rules for the separate states. Their action refutes such a doctrine. By the legislation of the past winter Virginia and Ohio, Pennsylvania and Minnesota are combined in the same passenger rate, though they vary as five to one, in density of population and travel. The subject is national, and the federal government with its national outlook can by organized investigation and accumulated experience best acquire the skill and knowledge necessary for its just and efficient regulation.

As to interstate industrial corporations, the subject is of much more recent development and the necessity for federal control is less urgent. It may well happen that many of the abuses in this field will disappear with the abolition of rebates and the other special privileges which such corporations have enjoyed at the hands of carriers. The evil arising from hostile state enactments may be remedied by a change of emphasis on this subject in the decisions of the Supreme Court. Heretofore that tribunal has been governed in such cases solely by a consideration of the nature of the corporate being. But the present tendency in corporate law is to look at rights rather than the nature of the being possessing them, and if the court shall adopt that view, it may yet hold that alienage alone is not a proper basis for discriminatory legislation; that legislation based solely upon that ground constitutes a denial of the equal protection of the laws. The late case of *American Smelting Co.* v. *Colorado* affords encouragement to expect such a change.

If, however, federal control shall be found necessary to correct the evils and protect the rights of interstate industrial corporations, authority for its exercise exists in the commerce clause of the constitution as already interpreted. It has been decided by the highest court that "The power to regulate commerce among the several states is vested in Congress as absolutely as it would be in a single government having in its constitution the same restrictions as are found in the constitution of the United States." That court has also held that as a means of executing this authority Congress may create corporations for the purpose of carrying on interstate commerce. One branch of that commerce is traffic or exchange among the several states, and if national corporations may be created for the purpose of carrying on that branch of interstate commerce which consists of transportation, as was done in the case of the Pacific Railroads, the same method may be adopted as to the other branch of interstate commerce which consists of traffic and exchange. Can a corporation created for this purpose be also authorized to produce the articles in which it deals? In thought, manufacture and commerce may be separated, but in business the former is always combined with the latter. No one ever manufactured except for the purpose of sale. Under the present régime of wide markets, large sales, and small profits, commerce has become the paramount feature even of manufacturing enterprises. The incidental powers which Congress may confer upon a corporation created for federal purposes were clearly defined in the litigation arising out of the United States Banks. There the federal feature was the collecting and disbursing of the national revenue. But to accomplish this result a corporation was created, authorized to do a general banking business and to establish branches for that purpose in the several states. Of the actual business transacted, the federal feature, though of capital importance to the nation, was a subordinate function of the corporation as a business concern. The opposition of the states was largely grounded upon this consideration. It was denied that they were agents. A resolution by the legislature of Ohio put the matter plainly: "We resist the shaving shops of a club of foreigners located among us without our consent." But the power of the federal government to create the bank and to exempt it from all local authority as to its entire business was vindicated in the fullest measure. Under the national bank act this authority has been carried much further. Usury and its consequences have been defined and all state criminal statutes affecting the transactions of these banks, or their agents or officers, have been held null and void. Now apply these well-established doctrines to corporations created for the purpose of carrying on that branch of interstate commerce which consists of traffic and exchange. Would they not fully sustain the authority of Congress to confer upon such corporations manufacturing as well as commercial powers? Would not the commercial activities of such a corporation which confessedly fall within the scope of the commerce clause of the constitution greatly surpass in importance the functions of the United States Bank which consisted in collecting and disbursing the public revenue? And if a bank created for that subordinate federal function might be given the power of carrying on a general banking business, why could not a corporation created for the purpose of carrying on interstate commerce, which would be a capital feature of its business, be at the same time authorized to produce either in whole or in part the articles which it applied to that commerce? It is said that *carrying on* interstate commerce is not the exercise of a federal power, as was the collection and disbursement of the public revenue, and that is conceded; but *regulating* interstate commerce is a federal power, and a corporation created as a means of such regulation may be freed from all state action that will interfere with the purpose of its creation. Surely if Congress as a means of regulating interstate commerce may create corporations to carry it on, it may endow them with all such powers as are fairly conducive to their success as business concerns, judged by the usual activities of corporations engaged in such commerce.

Our great corporations are now national in their character, and national and international in the scope of their operations. To regulate their formation is one of the most direct and efficient means of regulating their activities. For forty-five states to create corporations and the national government to regulate their most important business can not fail to result in inefficiency and conflict. Hitherto interests to be regulated have found advantage in the dual form of authority. It has enabled them to assert whenever either authority attempted their regulation that the power properly belonged to the other authority. We have now arrived at a state of knowledge and publicity which makes this kind of shuffling impossible. The nature of the subject to be regulated and not the shifting desires of the interests concerned must determine the place of authority.

Our first great conflict between the states and the nation was waged over the subject of banking and finance. No sooner were we started under the constitution than the need of a national agency in that field was discovered. But the local jealousy of the states prevented its establishment for more than seventy-five years. During that period we were subject to all the injury and confusion of wild-cat banking under state authority. Banking and finance, however, were not more national at that time than commerce and industry have now become, and the same conflict is again presented in this new field. We can get along with divided authority to-day on these subjects just as we got along with state bank notes. This nation can stand almost anything. But it is the duty of government in the exercise of its power to create conditions which are not simply tolerable, but those which are most conducive to the general welfare. A uniform authority in the field of interstate commerce and industry will be found as beneficent to-day as it was discovered to be in the field of finance and banking as the result of our first economic conflict. The problem of regulating these affairs has attained its present magnitude largely because the federal government has neglected to exercise its constitutional power over the subject in the course of its development. Until the interstate commerce act was passed in 1887 the negative power of the courts was the only federal control. Even by them till 1886 the states were sustained in their authority over interstate as well as domestic rates of carriers. The truth is that the national government has so long neglected its powers under the commerce clause of the constitution that now, when it tardily takes up its duties, it is charged by the states with usurpation.

The political revolution of 1776 required the creation of a central political power because it gave rise to great political concerns that could not be provided for by the several states. To-day as the result of an economic revolution quite as fundamental and far-reaching there are certain great business interests that have become national in their character and extent which can not be left to conflicting state authority. It is as unwise to stand timidly shrinking from the exercise of economic control now as it would have been a century ago to hold back from the exercise of political power through the fears of these who dreaded an adequate national government. We ought to look squarely at the nature and extent of our commerce and industry. Are they national? Ought they to be regulated by one or by fifty different sovereignties? If in their nature and extent they are national, and in justice to the public and the interests to be regulated ought to be subject to a single authority, then we ought not to hold back from the exercise of the necessary power simply because it would add to the activities of the federal government. We can not refrain from the exercise of necessary powers upon the ground that the federal government can not perform the work wisely and efficiently without confessing that that government is inadequate to perform the duties which the nature of things and the constitution alike devolve upon it. If national industry and commerce ought not to be subject to the jealousies and local interests of the several states, there is no alternative but to devolve their regulation upon the federal government. Between these two forms of regulation we must make our choice. The election is not between national regulation and some ideally perfect scheme; it lies between the single authority of the nation and the anarchy of the different states in combination with partial national control. The way, the duty and the power are plain. Unless domestic conditions such as in 1788 compelled the framing and adoption of the constitution, shall be impotent to compel the exercise of those powers granted by it in order that things which are national in their nature and extent may be controlled by national authority, there must be such an extension, not of constitutional power, but of the exercise of national powers already conferred as shall bring national commerce and industry under the single authority of the federal government.

One hundred years ago those who opposed the adoption of the constitution made "Consolidation" their cry of alarm. To-day those who oppose the control by the national government of the business affairs that have become national raise the cry of "Centralization." The one cry is as foolish as the other. On both occasions the opposition is guilty of that highest political folly which consists in hanging to a theory regardless of changed conditions in life. Centralization has already taken place out there in the world of commerce and industry. The only question remaining is, Shall the government take cognizance of the fact?

OUR CHANGING CONSTITUTION [1]

By Alfred Pearce Dennis

THE measure of the interpretation of our Constitution is found in the logic of personality, rather than in the logic of legalism. The unfolding of our national life according to this logic has involved three processes: first, new meanings have been written into the fundamental law by judicial interpretation; second, the unrebuked exercise of doubtful powers by the executive and legislative branches has extra-legally enlarged the sphere of governmental action; finally, through the spontaneous out-workings of our political genius, new rules, understandings, and convictions have been introduced into our constitutional system, without the intervention of direct governmental agency.

[1] *Atlantic Monthly*, 1905. Reprinted in part, by permission. Copyright.

I

Illustrations of the expansion of the Constitution by judicial interpretation may be briefly offered. Let it be borne in mind that the jurisdiction of federal courts is, by custom, limited to the determination of concrete cases. Federal judges do not decide abstract questions or settle disputed points of constitutional law unless such points are raised in a *bona fide* suit. It follows that judicial decision is ordinarily the second term of which legislative enactment is the first in the interpretative series. A decision adverse to a claim based upon the alleged unconstitutionality of a state or federal statute tends, of course, to enlarge the field of legislative competence, and to widen the scope of the written Constitution. Constitutional development has not followed the direct line of strict legalism, nor the haphazard line of pure circumstance, but rather the resultant of these forces. The logic of legalism and the logic of facts are never in exact accord. Congress, following out the logic of legalism, has power to declare war, and did declare war against Spain in 1898. Spain's sovereignty in Porto Rico and the Philippine Islands was extinguished as a result of the war. The United States succeeded to the sovereignty thus relinquished, and a kind of political relationship with the peoples of these islands has been imposed upon us which heretofore had not been deemed compatible with our legal scheme of political existence. According to the logic of legalism, it would seem that the Tagalogs and Moros, since they are subject to the jurisdiction of the United States, are possessed of the civil and political rights of United States citizens. The highest judicial authority, however, following a resultant between the logic of legalism and the logic of events, decides that the islands ceded to us by Spain have not been "incorporated into the United States." Hence it is perfectly possible for territory to be part of the United States in a geographical sense, without being an integral part of the United States; and that, in spite of the constitutional requirements as to uniformity of legislation, Congress can legislate pretty much as it pleases for the different territories, according to their varying requirements. As a result, then, of the decisions in the so-called "insular cases," it is judicially settled that the non-contiguous territories of the United States are to be governed in very much the same way as Great Britain governs her vassal states, — the Crown Colonies.

Again, under the commerce clause of the Constitution, federal authority over great commercial corporations chartered by individual states has been exemplified in the application of the Interstate Commerce Act. The Anti-Trust (Sherman) Act of 1890 did not in the view of its framers apply to railroads nor to reasonable restraints of trade, but the courts held that it did apply to railroads and to all restraints of trade, whether reasonable or unreasonable. The scope of federal activity was further widened in the "Northern Securities Decision," according to which the mere ownership of stock in an interstate railroad brings the owner into such direct relation to interstate commerce as to subject him to the plenary powers of the federal government. This decision, coming upon the heels of the Lottery case, marks an epoch in the history of federal centralization of power. Two important points were decided in the Lottery case: first, that the transmission of lottery tickets from one state to another is commerce, and therefore subject to federal regulation; second, that the power to regulate commerce includes the power to destroy it.

The inclination of the Congress and the President to give the Interstate Commerce Commission power to fix railway rates, subject to review by the courts, or the conferring of such power upon a new court created for this purpose, as under the provision of the Elkins Bill, are epoch-making proposals in the exertion of federal power through the elastic commerce clause. The creation of the Department of Commerce, with its Bureau of Corporations, marks another stage in the progressive unfolding of federal power over commerce. Mr. Garfield, Commissioner of Corporations, in his recent report, recommends that all corporations doing an interstate business shall be compelled to do so under a federal license. Under the proposed licensing act the national government may impose such conditions as to the organization, capitalization, and management of corporations as it may deem conducive to the public welfare. A proposition to take from the states the power to charter corporations engaged in interstate commerce, and to vest that power in the federal government, is already commanding a strong following. We hear little talk about the constitutionality of these measures. It is assumed, and rightly, that the courts would support the government in the exercise of these powers, although they are far beyond anything ever contemplated by the framers of the Constitution. The truth is, the courts will not, in interpreting the words of men who lived in the eighteenth century, place an injunction upon American progress in the twentieth century. While the great land-owning, ship-owning, or slave-owning individual was the most potent force in our economic life of a century ago, the great corporation is the most potent force in our economic life of to-day. These great artificial beings, the creatures of state law, have outrun the control of their creators. It is inevitable that the nation should take hold where state control has broken down. A hundred years ago the only media of interstate communication were coastwise sailing vessels and the occasional stagecoach that lumbered across state lines. But to-day steam and electricity are welding the states together, commercially and industrially. With the destruction of the states as industrial entities will follow, in the fullness of time, their destruction as political entities. Historically, federalism is like the grave: it takes, but it does not give.

II

The development of the commerce clause has been cited as an illustration of the expansion of the Constitution by judicial interpretation. Equally good illustrations may be found in the interpretation of the war power grant or the grant of the power to borrow money. We may pass, however, from this point to note that, while the Supreme Court is legally the ultimate guardian of the Constitution, the legislative and executive branches have frequently exercised wide powers of independence in interpretation. Illustrations may be offered, in the first place, of the expansion of the Constitution by legislative action without the actual intervention of the courts. This may proceed by affirmative action, as in the case of the congressional statute prescribing limited tenure of office for federal judges sitting in territorial courts. Or, secondly, the Congress, by refusing to act, can virtually nullify provisions of the organic law. For example, the *Congress has never provided adequate machinery for enforcing the extradition clause of the Constitution.* Governor Durbin, of Indiana, has steadily refused to surrender ex-Governor Taylor, indicted by a Kentucky court for complicity in the Goebel assassination. The Constitution provides that the governor of the asylum state shall "deliver up the fugitive on demand," but the Governor of Indiana pays no attention to the demand of Governor Beckham of Kentucky, and the Congress has provided no means for the execution of the constitutional mandate. It is possible, therefore, for a state governor to set himself up as a trial court, and arbitrarily refuse to surrender a fugitive from justice. Again, the provisions of the fourteenth amendment, penalizing by a proportional *reduction in representation* any state which excludes from the suffrage adult male citizens, is to-day as worthless as a counterfeit note drawn on a broken bank. The constitutional provision appears to be automatic, but no legal provision is self-executing unless the government provides the means. Again and again the Congress has refused to take affirmative action in support of the constitutional mandate. More than this, the fifteenth amendment is cynically nullified in its spirit, if not in its letter, by the constitutions of the Southern states. The Supreme Court recently refused relief to an Alabama negro seeking the suffrage denied to him by the constitution of that state, on the ground that the court lacked jurisdiction over the case as presented. Thus it happens that, when the disfranchised negro petitions the Congress for relief, he is told to go to the courts, because a legal question is involved; when he invokes the aid of the courts, he is told to go to the Congress, because a political question is involved. The truth is, the Congress and the courts recognize that the bitter experience of an entire generation stamps the *fifteenth amendment as a cruel error of national judgment.* Next to secession, it was perhaps the greatest political mistake of our

history. The South has long known it; the North is fast learning it.
American common sense, as represented in legislative and judicial
councils, goes to the root of the matter, and, by acquiescence in the
nullification of the written word, constitutes an unwritten amendment
to the organic law.

III

In the third place, important changes have been made in our constitutional fabric by executive interpretation. It is of interest to recall that
Jefferson, Jackson, Tyler, Buchanan, and Lincoln successively declared
that they did not regard as binding and final an interpretation of the
Constitution by the United States Supreme Court. Jefferson was not,
scrupulous in performing a legal duty as defined by the Supreme Court
in the celebrated *Marbury* v. *Madison* decision. Jefferson was also responsible for the Embargo Act and for the Louisiana Purchase, —
measures of doubtful constitutional standing. Jackson vetoed a bill for
rechartering the United States Bank, on the ground that it was unconstitutional, although the Supreme Court had previously decided to the
contrary. President Tyler, later on, endorsed Jackson's position in his
veto of a new Bank Bill. Mr. Buchanan, then a member of the House,
voted against the Bank Bill, declaring the legislator to be as independent
of the court as the executive. Lincoln impugned the constitutionality
of the Dred Scott decision, and, had he been President in 1858, it is
doubtful whether he would have employed the executive arm of the
Government to enforce the decision of the Court. In the manumission
of the slaves, and the suspension of the writ of habeas corpus, he made
no appeal to constitutional sanction. Legal limitations were brushed
aside in order that the life of the nation might be preserved.

Not a few of the discretionary acts of the present chief executive have
fallen within the shadowy realm of extra-legal powers. The following
so-called executive "usurpations" may be noticed: —

1. Ad interim executive appointments, the validity of which rested
upon a "constructive" recess of the Congress. The metaphysical subtleties involved in an appeal to the doctrine of infinitesimals baffled the
simple intelligence of the plain man, and the "constructive" recess has
been challenged as an unwarranted exercise of executive authority.

2. Executive order number 78, constituting the age of sixty-two a
prima facie evidence of disability in the adjudication of pension claims.
This act has been widely viewed in the light of the appropriation of
public revenues by executive decree, rather than by act of the people's
representatives in the Congress.

3. Mr. Whitelaw Reid's appointment as special embassador to attend
the coronation of his Majesty, King Edward VII, without the advice or
consent of the Senate.

4. The executive order excluding a great newspaper from the news of

the departments because that paper had published a silly canard about the President's children.

5. Intervention in the Panama affair, amounting, in the view of many thinking men, to a usurpation of the war power vested by the Constitution exclusively in the legislative branch.

6. The interposition of the President in the Pennsylvania coal strike through the creation of a commission to arbitrate a labor dispute.

7. The Executive "Agreement" with the Republic of San Domingo.

8. The creation by executive act of the office of Chief Engineer of the Irrigation and Reclamation Service, without the authorization of the Congress.

The exercise of these and other doubtful powers by President Roosevelt received no rebuke from the courts. From no responsible source came any suggestion of impeachment. Finally, the President received overwhelming vindication by the people at the polls. Hence the so-called usurpations are not to be regarded as usurpations at all. It all goes to show that executive and legislative officials (though this is true of the latter in less degree) are bound to the extent of their conscience and their political responsibility. As Walter Bagehot remarks, in one of the profoundest of political aphorisms: "Success in government is due far more to the civil instincts and capacity of our race, than to any theoretical harmony or perfection of the rules and formulæ of governmental conduct."

IV

Finally, radical changes, unrecognized as yet in the written law, but embodied in what may be called the organic "common law," have been wrought in the Constitution by custom, precedent, and the silent pressure of public opinion. The unfolding political consciousness of the nation reveals itself in spontaneous processes of growth, which without legal recognition are gradually transforming the body of written law. Nature's live growths rive even the rocks. Young and vigorous institutional plants thrust their roots into the crevices of crumbling constitutional walls, and at last overthrow them.

Our Constitution provides a theoretically perfect plan for the indirect election of president and vice-president. The demand of the popular consciousness for a direct choice has nullified this provision. Presidential electors have become mere pawns. They register, they do not elect. They must take what has been proposed at a convention and ratified by the people. Furthermore, while as late as 1824 presidential electors in the majority of states were chosen by the legislatures thereof, they are now, in all cases, chosen on a general ticket by a direct vote of the people. This practice, with rare exceptions, — as, for example, Maryland's split electoral vote in the last general election, — throws the entire weight of each state for the candidate whose list of electors happens to be carried.

The device of indirect election has thus gone to the constitutional scrap-heap. The growth of democratic sentiment has not only reduced the choice to a direct popular basis, but has hinged the decision on a vote by states.

In like manner, the growth of democratic sentiment is demanding the election of United States senators by direct popular vote, and we may look to see a progressive nullification of the legally prescribed plan of indirect election. The demand for formal amendment breaks fruitlessly against the determined opposition of the Senate itself, but the desired end is being sought through extra-legal channels. As, for example, in South Carolina, where a senatorial nomination in a primary election is considered binding upon the formal action of the state legislature. Under such a condition the legislature, like the electoral college, no longer elects, but merely ratifies the popular choice. In other states the legislature is not infrequently called upon to ratify a selection made by a knot of party bosses, in some back-parlor conference, weeks before the legislature convenes. Mr. Depew affably receives congratulations upon his return to the Senate three weeks before the convening of the legislative caucus nominally charged with the function of naming a junior senator for the state of New York. The old Frankish Mayors of the Palace were accustomed to pay elaborate homage to the kings of the Merovingian dynasty. Yet the king was a mere trapping of state, a glittering puppet, and the will of the enthroned monarch actually yielded in all important matters to the will of the uncrowned vassal. Thus it is that the body vested with independent choice may be reduced in great states, such as Pennsylvania, New York, and Indiana, to a mere ratification assemblage. Of the three branches of the government only one-sixth, in the beginning, was popularly elected; to-day one-half is popularly elected, and the sappers and miners of Democratic tendency are already beneath the foundations of another sixth, the Senate.

Again, the great national nominating conventions are absolutely unknown to the federal Constitution or statutes. The National Convention, made up of a thousand delegates, and as many alternates, elected by all sorts of process, not knowing one another, bound by no oath of office, is an absolute and final judge of its own procedure and its own results. Such a body, as in the case of the last Democratic Convention, passes through a four-day delirium of intrigue, oratory, and uproar, proclaims its creed and its nominees, and with adjournment goes down to a death that knows no resurrection. The conduct of public affairs, even when not veiled from the public eye, is humdrum enough. A convention, with its brass bands, its mad cheering, its high-keyed oratory, its thousands of spectators, and its frenzied enthusiasm, furnishes the most stirring, dramatic, and grandiose exemplification of public action which the political processes of this country afford. Yet of the conduct, function, and place of the convention in our political system the foreign student would gain not a hint nor suggestion from the entire body of our written organic law with all the commentaries thereon.

Equally without recognition in the organic law is the spoils system, the great foundation upon which party service rests. The practice of the executive to-day in appointments and removals is, barring the limitations of the Civil Service Law, substantially what President Jackson made it seventy years ago by the removal, during the first year of his administration, of two thousand placemen for political reasons. In recent years there has been a practical transfer of the appointing power in the case of postmasters from the president to members of the House. The appointing power is, of course, legally shared by the Senate. The president must take somebody's recommendation, and the custom of allowing congressmen the right to name postmasters implies a disposition on the part of senators to "go halves" on the spoils of office. Washington was called upon to appoint but seventy-five postmasters; this number has since increased a thousandfold, and it is absurd to suppose that any mortal can, on his own judgment and intuition, pick out suitable men for all these places. The president, in the majority of cases, can do no more than ratify an antecedent choice. In the *cause célèbre* of the recent Haverhill appointment, the President asserted a dormant prerogative and rejected the candidate for postmaster named by the local representative, Mr. Gardner. But even this exercise of so-called independence reduces to the acceptance of another's nominee. In this case Attorney-General Moody was given the right of way in nominating an official for his home city. The outpourings of Mr. Gardner on the occasion are of interest. He felt that he had been beaten by a series of moves not allowed under the rules of the game. He relied upon his "rights," and speaks of the "unwritten law" which vests in congressmen the right to name the postmasters in their respective districts. The representative from the sixth Massachusetts district received a stinging rebuke for bluntly insisting upon the observance of a custom which is tacitly recognized. In this respect he reminds one of Helvetius, who put into print in his book, *L'Esprit*, theories which contemporary thinkers had been content to advocate only in private. "They make so much ado about Helvetius," said Madame du Deffand, "because he has revealed everybody's secret." There is no reason other than the letter of the Constitution why postmasters should not be named by legislatively determined post-office districts, just as congressmen are chosen from legislatively defined congressional districts. The appointment of a postmaster who is *persona non grata* to the locality immediately concerned, as in the Indianola case, is foreign to our political habit, and one may assume that the attitude of the executive in this matter will tend even more to become one of mere acquiescence in a predetermined choice.

Again, one discovers no statutory basis for the custom which limits the choice of a congressman to the district in which he resides. American local pride rejects the notion that one's district can not be suitably represented by a local product; then, too, each district feels itself entitled to special legislative favors, and bases its hopes of realization upon a representative's familiarity with home needs, rather than upon the quality of his influence in legislative halls. The idea that Mr. Bryce, a Londoner, may acceptably represent the constituency of Aberdeen in the British House of Commons, is quite foreign to the average American's notion of representative government. This custom of limiting the choice of a congressman to the district in which he resides has entailed a distinct loss in the character of our representative body. An important state, and the nation, as well, were deprived of the fine legislative capacities of the late William L. Wilson, because a passing party upheaval changed the political complexion of the particular district in which the distinguished member from West Virginia happened to reside.

Without any sanction of positive law is the rule which declares the President ineligible for a third term, and the senatorial rule of confirming, without question, the President's cabinet appointments.

Again, both legislative houses are bound by a mass of rules which possess no legal sanction whatever. Invoking the rule of senatorial courtesy, Senator Hill was able, single-handed, and for purely personal and factional reasons, to defeat President Cleveland's excellent nomination of William B. Hornblower to the bench of the United States Supreme Court.

Unlimited debate in the Senate may now be regarded as an extralegal feature of our Constitution. This unwritten rule is defined by failures repeated through a hundred years to secure the adoption of a closure rule. Limitation of debate has been found necessary in the parliamentary bodies of England, France, Germany, Denmark, Belgium, Italy, Switzerland, and Canada. The United States Senate alone of all the great deliberative, law-making bodies honors no demand for the "previous question." The populistic outpourings of the Allens, Peffers, and Pettigrews, constitute a heavy price to pay for absolute freedom of debate, but perhaps not too high a price when one reflects that Senator Carter, invoking the equal protection of the unwritten law, held the floor of the Senate for ten hours during the last legislative day of the fifty-sixth Congress, and thus killed the River and Harbor Bill. By the failure of the bill, a saving of fifty million dollars was accomplished, and, as Senator Carter phrased it, "no injury was done to any living human being anywhere." In like manner, through the inflexibility of this unwritten rule, the whole fifty-seventh Congress, in its closing hours, was whiplashed by Senator Tillman over an old war claim of South Carolina's for forty-seven thousand dollars, which an auditor of the Treasury had appraised at thirty-four cents. Chairman Cannon of the Appropriations Committee denounced this transaction on the floor of the House in memorable words: "In another body," said he, "an individual member can rise in his place and talk for hours. . . . Your conferees had the alternative of submitting to legislative blackmail at the demand, in my opinion, of one individual, or of letting these great money bills fail. . . . In my opinion, another body must change its methods of procedure, or our body, backed up by the people, will compel the change, else this body, close to the people, shall become a mere tenderer, a mere bender of the pregnant hinges of the knee, to submit to what one member of another body may demand of this body, as a price for legislation."

Another extra-constitutional rule, which will undoubtedly prevail in future cases of ad interim gubernatorial appointments to Senate vacancies, was recently established in the Quay case. The Senate, by majority of one, decided that Mr. Quay was not entitled to his seat on a certificate of appointment issued by Governor Stone after the legislature of Pennsylvania had adjourned without making a choice. That the governor has no power to appoint in case the legislature fails to elect is a rule which may now be described as a principle of Federal "Common Law."

In like manner a binding customary rule provides that all appropriation bills shall originate in the House, although the written Constitution is silent upon the subject.

Equally without legal sanction is the Congressional Caucus, which silences the opposition of party dissenters, and secures unity of party action; or the unwritten rule of the Senate that seniority shall govern in the make-up of committees. Under this latter custom the most distinguished lawyer in the country probably could not reach the head of the Judiciary Committee until all party members who preceded him on the committee had retired from the Senate.

Finally we search the Constitution and statutes in vain to discover legal sanction for the tremendous legislative and political power now exercised by the Speaker of the House. The precedent which had the greatest influence with the men who sat with the Philadelphia Convention was that of the Colonial Speaker. He, like the Speaker of the House of Commons, was nothing more than an impartial moderator. The imperfect organization of the House, the rise of the party system, the vast increase in the amount of congressional business, have united to transform the speakership into a great political office. The central, vital weakness in our legislative system is found in its lack of unity and coherence. By processes of slow and inappreciable adaptation, our political genius applies empirical remedies to our constitutional defects, just as nature herself, by silent and inscrutable agency, applies to a wound or sore her processes of healing. Our income is raised by one set of men, our expenditures are applied by another. Government by standing committees means government by fifty-five jarring, petty leg-

islatures. A unifying influence in legislation is demanded, and partial
coördination is found in the paramount political and legislative control
now exercised by the Speaker. One admits that his power, through
recognition, seems tyrannical, that his authority to appoint all committees seems arbitrary, and that his control over the order of business,
as Chairman of the Rules Committee, seems dictatorial. But what
then ! The House acquiesces in "one man power," and there is a reason
for it. Macaulay observes that an army can not be led by a debating
club; neither can the House, which, without rigid discipline, would degenerate into a debating club, lead itself. Individuals, for the sake of
order and efficiency, must under military discipline surrender their
capricious, conflicting, casual wills to the will of a common superior,
just as, in the thought of Hobbes, the warring human atoms in "a state
of nature" confer, for the sake of peace and order, all their powers upon
a common coercive superior, called by Hobbes the great Leviathan, or
mortal God. The British House of Commons is able to govern because
obedience to leaders is of its essence. It lives in a state of perpetual potential choice of leaders, but leaders there will always be, and these leaders
must be obeyed. The penalty of disobedience is legislative impotence.
In a sense the House of Commons does not rule; it merely elects the
nation's rulers. This, in larger measure than is generally suspected, is
true of the House of Representatives. The three hundred and eighty-
six members who may occupy the floor constitute the House on parade.
The House at work is a disintegrate body, grinding away behind the
closed doors of fifty or more committee rooms. The House in session
is no longer the real legislative power, but rather the maker of the real
legislative power, — the Speaker and his appointees, the chairmen of the
great standing committees. Instead of a responsible ministry, as under
the British system, the House appoints a hierarchy, which in the present
state of evolution consists of four members, three a constant, and one a
variable, — the constant being the Speaker and his two party associates
of the Rules Committee, the variable being the chairman of the committee having jurisdiction of the measure which has been given right of
way by the Rules Committee. While the House has the constitutional
right to determine its own rules of procedure, it can not be maintained
that the Fathers intended to grant a power which should deprive the
popular legislative branch of its deliberate functions, or impair the free
representative character of the body itself. The transformation of the
popular branch has proceeded in obedience to the laws of our political
evolution. This development has been largely along extra-constitutional
lines, and, in the opinion of the writer, changes will continue to work
themselves out along the line of coördinating, with the legislative power
of the rulers of the House, a reciprocal measure of defined political
responsibility.

Who, ten years ago, could have divined the mighty changes wrought in our institutional fabric within the narrow limits of a single decade? To-day the thoughtful man turns to the future and wonders what is coming to the Republic. One notes the drift toward strong government and the growing disposition to appeal to Washington for the correction of all manner of public ills. The conclusion is borne in upon us on every side that out of the federal state is rising the unitarian state, just as out of the federation, — a band of states, — rose the Federal Republic, — a banded state.

The Constitution can be treated no longer as a written instrument defining the measure of American destiny, but rather as the sum of the political habits and convictions of the nation. This is not the place to deplore nor to approve. What is written, is written. *Litera scripta manet.* The written word does not change, but the consciousness of a progressive society, like that of the human organism, is always changing. Herein is a relation between a constant and a variable, — fixed law and changing life. Life can not be expressed in a formula or reduced to a syllogism. In a tempest the sea anchor, fixed in nothing more stable than the watery element, holds the ship to windward when otherwise the craft might be blown helplessly from her course. Our political development has followed the course laid down by the rigid, written constitution, but the anchor of limitations is fixed in an element which is itself shifting and unstable. The old conflict between the unyielding law and the living organism has resulted, as it must always result in any expanding life, in a victory for the organism. For the letter killeth, but the spirit giveth life.

SPEECH OF REPRESENTATIVE DE ARMOND FOR A CONSTITUTIONAL CONVENTION [1]

MR. DE ARMOND said:

Mr. Chairman: Listening to the remarks of the gentleman from New York (Mr. Perkins) upon the subject of an inheritance tax, my attention is directed also to the matter of an income tax, and to some things that are involved in the consideration of the two questions. All know that as matters now stand, unless through change in the personnel of the Supreme Court, leading to a change in its views and decision upon this subject, an income tax can not be imposed and sustained. There are a great many people of the nation, and I am one of them, who believe that a graduated tax upon incomes is a most righteous and most desirable tax. I quite agree with the gentleman from New York (Mr. Perkins), and with those taking a similar veiw, that an inheritance tax also is most desirable, and I hope the time is not far distant when we may have it established in this country.

[1] *Congr. Record,* Dec. 11, 1906.

In view of the fact, however, that an income tax is a mere experiment — not as to the qualities of the tax or its beneficial features, but as to the opinion of the court concerning its constitutionality — and inasmuch also as there are a good many other things that in the estimation of a good many people in this country would be wholesome as matters of legislation, which perhaps are not constitutional at this time, efforts are made from time to time to amend the Constitution, and such efforts will be continued almost indefinitely. When we reflect that no amendments to that great instrument have been made in more than a hundred years, excepting only the three which grew out of the civil war, and that excepting these civil war amendments and the one in relation to the electoral college, growing out of the contest between Jefferson and Burr for the Presidency more than a century ago, all the other amendments may be regarded as practically part of the original Constitution, we may safely conclude that the Constitution will not be amended in our day through the submission of amendments by the Congress.

The Constitution itself, however, provides another way of securing amendments to that instrument — that is, by the action in the first instance of the several States themselves (Article V).

There has been a great deal of agitation in the country from time to time, and there is perhaps a good deal now, over the proposed amendment of the Constitution in a good many important particulars. With some of this agitation and some of these movements I am in sympathy; with others I am not. A great many very good people, entitled to their views and entitled to a hearing upon them, are of the opinion that in a good many important particulars the Constitution ought to be amended. For instance, there are those who believe that it ought to be amended so as to provide for female suffrage. Others would have a marriage and divorce amendment. Some believe it should be amended with reference to the liquor traffic, or by way of prohibition of the liquor traffic. Many believe there ought to be a constitutional provision for the election of United States Senators by direct vote of the people. There are those who are of the opinion that the President and Vice-President should also be chosen by a direct vote. Some believe the Presidential term ought to be six years instead of four years, and that the President ought to be ineligible for reëlection as his own successor. Some people, particularly in the latitude of Washington, believe it is vastly important to have the Presidential term begin later in the season, so that inauguration day may fall at a time when the weather is more agreeable and fit for a pageant than it is likely to be about the 4th day of March. A great many people believe that Congress ought to be convened shortly after the election, instead of thirteen months after the Members of the House of Representatives are chosen. There are some who believe that provision ought to be made in the Constitution whereby the Government, under suitable regulations of law, might insure the lives of citizens of this great Republic. I am one of those who entertain that opinion. Life insurance by the Government could be made both safe and profitable; and what a boon to the people to get insurance at what it is worth! There are people who believe that by an amendment to the Constitution greater power, better-defined power, power that may be more easily exercised and more effectively employed, might be supplied for dealing with great trusts and other mighty corporate agencies of the land. I need not take the time of the House in enumerating the various matters concerning which amendments have been and are persistently urged and earnestly desired. I mention some of them merely as preliminary to the consideration of whether or not it might be advisable for the people of this country, by action of their various State legislatures, to call upon Congress to make provision for a constitutional convention, in which all the plans and schemes of amendment might be presented. Such a convention surely would be composed, in part at least, of the ablest men in the land. It would be a very great body of American statesmen and citizens. I believe the very fact of the assembling of such a convention — I believe, indeed, the preliminary discussions leading up to it or designed to bring it about — would be productive of much good in legislation in Congress and in the several State legislatures. The convention, I presume, would submit some amendments for the ratification of the people, and State conventions might follow, for considering and determining the adoption or rejection of the amendments submitted.

Now, I am not one of those who believe that the old Constitution is worn out, or that the ingenuity and statesmanship and patriotism of to-day would be likely to supply something which in its fundamental principles would be any improvement upon, or even as good as, that old instrument; but I am one of those who do believe that a constitution made more than a hundred years ago, when conditions were vastly different, when corporations were in their infancy, when our population was sparse, when wealth was not concentrated, when great agencies in government were not employed as they are employed now, before the day of the telegraph and telephone and the many triumphs of electricity, before many of the mighty inventions of to-day and yesterday were dreamed of; that a constitution made then may lack something now. I believe the makers did not embody in that instrument of matchless worth, our Constitution, all that might be or is now sufficient or desirable for present needs or to equip the people to meet the rapidly growing needs of the future of a great country. I believe a convention of American citizens, assembled for the purpose of considering various propositions to amend that Constitution, would be likely to submit some wholesome and timely amendments, perhaps a good many, but some, at least, which would meet the approval of the American people, and, by their sovereign will, be made part of the Constitution.

I believe there is enough of wisdom and patriotism and justice in the

American people, enough pride in their past, interest in the present, and hope of the future, to protect us against any possible danger that the Constitution might be impaired by the adoption of an unwise amendment. It requires three-fourths of the States, either through conventions or through State legislatures, to ratify any amendment to the Constitution. I can not believe that any amendment not deserving ratification, any amendment which really would not be an improvement, an enlargement, a perfecting, of the Constitution would meet with the approval of legislatures or conventions in three-fourths of the States of this Union. Of course, our action here, if any action is to be taken along this line, would be action only after the State legislatures, to the number of two-thirds of those in the Union, shall have called upon us for action. A good deal of time has been taken in committee and some in the House and in the Senate on various propositions to amend the Constitution. Every session these propositions are up. There are hearings before committees and occasional reports, sometimes lengthy and sometimes learned, upon this or that proposition, but no amendments are made, and no opportunity is given the people to consider whether or not any amendment should be made.

I am one of those who believe that there ought to be recurrence as frequently as possible to the judgment of the mass of American citizens. I believe that under our system of government it is wise every now and then, and quite frequently, to get at the sense of our people, affording them full opportunity to make themselves heard. There is a growing feeling, I think, and I think it is one that has foundation in real fact and real need, that very often legislation is too far away from the masses of the people; that their will is expressed in legislation too slowly and too imperfectly; that combined powers that can make known their wishes quickly, that exert their potent influence rapidly, that can concentrate at the very point where things are to be done, are more likely to prevail than the profound sentiments of the scattered citizenship of the country.

There are a great many people who believe that in our Constitution there ought to be provision made for what is popularly known as the Initiative and Referendum, by means of which the people themselves might directly suggest and initiate and directly pass upon legislation. I believe our Constitution would be improved by providing in it for this exercise of power by the people.

The whole problem of modern government, where the people seek to govern themselves, is involved in the one proposition of enabling the great masses of people, the 999, scattered and dispersed in their various vocations over the country, to make their power felt, register their will, and have done that which they desire to have done, in their own interest, for the welfare of the whole community and for the perpetuity of the Government. It is vastly important for the people that they be provided with the means of opposing effectively, and surely and swiftly overcoming those who have usurped authority, and those who by the concentration of wealth and by the powerful modern agencies for its creation and utilization in all sorts of ways, good and bad, are constantly pushing on to further their own interests and are constantly growing more heedless of the rights and interests of the plain American citizen. Now, if the Constitution could be amended so that the people will have more power, so that there may be quicker response to popular demands, so that there may be a correct and more authoritative registering of the popular will, very much will have been done toward insuring the perpetuity of government and preserving and enforcing the rights of our citizens.

An election was held last month for Members of the House of Representatives of the Sixtieth Congress. Unless there should be an extraordinary session called, the Members then elected will not assemble to discharge the duties of their office until ·December of next year — 1907 — thirteen months after they were elected. There really ought to be in the Congress of the United States, as there is in all of the State legislatures, an assembling of the newly elected body quickly after the election, while the Members are fresh from the people, whence they come with the authorization of the people, the command of the people, to do certain things and to refrain from the doing of certain other things; to make new laws; to amend or repeal old laws. A great many things happen in this country in the space of thirteen months, and Representatives who do not serve the people early, often do not actually serve them at all.

It is true that a Congress could be assembled, under the Constitution as it is, very much earlier than we meet. Instead of meeting on the first Monday of December, we could fix our meeting day at any time after the commencement of the Congressional term. Any time after the 4th of next March the Sixtieth Congress, by operation of law, if we saw proper to change the law with reference to the time of meeting, might be assembled. Somehow or other, I know not why, there seems to be opposition to any change, and the result is, Congress after Congress, we meet first in December, thirteen months after our election. We choose Members of the House of Representatives for two years, and thirteen months of that period are suffered to pass before the Representatives enter upon the discharge of their duties. This would appear passing strange if it were not so familiar and common, if it were not the order of things. It is strange that we do not amend the law, do the best that we can. But there could very easily be an amendment to the Constitution, if a convention were assembled to consider such things, by means of which Congress would be assembled soon after the election, speedily, in January or even in December following the election.

Then there is no reason why a Congress, after its successor has been chosen, should sit at all, except in extraordinary session, before the new Congress comes in — when there is, in the judgment of the President, an emergency for Congressional action before the new Congress can act.

There is no reason in the nature of things, there is no·reason in the essence of good government, why this Congress instead of the new Sixtieth Congress should now be in session. Those who declined reëlection or failed to secure it are supposed not to be so vigilant, so zealous, in the closing months of a term as those newly elected, who have the stimulus of a fresh baptism of popular favor, and something here for ambition to feed upon. I speak of this in generalities, because I know in many instances men whose terms are soon to expire have enough vigilance and are patriotic enough to be useful up to the very last hour of their service in a short session of Congress, when they know they will not be Members of the next Congress.

There can be no good reason why a Congress should be elected in November, for a period of two years, to assemble thirteen months later, and in a few months perhaps be involved in the throes of the on-coming campaign, a very large share of the membership being candidates for renomination and reëlection. Now, it may be supposed, and if we were not acquainted with the history of things and did not know how things go here, it would be supposed, that a change in the meeting time of Congress could be easily effected; but it can not be easily effected. We know that for years and generations, even, there have been efforts made without effect for a change, and perhaps other years and other generations may pass without its being accomplished. But I think it is very fair to assume that through a Constitutional convention this change at least might be made; and if the Constitution were amended in no other particular, if no other change were made in it, there would be enough of consideration for all the expense and all the labors of the convention if provision were made for assembling Congress speedily after election. To-day a constitutional amendment is necessary, because now the term begins on the 4th day of March, and, by shortening or lengthening one term, it should be made to begin in December or January next after the election.

· Now, I believe there would be wisdom in an amendment limiting the incumbency of the Presidential office to a single term. In some of the States the governor is ineligible to reëlection as his own successor, as in Missouri, where the treasurer likewise is ineligible.

When you look to the new State constitutions, there will be found many minor provisions which might, with great propriety, be incorporated in the Federal Constitution. For instance, a number of these constitutions enable the governor to veto items in appropriation bills. A bill may contain thousands of items, and the governor has the right to veto any one or any number of them and approve the bill as to the others.

I believe such a provision would be immensely beneficial. There are a number of abuses it would cut off, and the saving would be great. Too often it is only necessary to get an item, no matter how objectionable, into a great appropriation bill, and as the bill must go through and does go through, that item stands with the very best and the most necessary ones in it. The result is that combinations are invited, and sometimes, I fear, combinations are made, by which A assists B and B assists A, and the unholy alliance extends through the alphabet, with the result that probably two or three or a dozen or fifty or a hundred items are incorporated in the bill, not one of which, perhaps, has merit enough to stand alone or to win by itself upon its own merits. Now, if the President, when he comes to pass upon such a bill, could veto any item or items in it, there would be cut off the tendency to the abuse of combinations for the purpose of loading up bills, and in large part the possibility of success, because it might be assumed that most objectionable items would be vetoed.

Then I think the veto power itself ought to be limited, for I do not believe that the President's power in legislation ought to be equal to the voting power and the persuasive power of one-sixth of the membership of the House and one-sixth of the membership of the Senate. It is one thing for the President to veto a bill and it is another thing for that veto to be effective, unless one-sixth of the membership of this House and one-sixth of the membership of the Senate, added to a majority of each body, unite to override the veto. The real purpose of a veto, it seems to me, ought to be to invite the attention of the legislative body to supposed objections in the matter vetoed. It ought to be rather in the way of a holding up, a cautionary sort of proceeding. It ought not to require so large a vote to overcome a veto. It ought to be rather a check upon legislation, a challenging of the special attention of the lawmakers to the matter regarded as objectionable. "I do not believe this matter ought to pass. Please look into it more carefully; please give it reconsideration and see what your deliberate judgment about it is." But of late years there has been no particular abuse of the veto power, and a change in it is perhaps a matter of comparatively small importance.

But, as to the main proposition. Here we have a Constitution, one of the greatest and best ever brought into being by human brains; we have a Constitution framed in the infancy of the Republic, framed in the primitive days, before the great railroad had an existence, before great electric motors and telegraph and telephone were known; before the modern agencies called "trusts" had a being or were dreamed of; before the appearance of the millionaire as a common, every-day citizen; before the near approach of the billionaire; before the aggregation of hundreds and thousands of millions of dollars under single control; and it seems to me that in our progress, in the history of our nation and

49

of the world, we certainly have reached a time when it might be wise to assemble a convention to consider whether or not amendments could with profit be proposed to the great conservator of our liberties; and if they should be proposed, for the people deliberately, after their own manner, in their own fashion, to consider whether or not the Constitution should be amended.

Now, out of the discussion that would necessarily arise in a convention and after a convention certainly would come an awakening that could not be anything else than beneficial to the people of this country. There would be attention centered upon matters that are now overlooked and neglected. The people would have opportunity to assert their power and resume their control over some of the things, control of which has largely slipped from their hands. For instance, there is going on all the time now a conflict in opinion, and sometimes a conflict beyond opinion, between capital and labor, where serious questions as to the writ of injunction are involved. There has been a great deal of discussion and much uncertainty in a great many minds as to how the matter really stands. There is one school of thought that takes the view that the courts have the inherent power to determine what writs they ought to issue, and, if they decide they ought to issue particular ones, to issue them; that it is an inherent, necessary, preservative power and prerogative of the courts; that the court must say what is necessary to maintain its dignity and preserve its authority and execute its mandates, and that there is no power under the Constitution, no agency in the Government, to interfere with that exercise of authority.

Then there is another school of thought claiming that the courts, excepting alone the Supreme Court of the United States, being creatures of the law-making power, are within the scope of such laws as are made and such laws as may be made; that the question whether or not particular writs should issue, the circumstances under which they shall issue, if issued at all, are legislative questions and not judicial questions; that the power to make courts is the power also to unmake courts; that the right to confer, through legislative action, power upon courts carries with it also the constitutional right to circumscribe that power, take away part of it, and direct how it shall be exercised.

Now, that is an unsettled question in this country, with a tendency all the time in the courts to magnify themselves and to determine more and more and more that they have this power and that power, never given to them, as was foreseen by the wise men of the early day; a tendency ever toward magnifying the power of the courts and lessening the power of the legislative and executive branches when brought into conflict with them, and what is of far more importance, lessening in a good many instances the inherent and vital privileges and immunities of the people.

I believe a great deal of good might be done by a constitutional convention considering that among other questions. Shall our courts be final and supreme arbiters? Shall the courts determine what its powers are? Shall the court, independently of the Congress, determine when it shall issue a particular writ, who violates an injunction or a writ of prohibition or any other extraordinary writ, and what the punishment shall be — all determined by a single lifetime appointee — or shall the people, through those whom they elect to Congress from time to time and who are responsible to them, determine what the power of the courts shall be? Shall the Congress determine within what bounds the powers given shall be exercised, what powers they will give to the courts, and what powers they will withhold from them? I believe a question like this is worthy of the consideration of the ablest minds of the country, and I believe that a great constitutional convention would give to it, as to other great questions that would naturally arise and naturally be suggested, the consideration which they really merit.

Now, I believe one of the troubles of this country at this time in the conflict between labor and capital grows out of the assumption on the part of the courts of the right to issue certain writs when they have no right to issue them unless authorized by the law-making power to issue them. A court created by law possesses no power except what the law gives it. [Applause.] Those who can create can destroy, if they see proper to destroy; those who can grant power can withhold power. The question of whether or not a particular writ should issue in a particular instance — barring only the United States Supreme Court, created by the Constitution itself — certainly ought to be, it seems to me, a question to be determined, as all other questions of law making are determined, by the law-making body of the country — the Congress of the United States. And there ought to be some way of getting at undesirable judges, whether unfaithful or no longer efficient, and something more expeditious, something less cumbersome, something surer than the one remedy provided by the Constitution — impeachment — ought to be available. There ought to be something equivalent to removal by address. There ought to be some added sense of responsibility imposed upon every man who holds a judicial office in this country by life tenure.

Mr. STANLEY. Is it not true that that was one of the first defects pointed out in the Constitution within a few years after it was adopted? If my memory serves me correctly, Thomas Jefferson pointed out the danger of putting that power into the hands of the court.

Mr. DE ARMOND. Well, of course, Mr. Chairman, Jefferson's writings I think are full of warnings and admonitions and expressions of fear as to what may result from an encroaching judiciary.

Everybody in this country has respect for the courts, and in a body like this, where a large majority are members of the bar and a good many of them ex-judges, of course respect to the highest degree exists, but there is a tendency in the human mind and in human conduct to gather power, and, unconsciously perhaps — sometimes unconsciously and sometimes consciously — to usurp authority. You appoint a man judge for life, removable only by impeachment, a slow, tedious process, which, as the history of the country shows, usually brings no results. All he has to do is to avoid an offending on account of which he can be removed by the process of impeachment. A large number of his actions are not reviewable in higher courts. Either there is no provision for review or those affected injuriously are too poor to go to a higher court, The result is that there is a tendency all the time for the judge — assuming he is trying to do what is right and proper — if he thinks the case is one calling for a strong remedy to bottom his decision and justify his action upon the most extreme action, the most radical assertion of power, of any other court or judge whose ruling falls under his notice. He may go a little grain beyond any other one. Another case arises, and another judge goes further still, following and enlarging upon precedent; and so it goes, a constant, steady, gradual, and sure advance in the claim of power, in the assumption of power, in the exercise of power, with no unquestioned agency to check or correct. Now, take the matter of injunctions, if you please.

Mr. STANLEY. Will the gentleman yield for an interruption at that point? I am very deeply interested, and I would like to ask the gentleman it he does not think it would be wise, in cases of constructive contempts, where heavy fines and long terms of imprisonment may probably be imposed, to have the punishment inflicted by the intervention of a jury?

Mr. DE ARMOND. Mr. Chairman, I have heretofore expressed myself in favor of that, but I am trying to talk now about the fundamental principles rather than about the details of legislation.

The writ of injunction, of course, is an old writ. The courts assume to apply it to new facts, to new cases as they arise. The question comes up, and a most interesting question it is — it is one, in my judgment, that could be dealt with by legislation, but more effectively dealt with by a constitutional convention — when the new facts arise, when the new conditions are brought about, when there is supposed to be occasion for the application of an old principle to a new case — who is to say, who has the right to say, whether the old principle or the old writ shall be applied to the new state of facts, to the new condition of things? The judges assume that they have the right, and for a century in this country and more they have been steadily moving forward on that theory. My judgment is that the legislative body, and that alone, has the right to say whether when a new state of things arises, when new conditions develop, when new agencies are brought into play, this or that writ or this or that process shall be employed.

Now, take, for instance, the great development in railroad building and railroad operation. In the olden days, when the writ of injunction came into being, there were no railroads. No question arose as to whether there ought to be an injunction issued in a dispute between the mighty employer and the humble employee, because none could arise. There were no such conditions and no such situation at that time. In the process of time, by means of inventions, development of the country, growth of population, multiplication of corporations, vast increase in their power, functions, and ramifications, new questions arose, entirely different from the issues of the dead centuries. Yet the contention is that in order to determine what a court of its own power and right — its own inherent, necessary power, as they say, and its own constitutional and prerogative right — may do or shall do, the courts are justified in drifting away back to the pretended fountain of judicial power, the decisions of English judges and English courts, centuries ago, in cases having really no analogy, when you consider them properly, to the cases in which the principles thence deduced are now applied. Now, is it in the power of the courts to go on eternally in that way? Is it the right of the courts to determine when new conditions arise, when new agencies come into play, what they shall do, and how they shall do it, or is the determination within the power of the law-making body? My judgment is that the law-makers have the right to determine about it. Some people talk as if when you interfere with the courts in any particular, when you raise any question as to whether a court possesses power which different judges of the country assume to have and which they exercise, you are seeking to undermine the foundations of our Government and destroy property rights; invading the province wherein the courts stand as the guardians and protectors of everything that the citizen enjoys under the law.

Who make the laws? The representatives of the body of our citizenship itself, men selected for the very purpose of doing that very work, men responsible to their constituents for the way in which they do it or for neglect to do it. What reason is there to suppose that these men will not have as tender a regard for those upon whom they directly depend as will these lifetime judges who are not dependent at all upon the great body politic?

I did not mean to drift off into a discussion of this matter, because it is really foreign to the subject to which I wished to address myself. What I wished was merely to throw out the suggestion that I think the time has arrived when a constitutional convention might by action of Congress, stimulated and brought about under the Constitution by the State legislatures, be assembled to consider whether or not in some important particulars this great Constitution of ours might not be made better. This little discussion with regard to injunctions, by way of illustration, although it went much further than illustration, is an afterthought, and just simply happened.

NEW FIELDS FOR FEDERAL POWER [1]

"BEFORE many years," said in effect a conservative member of Congress the other day, "there will not be left a department of human life over which the national government does not somehow exercise control. "Great as have been the extensions of Federal functions within a comparatively few years past, there are enough others in contemplation to draw from their graves the statesmen who were arguing against internal improvements three-quarters of a century ago. In the President's last annual message there were no less than eight specific recommendations involving the exercise of new functions, or the assumption of new tasks, by the Federal Government. And if a list were compiled of the suggestions made along the same lines by bills now before Congress, or resolutions of public bodies — leaving out freak bills and constitutional amendments — it would probably be twice as long.

Railroad rate-making happens to be the most conspicuous proposal just at present. This is one of the things the National Government is asked to do because, unless it undertakes the task, it will not be performed at all. The States could not secure the same results even if they all coöperated to the full. The same may be said, of course, regarding the proposed regulation of express companies and national supervision of insurance. Other measures, widely differing in subject-matter, fall into the same general class, because they propose that the government shall do something not done by anybody at present, or at least not done efficiently. Such, for instance, are the protection of Niagara Falls — in which the Federal power over boundaries may be invoked — the preservation of the Great Lake fisheries by international agreement, and Commissioner Sargent's much discussed scheme for deflecting the stream of immigrants to those sections of the country where they are wanted.

Next may be classed the proposals which are urged on the ground that the Federal Government should step in merely to give the several States a chance to regulate their own affairs. These, for the most part, grow out of changed conditions. Centers of production and consumption have come to be so far apart, transportation so easy, and traveling so incessant, that local regulations, once amply sufficient, have proved, in many lines, to be little better than farcical. The Pure Food bill owes much of its backing to the fact that a State with good food laws is now at the mercy of one with bad laws or none, which can flood it with impure products; the prohibition communities never cease asking for Congressional action that will undo the "original package" decisions and help the State authorities to stop liquor in transit the moment it

[1] *The Nation*, 32: 131.

crosses the line. Other bills favored by the same interests wish a law that will make the records of the internal-revenue office more useful in the prosecution of illicit liquor-sellers. The national quarantine law, which, as always after the threat of an epidemic, is being strongly urged this year, would similarly save the neighboring States from the consequences of the laxity of any one. And President Roosevelt's recommendation, that the criminal process of each State be made to run throughout the entire country, bears somewhat the same relation to moral health.

Finally should be mentioned those instances in which national action is urged chiefly to secure uniformity of system in some department. The practical restriction of naturalization to the Federal courts, as recommended recently by a commission, is one example, and another the partly completed extension of national trade-mark legislation; while the national child-labor law, strongly pushed by a State labor commissioner recently, though without citation of the constitutional provision which would authorize it, is a type of many benevolent measures so advocated. Though some of these have been actively opposed and some kept from passage for many years, the argument, on abstract principles, of danger from the assumption of additional functions by the Federal Government is almost never heard. In fact, it is remarkable how much support such measures have in the old region of jealous States-rights sentiment. The national quarantine is distinctively a Southern measure, the liquor shipment bills are most strongly advocated there, and as for pure food, two Southern States are the only ones which, by a provision of their State law, have made the food standards of the Secretary of Agriculture go into effect within their borders as fast as promulgated. So a number of Southern as well as Northern States have voluntarily turned over their quarantine stations to the Public Health and Marine Hospital Service.

Efficiency has come to be the controlling argument in most of these cases. Our National Government has a way of getting things done — not economically perhaps, but efficiently — that the States simply stand by and envy. The illicit liquor-seller, who defies the sheriff and the chief-of-police, would not dare to run for a week without paying his Federal tax. The Federal officer, in any line of work, is freer from hampering local influences and is apt to be backed up more firmly in doing his duty. The present advocacy of Federal control as a general panacea is really not so much an indication of changing Constitutional views, as a tribute to the relatively effective way in which power is applied from Washington.

FROM A MEMORIAL ADDRESS ON THE BATTLEFIELD OF GETTYSBURG

By Representative James A. Tawney [1]

" I do not plead for States rights. I plead for the right and the duty of the Federal Government to protect itself and its Treasury against the encroachments of the States and private interests upon its powers, its duties, and its revenues."

*   *   *   *   *   *   *   *

In the early part of the nineteenth century there was fear and danger that the Union of the States was as a rope of sand and would fall apart. To-day there is more reason to fear that the several States and the local self-government which they represent will, for all practical purposes, disappear from our politics as distinct entities and be swallowed up in one all-embracing Federal power. The States not only seem inclined to allow, but in many instances are anxious voluntarily to surrender, to the Federal Government the discharge of duties and the exercise of powers and privileges reserved to them by the Constitution, especially when the exercise of those powers involves the expenditure of money. They are also to-day either soliciting or acquiescing in a degree of Federal supervision over their domestic affairs that less than half a century ago would have led to revolution had the Federal Government attempted to force such supervision upon them.

Much of the Federal legislation now being enacted, especially that creating new services in respect to the local affairs of the people, would not twenty-five years ago have been tolerated by the States at whose instance, through their Representatives in both Houses of Congress, such legislation is now demanded. Even private interests, interests entirely outside of State and Federal governmental functions are, through the activities of the Federal bureau chiefs, aided by the people of the States, seeking Federal legislative authority and Federal appropriations with which to develop local industries for the benefit of private enterprise.

The recent surrender by the Southern States of the exercise of the right reserved to them by the Constitution to maintain control, and regulate local quarantine, primarily because of the expense incident to the maintenance of an efficient State quarantine; the practical surrender to the Federal Government recently made by the State of Maryland of sovereignty over her oyster beds, that the State might be relieved of the cost of an accurate and necessary survey; the Federal inspection of the products of private manufacturing establishments and the sanitary in-

---

[1] Delivered May 30, 1907. Reported in the *Congr. Record*, May 16, 1908.

spection and control of the establishments themselves; the Federal inquiry into the physical, mental, and social conditions surrounding women and child labor in all local industrial occupations, with a view ultimately to securing national legislation to regulate domestic occupation; the inspection of cattle, of insects, and of all agricultural products; the investigation of soils, in which the Federal Government has no interest; the care and disposition of timber on State lands set aside by the States as forest reserves; the actual breeding of horses and cattle, primarily for the benefit of the few fancy stock raisers of the country; the making of topographic and geological surveys of States in which the Government does not own a foot of unoccupied mineral or agricultural land; the making of topographic surveys of cities and counties, primarily for the benefit of municipalities, private owners of waterworks, and interurban and other electric railways; the free testing of coal by the Federal Government for the benefit of private owners of coal mines to determine its quality in heat units and the best and most economical utilization of the by-products; the free testing of building materials for the benefit of private individuals, contractors, and consulting engineers; the work of gauging streams that are nonnavigable in States where the Federal Government owns no land and therefore has no jurisdiction or control over the streams gauged, a work which, as testified to by the former Director of the Geological Survey, is performed for the benefit of municipalities and "primarily for the benefit of prospective investors in water powers." These and many other undertakings which belong exclusively to the States or private interests to do and to pay for, but which have been authorized by Congress and must be paid for from appropriations made from the Federal Treasury, exceed the legitimate functions of the Federal Government as conceived by the founders of our political institutions and as declared by them in the Constitution of the United States.

To illustrate the unprecedented growth of Federal supervision and control over the local affairs of the people at the solicitation or with the consent of the States, I will call your attention to the extent of the special agent and inspection service ten years ago and at the present time. It is through this service that supervision and control over the domestic affairs of the people is exercised by the Federal Government. In 1896 the inspectors and special agents, including those employed in the Treasury, the Post-office, and the Interior Departments, where that service is legitimately employed in protecting the revenue, the mails, and the public domain, numbered, all told, 160, and this service cost the Government in 1896, in round numbers, $1,300,000. In 1907 we are employing an army of three full regiments of inspectors and special agents — 3,000 men — and this service is now costing the American people about $9,000,000, while the full quota heretofore authorized has not yet been appointed or appropriated for. The number of men employed in this service in 1907 is therefore more than eighteen times greater than in 1896, and the cost has increased about 700 per cent in ten years.

We hear it said by some that whatever enters into or concerns inter-state commerce and whatever affects the welfare of the people of more than one State logically falls within the provisions of the National Government, and this is made the apology for such authorizations and expenditures as I have referred to and for many other demands upon the Federal Treasury which the Congress has not yet seen fit to grant. But can you name a single important matter which does not affect the people of more than one State? Is there any phase of any great industry which does not come within the scope of interstate commerce? In short, is there any important private undertaking these days which can not upon some such pretext be brought within control of the Federal power? And yet, my friends, this is the tendency of the times, the growth of which during the last decade can be comprehended only by a careful analysis of national legislation and the aggregate annual expenditures of the Federal Government. If this tendency is not checked and the States continue to surrender the exercise of their reserved powers, or fail to exercise them in harmony with the interests of their sister States, then the Federal Government, as a dernier ressort, may be compelled to assume practical control over the States and the affairs of their people. In that case, with the vast and varied local and national interests of a hundred or a hundred and fifty millions of people, how long would it be before the task of government would become so complex and the financial burden so stupendous that of its own weight our splendid system of government would fail?

I grant you that it is more difficult now than formerly to draw a line between Federal and State authority, and between Federal and State expenditures; but it is not an insurmountable obstacle to the continuance of our dual system of government, nor should this difficulty be made the pretext for the Federal absorption of the functions of the States in respect to local self-government. But I would call your attention to the fact, and endeavor to impress upon you the direction in which all this is tending. The inclination on the part of the States to let the Federal Government exercise the rights reserved to them is greatly weakening the powers of the States. What is infinitely worse, it is weakening the respect of the people for the authority of the States. It is also causing the people to ignore and forget all those wise considerations which led the founders of our Government to provide for local self-government by reserving to the State all governmental powers not expressly conferred by the Constitution upon the Federal Government.

It has been suggested that the reason for this practical change in our system of government is to be sought in the imperialistic aggressiveness of the party now in control of the National Government. But, my friends, let us not deceive ourselves with shallow reflections. The real reason lies deeper than this. The tendency on the part of the States to surrender the exercise of powers belonging to them and the willingness of the Federal Government to assume such exercise, together with the burdens incident thereto, is not peculiar to any political party nor to any particular section of our country. It exists in all parties and in every section of our fair land. Let him who doubts this statement examine the record of the vote of the representatives of the people in the House and the record of the vote of the representatives of the States in the Senate. He will find that when there is a demand, either from the people or from the States, for the authorization of a new Federal service, a service which belongs to the States or to private interests to do, and an appropriation from the Federal Treasury to pay for the same, there will almost always be found in both Houses of Congress a majority composed of men of all parties and from all sections of the country who do not even pause to inquire whether the proposed authorization and expenditure falls within the legitimate function of the Federal Government. Their only concern is whether the revenues will be equal to the consequent increased appropriations; and even this consideration has but little weight, especially if their State or any of their people are to be the beneficiaries.

The true reason, my friends, why the people are willing to let the National Government perform and pay for so many things which properly fall within the obligations of the States is found in the fact that they do not realize that they are themselves paying for the things which the National Government pays for. The Federal revenue is secured by indirect taxation, while the money in the treasuries of the several States is secured by direct taxation upon the property of the people.

When any State increases its appropriations for any purpose, every legislator knows that that means an increase in the direct tax upon the people. Moreover, he knows that the people know this and that they watch with zealous care the tax rate which they must pay in cash from their own pockets. The legislator is slow to expose himself needlessly to the criticism and disapprobation of his constituents. Therefore needed legislation is postponed because of the expense it involves, and the Federal Government is appealed to, whenever possible, through the President, through the people's Representatives in Congress, and through the various Departments and bureaus of the Government. From my experience I can say that the Departments and bureaus of the Federal Government are at all times eager to enlarge the sphere of their activities and powers by taking on new services and securing increased appropriations. When popular demands are strong enough and it has become obvious that the States will not severally or jointly undertake obligations belonging to them, though seriously needed, the experience of the last ten years shows that the Federal Government, through its legislative

and executive departments, is only too willing to undertake such responsibilities and relieve the States of the burdens they involve.

My friends, our dual system of Government is threatened to-day by the tendency of the States thus to put upon the National Government the burden of administering their local affairs, and this tendency is constantly increasing as the result of the failure on the part of the States to perform their functions of local self-government, and in this failure they are encouraged by a sentiment created by the press of the country, teaching the people to believe that if the State legislatures do not act, "the question as to whether such legislation belongs in the field of the Federal Government will sink to a purely academic question."

I do not plead for States rights. I plead for the right and the duty of the Federal Government to protect itself and its Treasury against the encroachments of the States and private interests upon its powers, its duties, and its revenues. Where will this tendency end? To what result, think you, does it naturally and inevitably lead? Whither are we going in this centralization of Federal power and mutilation of local self-government? I lay no claim to prophetic powers, but I bring to you the thought of many of the ablest men in the public service to-day, when I say that we are unconsciously drifting toward a highly organized, bureaucratic form of Federal Government, such as has become the bane of most of the Old World governments of Europe. We are, either consciously or unconsciously, being drawn away from the simple and sublime ideals of local self-government, which not only gave shape to, but enabled us to adopt, the Constitution and have given unique significance to our political history up to the present time.

The remedy for this tendency, which we can not much longer look upon with indifference, lies in the simple application of the golden rule by each State to itself.

The only possible remedy lies in each State taking upon itself the burden of enacting all needful legislation and administering its own affairs within the rights and powers which it possesses, and in each State so legislating and administering its affairs that other States may do likewise without injury to any. The individual State should not only rise to the legislative needs of its own people in respect to local self-government, but should also consider what is deemed needful for the people of other States and act accordingly. Unless this is done, unless the States can thus join hands in the wise discharge of all the obligations devolving upon them under our dual form of government, it is inevitable that some of the fundamental features of our present system of government must sooner or later be abandoned. For it is certain that a people, believing as we do in self-government, will not long tolerate a condition of affairs in which the States fail either to exercise the rights reserved to them for the benefit of their own people or to exercise these rights in harmony with each other and for the best interests of all.

It has been said by a member of the Senate of the United States that such unity and harmony between the States is not possible; that it can not be attained without the interference of the Federal Government. This may be true; but, my friends, no such doubt entered the minds of the makers of our Constitution, or was ever expressed by them or by anyone else until within the last decade. They had supreme confidence in the power of the States to legislate in harmony with and for the best interests of the country as a whole. If their confidence was unfounded, if we must, with the further development of our industries, our commerce, and our political institutions, fall back upon the strong arm of the Federal Government to support and sustain us, then must the political significance and importance of our State boundaries become less with time and the splendid conception of local self-government, which has guided and restrained our lawmakers heretofore, be proven a failure.

The vital question, therefore, which confronts the American people to-day is, whether our dual system of government, in the form conceived and established by its founders, is ultimately to be wrecked upon the rock of a highly centralized bureaucratic Federal authority, or whether it can endure in the form originally created as the nation moves on to greater heights of development in industry, in wealth, in power, and in international influence.

Here, then, let us renew that high resolve, uttered upon this spot forty-four years ago, by the immortal Lincoln, that this Government "of the people, by the people, and for the people," in the form in which it was conceived by the founders of the Republic, in the form that has made us superior to all governments in the past, in the form for which brave men laid down their lives upon this and many other historic battlefields, shall not perish from the earth.

FROM AN ADDRESS BY REPRESENTATIVE J. S. WILLIAMS, ON "FEDERAL USURPATION" [1]

EVERY governmental abuse is based upon some plea or pretext and the usurpation of power by government is generally based upon "necessity," the tyrant's plea. This real or fancied necessity generally grows out of war.. This has been especially true with regard to legislative and executive usurpations by our Federal Government. Real or fancied war necessities are and ever will remain the chief pretexts for Federal usurpation. Amidst the universal plaudits which he has received and deserved, there are few people left ungracious enough to give sufficient emphasis to the part which Abraham Lincoln and his Cabinet had in changing the spirit, if not the form, of the American Government. The doctrine

[1] Delivered before the American Academy of Social and Political Science. Reported in the *Congr. Record*, June 3, 1908.

of "war powers" came into being, and after war had passed and peace had come the usurpations following from the exercise of the so-called "war powers" furnished precedence for their continuance and for other usurpations like them. As has always been said *inter arma leges silent;* there are undoubtedly certain powers which have been recognized to belong to all governments with forces operating during war in the field and in the enemy's country beyond those which are conceded to the same governments at peace and at home.

During the war between the States the Executive first asserted and Congress afterwards attempted to confer upon the Executive the right to suspend habeas corpus, not only in the territory which was within the boundaries of the Confederacy, but in the States which had remained in the Union. Things went so far that the writ of habeas corpus was suspended on the order of a lieutenant-general, acting under general authority conferred by proclamation of the President.

The Secretary of War and the Secretary of State, on bare orders, based upon no affidavit even, much less indictment, arrested and confined citizens of the loyal States and spirited them off to prison. Federal marshals and police did the same thing. All this, too, prior to the act of March 3, 1863, whereby Congress attempted to confer the power and the right to suspend the writ of habeas corpus, a power vested by the Constitution, according to all judicial construction, in Congress alone. Under a proclamation of the President, amongst the classes to be thus treated were described those who "magnified the resources of the enemy" and those "inflaming party spirit among ourselves." It seems almost incredible now that men could have been taken out of their beds at night and carried away to prison, without even affidavits, by ignorant marshals, who determined for themselves the questions whether or not those seized and imprisoned were guilty of disloyalty, especially when disloyalty was defined in such vague terms as "magnifying the resources of the enemy," "underrating our own," or "inflaming party spirit amongst ourselves."

Fortunately for the future of our republican institutions, in December, 1866, in the case of ex-parte Milligan (4 Wallace) the Supreme Court pronounced these proclamations of the President unconstitutional and the act of Congress so, except in so far as it was in its provisions "confined to the locality of actual war" and not elsewhere, and to places "where courts are not open."

There are those who believe that the branch of the Government most guilty in the field of Federal usurpation is the judiciary. This is not true. Upon the whole, the courts have been a bulwark of protection for the natural rights of the individual and for the reserved rights of the States. Judicial usurpations which have been successfully accomplished have not been a tithe of those which have been unsuccessfully attempted by the Federal Legislature or the Federal Executive. The Ku Klux act, which would have carried the Federal authority into every man's home within the States in the enforcement of ordinary criminal law; the civil rights act, which usurped to the General Government nearly all of the police powers of a State and the control of the social affairs of the citizen, are illustrations of attempted Federal usurpations set aside by the courts.

During the period immediately after the war between the States Congress fought most viciously against the courts, frequently attempting by acts of Congress, and sometimes successfully, to prevent appeals to the Supreme Court of the United States. A book might be written, and a very interesting one, too, upon usurpations flowing out of the civil war and out of the supposed necessities of a reconstruction of the Southern States.

Some of the usurpations that owe their real existence to the civil war still remain to plague us; for example, the legal tender case. The Constitution deprived the States of a power which was inherent in their sovereignty, but which had been found to be greatly abused — to emit letters of credit and issue paper currency. Hamilton himself contended that not only was this power not granted to the Federal Government, but that in spirit it was actually prohibited to it. Nobody ever did, or does now, doubt the right of the Government to issue a note as evidence of indebtedness when it has not the money wherewith to pay. But nobody up to the civil war had ever, for one moment, dreamed that the Government had a right to levy a forced loan upon the people by making its notes a legal tender for the payment of debt. This legacy, however, is not justly attributable to the judiciary, but to the President and the Senate. You are familiar with the manner in which this result was arrived at. After a first decision by the court declaring the legal-tender act unconstitutional, the addition of a new judge to the number on the bench and the appointment of another new judge to fill a vacancy, meantime caused by death on the old bench, accomplished a reversal.

It requires no imagination, but a plain survey of the field only, to realize what an immense capitalistic and centralizing influence the judicial construction into the Constitution of this power which was never granted — the power to make of Government notes a legal tender to take the place of gold and silver — has vested in the Federal Government.

John Marshall, in the case of McCullough against Maryland, had early in the history of the country upheld the power of the Federal Government to charter a national bank of issue, although a proposition in the Constitutional Convention to confer such power had been expressly offered and expressly voted down. The opinion in the case upheld the bank as a "fiscal agency" of the Government, and as such it was declared that it could not be taxed by a State, because such a power of taxation would carry with it to one sovereignty the power to destroy the fiscal agencies of another. And yet, long afterwards, when the law to establish the present national banking system, in order to strengthen the credit of the Government and to increase the price of its bonds, carried a pro- vision to tax State bank issues 10 per cent, it being admitted that this tax was levied not for the purpose of revenue, but for the purpose of stamping State bank issues out of existence, the court cavalierly flung aside its former doctrine that one sovereignty could not tax out of ex- istence the fiscal agencies or chartered instrumentalities of another, and held, in substance, by sustaining the constitutionality of the 10 per cent tax, that it could. The power to "issue 'money' directly to the people" in the shape of legal-tender Treasury notes, and the power to confine the function of bank-note issuance to national banks and to monopolize its regulation have together given to the Federal Government that power and influence over *finance and business* which make other usurpations, whenever all three branches of the Federal Government are desirous of making them, irresistible by the States or by the people thereof.

The early assertion by Congress of the power to levy import duties not simply as taxes for raising revenue, but for the admitted purpose of hothousing into prosperity at the common expense such industries as, in the opinion of Congress, it is for the common interest and the general welfare to hothouse, has given a whip handle, if not a mastery, over the *manufacturing* interests of the country to the Federal Government. The control of finance and of manufactures thus usurped, together with the immense powers actually vested by the Constitution itself in the Federal Government, under the treaty-making clause and under the interstate commerce clause, constitute our Government of to-day a Government stronger than any that Hamilton and his compeers ever dared attempt to inaugurate in the Constitutional Convention — stronger than Marshall even ever dreamed of construing or wanted to construe into existence.

This is true even when you consider alone the *real* power of Congress under the interstate commerce clause when exercised *honestly* and gen- uinely for the sole constitutional purpose of the regulation of interstate commerce. When you consider the cases where this power has been abused as a means to accomplish ends not contemplated by it, this con- clusion is stronger.

What has been actually accomplished, however, by legislation regulat- ing, or pretending to regulate, interstate commerce is nothing compared to what is proposed. A brilliant young Senator from Indiana proposes to control child labor within the States, through the interstate commerce clause, by denying to products manufactured within a State interstate transportation when produced by child labor, though employed in ac- cordance with the laws of the State of their manufacture. If Congress have power to do this, it has also power to say that no products shall be carried in interstate commerce if produced where labor is employed for longer than eight hours a day. If it have the right to do either, it has an equal right to say that no man or woman shall travel upon an interstate passenger ticket who has been divorced according to State divorce laws which do not meet with the approbation of Congress.

Early in the history of the country the story is told that the House of Representatives sent to the Senate a bill to regulate and work certain copper mines, and Mr. Jefferson, in his playful but philosophical manner, said that their method of deriving from the Constitution their power was about this: Congress has a right to provide for the common defense; ships are necessary for the common defense; copper is necessary to finish ships; mines are necessary to be worked in order to get copper, and, therefore, Congress has a right to work copper mines within the States; and added that anybody who had ever followed the reasoning in "the house that Jack built" could readily understand and would be convinced by the argument.

By parity of Indiana Senatorial reasoning Congress might enact a force bill under the interstate commerce clause, basing it upon the right of Congress to say what should or should not enter into interstate commerce as freight or as passengers. It might, therefore, say that any man elected to Congress unless elected in accordance with a certain law passed by Congress, should not be permitted to travel in interstate commerce, and therefore should not be permitted to leave his State and come to Washington to take his seat as a Representative. I know, of course, that the *reductio ad absurdum* is not the safest of arguments, but it sometimes makes things ridiculously clear.

Add to all this power over finance, banking, commerce, manufactures, the immense spread of the activities of the Department of Agriculture. It is furnishing seed to the farmers, it has established a stock farm in one of the States for the purpose of breeding "a standard national horse," and the right is about being asserted of entering into a State, with or without its consent, to construct roads not only between the States, but *within the States*. With their construction will come the assertion of the right to control, if not to police them.

The undoubted right of Congress to so regulate interstate commerce as to stop the spread of disease by it, from State to State, amongst men, animals, or plants, is as yet being driven only to its utmost, but will finally be driven beyond its utmost, legitimate application. That the operations of the great Department of Agriculture are beneficent there can be no doubt. The few millions appropriated each year for that Department accomplish more good than ten times as many millions appropriated for some other purposes.

But it does not follow that, because a given work is wise and beneficent the Federal Government has the right, or even by amendment to the Constitution should have the right, to do it, nor does it follow that because the Federal Government does beneficently carry it on, that it could not have been carried on quite as beneficently by the States, if the Federal Government had stayed out of the business. In connection with agriculture, for example, I for one believe that if the Federal Government had never undertaken to do anything at all with it the general condition of agriculture in the country would yet have been quite as good as it is, perhaps better, because then the States would have established magnificent agricultural departments, with experimental stations, training schools, and all that; would have vied with one another, from New York to California, in doing the work, each actuated by the motive of excelling others in the prosperity to be brought about by improving the basic art — agriculture. Those taught to lean upon others for support forget how to lean upon their own backbones.

The Department wants the Federal Government to go further yet and to inaugurate and maintain in the States technical, agricultural, and manual training schools, with what measure of Federal control it has not thus far seen fit to indicate.

Take, as the next illustration, the gradual assumption of power to the Federal Government in connection with works of irrigation. That Congress has a right to irrigate the public lands so as to make them valuable and so that the proceeds of their sale may inure to the interest of all the people there can be no doubt. Growing out of this right Congress has taken hold of the work of irrigation everywhere, on private lands as well as on public domain. It has added to that the kindred subject of drainage, because, undoubtedly, if Congress have power to put water on lands outside of the public domain, it has an equal power to take water off of lands outside of the public domain. The departmental work does not seem to have received even a momentary check from the decision of the Supreme Court in the great case of Kansas against Colorado, in 206 U. S., where the court says, after examining in detail all the enumerated grants of power to Congress, that "no one of them, by implication, refers to reclamation of arid lands."

In some cases where Congress has usurped power and where the courts have subsequently set aside the acts of Congress as unconstitutional the wrongs perpetrated under the acts have been perpetuated. Retaining in the Federal Treasury the money received under the "captured and abandoned property act " is an instance in point. After the general amnesty proclamation of the President, it became evident that the money lying in the Treasury from the sale of "captured and abandoned property," would have to be restored to the Southern people who had owned it. A rider on an appropriation bill of July 12, 1870, undertook to annul, and Congress, by refusing to appropriate the money out of the Treasury, practically has annulled the subsequent decision of the court to this effect. Millions of dollars are now lying in the Treasury accumulated there under this act of Congress, which the court subsequently held to be a special fund to be repaid to the owners of the property. There is no way of getting it out, however, because, as the court properly says, it requires an act of Congress to appropriate money once covered into the Treasury out of it again. Here is a case where Federal legislation has been adjudged invalid and unconstitutional, and yet where the people injured by the usurpation have suffered the effect of it until they died and where their heirs or assignees are suffering yet. The money in the Treasury derived from the cotton tax, and still kept there, is another instance almost in point.

I have referred to the war between the States as a source of much Federal usurpation. The Spanish-American war might be referred to in the same connection. The Constitution of the United States provides for the separation of the judicial, executive, and legislative functions. In the Panama Zone the Executive alone has been and is exercising not only executive, but legislative functions. When a resolution was introduced into Congress, and passed by it, asking "under what authority of law" the President was doing this, the answer came that it was under authority of certain acts of Congress, their dates being recited, and under authority of a treaty with the so-called "Republic of Panama," as if either an act of Congress or a treaty could confer upon the Executive the right to exercise judicial or legislative powers, in the teeth of an express constitutional prohibition of their consolidation.

Our experiment with schemes of crown colonialism in the Philippines now, and for a while in Porto Rico, was so stupendously alien to the spirit of all our institutions as to be at once horrible and amusing. Department law clerks sent out as proconsuls are learning in the Philippines and in Cuba to-day lessons which will return to vex the Republic at home. You need not expect that what is learned there will be forgotten here. In Rome the Imperator was first a field officer in Gaul or Asia or in other conquered territory. Then there came the exercise of powers as Imperator in Rome itself. Marius and Sulla as well as Julius Cæsar were virtually emperors long before Augustus Cæsar had founded what we now call the "Roman Empire."

Peace is important to all peoples. I sometimes think that two-thirds of the energies of all the statesmanship in the world might be profitably employed in the maintenance of peace throughout the world. But if important to other peoples, it is doubly so to us with our peculiar dual government, the balance of which is so nicely adjusted and so vital and which is always shaken by the sequelæ of war. We never know beforehand what these sequelæ are going to be. You hear much of "the horrors of war." The greatest of all these horrors is the murder of free institutions, and especially of local self-government, the only possible field for development of individual manhood.

The spirit of absolutism necessary to crown colonialism will be found to be contagious. Accustomed to it in all its spirit in our daily administration of colonial affairs, the public will gradually become accustomed to the insidious introduction of its features at home. No free government can successfully control alien and unassimilable peoples, except by the violation of the fundamental principles of free government itself. Our forefathers recognized this when they placed the Indian tribes on the footing of foreigners, to be dealt with by treaty.

The mailed fist, well exercised to its task, is dangerous, ultimately, to liberty of citizens much more than it is even to subject peoples. The system will some day drag down England herself by the exhaustion of her sons and her revenues in maintaining her hold upon India. The inauguration by us of the system in the Philippine Islands, unless once we have the good sense to put the people of the archipelago upon their own feet, teach them to stand alone, and leave them standing afterwards, will have the same effect for us in the long run. It is even now furnishing the excuse of great armaments, naval and military, and the Philippines constitute to-day the one point of unnecessary and unnatural contact out of which great wars may, if not must, ensue.

These Federal usurpations are going on not only through the Executive and the legislative, but, insidiously, gradually, unmarked, by bureaucratic operation, through the administrative rulings of the Government. Charles I lost his head and James II his throne because of executive and administrative suspensions of acts of parliament. The American people have become so accustomed to the suspension of laws by mere nonenforcement by the Executive, or some obscure bureaucrat under the Executive, that you perhaps could not excite real alarm in the minds of five men by a full recital of them all. The Executive sits in judgment every day on the wisdom of statutes.

Mr. Shaw while Secretary of the Treasury took money *already covered into the Treasury*, and under the guise of depositing it virtually loaned it to such banks as he chose without interest. This notwithstanding Article I, section 9, clause 7, of the Constitution, which says: "No money shall be drawn from the Treasury but in consequence of appropriations made by law."

The same Secretary of the Treasury quietly construed the disjunctive "or" in a law passed by Congress to have the meaning of the conjunctive "and," so that when Congress had by law said that those receiving deposits of public money — not deposits of money already covered into the Treasury, remember — but deposits of money collected from internal revenues and not yet covered into the Treasury — should deposit as security United States bonds "and" other bonds, that it meant "or" other bonds. Upon this he quietly issued a ukase to the effect that he would receive such securities as "complied with the savings-bank laws of New York and Massachusetts," and would dispense with the deposit of United States bonds altogether, in his discretion. The discussions in Congress at the time that the law under whose alleged authority he acted was passed show the reasons for the original act. People forget now that there was a time when United States bonds were not at par.

It was wise, therefore, upon the part of Congress to provide originally that the Secretary of the Treasury might require other security as *additional* to that of national bonds in order that the security might always be equal in par value to the money loaned. I need not dwell upon the total torturing of the original meaning by the Secretary's decision. Secretary Cortelyou ruled later on that, under the provisions of a law permitting the issuance of Treasury certificates "when necessary to meet public expenditures," he was enabled to issue these certificates to get money in order to help the banks by free loans in a panic.

An administrative board of the United States, engaged in the business apparently of seeing to it that due "protection" is rendered to "American industries," and finding that there was no tariff on frog legs, which were being imported into our territory to the detriment of the great American industry of bullfrog raising, gravely ruled that they were taxable under the clause which put an import duty upon dressed poultry.

What has been accomplished in the way of Federal usurpation by the National Legislature and Executive and either set aside by judicial authority or left to stand and stay to plague us yet does not constitute a tithe of what we are to expect if some recent utterances by great and popular men are to be taken at their face value.

The President in his Harrisburg speech, delivered in the month of October, 1906, says: "In some cases this governmental action must be exercised by the States. In others it has become increasingly evident that no sufficient State action is possible, and that we *need* through *Executive action*, through *legislation*, and through *judicial interpretation and construction*, to *increase* the power of the Federal Government. If we fail thus to increase it we show our impotency."

Mark the language. "We need — that is the old familiar tyrant's plea — necessity." To do what? To "increase" the "power of the Federal Government." The very verb "increase" is the President's word and is a confession that the Federal Government does not now possess the powers desired to be annexed — a confession, therefore, of deliberately contemplated usurpation. And to increase power how? Not by amending the Constitution, even though we had to amend the amendatory clause in order to make the work of amendment easier, but "by Executive action," and, "by legislation," both of them necessarily, if there be an "increase" of power, violative of the constitutional limitations upon "Executive action," and upon Federal legislation. It can not be too often repeated that this is true, or else the word "increase" would not have needed to be used. And third, and more insidiously still, by express executive injunction there should be and must be "increase" by judicial interpretation and construction. By the Soul of all Insidious Revolution! Mark the quoted words well in your memories!

Secretary Root, in his New York speech in December, 1906, evidently following up a deliberately laid scheme and purposely supplementing the President's speech in Harrisburg in October of that year, uses this language: "Sooner or later constructions *will be found* to *vest* power where it will be exercised, in the National Government." Secretary Root is a lawyer. He knows what the verb "vest" means. His language is to "*vest* power." "Vest" means to give — to deposit a new power, not to apply an existing one to new conditions. His ground and excuse and reason for "vesting" it is that it must be "placed" where it will be "exercised." The necessary inference is that it is *now* vested or placed in the States and that they ought to be *divested* of it, *because* they do not "exercise" it. IIis method of "vesting" power again is, like the President's method of "increasing" it, not by amendment to the Constitution, whereby the people themselves can redistribute the powers, which are theirs, and which they originally distributed between our dual sovereignties, but by "constructions" which are to *be "found!"* "Found" by whom? By the very men who are to exercise the powers construed into being by being "found."

An American citizen does not take an oath of allegiance to any government. His oath of allegiance is to the Constitution. Every officer who serves the Federal Government, from the President down, whether he be Cabinet officer, judge, Senator, or Representative, takes this oath. It is now proposed that the Executive officers of the Federal Government shall "vest" power in themselves "by construction," to be "found," and that they shall "increase" their power "through Executive action." Think of it! And yet in all this broad land no hint or suggestion of impeachment!

This method of amending the Constitution does not require a two-thirds majority in each House nor three-fourths of the States in confirmation of it. It is easy. It requires nothing but momentary forgetfulness of an oath registered in the chancel of God. It is not dangerous. It may, perhaps, even be applauded, if the thing sought to be done be popular with the populace.

What is more, the President proposes to "make good" — a phrase he is fond of. I have not time to refer to all the circumstantial evidence in support of this statement, but run over in your minds recent history — Root's part in it in the Philippines; the acts of our proconsular agents; the present condition of things in the Canal Zone, and the frequent chidings by the President of the Federal judges where they do not decide to suit him, showing a purpose of bending and warping the personnel of the Supreme and other Federal courts to an incorporation of his policies, where unconstitutional, by "judicial construction," as a part of the authority of the Federal Government. No lawyer not entertaining an opinion favorable to these policies can go upon the bench unless he succeeds in fooling the President or unless the President fools himself as to his legal opinions. Daniel Webster was right when he said that "the judicial power can not stand for a long time against the Executive power." The present President has already during his tenure of office appointed one-third of the Supreme Court and over one-half of the subordinate Federal judges.

Judges on the district and circuit bench, although they hold their offices "during good behavior," feel ambition like other men and would like to fill vacancies upon the Supreme Bench, as they arise. They can pursue no course better calculated to bring about that result than to let it be known by their decisions as subordinate judges that they share the President's opinions, and among others, perhaps chiefly, his opinion of the rightfulness of "increasing" Federal power " by construction."

The difficulty of amending the Constitution is the excuse at heart for most Federal usurpations, this with and even more than, the alleged "inaction of the States." It was well that at the beginning the practice of amendment should have been made extremely difficult. The thing was to put the Government upon its feet and "teach it to march," as the French say; to stop experiments with the framework until the people had become accustomed to it. We have reached the point now where there are many amendments that ought to be made to the organic law; first, because they are highly beneficent in themselves; secondly, because we want to do away with this excuse and pretext of usurping power "in order to do good." It has been said that the Federal Constitution can not be amended except as the result of some great cataclysm, or foreign or civil war. It is true that it is very difficult, indeed, to amend it — so difficult as to be, under ordinary circumstances, almost impossible. If you have a system which is too difficult of legitimate change, you therefore invite illegitimate change — or usurpation.

Changes by amendment. The first clause in the Constitution that ought to be amended is the amendatory clause itself. Amending the Constitution ought to be difficult, but not so difficult as it is now. It would seem that to require a majority of 10 per cent over one-half in each House, voting for two successive Congresses to submit an amendment, would be a requirement sufficiently difficult in the initiative. This would require at present 51 Senators and 215 Congressmen, and as that vote would be required in two successive Congresses, the scheme would give the people time to think between the two Congresses and an opportunity to pass upon the proposed amendments tentatively when they came to elect the Members of first Congress after the one proposing the amendment. If to this were added that the proposed amendment should not become a part of the fundamental law unless it shall be ratified both by a majority of the people and by a majority of the States, the practice of amendment would not be rendered so easy as to lead to many propositions of amendment, and still would be made easy enough to encourage a hope upon the part of those who wish to preserve our institutions, that they need not be destroyed because of the very organic difficulty of changing them.

It is not, however — note ye well — in this way that either President or Secretary proposes to go about the introduction of reforms or a redistribution of governmental powers. It is not proposed that it shall be done deliberately by amendment upon the initiative of the National Legislature and by the confirmation of the people in the States, but that powers are to be "vested" in the Federal Government, and the Federal Government, and that Federal powers are to be "increased" by "constructions," which are *"to be found;"* and by "Executive action" and "by legislation" and by a judicial reading into the instrument of that which is confessed, by the very language used, not to have been written into it.

There has been a recrudescence of federalism here lately alarming in its proportions. We begin to hear a great deal once more about "inherent powers," about "powers ordinarily exercised by sovereign nations," and therefore, as it is claimed, to be exercised by the Federal Government and about affairs of "national concernment." This latter phrase would include murder, theft, divorce — almost everything pertaining to morals or health. The President talks about court decisions which have left "vacancies," "blanks" between Federal and State powers, and wants these vacancies and blanks filled, occupied "by Executive action," by "legislative action," and "by judicial construction." How absurd! No decision of any court could possibly have ever left a blank or a vacancy between the powers to be exercised by the Federal Government and the powers to be exercised by the States. The moment the court decides that a given power is *not* one of those granted to the Federal Government, either expressly or by proper and honest implication, that moment the court has decided *e converso* that it *is* a power reserved to the States or to the people by virtue of the tenth amendment.

Much has been written about what is meant by the phrase "or to the people" in this amendment. In my mind it is clear; the powers not delegated are reserved either to the States or "to the people" *for redistribution*, as they may choose, by amendment of the Constitution. Both State and Federal governments are their servants, not their masters. The people of the United States, acting within their respective States, have reserved the right of further distribution of governmental powers. Again, individuals have also certain natural and inalienable rights, to which reference is likewise made in the phrase. These are by nature "reserved to the people," as individuals, as rights not to be touched either by State or by Federal Government — by any governmental or political agency whatsoever. That man does not understand the nature of American institutions who thinks that arbitrary and unlimited power is vested anywhere under our system, even in a majority of the people themselves, acting through any government or of themselves. There are things which under our system a majority can not do, whether they are right in their opinion to be done or not; thus high was the sacredness of individuality held by our forefathers!

I was talking a moment ago about the influence of the Executive over the judiciary — quoted Daniel Webster to the effect that the judiciary "could not long stand against the influence of the Executive" — and yet the spirit of the time is such that it has been gravely proposed in a bill introduced in the House to make this influence still greater. That bill, introduced on January 4, 1907, provides that the President may, "whenever in his judgment the public welfare will be promoted by the retirement of a judge," retire him and appoint somebody else, "with the advice and consent of the Senate," who shall take his place in the exercise of judicial functions. This would give to the President and to the Senate of the United States absolute control over the judiciary.

Our executive department has carried the Root doctrine into its dealings with Congress. Where Congress will not enact legislation that the Executive wants and loses patience about, some administrative department construes it to exist. This was the case in the graded-age-pension ukase, issued by the Commissioner of Pensions. A bill has been pending in Congress to accomplish the precise result; Congress would not pass it; the Executive, through the Commissioner of Pensions, amid popular applause, construed it into existence.

When, later, it was proposed upon a general appropriation bill to insert a clause enacting into law the graded-pension system thus promulgated, the point of order was raised that the motion could not under the rule be entertained by the House when a "general appropriation bill" was under consideration, because it was "contrary to existing law." In other words, that the amendment containing the very language of the ruling of the Commissioner of Pensions was confessedly a change of existing law. This point of order was sustained. Sustaining it was an admission of the fact that the Executive order had promulgated a new law — that a branch of the executive had legislated. If, on the contrary, the point of order had not been sustained, then the very fact of the adoption of the amendment would have been a confession of the fact that Congress *needed* to act *in order to make lawful* that which by Executive order had been promulgated.

Again, a treaty with Santo Domingo was pending before the Senate of the United States which the Senate for a long time refused to confirm. The Executive, being determined to have its own way, Senate or no Senate, did, as a historical fact, for two years before the ratification of the treaty by the Senate, execute the terms of the treaty.

Yet, again, the President at one time having a nomination of a certain South Carolina negro named Crum pending in the Senate, and the session having come to an end without action on it, and thereupon an extraordinary session having been called to begin at 12 o'clock on the very day upon which the former session expired, Secretary Root and the President between them construed into existence what they called "a constructive recess" — that is, that between the beginning of 12 o'clock and the end of the same 12 o'clock on the same day there had been a "constructive recess," and that this being the case, the President had a right to reappoint this proposed appointee during this so-called "recess." He did reappoint him thus contrary to law, and the Senate was subsequently coerced or persuaded to confirm him.

The logical inconsistency of public opinion in America was never better shown than with regard to this incident. The President's construction into existence of a "constructive recess" for the purpose of saving his right of appointment aroused no indignation, although it was the act of one man. He had, however, set a precedent which soon found imitators. If there had been a recess, then Members of Congress were entitled to mileage for the recess or, rather, the new session following it. They therefore very logically, according to the precedent set by the Executive (although of course very wrongfully, but no more wrongfully than the President) voted themselves mileage for the "recess."

A storm of disapprobation from the throats of the people and the columns of the newspapers swelled to heaven. The Senate voted the extra mileage out, and President, people, and all "congratulated the country." The man who imagined the iniquitous thing and acted upon it secured the result that he aimed at and was little, if at all, criticized. The very Senate that voted extra mileage out of the law upon the ground that there had been *no* constructive recess finally confirmed the appointee whom the President had hurled back at them upon the opposite theory that there *had been* a constructive recess.

Franklin Pierce in a recent book, that ought to be taught in every school and college where civil government is taught, a book entitled "Federal Usurpations," from which I have drawn much for this speech, says: "Social evolution progresses actually with the importance of the citizen over the State and decreases in the proportion of the importance of the State over the people." All these propositions of adding to the powers of government by "Executive action" and "legislative action" and "judicial construction" and "constructions to be found" leave that great truth out of sight. I know of no people who have too little government. We do not want an America like Sparta, where the State was all and man was nothing. We want no Rome, even, where responsibility was so entirely devolved upon government that when government itself grew weak there was no initiative left among the people even to resist invasion — a herd of helpless sheep they were.

Our weight of political machinery is increasing all the time. Not many years ago there were about 200 special agents — in other words, detectives and spies — in the employ of the Government. There are over 3,000 now, taking the places of ordinary Government officials, going up and down the land hunting up, by detective methods, violations of Federal statutes. A detective is like an expert in the medical profession. He generally finds what he is seeking. God never made a throat or a nose to suit a throat and nose expert; he never made a pair of eyes to suit an eye specialist. The Department of Justice uses a great many of these detectives. When you begin to inquire under what authority of law, it is difficult to procure an answer. That Department seems to borrow them from the Treasury Department. In other words, they are detailed from the Treasury Department to do work for the Department of Justice. The law appropriating for them in the Treasury Department appropriates for them for certain express purposes — chiefly for ferreting out and procuring punishment of counterfeiters and violators of the internal-revenue and customs laws. They are being used for a hundred purposes — peonage is the immediate fad; public-land stealing was the fad a few months back. In so far as special agents are being used for the purpose of investigating trusts and bringing them to book, there is express authority of law independently.

Judge George Gray well says in a recent speech that in Rome when a Dictator was appointed, his instructions were "to take care that the State receive no harm." This was a pretty broad authority. Mr. Bryce, the author of "The American Commonwealth," a book which has done much harm, seems to think from what he says that by a sort of construction or implication our Presidents, in times of acute peril may, or must, act on a like instruction. The present President does not seem to think that it is necessary to wait for a time of acute peril, but that the instruction is good "for any old time."

When the New York constitutional convention adopted the Constitution of the United States, it adopted it with the proviso that there should be no extension of power "by legal fiction." This was to prevent usurpation of Federal power by construction. How far the power of legal fiction may carry a system of laws may be realized when it is remembered that from the twelve tables of ancient Rome there grew up by construction and legal fiction the *corpus juris civilis*, and that from a lot of old customs there grew up by court precedents the great body of our "common law," or *lex non scripta*. The only restraint that we have upon Executive usurpation is judicial constraint and impeachment, and the only restraint on judicial usurpation is the power of impeachment by the House of Representatives before the Senate acting as a grand court of impeachment. It requires two-thirds of the Senators to convict, and the sole penalty is deprivation of office.

*   *   *   *   *   *   *   *

I shall not say much more, however, about judicial usurpation, because there has not been as much of usurpation by that branch of the

Government, either attempted or consummated, as by the other two. Upon the whole, our judiciary has rather preserved the Constitution from popular passion and impulse, from party spirit and sectional hate, and in proportion as Congress and the Executive grow wilder, it sets aside from year to year a larger and larger proportion of their acts. During the entire period before the civil war it had set aside only two or three general acts. Just how many multiples of that number have been declared unconstitutional since I can not now say, but we have grown accustomed to the Supreme Court's checking up Congress and the President every now and then, and the prayer of every good American is that it may do so "more and more unto the perfect day."

Yet even the judiciary has made some apparently queer decisions lately. In Mankichi's case, which came up from Hawaii, there had been no indictment nor any unanimous verdict of twelve men — in our constitutional sense a jury verdict — against the prisoner, and yet the Supreme Court affirmed the case upon the ground that the laws of Hawaii, when annexed to the United States, had not required an indictment and had made provision for a jury that did not find a verdict by unanimity, but by majority. Upon what principle, the court arrogated to itself the right to say just which fundamental constitutional principles should go with the Constitution to Hawaii simultaneously with annexation, and which of those fundamental notions should remain behind — to go later or not at all — presents a curious study.

The gradual growth of injunctions in Federal courts constitutes the chief thing to complain of in connection with that branch of our Government. Originally the equitable right of injunction was issued only when the law remedy was inadequate because of damages immediate and irreparable, and it did not apply to crimes. *In Lennon's case* (166 U. S.), however, men were actually enjoined from refusing to haul cars of a railroad and from leaving the employ of the railroad, while under the charge of a receiver appointed by a Federal court, on the ground that their quitting the employment "crippled the railroad's operation," and I believe, if I remember correctly, also upon the ground that it interfered with interstate commerce. This injunction was issued in spite of the thirteenth amendment, which forbids "involuntary servitude except from crime."

If everything that can be construed to be an interference with interstate commerce is to be taken as a just ground for an injunction, then a man who shoots another riding on an interstate ticket from Philadelphia to New Orleans would, as far as I can see, subject himself to Federal judge-made penalties, instead of being simply tried by a jury for murder, according to the laws of the State of the place where he committed the murder. Even when United States penal statutes exist, where a man can be arrested upon affidavit and rendered harmless, the Federal courts still issue injunctions.

The assertion of the power to inflict penalties for indirect contempts — constructive contempts, contempts committed out of the view of the court — punishments which carry deprivation of liberty and deprivation of property without a jury trial is another abuse.

These things encourage a spirit of anarchy.

Every man, if possible, ought to have a trial by jury.

Injunctions are issued on *ex parte* hearing, on mere affidavits without notice even to the defendant, and on reference of questions of fact to one referee. Upon such evidence as that, and such findings of fact as that, before any real trial, the enforcement of State laws, passed deliberately by State legislatures and approved solemnly by State executives, are enjoined. The plea generally is that the State law is "confiscatory." Of course, when upon a hearing properly had, after due notice to both sides, and a proper investigation of the facts, State legislation is found to be really confiscatory, it must be set aside by permanent injunction, as conflicting with the Constitution of the United States. But that is not the question here; the question is whether the temporary restraining order issued *ex parte* upon mere affidavits and so-called ascertainment of fact by a master in Chancery, very little acquainted with the subject-matter and very little able to judge of it, should prevail to annul a State statute.

Let us notice a tendency to usurp Federal power under the treaty clause. Calhoun says that treaties are the supreme law of the land "provided such regulations" (in treaties) "are not inconsistent with the Constitution." I quote Calhoun, because he went further than almost anybody in maintaining the "plenary power of the Federal Government to regulate our intercourse with foreign powers."

If the treaty attempt to treat concerning some subject-matter the regulation of which is not delegated to any branch whatsoever of the Federal Government, then that treaty is "inconsistent with the Constitution," as being inconsistent with the purpose for which the Federal Government was formed. If it attempt to treat of some subject-matter the regulation of which is delegated to any branch of the Federal Government, I care not which branch, I admit the "plenary power of the Federal Government" thereby exercised. That the treaty can give an alien equal rights with the citizen, even within a State, concerning a subject-matter that the Federal Government would otherwise not control I do not doubt, but that it can give him superior privileges to a citizen I deny. If by treaty with Japan, for example, California can be forced to admit Japanese, or by treaty with China it can be forced to admit Chinese, to the same schools with white children, then by treaty with Haiti or Santo Domingo negroes from those islands could be admitted to the same schools with white children in Mississippi, let us say, where native-born negroes, citizens of the United States, can not attend white schools.

The President in a Massachusetts speech is quoted as saying: "States rights ought to be preserved when they mean the people's rights, but not when they mean the people's wrongs."

In God's name, who is to say what are the people's rights and what are the people's wrongs? If I undertook to answer the question, I should say: "The people themselves." And then, if I were asked further how they were to say it, or have said it, how they were to draw the line, or have drawn it, how they were to prescribe the people's rights and prescribe the people's wrongs, I would say in the fundamental organic law, the Constitution of the United States and in the constitutions of the several States, which are *the prescribing voice of the people themselves*, saying both to the Federal Government as contra distinguished from the State governments: "Within these boundaries thou must travel," and saying to the State governments, the *residua* of governmental authority: "Thus far and thus far only in the United States shall any governmental authority over man ever go."

We are running mad. The latest proposition is to have a law for Federal registration of automobiles, on the ground that automobiles do sometimes cross State lines.

It is proposed by the President to charter and by Mr. Bryan to license corporations chartered by the States before they can enter into interstate business.

The President's latest astounding proposition is to leave a branch of the executive government to distinguish between "good trusts" and "bad trusts," marking out one for a license to do business and another for extirpation. What a campaign-contribution breeder that would be! How the combinations and trusts — the present substantive law being cunningly retained in the plan — would run over one another in contributing to the campaign funds of whichever party happened to be in power, in order to bias the executive department of that party in finding them "good" and not "bad!"

I have referred once before to administrative or bureaucratic usurpations of Federal power as being most dangerous of all, because most insidious and least seen by the average citizen. I wish that some of you, who have time to do it, would study the case, referred to by Franklin Pierce, by Juy Toy, a Chinaman (reported in 198 U. S.), who was born in the United States, went to China on a visit, and came back; was sentenced to deportation as an alien by the Immigration Commission, and whose sentence was affirmed by the Secretary of the Treasury. In some way the poor devil managed to communicate with a lawyer and to avail himself of habeas corpus proceedings.

The referee found Toy's statement that he was born in America to be true. The case finally got to the Supreme Court. That court decided that the question of fact as to whether he was or was not a native-born citizen of the United States had been decided by an administrative tribunal authorized to try it and that that finding was final and conclusive;

in other words, that it made no difference whether, as a matter of fact, Toy was a natural-born citizen or an alien, he was banished, and that was all there was to it!

It is not alone in connection with this case that the courts have held that they could not take cognizance of the conclusions reached by executive and administrative tribunals and that no appeal to any court would lie, but in other matters as well.

For example, the power at present reposed in the Post Office Department when issuing fraud orders, although it has not as yet been as seriously abused as it may be, is a power out of which the destruction of the entire principle of the freedom of the press may flow, especially when dealing through it with dangerous and unpopular classes. The Department may to-morrow, if it choose, cut off the *New York Times* or the *North American Review*, or *Collier's Weekly* from the right to be transmitted through the mails, under a fraud order. If it chose to do so, there would be no appeal to any court. It could furthermore, if it chose, refuse by a fraud order to permit any mail to be delivered to either of them or to me or to you. It could do this upon the report of detectives in the Department, and perhaps the first we would know of it would be from missing our mail. Moreover, upon complaint and inquiry as to the exact point in which we had offended, the Department might furthermore return the answer that it was not "practicable to make reply" to our inquiry.

Franklin Pierce, at any rate, quotes a case in the book to which I have referred, where certain printed matter was excluded from the mail on the ground of "obscenity." The Department was written to to specify in what respect and how and where there was anything obscene in the printed matter, and it is quoted to have replied that it was "not practicable" to answer the inquiry.

It is not to the purpose to reply that the Department *would* not do what I have supposed. That it *might* is a sufficient danger to human liberty.

In the case of South Carolina against the United States (199 U. S.) the Supreme Court says of our Constitution — which, I repeat, is the only sovereign in America except the people themselves acting in a prescribed way while exercising the power to amend and change it — the Supreme Court says of that Constitution, that it "speaks not only in the same way, but with the same meaning and intent with which it spoke, when it came from the hands of its framers and was voted on and adopted by the people."

That phrase ought to be memorized by every schoolboy who is studying "civil government" in every public school. Whatever the British constitution may be — unwritten, not exactly definable — the American Constitution is an instrument of written, prescribed, fixed sentences, phrases, and words, that do not dance about kaleidoscopically upon the printed page, and bear different meanings to-day and to-morrow, but mean just what they meant when they were uttered, although to-day, of course, they may be applied to very many conditions and instrumentalities that did not exist then. "Whenever an end aimed at is constitutional then all proper means to that end are also constitutional."

The great Federalist judge himself, John Marshall, uttered those words. The converse to that is not true, to wit, that whenever a certain *means* is constitutional, therefore the *legislative end* aimed at is constitutional. Congress has a right, for example, to regulate interstate commerce; but if the end aimed at be not in verity the regulation of interstate commerce, but be the regulation of child labor, or manufacturing, or education, or the suppression of ordinary crimes within a State, and the interstate commerce clause of the Constitution be resorted to merely as a means to the accomplishment of one of these latter ends — which end is in itself unconstitutional — then the thing sought to be done is exactly the opposite of that which John Marshall said could be constitutionally done.

One of the features most precious in our dual system of government consists in the very fact that there are so many State governments, in so many different climates, with so many different sorts of population, so many different systems of agriculture, such diversities of pursuits and occupation, of heredity and environment, that they enable our laws through the instrumentalities of the State legislatures to be adapted to the needs of the communities. Thus the States become great experimental fields. South Carolina can experiment with a dispensary law. If damage ensue, it is limited to South Carolina.

The people of the balance of the States can watch it without harm and learn lessons; find out if it is to be imitated or if it is to be avoided. If Oklahoma wants to make an experiment of governmental guaranty of bank deposits, the balance of the Union can watch the experiment with interest and with profit; without loss no matter how it turns out. If Oregon wishes to try the experiment of *initiative* and *referendum*, the same observation is applicable. All of us can watch the experiment of woman's suffrage in Colorado and some day imitate it or else learn to avoid it. And so with infinite diversity of surroundings and influence, with emulation existing between localities, the Federal Government does not need to experiment. In other lands experiments, if harmful, are not national hurts.

The very maxim, "E pluribus unum," is a Federal maxim. We must preserve not only the "one," but we must preserve, with equal care and jealousy, the integrity of the "many" governments which constitute our system — an "indissoluble union of indestructible States" — a "Republic of lesser republics."

May God grant that Jefferson prove right and Macaulay prove wrong, and that this constitutional, democratic, representative, Federal Republic of ours prove not a failure, as it assuredly must prove, if individual self-government based on the "self-denying ordinance of a majority" — the Constitution — denying absolutism to themselves even, and if local self-government or home rule based on the reserved rights of the States be lost sight of by us or by our children.

Remember these words of George Washington:

"This Government, the offspring of our own choice, uninfluenced and unawed, adopted upon full investigation and mature deliberation, completely free in its principles, in the distribution of its powers uniting security with energy, and *containing within itself a provision for its own amendment*, has a just claim to your confidence and your support.

* . * * * * * * *

"The basis of our political system is the right of the people to make and to alter their constitutions of government. But the constitution which at any time exists, *till changed by an explicit and authentic act of the whole people*, is sacredly obligatory upon all."

Spell "Nation" with a capital N, and spell "State" with a capital S, but, above all, spell "Individual" with a capital I, just twice as large. Be jealous of all government and of all increase of the weight of governmental machinery.

SPEECHES OF REPRESENTATIVES SHERLEY, COCKRAN, AND OTHERS ON FEDERAL POWERS[1]

MR. PAYNE. Mr. Speaker, I do not desire to discuss this resolution at any length, as the matter was fully discussed at the last Congress, in reference to the agricultural appropriation bill, which came over here with a revenue amendment attached by the Senate. On that occasion the precedents were stated to the House, and on a yea-and-nay vote only three or four gentlemen voted against it, and that because of their doubt as to whether the bill really contained a revenue clause or not. The bill was sent back to the Senate, and the Senate acquiesced in the decision of the House, and withdrew the amendment from the bill. Now they send over here a bill which is purely a measure of taxation. They propose that the 2 per cent bonds to be issued for the construction of the isthmian canal shall be taxed the same as other bonds for which provision of law is made that they shall be used as a basis for the currency of the national banks. They reduce the tax on those bonds, to be sure, but the bill authorizes a tax. This is a tax bill pure and simple. The Constitution has provided for the origination of these bills in the House of Representatives. The framers of the Constitution thought there was a reason for this. The House has contended immemorially, they have always contended that they have the right, and they have asserted the right time and again to institute revenue measures. They have the only jurisdiction in the Congress of the United States where these measures may be originated. Therefore, I ask the House to adopt this resolution; and in that connection I do not care to take up the time of the House by debate now. I may desire to extend my remarks citing some of the precedents; but the Constitution is so familiar, and this clause of the Constitution is so familiar that I do not think it is necessary for me to recite them for gentlemen to vote intelligently upon this resolution. [Loud applause.]

Mr. WILLIAMS. Mr. Speaker, this comes to me rather suddenly, and is rather an astonishing thing. I saw in the morning papers that the Senate had taken this action, but I thought they had taken it en route to settlement and the passage of a bill "for the construction of an isthmian canal." This matter comes back entitled "An act to provide for the construction of a canal," etc., but there is nothing in it at all except a provision for putting certain bonds in another class; and in my opinion it is undoubtedly a violation of the privileges of this House, as given to it by the Constitution of the United States. [Loud applause.] I believe that the position taken by the gentleman from New York is correct, and I think we ought to pursue either the course suggested by him or some other course that would indicate our opinion to the effect that it is a breach of the constitutional privileges of the House. I see no objection at the first blush to the resolution as read:

Resolved, That the bill S. 1475, in the opinion of the House, contravenes the first clause of the seventh section of the first article of the Constitution and is an infringement of the privileges of this House, and that the said bill be taken from the Speaker's table and be respectfully returned to the Senate with a message communicating this resolution.

[Loud applause.]

Mr. PAYNE. If there is no debate upon this question, I shall ask for a division, in order that we may have a rising vote and a count on this subject. I do not care to ask for the yeas and nays, but simply call for a division.

The question was taken on agreeing to the resolution; and on a division there were — ayes 357, noes none.

So the resolution was unanimously agreed to.

On motion of Mr. Payne, a motion to reconsider the vote by which the resolution was agreed to was laid on the table.

Mr. PAYNE. I now move that the House resolve itself into Committee of the Whole House on the state of the Union.

The motion was agreed to.

DISTRIBUTION OF PRESIDENT'S MESSAGE

The House accordingly resolved itself into Committee of the Whole House on the state of the Union, Mr. Butler of Pennsylvania in the chair.

The CHAIRMAN. The House is in Committee of the Whole House on the state of the Union for the further consideration of House resolution 42, and the gentleman from Kentucky is recognized.

Mr. SHERLEY. Mr. Chairman, it is never pleasant to find one's self in the position of Mahomet's coffin, suspended between heaven and earth, but I was very glad to yield the floor that this committee might rise, in order that the House might maintain its constitutional rights. It is so seldom that a member of this body has a chance to protest against the constant disregard of the constitutional rights and dignities of the House that I am always willing to yield the floor for any such purpose. [Applause.]

To return to the subject of discussion, I know of no more immoral practice than that which has grown up in the House of Representatives of using the taxing power for other purposes than the raising of revenue. It may be that in other countries the taxing power has been necessary as the weapon of liberty, either by denying appropriations or by taxing particular things, but in America the theory of our Constitution has been, and still is, that through other means the liberties of the people are guaranteed, and the taxing power was given only for the purpose of raising revenue. So, when you find upon this floor serious discussions of the reference of a bill to the Ways and Means Committee, upon the implied, if not the openly expressed, opinion that the taxing power shall be used not for the purpose of revenue, but for the purpose of doing something that otherwise Congress could not do, and that it was not intended that Congress should do, I, for one, propose to protest. Therefore, I am opposed to the reference of this matter to the Ways and Means Committee. I am also opposed to the reference of it to the Interstate and Foreign Commerce Committee. It is conceded by the distinguished chairman of that committee that the Supreme Court will have to change its mind in order for this Congress to have jurisdiction under that clause of the Constitution. He enters the domain of prophecy and says that they will do it. It may be that he agrees with Mr. Dooley, who, in the discussion of the insular cases, said to Hennessy that he was in some doubt as to whether the Constitution followed the flag, or the flag the Constitution, but it was evident that the Supreme Court followed the election returns. [Laughter.]

It may be that he considers the clamor now being raised throughout the land for the regulation of insurance companies by the National Government will have sufficient effect that, in the event of national legislation, the Supreme Court will sustain it and overrule itself. About that he may be a better judge than I am, but it is apparent to every Member on this floor that the discussion had for the past two days shows that it is the overwhelming judgment of the House that, as the Constitution is now interpreted, we have no such jurisdiction; that if we are to legislate on this subject, we must discover some other provision of the Constitution than the commerce clause.

Now, we have a great committee in this House, a committee that not only reports bills for legislation, but is also the judicial adviser of the House. The Committee on the Judiciary is supposed to be made up in its membership of the ablest lawyers in the House. They are there for the purpose of not only originating legislation, but they are there for the purpose of instructing the House upon questions of constitutional power. What more proper than to do what the Senate has done, make reference of a matter of this kind to the Judiciary Committee, that they may report back to the House whether, in their judgment, this House has jurisdiction, and if it has jurisdiction, the extent of it. Shall we determine now that one or the other of these committees may have this matter without a proper investigation? If the House is to now determine that fact, then, on the knowledge that the House has of the decisions of the Supreme Court, it ought not to refer this to any committee, because this House knows that it has been expressly declared that there can be no interstate commerce in insurance. Of course it can be reached collaterally, but is n't it a humiliating spectacle, is n't it such a spectacle as has been responsible for a whole lot of trouble in America, that men sworn to support the Constitution, representatives of a great body of the Government, are willing to disregard its plain limitations, and by subterfuge, under the taxing powers, do that which in their hearts they do not believe they are entitled to do? The fact that the House has done it, the fact that we have got precedents for it, only makes it worse. It only shows how one thing leads to another. The other day a statement was made in the other branch of the National Legislature that that provision in the law creating the Bureau of Commerce and Labor, relating to insurance, crept in there without the knowledge of that body; that had they had knowledge of it, there would have been a pronounced protest; and now we have a marked illustration of the danger of a precedent.

The President of the United States in his message says that because Congress has given to the Bureau of Commerce and Labor the power to make certain general investigations and inquiry as to insurance, therefore we have presumptively declared that it is a matter proper for national governmental control, and that declaration is used as a lever to make us go a step further. I understand that some member of the Judiciary Committee will offer an amendment referring this matter to that committee, and I hope that that amendment will prevail.

Now, Mr. Chairman, I desire to turn from this discussion of a narrow proposition to the discussion of a broader one. I believe the House will bear me out in the statement that I have never taken a partisan, captious position on the floor. I do not propose to do it now, but if I should let pass by in silence certain portions of the President's message without a protest, I should consider that I had no reason to be upon this side of the aisle, that I ought to go over to the other side. If I am to assume the position that seems to be taken by some, of out-heroding Herod, then I propose to go into Herod's camp where I can do it effectively, and not remain outside of it. I want to protest against that modern theory so pronouncedly and ably stated in the President's message that because a thing is big therefore it must come within the national jurisdiction. It is true that this whole country has been stirred from one end to another by the disclosures in regard to life insurance. It is also true that every one of those disclosures have been made known to the public by State agency and not by the National Government. It is true that the Supreme Court of the United States in deciding the case of Paul against Virginia, in deciding the cases that followed after that, plainly indicated that the States had complete — not only complete, but exclusive jurisdiction over the subject. Yet we have sent us a message saying that the time has arrived where it is evident, in the judgment of the people, that the States can not manage these things and that we must come to the National Government.

The President in his message says:

The fortunes amassed through corporate organization are now so large, and vest such power in those that wield them, as to make it a matter of necessity to give to the sovereign — that is, to the Government, which represents the people as a whole — some effective power of supervision over their corporate use. In order to insure a healthy social and industrial life, every big corporation should be held responsible by, and be accountable to, some sovereign strong enough to control its conduct.

  * * * * * * * *

The makers of our National Constitution provided especially that the regulation of interstate commerce should come within the sphere of the General Government. The arguments in favor of their taking this stand were even then overwhelming. But they are far stronger to-day, in view of the enormous development of great business agencies usually corporate in form. Experience has shown conclusively that it is useless to try to get any adequate regulation and supervision of these great corporations by State action. Such regulation and supervision can only be effectively exercised by a sovereign whose jurisdiction is coextensive with the field work of the corporations — that is, by the National Government. I believe that this regulation and supervision can be obtained by the enactment of law by the Congress. It this proves impossible, it will certainly be necessary ultimately to confer in fullest form such power upon the National Government by a proper amendment of the Constitution. It would obviously be unwise to endeavor to secure such an amendment until it is certain that the result can not be obtained under the Constitution as it now is. The laws of the Congress and of the several States hitherto, as passed upon by the courts, have resulted more often in showing that the States have no power in the matter than that the National Government has power; so that there at present exists a very unfortunate condition of things, under which these great corporations doing an interstate business occupy the position of subjects without a sovereign, neither any State government nor the National Government having effective control over them. Our steady aim should be by legislation, cautiously and carefully undertaken, but resolutely persevered in, to assert the sovereignty of the National Government by affirmative action.

    *   *   *   *   *   *   *   *

And again:

The great insurance companies afford striking examples of corporations whose business has extended so far beyond the jurisdiction of the States which created them as to preclude strict enforcement of supervision and regulation by the parent States. In my last annual message I recommended "that the Congress carefully consider whether the power of the Bureau of Corporations can not constitutionally be extended to cover interstate transactions in insurance."

    *   *   *   *   *   *   *   *

That State supervision has proved inadequate is generally conceded. The burden upon insurance companies, and therefore their policy holders, of conflicting regulations of many States, is unquestioned, while but little effective check is imposed upon any able and unscrupulous man who desires to exploit the company in his own interest at the expense of the policy holders and of the public. The inability of a State to regulate effectively insurance corporations created under the laws of other States and transacting the larger part of their business elsewhere is also clear. As a remedy for this evil of conflicting, ineffective, and yet burdensome regulations there has been for many years a widespread demand for Federal supervision. The Congress has already recognized that interstate insurance may be a proper subject for Federal legislation, for in creating the Bureau of Corporations it authorized it to publish and supply useful information concerning interstate corporations, "including corporations engaged in insurance." It is obvious that if the compilation of statistics be the limit of the Federal power, it is wholly ineffective to regulate this form of commercial intercourse between the States, and as the insurance business has outgrown in magnitude the possibility of adequate State supervision, the Congress should carefully consider whether further legislation can be had.

The President's reference to the reasons that controlled the makers of the National Constitution in framing the commerce clause is, I suggest in all humility, not historically accurate. The fact is, the convention of Virginia and Maryland was called — the convention that led up to the subsequent convention which adopted the Constitution of the United States — for the purpose of trying to arrive at some method of settling the conflicts that arose as to the commerce on the rivers and waters that divided those two States and to arrive at some method by which States would not be able to hamper and handicap the commerce of other States.

As a result of that convention came the national convention that adopted the Constitution. Now, the commerce clause has two provisions in it. They are in the same sentence, but they are distinct in the sense that they were put into the Constitution. One of them relates to the power of Congress over foreign commerce; the other relates to the power of Congress over interstate commerce. It was desired at that time that the United States of America might have a weapon that she might use against England, who was then fighting her commerce on the high seas. It was expected that the United States of America should use its power through that provision against other nations, but that part of it which relates to the States was put into the Constitution for the purpose of preventing the States from discriminating against the commerce of their sister States. It was put in there for the purpose of keeping commerce free, not for the purpose of shackling it. Yet to-day, and for many years past, it has been made the pretext for giving power to the National Government to hamper and control. Now, I trust I am not a man who looks backward. I hope I am not speaking of the tender grace of a day that is dead, but I do feel that half of the evils that confront the country to-day confront it because we have disregarded the fundamental theory of our Government. I believe the way to govern best is not only to govern least, but to govern as near as possible at home. [Applause.]

That is my kind of Democracy. That is the reason I am where I am. If we could make the people of the States realize that of necessity under the Constitution 95 per cent of the things that relate to life, liberty, and property belong to the States, and unless we change the organic law must remain with the States — if we could make them realize that therefore they must make their own State governments effective in order to deal in nine cases out of ten with those matters that affect life, liberty, and property, we might hope to solve our problems. But what has been the result? Largely as a heritage of the civil war, largely as a result of the acceleration that was given to the national power due to the emergency that that conflict brought about, we have had the spectacle that whenever a condition requiring a remedy arose in a State, the people, instead of trying to solve it there, come to the National Government and undertake to have the power under the Constitution stretched so as to bring the matter within the national domain.

The people, simply because the National Government seemingly acts, think that it always acts better. They think it acts better because they know less about its actions. They get a knowledge of what it does simply from the men who do it. The newspaper accounts which go out nine times out of ten necessarily go from the very source that has done the act which is to be reviewed by the people. Naturally the report going out is favorable, and they get the notion that if the action is by the National Government it will be better action. Maybe it is better, but, gentlemen, there is no reason why it should be as good. There is not a power contained in the Constitution of the United States in regard to most questions arising that is not contained in even greater measure within the State. Tell me that States composed of millions of people, bigger than some of the great nations of the world, are not able to have proper officers, capable of proper legislation, solving these problems, and what is equally important, capable of enforcing the law! I will not admit it.

This tendency toward centralization has gone on until, from having started out a hundred years ago in fear of the Executive, we have become afraid of the legislative bodies, from a fear of the National Government, to now a total disregard of State power. The people have a distinct contempt for the State legislatures, and they have more or less contempt for the National Legislature. It has become so that a member of the State legislature has to almost prove aliundi that he is an honest man and a man of good ability. Gentlemen, you get the service you expect. The people have restricted them; they have hampered them. Recent State constitutions have restricted the meetings of the legislatures to once in two years. They have restricted that meeting to sixty days or some short period. In a special session they are restricted to considering what the governor desires shall be considered. All these are indicative of the fact that the people are fearful of these bodies. The result is we have brought on this floor great questions not properly here, and *we have to spend nine-tenths of our time in determining not what we ought to do, but how we can do it.* If the theory of the National Government being not only supreme, but all-embracing, if the theory as voiced by the President in his message is right, then I for one agree to the suggestion made in that message when he said that if we can not do these things, if we can not take charge of this insurance matter, we ought to amend the Constitution. I go further and say that if we are going to attempt this and similar things, if we must take care of them here, then I am in favor of abolishing State government. I would a great deal rather see this body dealing with what it should do instead of always having to consider whether it can do it. That is common sense. If this idea of concentration is right, if centralization of power is right, then let us go on and carry it out. It is true we will be giving the lie to the theory which has prevailed in America since the beginning; it is true we will be running in the face of Anglo-Saxon history.

If it is true the time is coming when we are to have such power not only given the National Government, but are also to have given to the executive arm of the Government the right to handle everything under the sun, from football up, let us abolish the State government outright and make a clean job of it. Look how this idea of centralization is working right here among us. Look how it is working with the two bodies of Congress. One body, because it was smaller and because it had in a sense executive power, in that it could pass upon Presidential appointments, has grown and grown, until to-day this body is practically ignored, and we had the spectacle a few moments ago of that body, in plain contravention of the Constitution, undertaking to pass a bill that only could originate here. It is simply a further tendency toward centralization. You are not only concentrating the States out of their power, but now you are beginning to concentrate the different bodies of the National Government out of theirs. Against that, as a Democrat, as a believer in the history of my nation, I protest. It is for this reason I have taken advantage in this body when the President's message was up for discussion to voice my protest. I had been in the hope that some man abler than I, some man longer in the service of the House, might have felt called upon to do it, but in the absence of that I felt I should be untrue to those motives which actuate me, to the position I occupy in this House, if I did not protest.

Mr. DRISCOLL. Does the gentleman yield for one question?

Mr. SHERLEY. Certainly.

Mr. DRISCOLL. I have enjoyed the address so far very much, but I wish to ask the gentleman if it is not true, in his judgment, that gentlemen from the Southern States — Democrats from the Southern States — have a marked tendency to yield up their ideas of State rights in order that their States or their districts may get some benefits or emoluments out of the United States Government? Is not that the marked tendency with Democrats in the House?

Mr. SHERLEY. The gentleman has asked me a frank question. I will answer it frankly. It is true that in the past the ark of the covenant of local self-government has rested among the Democrats of the South. It is true to-day, unfortunately, that there are some of them, breaking the traditions, as I conceive them, of the party and of the country, who have wandered away after the fleshpots of Egypt. But, gentlemen, what is true in one instance on this side of the House is true in nearly all instances of that side of the House. [Applause on the Democratic side.] That is my answer to the gentleman.

I realize that in a large measure I stand in some particulars alone on the floor even as a "voice crying in the wilderness." I realize that the American people, from having been a very sober people, slow to form an opinion, have become a mercurial people, with opinions over night. I realize that in men's memory history goes back to the last edition of the paper of the day before, and their view of the future goes forward to the first edition of the day after. I realize that any clamor that happens to be loud enough may not only get the ear of individual Members, but it may get even the ear of the Executive of the nation; and because there is now a clamor we have sent to us a message saying that we must try and find a way in and out of the provisions of the Constitution to do certain things, and then if we can not do them we must do away with the Constitution in order to do them.

The message makes the surprising statement that the States are unable to control insurance. On what theory is that made? Does not every man know that if you had thè right sort of law, and, what is better still, the right sort of enforcement of the law, in the States that the power exists there to control insurance and control nine-tenths of our other troubles?

The President speaks of the fact that overcapitalization is the worst evil in connection with big corporations. Does not every man who is the least of a lawyer know that it is in the power of a State that creates the corporation to prevent overcapitalization? It can put all of the restrictions upon it that it pleases.

Now, it may be a sufficient answer to you — it is not a sufficient answer to me — to tell me the State has not done it. I say what we must do in this country is to awaken the people to a realization of that power at home; demand that a man shall exhaust the power that is given to the States before he comes to the nation. Why, if the President's theory is true, then there is not a city in the Union that should not be put under the control of the State government, because they have all been notoriously badly managed. Now, if the fact that they are badly managed, if the fact that the people of the city do not manage them right, do not elect the proper sort of officials to the common councils, is sufficient reason, then by a parity of argument the State should take control of the cities, and you should have them managed by your legislatures and the governors of your States. You only need to examine the proposition to see how it strikes at the fundamentals of this Government. Take the history of England and see what has been done in her city governments. It is true that Parliament is all powerful, and always has been, but it is also true that there is more local government there to-day than there is here, despite our boast. They send men of the highest ability to the common councils of their cities; put in men capable of occupying any position in any legislative body, and as a rule all of these cities are efficiently and capably managed, and they do not need to appeal to Parliament.

If the cities and the States should send into public life the right sort of men, making it worth while for a man to be independent, and keeping him in his position when he does show independence — if they would do that, you would find nine-tenths of the questions that trouble the Government would no longer be sent up here to trouble us. Every man in this House knows that the size of this House, the amount of business that comes here, practically prevents real judicial consideration of questions. [Applause.] The day has gone by when the House of Representatives can intelligently do affirmative work. There is no man here but who in his heart of hearts knows this to be true. What has been the result? You send important measures to a committee; you put into the hands of a few men the power to bring in bills, and then they are brought in, with an ironclad rule, and rammed down the throats of Members, and then those measures are sent out as being the deliberate judgment of the Congress of the United States; but no deliberate judgment has been expressed by any man. Now, if you are going to bring in additional to that other problems that you think should receive consideration, where are you going to end? Will it not have a tendency to end altogether in a government of bureaus? No man that will be frank in the statement of his opinion but knows that that is true. We all admit and we all admire the ability of the President; we realize his purpose is a high and lofty one, and yet we permit ourselves to sit silent, voicing no protest against a message to Congress that contains more of centralization than any other message that was ever written to the American people. [Applause.]

Mr. GROSVENOR. Will it disturb the gentleman if I make a suggestion or two along the line of his argument?

Mr. SHERLEY. Not at all.

Mr. GROSVENOR. Has the gentleman from Kentucky considered in his evident study of this question how you would establish two jurisdictions, two supreme authorities — one supreme in the State and one supreme in the United States — so as to administer in the form of regulation or taxation or prescription the duty of a corporation, it being an instrumentality of the States in some industry or in any other branch or business, so as to have both jurisdictions operating upon that corporation at the same time; and would it necessarily in the long run oust the State jurisdiction absolutely and put the whole power in the General Government? I am on the side of the gentleman; I am a Democrat in the matter of the rights of the States to control their own local institutions, and have always been so. [Loud applause on the Democratic side.]

Mr. SHERLEY. I am glad to have such able support, and in answer to the gentleman's question I will also try to be as frank as the gentleman was in propounding his question. No lawyer — no real lawyer — who has ever advanced beyond the mere citation of cases and gone into the philosophy of the law but what knows that the problem offered by a dual system of government is one of the most difficult problems ever offered to a people. And a further difficulty in that problem has been caused in large part by the extension of national control to the exclusion of State control, because of the temporary inefficiency of State governments. But the main idea that I wish to convey is this: Not that we do not realize the great inherent difficulty, that we do not recognize that there are many questions that lie on the border line of the jurisdiction of the two governments, questions about which men must differ and about which the courts have differed, and that when these questions come up it must follow that one or the other of these governments will get the jurisdiction to the exclusion of the other, according to the trend of the times, and frequently the practicability of its dealing with the question, but that as to those things that are clearly within the State's power and can be controlled by the State, that when no effort is made by the State to remedy the evil that that neglect should not be made an argument and an excuse for this Government, the National Government, entering the domain. Now, here is a practical illustration in the insurance matter. Here is a matter that has come to the attention of the people — this corruption, this wrong-doing — by virtue of a State investigation. Our States are just beginning to awake to a long-neglected duty, beginning to investigate and to formulate laws to control the situation. I undertake to say that if persevered in the States will be successful. The condition arose simply because the States have been neglectful of their duties in the past, and now we are told that we should, in advance of any results growing out of the States' activity, take the matter from them, notwithstanding the evil that inherently follows an entrance by the National Government into the State domain. It is not only true physically and mentally, but true governmentally, that a power unused becomes weakened and will in time be destroyed.

Let any part of the anatomy of man cease to be exercised and used and that part goes into decay until it finally disappears. Let the quality of local government, let that power which rests in the States, fail to be used; let the people forget that they have in their own hands the power to remedy evils; let them forget that after all it depends upon the moral atmosphere of the people themselves, their desire to enforce the laws that they pass — let them forget that and come constantly to the National Government for aid, come up here away from the place of the evil, and you will find that the ability to solve problems at home will die because of disuse. [Applause on the Democratic side.] Gentlemen, we make too many laws; we enforce too few. The trouble is that out of hypocrisy, out of cant, which seems to be a part and an attribute of the Anglo-Saxon, we are willing to pass laws that we do not believe in. There comes a clamor, and we yield to the clamor for fear of our jobs, and we put the law on the statute book when we do not think it ought to be there. Even although it remedies a particular evil, we know that it carries in its train many other evils. Then having put it there we wink at its being ignored. ·
Why, gentlemen, we pass every year numerous temperance laws and then permit them to be dead letters, because we have been cowards and were afraid not to pass them, and yet do not want them enforced. If the people will enforce the law, if we can have the enforcement of the law against the high as well as the low, we will solve many of our problems without any need for new legislation. Nothing has come ·out in the insurance investigation that the State of New York can not handle, and most of the problems can be handled on the criminal side of the law docket. [Applause.] It is a question whether the people of New York will have the courage, but if they do not have it that is no reason why we should take up their burden. We must send back word to them,

"You must solve your problems at home. If you do not do it, they will not be solved." [Applause.]

Mr. Chairman, I reserve the balance of my time.

* * * * * * * *

Mr. COCKRAN. This debate has taken a range far beyond a mere question of procedure in the House. It has touched a most important question of Federal jurisdiction. It has done more. It presents a question affecting the very existence of republican government and our power to take effective action for its preservation.

A most interesting contribution to the discussion has just been concluded by the gentleman from Kentucky [Mr. Sherley]. With the object which he had in view I sympathize most heartily. The method by which he pursues it I think is open to question. The gentleman from Kentucky [Mr. Sherley] has bemoaned the decline of State governments and the decay of representative bodies, including this one — two features of our evolution which I believe to be ominous in the last degree. But the gentleman says that he is opposed to any use of the taxing power as a means of enforcing authority by this House over important questions affecting the public welfare. So far as I could understand his argument, he stated that while this taxing power had been the effective weapon by which representative bodies had established their authority in the past, for some reason or other not made quite clear to me, and I fear not quite clear to the House, it was not proper or judicious at this day to invoke it for the preservation of the authority which had been established by its exercise. I have observed through all this discussion on the part of gentlemen who have opposed the reference of this question to the Committee on Ways and Means a disposition to treat the taxing power of this body as though it were a mere power conferred by law on some city or village government to levy an assessment for the support of a municipal department. It is important and, I think, essential to remind gentlemen that this power of taxation vested in the House of Representatives by the Constitution is the weapon by which all the importance of legislative bodies has been established.

If the conception of the gentleman from Kentucky [Mr. Sherley] and other gentlemen who have spoken on this subject be correct, then that provision of the Constitution which places in our hands the exclusive right to originate revenue bills is a mere idle expression — superfluous, meaningless, unimportant. Sir, I do not believe any line of the Constitution is either superfluous or meaningless. There are weighty reasons why that power has been bestowed on us. Sir, I think anybody familiar with the debates in the convention where our Constitution was framed will concede that through all the discussions it was assumed that this body would always be the important feature of our Government, and its importance in the judgment of the framers was assured when the taxing power was placed in our hands. If we are but a board of aldermen to decide whether the rates levied to support some city or village government should be 1, 2, 3, or 4 per cent on the assessed value of all its property, then the power to originate revenue bills might have been placed at the other end of the Capitol without in the slightest degree affecting the importance of this body. But, sir, because all the successful battles for liberty have been fought with that weapon, it was intrusted to us by the wise men who established this Government, in the belief that privileges which heroes had won in the field patriots would conserve in the council chamber. That power of taxation we have a right to exercise absolutely according to our own discretion. As we use it our consequence and our dignity will stand in the structure of our Government. The gentleman from Kentucky [Mr. Sherley] bemoans very properly the fact that legislative bodies have sunk into contempt while the body at the other end of this Capitol, which has some share of executive power, has risen steadily in importance, and he assigns the reason for it correctly. The reason is that the Senate of the United States exercises to the full every function and power the Constitution has placed in its hands. Every day witnesses not a recession or concession, but a new and further assertion of authority. Only this morning we in this Chamber felt bound to rise unanimously and declare that this last intrenchment of our power, this exclusive right to originate revenue bills, should not be broken down without at least a protest from ourselves. Yet the gentleman from Kentucky [Mr. Sherley], while recognizing and, indeed, deploring the growth of the Senate and bemoaning the decay of the House of Representatives, tells us in the same breath that he disapproves any use of the one power, the one weapon, by which our consequence can be established.

Mr. SHERLEY. Will the gentleman yield?

The CHAIRMAN. Does the gentleman from New York yield?

Mr. COCKRAN. Certainly.

Mr. SHERLEY. I differ simply because I do not believe that is the only power by which the House can assert its dignity and do not think the makers of the Constitution intended it should be the only power.

Mr. COCKRAN. Mr. Chairman, I suppose, of course, that was the gentleman's view or he would not have made the speech he did upon the floor, but the fact remains that he has bemoaned the waning dignity of this body and he has deplored, or, I believe, criticised, the growth of the other. My object now is simply to supply an explanation of what he considers a calamity and to suggest a method by which it can be repaired. With singular force he declared that powers which are not exercised are powers which are declining, that powers unused are perishing powers. The power to arrest our decay and reëstablish our consequence is ours, yet that is the power which the gentleman even now declares is not a proper or legitimate one to be used in maintaining our authority and our dignity. While that power is vigorously asserted there is no subject within Federal control on which we may not exercise the dominant influence, aye, sir, that we were not intended to dominate by the framers of our Constitution. The mere grant of this exclusive right to originate revenue bills shows that we were intended to be the principal feature of this Government. If we have declined and decayed, it is not for lack of power, but through failure to exercise the powers which are ours. The power of the English House of Commons theoretically is very little. Theoretically it is vastly inferior to that of the Lords; practically it is paramount through its control of the purse. Under the feudal system representative bodies had no power except the right to levy taxes. They had no right even to consider any other question unless it was expressly submitted by the sovereign through officers of his own selection and household, known as "lords of the articles."

The gentleman deplored a recent tendency of State constitutions to limit subjects which State legislatures can consider when called in extra session to those which the governor might submit to them. You see, sir, there is nothing original in personal government. There is nothing original in the forms by which distrust of popular government seeks expression. That tendency, which the gentleman deplored, is but a revival here in this land of the power exercised through lords of the articles under feudal institution, when the sovereign treated the legislature, parliament, or council simply as a body whose advice he might ask on certain matters, but whose authority, except upon taxation, he did not concede. The power over the purse alone was always conceded to the representatives of the people; and yet upon this slender foundation the stately structure of the British House of Commons has been erected, which dominates the entire English system, and which furnished the framers of this Constitution with a model for the establishment of this body.

Mr. SHERLEY. May I interrupt the gentleman again?

Mr. COCKRAN. Certainly.

Mr. SHERLEY. Is it not true the use of the power over the purse was in respect to appropriations, and not to do an arbitrary and unconstitutional thing?

Mr. COCKRAN. No, sir; the gentleman must study history a little more carefully. On the contrary, the power which was used most frequently and most effectively was the very power of which this House has deprived itself by special rule, the power to impose conditions on appropriations, to impose taxes on domains, privileges, monopolies, and other features of their political system which they considered dangerous to the prosperity or the liberty of the citizen.

Mr. SHERLEY. Does not the gentleman know that the National Government has no police power and it has been so declared, and does the gentleman not believe that the use of the taxing power for police purposes is unconstitutional to-day?

Mr. COCKRAN. Mr. Chairman, I am not conceding that this is a police power. The gentleman undertakes to anticipate the point at which I am aiming, and being doubtless innocent of the course of reasoning which I am pursuing, is naturally ignorant of the end which I seek to attain. [Laughter.]

I trust the gentleman will possess his soul in patience and at the end of a 'very few minutes he will understand precisely the character of the proposition which I am seeking to establish. I say, Mr. Chairman, that this body now possesses sufficient power to establish its consequence and its predominance if we choose to exercise it. There is but one change, one amendment that in my judgment could possibly increase its efficiency in legislation or its capacity to defend itself, and that concerns simply the term for which its Members are elected. Where a Member is chosen practically for two sessions and by the operation of our constitutional system one session must be held after the election of his successor, it necessarily happens that the very day on which he takes his seat upon this floor and begins the discharge of his duties he is at once thrust into the throes of a contest for reëlection. No man can perform his duty here wholly and efficiently when every day his mail is charged chiefly with information, representations, remonstrances, and appeals that concern not the public business at hand, but the prospect before him in his own district. [Applause.] If this democratic body is ever to acquire and exercise the measure of power which the builders of this Government believed it should possess in order that this constitutional system may be safe and prosperous, there should be at least one or two sessions in which Members could devote themselves to their public duties free from the distraction of a campaign for reëlection. Apart from that there is no effective power the Constitution could bestow on us that it has not already bestowed when it gave us the taxing power.

If we have no importance, it is not because we lack power, but because we have put away the great power which has been conferred upon us. And strange as it may seem, the gentlemen who are the most solicitous about the Constitution, the gentleman who describes that instrument as the sacred ark of the covenant — I think I am using the exact words of my friend from Kentucky — condemns as vicious a use of its most important feature, the one on which depends the importance of the body of which he is already a distinguished member and certain in the near future to become one of its most brilliant ornaments. [Applause.]

Now, Mr. Chairman, the suggestion which I would like to place before this committee is that there are various provisions of the Constitution which may be invoked to deal effectively with the abuses grown out of the maladministration of these insurance corporations. But before we consider the remedy which should be applied, let us for a moment consider the nature of the difficulty which confronts us. I believe that on any subject fairly within the authority of the Federal Government — any subject over which the Federal Government has jurisdiction — this House has the right to exercise the taxing power in any way it pleases for the maintenance of its own authority and the enforcement of its own views as well as for the general welfare of all our citizens.

For no other purpose was the taxing power — the right to originate revenue bills — confided to us. I am perfectly willing to admit that we should not undertake to establish jurisdiction by extending arbitrarily the taxing power into fields not properly belonging to the dominion of Federal authority.

Mr. SHERLEY. How does the gentleman explain the case of Dewitt?

Mr. COCKRAN. I beg the gentleman will not interrupt now by asking me to explain special cases. I entreat the gentleman to realize that, after all, he is but one Member of this House, though probably the best among us all, and I am addressing a collective body of which at least 250 Members are present. I can not in the course of this discussion meet every possible difficulty that may arise in the gentleman's mind. If he will allow me to finish, and make note in the meantime of any question that he chooses to ask, at the end I will be glad to spend an hour or two hours in cheerful and, I hope, improving colloquy with him. [Laughter.]

Now, a more important matter, Mr. Chairman, than satisfying the scruples, or shall I say attempting to follow the interesting speculations of the gentleman from Kentucky, is a definite statement of the precise question presented to this House.

We have heard much about the difficulty of dealing with the matter of insurance. From the beginning it seems to have been assumed that the existence of large corporations, each prosecuting its business in several States, and all the corruption and vice in the management which have recently been laid there, are in some way or other inherent in every insurance system, and that the only reform possible is to provide some means of regulating them. The gentleman from Kentucky [Mr. Sherley] pleads for a State regulation; the gentleman from Illinois [Mr. Mann], if I understand, pleads for a Federal regulation. Now, I think it is possible to exercise the power of this General Government so as to remove completely the conditions which have produced the sinister fruits of corruption which we all deplore. If that can be accomplished, then it is clear no regulation of a Federal character anyway will be necessary or advisable.

* * * * * * * *

Mr. DRISCOLL. There is another idea, simply a suggestion, which I would offer for the consideration of this committee. I quite agree with the gentleman from Kentucky [Mr. Sherley] that there is a marked tendency of late toward paternalism, or paternal government, and I am not a strong advocate of that form of government. I agree with him that the central Government is growing stronger day by day relatively to the strength of the several State governments. Every dollar spent for canals, every dollar spent for irrigation, every dollar spent for the improvement of rivers and harbors, every rural delivery carrier started on a route tends to enhance the power of the National Government relatively to the power of the governments of the several Commonwealths. But this argument does not apply especially to the Republican party. There is a marked tendency on the part of gentlemen, Members of this House, Democrats from Southern States, to surrender the doctrine which they inherited from Calhoun and to abandon their ideas of States rights in order that they may get a little pork in the barrel, or that they may get some benefit from the central Government for their several States or districts.

The Democratic party in the State of New York only a few years ago introduced a plank in its platform for ownership of the anthracite mines. On the 7th of last November a Member of this House on the Democratic side ran for mayor of New York on a municipal-ownership plank and received a very large vote, and possibly on a fair canvass and honest count he was elected. I say possibly because I venture no opinion as to the merits in that contest. There are in our country many advocates of Government ownership of railways, telegraph and telephone lines, and, in short, in favor of governmental or municipal ownership of all property employed in the production and distribution of the necessaries of life. The signs of the times all indicate that there is a marked tendency toward paternal government, and I do not know of any business where paternalism would be as wise or beneficial to the people as in life insurance. This is offered merely as a suggestion. It may come up as a matter of serious consideration by and by. With the central government as the life insurance company, as the underwriter of all policies, all the expenses of the vast competition which is now being waged between the several companies would be saved. Those expenses are very heavy. The commissions and other expenses in securing new insurance are very large. As a result the cost of insurance in the great life companies is nearly as much again as it ought to be. It is nearly as much again as the real risk would justify. If the expenses of competition and the extravagance and waste in those large companies were eliminated; insurance could be sold for about one-half what it costs now, because not more than one-half the income is paid out as actual benefits for loss.

*   *   *   *   *   *   *   *

Mr. SHERLEY. Mr. Chairman, I do not know that I desire to add much to what I said earlier in the day, but certain remarks made by the distinguished gentleman from New York [Mr. Cockran] have made it seem to me proper that I should say a few words. The House always listens with great delight to the gentleman, and wisely so, and yet I never hear him make a speech without being reminded of a story that was once told by Huxley, when he said that "Herbert Spencer's conception of a tragedy was the destruction of a syllogism by a fact." And when the distinguished gentleman declined to yield to me on the ground that he would illustrate the tendency and purpose of his speech if I would only be patient, I could not help but think that he was considering the possibility of a destruction of one of his syllogisms by a fact. And it was just such a fact that I think necessary to bring to the attention of this House.

The point that I made in my speech, and that I desire to emphasize because of the very eloquent denial of it made by the gentleman from New York [Mr. Cockran] is this: That there can be no more immoral practice than for members of a legislative body to use the taxing power, which is given them for the sole purpose of raising revenue, for some other and ulterior purpose. I not only maintain that, but, despite the fact that my reading may not be as extensive or along the same line as that of the gentleman, I maintain that where the taxing power has been used in support of the liberties of the English people it has been used along the line of a denial of appropriations rather than the line of diverting it from its real purpose into other purposes not germane to revenue raising.

But if that be not historically true the gentleman overlooks the distinction — that in England there is not the limitation of power that there is in regard to our National Government. Here the taxing power is expressly given for one purpose and one purpose only, and the Supreme Court has had occasion repeatedly to declare that police power did not exist in the National Government.

The point I wanted to make, and that I desire to emphasize, is that if the States do not use their power, then by not using it they will cease to have the capacity to use it, and as a result of that we will see a concentration and centralization such as the world never saw before. And in that connection it is a curious fact that the loudest advocates to-day for national control are the same distinguished gentlemen whom the gentleman from New York described in such glowing and accurate terms. They are the presidents of the life insurance companies themselves.

*　　*　　*　　*　　*　　*　　*　　*

My position about that is my position about the great subject of government in general. Because I have seen the people fail, because I have seen abuse prosper, because I have seen the wicked and the powerful flourish as the green bay tree, it has not made me believe less in the people, but only more. The day may be postponed, but the day is not going to be brought nearer by saying to the people, "You must not use your power." It is not going to be brought nearer by concentrating the power a long way from home. It is going to be brought nearer and made more certain by making the people realize that in their own hands, on their own heads, the sin and the saving lies. They must go to work themselves, and they must do it through their agencies at home. [Applause.]

Mr. COCKRAN. I would like to ask the gentleman from Kentucky [Mr. Sherley] if the power of the Federal Government is any less the power of the people than the power of the town, the power of the county, or the power of the State?

Mr. SHERLEY. I shall answer the gentleman in this way, and when I have answered I shall not further detain the House by this dissertation between the two of us, because I remember the gentleman's suggestion that I should not have the egotism to think that I constitute the House or that my private views and an explanation of them was the only matter of discussion. I will answer the gentleman in this way, that my conception of government, and the Democratic conception of government, has been, first, that that government which governs least governs best; second, that that government which stays closest home to the people is most democratic and less liable to abuse, less liable to get beyond control. It is easier for the people of the State of New York to know something of their State government than it is for them to know something of their National Government. It is easier for the people of Kentucky to know more about their State government than they do about the National Government. The fact that they do not know it is not a contradiction of my statement. They could know it. This I know, that when this country started on its career the State legislatures contained the ablest of men; that the time was when men resigned from the National Congress to take a seat in their State legislature. That may have been a false position, but it is not half so false a position as that which to-day makes your State legislature a disregardable body, and to which are sent men who are not capable of broad statecraft. And I say to you if there is any hope for the redemption of America, though the picture be as black as the gentleman has painted it, the hope lies in going back to the people and letting them learn the old lesson that they can not shirk responsibility, can not shift it off to another forum and expect relief; they must get it at home, and that thought was the cause of and excuse for my speech this morning. [Applause.]

Mr. WILLIAMS. Mr. Chairman, it is great good fortune to have listened to two such addresses as we have heard to-day, one from the gentleman from Kentucky [Mr. Sherley], containing a clear analysis and sound and philosophical exposition of the status of this question in its relation to the Federal and the State governments — a statement of a lawyer, founded upon law, cool and clear; the other, an eloquent denunciation of wrong and vice and criminality in high place and an exposition of the underlying ethics, ·excelled by nothing that I have ever heard upon this floor. The gentlemen from New York and from Kentucky agree in their conclusion, to wit, that the Federal Government has no jurisdiction over the subject-matter of insurance. Now, Mr. Chairman, these speeches have been a public benefit, but they have been to some extent a personal injury, because they have cut out from under me many of the things that I desired to say, because these gentlemen have said them better. I shall, however, begin by saying that I agree with the gentleman from Kentucky [Mr. Sherley] that what the Irish call "home rule" is, as a rule, the most honest rule. [Applause.] It is honest for the reason that the men who are the "rulers," so called, the men in whom power is lodged, are neighbors of the men who lodge it, personal acquaintances of theirs — their characters intimately known — and because they exercise the power under the eyes of their neighbors and friends, who can at intervals withdraw it. I believe in it in an ascending scale, leaving power — in as far as can with safety be left — first to the individual, second to the family, third to the town, fourth to the county, fifth to the State, and sixth, and then only when the Constitution expressly or by necessary or obviously proper intendment delegates it, to the Federal Government. Now, the gentleman from New York [Mr. Cockran] has correctly said that all the liberties of the English-speaking people were founded upon the assertion by the legislative body of the taxing power. That is true; and while he can argue by analogy to some extent between the British House of Commons and the American House of Representatives, he must remember the distinction between the two. While it is absolutely true that the House of Commons exercised its taxing power for the strengthening and enforcement and execution of the power which it had — a legislative power — it is also true that the British House of Commons had an unlimited and original and inherent legislative power and therefore the exercise of the taxing power in order to execute that legislative power was totally a different and a larger thing than ought to be the exercise of the taxing power by the House of Representatives, which has only a limited power, a delegated power.

Mr. Chairman, it can never happen that the power to tax can give jurisdiction over a subject-matter of taxation when dealing with the subject-matter is neither delegated to the General Government nor prohibited to the States. You must first have the jurisdiction over the subject-matter. Then there follows, as the auxiliary or enforcing clause, the power to tax, not only to raise revenue, but, if actual need be, to enforce the power. If you have the power over the subject-matter, you may tax, not only to bring a revenue, but to execute the power, if that be an obviously proper or necessary means to the end of exercising the power. For example, if the Federal Government has the power to forbid certain things, it may forbid them by taxation, let us say. I do not think the distinguished gentleman from New York [Mr. Cockran] intended to leave the impression which he left upon the mind of the gentleman from Kentucky [Mr. Sherley], to wit, that the Federal power had any specific, substantive power of taxation independently of all other powers granted or denied in the Constitution of the United States. The power to deal with the subject-matter must be there first. You ought never to form a nexus between a subject-matter over which you have no constitutional power and the Constitution itself by the assertion of it through the taxing power. Taxes are always means to an end, not in themselves an end. The end itself must be constitutional.

Now, I am perfectly aware of the fact there is a little weight in the Supreme Court decisions that would seem to squint the other way if unstudied, but it amounts to nothing if studied. Here is the Supreme Court of the United States stating in effect that it would not undertake to investigate the motives of Congress when exercising the taxing power. In other words, it is a compliment to Congress, to the legislative body from a coördinate branch, stating that it would not attribute to it the bad motive of obtaining jurisdiction simply by the assertion of the taxing power. It takes for granted integrity of motive, intellectual integrity. Now, Mr. Chairman, there are two forms of centralization by the Federal Government, one of which I am afraid we can not help and the other one we can help, I think. That centralization which proceeds from the exercise of clearly delegated power is a form of centralization which, I fear, must go on. In so far as Congress has not already exercised to the full its clearly delegated power it will in the course of history exercise it. Nor is there anything undemocratic in maintaining in full integrity the expressly delegated powers of the General Government. Jefferson said as much.

The other form of centralization, which is always vicious and an usurpation, is to assert Federal jurisdiction by a pretext, whether it be by the mere pretext of interstate commerce where no interstate commerce exists or whether it be by the pretext of the taxing power asserted as a connecting link with the trust that the court will not examine our motive; it is all the same; it is vicious and an usurpation. Now, let us come to this particular question, Mr. Chairman. The Supreme Court has spoken in this case and it has declared that insurance is not commerce of any sort and especially is it not interstate commerce. That disposes of the question as to whether there is any jurisdiction under the rule in the Committee on Interstate Commerce. To what committee it should go I myself am a little in doubt. My opinion was that it ought to have gone to the Committee on the Judiciary with instructions to investigate the jurisdictional power of the Federal Government and to report to this House, but the Chairman of the Committee on the Judiciary not having made a fight for the jurisdiction and the committee making none, we are faced with the alternative of sending it to the Interstate and Foreign Commerce or the Committee on Ways and Means.

* * * * * * * *

Now, Mr. Chairman, that the Members of the House may catch the reason for the distinction I have made, I will say that the Committee on the Judiciary has jurisdiction for the purpose of reporting to the House whether or not the Federal Government has jurisdiction. But, if they were to report to the House that the Federal Government did have jurisdiction, then the Judiciary Committee would not be the proper committee to deal with the subject-matter, because that would depend upon what ground they placed the constitutional jurisdiction of the Federal Government. If they placed it, for example, on the ground that it was interstate commerce, then the matter would go to that committee; if they would place it upon the ground that the exercise of the taxing power made a jurisdiction — an inconceivable thing for a lawyer to do — then it would go to the Committee on Ways and Means; if they said the Federal Government had no jurisdiction at all, then that would settle the matter. That is the reason why I would not vote for a general committal to the Judiciary Committee, while I would vote for a committal to the Judiciary Committee with instructions to report upon our jurisdiction. Now, let me proceed.

Mr. STEENERSON. Does not the message itself submit the question to the House simply? I find on page 16 the following:

I repeat my previous recommendation that the Congress should also consider whether the Federal Government has any power or owes any duty with respect to domestic transactions in insurance of an interstate character.

Is not the question submitted by the message, whether or not we have the power, and would a simple reference be a reference of that question?

Mr. WILLIAMS. It would not. Unless it is a committal requiring investigation and report on the question of jurisdiction, then it is a committal for legislation as well. The President is no lawyer, I will say, in answer further to the gentleman. He admits that he is not. That is one of the things which he is not, which is accompanied by an admission on his part to that effect. There are not many things of that sort. [Laughter.]

Now, Mr. Chairman, to go further in connection with this taxing power nexus between the subject-matter and the Constitution of the United States, just suppose you could have jurisdiction over any possible subject-matter simply because you had the power of taxation, where would it stop? Why, it would be a blanket clause that would cover everything. Congress might to-morrow pass an act ordaining a direct tax upon lands and apportioning it between the States, and then, inci-

dental to the power of taxation (if any power is to be exercised as incidental to taxation, when really taxation is itself only incidental to other
and substantive powers, or itself substantive only to raise a revenue),
the Congress could go on and in the same act enact the Henry George
system of single tax. It could do anything, I do not care what. It
could to-morrow tax barrels, and then it could legislate that the barrel
should hold only so much, or should not hold less than so much, or
should have so many hoops, or should contain nothing but water. The
minute that gentlemen, on this side of the Chamber especially, ever
surrender the idea that the taxing power can make a nexus between the
subject-matter and the Constitution where no other nexus exists, then
we have surrendered to federalism, and we might as well go out of
business, because we as a party would have no right whatsoever to
exist. [Applause on the Democratic side.]

Now, Mr. Chairman, I want to talk a little about the subject-matter,
although my friends from New York and Kentucky have left me no
opportunity to grow eloquent upon the crimes and abuses of the present
conditions, nor the advantages of preserving inviolate the reserved
rights of the States as the sheet anchor of individuality and local
self-government.

Mr. Hepburn rose.

The CHAIRMAN (Mr. COCKS in the chair). Does the gentleman from
Mississippi yield to the gentleman from Iowa [Mr. Hepburn]?

Mr. WILLIAMS. Certainly.

Mr. HEPBURN. Will the gentleman permit me an interruption?

Mr. WILLIAMS. Yes.

Mr. HEPBURN. The gentleman from Mississippi has already spoken
with relation to the taxing power and to the power that might be exercised under the commerce clause of the Constitution. The gentleman
from New York [Mr. Cockran] has suggested that there is another power,
lodged in the fourth section of the fourth article of the Constitution, that
each State shall be guaranteed a republican form of government. Will
the gentleman, before he leaves this branch of the subject, give us his
views as to the power that the Government of the United States may
have to control an insurance company through its undoubted power to
secure to a State a republican form of government?

Mr. WILLIAMS. I will reply by saying that a republican form of government does not mean an honest government or incorrupt government,
as all of us have ascertained in these latter days, and that the constitutional guaranty of a republican form of government is not a guaranty of
honest administration of government. It is a high tribute to my friend
from New York, his morals and his high ideals of republican government, that he should have led to an unconscious confusion of the two in
that matter. There are a great many sorts of republican governments.
Historically we find that there have been democratic republican govern-

ments like that of Athens, aristocratic republican governments like that of Sparta, plutocratic republican governments like that of Venice, and a mixed-up republican government like that we have — a republic of lesser republics, with two different sets of republican governments working along different lines with the power of the people over both checked — materially blocked in the Federal Government — by the Senate, and checked by the absolute veto of the Executive, neither of which is consistent with a pure democracy, but both quite consistent with a republican form of government. Undoubtedly what our forefathers meant by the phrase was a government of law and not a government of one-man power — a monarchy, or any arbitrary government — a government in which the people, or at least those of them competent for governing, should be the source of power and law, the form of its expression. They had just come out from under the Monarchy of England.

Mr. COCKRAN. If the gentleman will·permit me, I did not discuss the corruption of the Government in regard to that. The point I made was about a trust where the parties to the trust could not scrutinize the methods of administration, and a fund which must grow, without any possibility of distribution, were both elements in conflict with the judicial system established by every State and inconsistent with the security of republican government, which had nothing to do with its growth.

Mr. WILLIAMS. Let me state what I understand by corruption, because your supposition involves necessarily a presumption of corruption controlling or annulling government of the people. It presumes the case of one man, or a few men, who had immense amounts of money, enough to buy everything, that the people themselves had lost their vote and their voting power because that one man or that one corporation controlled everything and voted everybody by influencing or buying the voters, or else by influencing or buying legislators, judges, or juries. That would undoubtedly be corruption, but it would be corruption under spirit "a republican form of government." The republican governmental might have departed, true enough. If there were any law that gave that man or corporation the sole power, that would not be a republican form of government; that would simply be a corrupt monarchical form of government. If you let the State of New York alone; if you leave it to itself; if you carry the government right to the door of her people and let them alone, they will root up and eradicate this evil. They won't have it long. Where you carry responsibility you give experience, and where experience is gained you find ability, and with both you have watchfulness, and with watchfulness virtue, courage, and honesty. That has always been the case. [Loud applause.]

XVI

THE NATIONAL CONVENTION

THE REPUBLICAN CONVENTION OF 1880 [1]

[The two subsequent articles are among the most interesting accounts ever given of National Conventions. Senator Hoar, from whose autobiography the first account is taken, was the permanent chairman of the Republican Convention of 1880, which he describes. Mr. A. P. Dennis was a delegate to the Democratic Convention of St. Louis in 1904.]

THIS convention was menaced by a very serious peril. A plan was devised which, if it had been successful, would, in my judgment, have caused a rupture in the convention and the defeat of the Republican Party in the election. The Chairman of the Republican National Committee was Don Cameron of Pennsylvania, then and for some years afterward a Senator of the United States from that State. He was an ardent supporter of President Grant and had been Secretary of War in his Cabinet, as his father had been in the Cabinet of President Lincoln. Like his father before him, he had ruled the Republican Party of Pennsylvania with a strong hand. He was not given to much speaking. He was an admirable executive officer, self-reliant, powerful, courageous, and enterprising, with little respect for the discontent of subordinates. He was supported by a majority of the delegates from Pennsylvania, although Blaine, who was a native of that State, had a large following there. The New York delegation was headed by Roscoe Conkling, who had great influence over Grant when he was President, and expected to retain that influence if he became President again. The Maryland delegates were headed by J. A. J. Croswell, who had been Postmaster-General more than five years in Grant's two Administrations. On the Massachusetts delegation, as I have said, was Governor Boutwell, Grant's Secretary of the Treasury during nearly the whole of his first term, and on that from Illinois John A. Logan. These men had a large following over the whole country. There were three hundred and eight persons in the convention who could be counted on to

[1] From the *Autobiography* of Senator Hoar (Vol. I, 388), reproduced by permission of the Publishers, Chas. Scribner's Sons, New York. Copyright.

826

support Grant from beginning to end, and about a dozen more were exceedingly disposed to his candidacy. The State Conventions of the three largest and most powerful States, New York, Pennsylvania, and Illinois, and possibly one or two others, that I do not now remember, had instructed their delegates to vote as a unit for the candidate who should be agreed upon by the majority. Grant had a majority in each of these States. But there was a minority of 18 in Illinois, 26 in Pennsylvania, and 19 in New York, who were for other candidates than Grant. If their votes had been counted for him it would have given Grant on the first ballots 367 votes, 13 less than the number necessary for a choice. As his votes went up on one of the ballots to 313, it is pretty certain that counting these 63 votes for Grant would have insured his nomination. But there were several contests involving the title of their seats of 16 delegates from the State of Louisiana, 18 from Illinois, and three others. In regard to these cases the delegates voted in accordance with their preference for candidates. This was beside several other contests where the vote was not determined by that consideration. Now if the vote of Illinois, Pennsylvania, and New York had each been cast as a unit, in accordance with the preference of the majority of the delegation in each case, these 37 votes would have been added to Grant's column and subtracted from the forces of his various antagonists; and the 63 votes of the minority of the delegations in these three States would also have been added to the Grant column, which would have given him a total vote of more than 400, enough to secure his nomination. So the result of the convention was to be determined by the adoption or rejection of what was called the unit rule.

Don Cameron, the Chairman of the National Committee, left the Senate for Chicago about ten days, I think, before the day fixed for the meeting of the convention. It was whispered about before his departure that a scheme had been resolved upon by him and the other Grant leaders, which would compel the adoption of the unit rule, whatever might be the desire of the convention itself. It was his duty, according to established custom, to call the convention to order and to receive nominations for temporary presiding officer. He was pledged, upon those nominations, as it was understood, to hold that the unit rule must be applied. In that way the sitting members from the disputed States and districts would be permitted to vote, and the votes of the three States would be cast without dissent for the Grant candidates. When the temporary President took his place he would rule in the same way on the question of the choice of a permanent President, and the permanent President would rule in the same way on the conflicting votes, for the appointment of committees, for determining the seats of delegates, and finally the nomination of the candidates for President and Vice-President. If the minority claimed the right to vote and took an appeal from his decision, he was to hold that on the vote on that appeal the same unit rule was to apply. If a second point of order were raised, he would hold, of course, that a second point of order could not be raised while the first was pending. So the way seemed clear to exclude the contesting delegates, to cast the votes of the three great States solid for Grant, and compel his nomination.

But the majority of the National Committee, of which Cameron was Chairman, was opposed to Grant. They met, I think, the day before the meeting of the convention to make the preliminary arrangements. Mr. Cameron, the Chairman, was asked whether it was his purpose to carry out the scheme I have indicated. He refused to answer. A motion was then made that the Chairman, after calling the convention to order, be instructed to receive the vote of the individual delegates without regard to the instruction of the majority of their delegation. Cameron refused to receive motions on that question, saying that it was a matter beyond the jurisdiction of the committee. A large part of the entire day was spent in various attempts to induce Cameron either to give a pledge or permit a resolution to be entertained by the committee, instructing him as to his action. He was supported by Mr. Gorham, of California, who I believe was not a member of the committee, but was present either as Secretary or as Amicus Curæ. He was an experienced parliamentarian, and for a long time had been Secretary of the Senate of the United States. The discussion for the majority was conducted largely by Mr. Chandler, of New Hampshire, afterward Secretary of the Navy, and later Senator. After spending a large part of the day in that discussion, some time in the afternoon an intimation was made, informally, and in a rather veiled fashion, that, unless they had more satisfactory pledges from Mr. Cameron, he would be removed from the office of Chairman, and a person who would carry out the wishes of the committee be substituted. The committee then adjourned until the next morning. Meantime the Grant managers applied to Colonel Strong, of Illinois, who had been already appointed Sergeant-at-Arms by the committee, and who was a supporter of Grant, to ascertain whether, if the committee were to remove Cameron and appoint another chairman, he would recognize him as a person entitled to call the convention to order and preside until a temporary Chairman was chosen, and would execute his lawful orders, or whether he would treat them as without effect and would execute the orders of Cameron. He desired time for consideration, which was conceded. He consulted Senator Philetus Sawyer of Wisconsin, who was himself in favor of General Grant, but who desired above all things the success of the Republican Party, or was not ready for any unlawful or revolutionary action. Mr. Sawyer was a business man of plain manners, and though of large experience in public life, was not much versed in parliamentary law. He called into consultation ex-Senator Timothy O. Howe, of Wisconsin, formerly Senator from that State, and afterward Postmaster-General under Arthur. He was a very able and clearheaded lawyer, and had a high reputation for integrity. He advised Mr. Strong that the committee might lawfully depose their Chairman and appoint another, and that it would be his duty, as Sergeant-at-Arms, to recognize the new Chairman and obey his lawful orders. Strong was under great obligations to Sawyer, who had aided him very largely in business matters, and had a high respect for his judgment. He gave his response to the Grant leaders in accordance with the advice of Mr. Howe, in which Senator Sawyer concurred. They had intended to make General Creswell the President of the convention. But finding it impossible to carry their plans into effect, in order to prevent the severe measure of deposing the Chairman of the committee, they consented that the assurances demanded should be given. There was then a negotiation between the leaders on the side of Grant and Blaine for an agreement upon a presiding officer. It was well known that I was not in favor of the nomination of either. Senator Hamlin, formerly Vice-President and then a Senator, proposed my name to Mr. Conkling as a person likely to be impartial between the two principal candidates. Mr. Conkling replied that such a suggestion was an insult. Hamlin said: "I guess I can stand the insult." But on consultation of the Grant men and the Blaine men it was agreed that I should be selected, which was done accordingly. I was nominated orally from the floor when Mr. Cameron called the convention to order, and chosen temporary President by acclamation and unanimously. As proceedings went on it was thought best not to have any division or question as to a permanent Chairman and it was at the proper time ordered, also without objection, that I should act as permanent President.

But the Grant leaders were still confident. They felt sure that none of their original votes, numbering three hundred and more, would desert them, and that it would be impossible for the rest of the convention, divided among so many candidates, to agree, and that they would in the end get a majority.

I was myself exceedingly anxious on this subject. I also felt that if the followers of Grant could get any pretext for getting an advantage by any claim, however doubtful, that they would avail themselves of it, even at the risk of breaking up the convention in disorder, rather than be baffled in their object. So the time to me was one of great and distressing responsibility. The forces of Grant were led on the floor of the convention by Roscoe Conkling, who nominated him in a speech of great power and eloquence. The forces of Blaine were led, as they had been in 1876, very skillfully by Senators Hale and Frye. Garfield was the leader of the supporters of Mr. Sherman. One of the greatest oratoric triumphs I ever witnessed was obtained by Garfield. There had been a storm of applause, lasting, I think, twenty-five minutes, at the close of Conkling's nominating speech. It was said there were fifteen thousand persons in the galleries, which came down very near the level of the floor. The scene was of indescribable sublimity. The fate of the country, certainly the fate of a great political party, was at stake, and, more than that, the selection of the ruler of a nation of fifty millions of people — a question which in other countries could not have been determined, under like circumstances, without bloodshed or civil war. I do not think I shall be charged with exaggeration when I speak of it in this way. I can only compare it in its grandeur and impressiveness to the mighty torrent of Niagara. Perhaps I can not give a satisfactory reason for so distinguishing it from other like assemblies that have gathered in this country. But I have since seen a great number of persons from all parts of the country who were present as members or inspectors, and they all speak of it in the same way. A vast portion of the persons present in the hall sympathized deeply with the supporters of Grant. Conkling's speech, as he stood almost in the center of that great assembly on a platform just above the heads of the convention, was a masterpiece of splendid oratory. He began:

> And when asked what State he hails from,
>   Our sole reply shall be,
> He comes from Appomattox,
>   And its famous apple-tree.

It was pretty difficult for Garfield to follow this speech in the tempest of applause which came after it. There was nothing stimulant or romantic in the plain wisdom of John Sherman. It was like reading a passage from "Poor Richard's Almanac" after one of the lofty chapters of the Psalms of David. Garfield began quietly:

"I have witnessed the extraordinary scene of this convention with deep solicitude. Nothing touches my heart more quietly than a tribute of honor to a great and noble character. But as I sat in my seat and witnessed this demonstration, this assemblage seemed to me a human ocean in a tempest. I have seen the sea lashed into fury and tossed into spray, and its grandeur moves the soul of the dullest man; but I remember that it is not the billows, but the calm level of the sea from which all heights and depths are measured. When the storm has passed and the hour of calm settles on the ocean, when the sunlight bathes its peaceful surface, then the astronomer and surveyor take the level from which they measure all terrestrial heights and depths.

"Gentlemen of the Convention, your present temper may not mark the healthful pulse of our people. When your enthusiasm has passed, when the emotions of the hour have subsided, we shall find below this storm and passion that calm level of public opinion from which the thoughts of a mighty people are to be measured, and by which their final action will be determined.

"Not here, in this brilliant circle where fifteen thousand men and women are fathered, is the destiny of the Republic to be decreed for the next four years — not here, where I see the enthusiastic faces of seven hundred and fifty-six delegates, waiting to cast their lot into the urn and determine the choice of the Republic; but by four millions of Republican firesides, where the thoughtful voters, with wives and children about them, with the calm thoughts inspired by love of home and country, with the history of the past, the hopes of the future, the reverence for the great men who have adorned and blessed our nation in days gone by, burning in their hearts — there God prepares the verdict which will determine the wisdom of our work to-night. Not in Chicago, in the heat of June, but at the ballot-boxes of the Republic, in the quiet of November, after the silence of deliberate judgment, will this question be settled."

Conkling, while executing the admiration of all men for his dexterity and ability, lost ground at every step. He made a foolish attempt to compel the passage of a resolution depriving of their rights to vote delegates who refused to pledge themselves to support the choice of the convention whoever it might be. His speech nominating Grant contained a sneer at Blaine. So, while he held his forces together to the last, he made it almost impossible for any man who differed from him in the beginning to come to him at the end. On the contrary everything that Garfield said was marked by good nature and good sense. I said on the first day of the convention that in my opinion if the delegates could be shut up by themselves and not permitted to leave the room until they agreed, the man on whom they would agree would be General Garfield. This desire became more and more apparent as the convention went on. At last, on the thirty-sixth ballot, and the sixth day of the convention, the delegates who had previously voted for other candidates than Grant, began to wheel into line for Garfield. Garfield had one vote from the State of Pennsylvania in previous ballots. But on the thirty-fourth ballot in Wisconsin, the last State to vote in alphabetical order, had given him her sixteen votes, and on the thirty-sixth ballot she was joined by the delegates who had voted for other candidates than Grant. Grant held together his forces till the last, receiving three hundred and thirteen votes on the thirty-fifth ballot, and three hundred and sixty on the thirty-sixth. It was a sublime movement, which it was hoped would determine the destiny of the Republic for many years, a hope which was cruelly disappointed by Garfield's untimely death. It was, as might be well believed, a movement of sublime satisfaction to me. Garfield had been my friend for many years. I had sat close to him in the House of Representatives for three terms of Congressional service. He had been my guest at my house in Worcester; and I had been his colleague on the Electoral Commission in 1876. He had been educated at a Massachusetts college. He was of old Middlesex County stock. We were in thorough accord in our love for New England, our firm faith in her hereditary principles, and our pride in her noble history.

Garfield had been charged, in accepting the nomination for the Presidency, with having been untrue to the interests of John Sherman,

who was the candidate of Ohio, and whom Garfield had supported
faithfully through every ballot. The charge is absolutely unjust. Mr.
Sherman's nomination was seen by everybody to have been absolutely
impossible long before the final result. I was in constant consultation
with leaders of the different delegations who were trying to unite their
forces. There never was any considerable number of those persons
who thought the nomination of Mr. Sherman practicable, notwithstanding the high personal respect in which they held him. At the close
of the thirty-fourth ballot, when Garfield received seventeen votes, and
the following incident took place:

Mr. GARFIELD of Ohio: "Mr. President——"
The PRESIDENT: "For what purpose does the gentleman rise?"
Mr. GARFIELD: "Rise to a question of order."
Mr. GARFIELD: "I challenge the correctness of the announcement. The
announcement contains votes for me. No man has a right, without the consent
of the person voted for, to announce that person's name, and vote for him, in
this convention. Such consent I have not given."
The PRESIDENT: "The gentleman from Ohio is not stating a question of
order. He will resume his seat. No person having received a majority of the
votes cast, another ballot will be taken. The Clerk will call the roll."

This verbatim report is absolutely correct, except that where there is
a period at the end of Mr. Garfield's last sentence there should be a
dash, indicating that the sentence was not finished. I recollect the incident perfectly. I interrupted him in the middle of his sentence. I
was terribly afraid that he would say something that would make his
nomination impossible, or his acceptance impossible, if it were made.
I do not believe it ever happened before that anybody who attempted
to decline the Presidency of the United States was to be prevented by a
point of order, or that such a thing will ever happen again.

During the thirtieth ballot a vote was cast by a delegate from the
Territory of Wyoming for General Philip H. Sheridan. General Sheridan, who was upon the platform as a spectator, came forward instantly
and said: "I am very much obliged to the delegate from Wyoming for
mentioning my name in this convention, but there is no way in which I
could accept a nomination from this convention, if it were possible,
unless I should be permitted to turn it over to my best friend." The
President said: "The Chair presumed the unanimous consent of the
convention to permit the illustrious soldier who has spoken to interrupt
its order for that purpose. But it will be a privilege accorded to no
other person whatever." The General's prompt suppression of this
attempt to make him a candidate was done in a direct and blunt sol-
dierly fashion. I did not think it best to apply to him the strictness of
parliamentary law; and in that I was sure of the approval of the convention. But the precedent of permitting such a body to be addressed

under any circumstances by a person not a member would be a dangerous one, if repeated. Perhaps I may with propriety add one thing of personal nature. It has been sometimes charged that the delegates from Massachusetts were without great influence in shaping the result of this convention. They moved, and carried, against a formidable opposition, the civil service plank, which embodied the doctrine of civil service reform as among the doctrines of the Republican Party. Of whatever value may be attributed to the humble services of the President of the Convention, they are entitled to the credit. They had, I think, more to do than any other delegation with effecting the union upon Garfield. Of course the wish of Mr. Blaine had very great influence indeed. I think he preferred Garfield to any other person except Robert Lincoln, of Illinois, of whom he spoke to me as a person from whom it would be impossible to keep the votes of the colored delegates from the South, and who would be, by reason of the respect felt for his father's memory, highly acceptable through the country. But Mr. Lincoln, under the circumstances, could not have got the support of his own State, and without it it seemed unwise to attempt a union upon him.

THE DEMOCRATIC CONVENTION OF 1904[1]

By Alfred Pearce Dennis

In the last national campaign no political maxim fell with greater unction and finality from the mouths of Democratic orators than the apothegm: "Our government is one of laws, not men." To the mind of the foreign student legalism is of the essence of American political institutions. The competence of executive officials, both federal and State, is not only strictly defined by the organic law but further limited by the prescriptions of statutory enactment. Legislative bodies in turn are strictly subordinate under the provisions of organic law; they can not step outside the legal bounds defined by written constitutions. Every executive official in the land, from the occupant of the White House to the hog-reeve of a New England village, is strictly limited in the scope of his administrative duties by laws which he is powerless to alter. Every law-making body, in turn, from the national Congress to the pettiest city council, is restrained in its legislative competence by the limitations of laws which it may not change. As one notes the immense mass and particularity of our statutory law and the network of minute restrictions cast about legislatures by the fundamental law, one naturally concludes that American governmental doctrine is but an amplified affirmation of Job's theory that "man is born unto trouble as the sparks fly upward," and that, if he is to be saved, it is not to be through his

[1] From the *Political Science Quarterly*, June, 1905.

own goodness of heart or personal discretion, but through the external compulsion of unyielding law.

In view of the legalism that pervades our political processes, one is amazed to find that the great bodies which name our presidents are subjected to no external legal control. The idea of a nominating convention is neither a political inheritance nor a conscious contrivance. It is an evolutionary product; it is a development of the party system, just as the party system, in turn, is the product of a decentralized administrative system. A multitude of men must be selected to express and also to execute the will of the State. Our theory of government separates the functions of expression and execution. The harmonious working of the governmental system demands the coördination of the two. The means of coördination, as is clearly shown by Professor Goodnow in his *Politics and Administration*, has been found in an extra-legal institution, the political party. The national convention, which represents the supreme expression of the will of the party, is, like the party itself, an extra-legal institution. Great changes, unrecognized by the law and unenforced by the courts, have been wrought in our institutional fabric through the unfolding processes of national life. The national convention, an unfathered institutional waif, may at no distant day be formally adopted and placed under the control of the national government. Much may be said for the formal recognition and legal control of this robust extra-legal institution, if the national convention is to represent the best thought and the highest motives of the party which calls it into being.

The conduct of the last Democratic national convention furnishes strong presumptive evidence that the evolutionary process will not stop at the present point, but that changes in the direction of increased dignity and deliberation will be demanded of the great bodies which nominate our highest governmental magistrate. That the St. Louis convention was, in any true sense, a deliberative body will be denied by any close observer of its proceedings. A thousand delegates and an equal number of alternates elected by various processes — many of the alternates actually present by no process at all — met in the hottest month of the year in the pit of an oven-like building in one of the hottest cities of the border States. Crowded in with delegates and alternates at the bottom of the pit were reporters, amateur policemen, and hangers-on of every description. Ten thousand spectators filled the huge galleries, and a motley throng of jostling, perspiring humanity jammed the aisles and exits — the whole comprising the *dramatis personæ* in a serio-comic four-act extravaganza, known as the St. Louis convention. Strictly speaking, there were no spectators; all were actors. If not privileged to occupy the center of the stage, each person present was privileged to occupy a place in that assemblage which theatrical folk describe, without differentiation, as the "mob." It is all the same whether soldiers, village clowns, or chorus girls compose this assemblage. The mob is an indispensable adjunct in the representation of a great spectacular piece. In the St. Louis Coliseum the mob overplayed its part. It was not content to occupy the background, but again and again persisted in usurping the functions of the real actors in the foreground who had come upon the stage with speaking parts.

As a delegate to the convention, the writer ventures to record some personal impressions of the conduct of that body, and briefly to add a conclusion or two as to the bearing of it all upon future methods of selecting presidential nominees.

The prologue of the drama was spoken by Mr. John Sharp Williams, temporary chairman of the convention. Even in a real play not much attention is given to the prologue. The arrival of late-comers, the arrangement of seats, the buzz of conversation go on. Playgoers begin to settle down and give attention when the curtain rises and the real action begins. After a few minutes of curious interest in Mr. Williams, the mob fell to discussing its own affairs. The speaker's voice, overtaxed in the effort to make itself heard above the confusion, broke down almost entirely, and after the first ten minutes was scarcely audible even to the front-benchers. The address as printed is sensible, well-phrased, and keen in argument, but as delivered the speech was a failure. It was trying, even for delegates, to sit for an hour and forty minutes watching the moving lips and occasional gestures of a distant speaker, and to fail utterly to follow the thread of his argument. The mention of Mr. Cleveland's name infused a tonic property into the dreary proceeding. The cheering of near-by delegates was taken up by others, reached the galleries, and continued without cessation for thirteen minutes.

At the conclusion of Mr. Williams's address the committee on credentials submitted its report. Two points of interest are to be noted in this connection: first, the ruling of the chair that it is not within the power of the committee on credentials to admit delegates from the Philippines, inasmuch as these islands are declared by the Supreme Court not to be a part of the United States; and second, the adoption by the convention of the committee's majority report seating the Hopkins delegates from the State of Illinois. At this stage Colonel William J. Bryan appeared for the Harrison contesting delegates and moved the adoption of a minority report. His address aroused the galleries to a frenzy of enthusiasm. *Per se* the appeal was a powerful one, and it is safe to assert that the majority of the delegates were convinced that the cause Colonel Bryan championed was relatively if not absolutely righteous. And yet, on the balloting, delegation after delegation voted to validate the credentials of men who were obviously not entitled to them. There were two reasons for this. First, the feverish dread of a "Bryan stampede," and second, the desire to rebuke the obvious attempt of the mob to run the convention. Ten thousand people had cheered Colonel Bryan wildly and irresponsibly during the hour he held the platform, and this same crowd had refused to listen three minutes without derisive shouts and interruptions to the men who vainly endeavored in the hubbub to present the other side of the case. It was later, in the Committee on Resolutions, that Colonel Bryan won his most signal victory. On the convention floor, where he was deliriously supported by a vulgar claque that refused his opponents a decent hearing, and on an issue for which he was thrice-armed because of the justice of his contention, Colonel Bryan was beaten by a vote of 647 to 299.

With the adoption of the report of the committee on permanent organization, Hon. Champ Clark, as permanent chairman, read a long and rambling speech, which had a sedative effect upon his fellow Missourians in the galleries, who could but imperfectly hear it, and a benumbing effect upon those near-by delegates who had not left their seats before its conclusion. This was the end of the second day's labor of the convention.

While waiting for the report of the committee on resolutions, the convention occupied the morning session of the third day in roll-calls for the formal selection of the new national committee and the naming of honorary vice-presidents. .During a lull in this time-killing employment some one called for a speech from Captain Richmond Pearson Hobson. Captain Hobson possesses an impressive mien and a resonant bass voice. "We want no Cromwell in this land of liberty!" he loudly declared. Here was relief from the tedium of business and from the strain of listening to speeches which could not be heard. The crowd in the galleries sank restfully back into their seats and gratefully gave ear. "I can see," cried the man of arms in notes of bugle clearness,

the plains of Illinois as the infantry assembles. I can see the hill-tops of the Hudson and the Mohawk, where the artillery is located. I look to the ranks of Democracy when our battle-flags are unfurled. I see a Wellington take up the standard of Democracy; yes, from New York to Illinois, and from Illinois to California, the battle lines are extended. Here are our armies; let us make the Republicans give name to the battle field — let's make them call it Waterloo!

Now the cold-eyed cynic might possibly regard this performance as a perfect and exact illustration of the forcible-feeble style of oratory, but the piece pleased the audience mightily. With the exception of Colonel Bryan no man who addressed the convention was hearkened to with more deferential attention than was Captain Hobson.

The all-night session which resulted in the nomination of Judge Parker opened with the reading of the platform by Senator John W. Daniel. The Coliseum was thronged, but there was nothing spectacular about the platform, and the mob was there for a spectacle. Every man seemed free to wander as he willed. Informal social caucuses met here and there. A hum and a buzz as of five hundred afternoon tea-parties filled the great hall. On, on, read the speaker, never faltering, never raising his voice, never heard. He might have been describing the mural decorations of the imperial palace at Pekin or the habits of the Mississippi river catfish, for all his auditors knew or cared. At the close no one expressed approval or disapproval of the party creed thus formally enunciated. Of the character of the platform the delegates and mob alike could form no opinion from the evidence laid before the convention.

With the adoption of the platform an all-night carnival of oratory began. Eight names were formally placed before the convention, with a total of thirty-five nominating and seconding speeches. The majority of these speeches were stupid and tiresome. The cheap grandiloquence of the panegyrical orator ordinarily rose to its height with the enunciation of the favorite son's name at the end of the speech. There were some notable deviations from the prevailing type of convention declamation. Hon. Martin W. Littleton proved himself a master of the difficult art of convention oratory. In his address naming Judge Parker, Mr. Littleton's voice rose to clearness and strength; his words certainly stirred the imagination if they did not convince the understanding; and his speech really infused an element of genuine enthusiasm into the Parker demonstration which ensued. The ponderous oratory of Mr. D. M. Delmas, who placed the name of Hon. William R. Hearst before the convention, proceeded with the stately gravity and inexorable sequence of the cosmic process itself. But the piece dragged after five minutes, and few gave heed except those who felt it their business to do so. Of the Hearst seconding speeches, that of Mr. Clarence Darrow, of Chicago, was refreshing in its obvious sincerity. With the impetuous vigor of a Mirabeau he urged the convention to pause before placing men in charge who, in past time, had scuttled the Democratic ship. Quite out of the ordinary, too, was Hon. Champ Clark's good-natured nominating speech for Senator Cockrell. "This is a 'great historical occasion," he began, "and I am about to make a great historical speech." "They say that Roosevelt is a brave man," he declared in conclusion, "but old man Cockrell is as brave as he." In fine contrast to this speech was the dignified and impressive speech of General Collins, presenting the name of Hon. Richard Olney, of Massachusetts. In a voice adequate to the trying occasion he appealed in a brief, sententious and sincere argument to the intelligence of the convention. His words were followed by the delegates with the closest attention. Two more hours dragged wearily by, as orator after orator rose in the call of states. It was past four o'clock in the morning when Wisconsin was reached on the roll-call and Colonel Bryan strode to the platform. It was for this that fifteen thousand men and women had remained steadfastly in the uncomfortable seats and the vitiated atmosphere of a veritable fire-trap all the long night. The most ingenious stage director could not have planned a more theatrical setting. Earlier in the night Nebraska had given way to Wisconsin, which presented the name of Wall. Wisconsin now yielded to Nebraska, and thus gave Colonel Bryan the last word. A passionate cry burst from the lips of the multitude as the great champion of social democracy advanced to the platform. The appearance of the man heightened the dramatic effect of the scene. The marks of battle and of sleeplessness were upon him. His face was ashen, the lips compressed to a thin line, the eyes sunken in their sockets; the voice was husky and the figure drooped with fatique. He began to speak. A passion of soul seemed to communicate its fire to the spent body. The dull eyes of the speaker glowed with an almost fanatical earnestness. The gestures fell in quick, nervous rhythm; the voice, gaining in strength, rang out clear. The man seemed essentially a preacher, the embodiment of force and earnestness, with all the fire of a Whitefield and the passion of a Chrysostom.

Eight years ago [he said] a Democratic convention placed in my hands the standard of the party, and gave me the commission as its candidate. Four years later that commission was renewed. I come to-night to this Democratic convention to return the commission, and to say that you may dispute whether I fought a good fight, you may dispute whether I finished my course, but you can not deny that I have kept the faith.

With tense, drawn faces and streaming eyes men hung upon the words of the orator, as with studied pathos he reviewed the causes of his defeat and asserted that, though men of the party had deserted him in time of need, he himself would remain true to the principles of his party. As he closed with a summing up of the whole case against Parker's nomination, the sunlight of another midsummer's day was streaming through the windows of the convention hall, dimming the feeble electric lights and throwing the great yellow-decked roof into shadow. An outburst of frenzied cheering, elemental and uncontrollable like the roaring of the sea, rose from the ranks of the mob, while from the floor of the great hall, littered over with papers, the dust rose under the trampling of many feet as the smoke of battle rises from a crowded, hard-fought field. No stage could provide such a setting. No playgoing audience could afford such psychic possibilities. Nerves, racked and worn by nine hours of speechmaking, responded to a supreme stimulus, not in the conventional language of applause but in the incoherent language of hysteria. It was a study in mob psychology; a scene which witnessed once is unforgettable. At last the tumult and the shouting dies; the call of States begins; Judge Parker is nominated on the first ballot. Colonel Bryan's impassioned appeal had not changed the vote of a single delegate.

An interesting point of order was raised during the roll-call of States and decided by the presiding officer. When the State of Ohio was reached the chairman of the delegation announced a vote of 46 for Parker. A demand was immediately made for a poll of the delegation. The delegation was polled and the result announced: Parker 28, McClellan 9, Hearst 6, Cockrell 2, Olney 1. The point of order was now raised by a member of the delegation that the Ohio state convention had no right to instruct the delegates to vote as a unit, inasmuch as the district delegates had received their credentials from conventions held prior to the time of holding the state convention. The point of order was overruled by the chair in these words:

By express rule of the Democratic convention, the delegates come from a state and not from districts. Under the call for delegates to the convention each state is allowed as many delegates as it has senators and representatives multiplied by two, and these delegates are the delegates of the state and not the delegates of the districts, no matter how chosen.

It was therefore ordered that the entire vote of Ohio be recorded for Parker, although his actual strength was but 28 out of 46 votes. This ruling illustrates anew the distinctive difference between the practice of a Democratic and that of a Republican national convention. There is an intimate relationship at present between this so-called unit rule and the two-thirds rule of the Democratic convention, though there is no connection in origin between the two rules. So long as the unit rule is upheld, the two-thirds rule will also prevail. Suppose, as was suggested last spring in conservative circles when the Hearst boom began to assume portentous proportions, that the two-thirds rule had been abrogated by the convention, on the general theory that it is an undemocratic principle to give a faction of one-third the legal right to defeat the choice of the majority. Such a change might actually confer upon a minority not only the negative power of defeating a nomination but the positive power of making a nomination. A number of large states with pretty evenly divided delegations might so combine as to control, under the unit rule, a majority of the votes in the convention. A candidate might thus be nominated who was really the choice of only a small minority of the delegates, were the two-thirds rule abrogated and the unit rule retained. Again, great Republican states, such as Pennsylvania, Massachusetts, Ohio, Illinois and Iowa, might successfully combine and effect a nomination under a bare majority rule and yet not contribute a single electoral vote to the success of the candidate so nominated. Thus the perpetuation of the two-thirds rule rests upon the continuance of the unit rule, and the perpetuation of the unit rule is due in large measure to the traditional attitude of the Democratic party on the question of state sovereignty. In Democratic theory, each state controls its delegation. The Democratic convention recognizes an authority higher than itself. The Republican convention does not. The Republican convention has never allowed the states to use the unit rule. A clear statement of the

Republican doctrine was made by a delegate from Kansas in the convention of 1876, when the question was raised as to the acceptance of a unit vote from the state of Pennsylvania.

The principle involved in this controversy is whether the state of Pennsylvania shall make laws for this convention or whether this convention is supreme and shall make its own laws. We are supreme. We are original. We stand here representing the great Republican party of the United States, and neither Pennsylvania nor New York nor any state can come in here and bind us down by their caucus resolutions.[1]

One further fact, however, is to be noted with respect to the unit rule of the Democratic convention. In case no instructions are given by a state to its delegation, the convention assumes authority and allows each individual in the delegation to vote according to his preference. For example, in the St. Louis convention, Nebraska's vote was announced and recorded as follows: Hearst 4, Cockrell 4, Pattison 4, Miles 1, Wall 1, Gray 1, Olney 1. The unit rule of the Democratic convention is not an affirmative rule at all. It is simply an acknowledgment that the states may bind their delegations if they so choose. Despite the immense amount of newspaper clamor for the abrogation of the two-thirds rule, and the protests and objurgations of the minority Hearst members on such split but instructed delegations as those of Ohio, Indiana and Massachusetts, the fight for the modification of the rules was never at any time strong enough to reach the convention floor. As a corollary to the unit rule, the St. Louis convention, through the ruling of its chairman, upheld the traditional Democratic doctrine that the chairman of an instructed delegation is entitled to cast the entire vote of the delegation whether the delegation is fully represented on the floor or not.

Little need be said of the proceedings of the convention subsequent to Judge Parker's nomination. The text of the telegram as sent by Judge Parker to Hon. Wm. F. Sheehan is as follows:

I regard the gold standard as firmly and irrevocably established and shall act accordingly if the action of the convention to-day shall be ratified by the people. As the platform is silent on the subject, my view should be made known to the convention, and if it is proved to be unsatisfactory to the majority I request you to decline the nomination for me at once, so that another may be nominated before adjournment.

Great excitement prevailed when reports of the Parker telegram leaked out early Saturday afternoon. Newspaper extras proclaimed that Parker had declined the nomination, and garbled versions of his actual message were hawked about everywhere. The air was charged with uncertainty, bewilderment, and expectancy when the delegates assembled for the

[1] Carl Becker, "The Unit Rule in National Nominating Conventions," *American Historical Review*, V, no. 1, p. 81.

final session. The Bryanites affected to regard the message as a cunning trick of the Hill-Belmont-Sheehan combination. Senator Tillman violently denounced the message as an attempt to dictate and as an insult to the entire convention. The majority of the New York and New Jersey delegates seemed genuinely pleased with the message, but no one was jubilant. The situation was a most delicate one and fraught with immense hazard. The opinion of many thoughtful delegates at the time could have been aptly expressed in a later remark of Colonel Bryan's: "It is a manly thing for a man to express an opinion before the convention adjourns; but it would have been manlier to have expressed it before the convention met." The southern delegates appeared most deeply stirred by the telegram; their anxiety and doubt were strung to an intensity almost savage. Southern leaders were therefore put forward to pacify them. After some hours' work Tillman was quieted and induced, in conjunction with Williams and Vardaman of Mississippi, Daniel of Virginia and Carmack of Tennessee, to play the rôle of pacificator. The anger of the hotspurs began to simmer down. A notable speech at this critical juncture was made by a northern man, Hon. Charles S. Hamlin of Massachusetts. Mr. Hamlin as a member of the platform committee had labored indefatigably for a gold plank. That effort had been defeated by a vote of 35 to 15. Mr. Hamlin explained why the minority had not carried the fight to the convention floor, and closed with an eloquent plea for despatching a message prepared by John Sharp Williams to Judge Parker. The "Williams message," which virtually endorsed the position taken by the nominee in his telegram to the convention, read as follows:

The platform adopted by this convention is silent upon the question of the monetary standard, because it is not regarded by us a possible issue in this campaign, and only campaign issues are mentioned in the platform. Therefore there is nothing in the views expressed by you in the telegram just received which would preclude a man entertaining them from accepting a nomination on said platform.

It was at this juncture that Colonel Bryan rose from a sick-bed, entered the convention, and began a tedious and futile protest against sending the Williams telegram. Two rambling speeches were made, the last closing with the impossible suggestion that a sort of catechismal message be sent to the nominee, seeking explicit answers to several specific questions. The convention was not in the mood of the night before. Here were a lot of earnest men striving for harmony, willing to sink individual preferences, sick of factional rancor and impatient to conclude the work of the convention. The speaker recognized that his appeal fell upon cold if not resentful ears. He accordingly withdrew his amendment and thus escaped a crushing vote of disapproval. The motion to send the Williams telegram was carried by the overwhelming vote of 794 to 191.

At one o'clock Sunday morning Hon. Henry G. Davis was nominated for vice-president. The excitement over the Parker telegram had been absorbing. A benumbing fatigue dulled all further interest in the proceedings and imposed an effective closure rule upon discussion. "Word was passed around" that Davis was the man to be voted for. The writer heard little talk of superannuation, and in general little discussion of availability or fitness. When the roll was called, chairmen of delegations wearily rose and mechanically uttered the name of Henry G. Davis. At no point did the convention so absolutely divest itself of the character of a deliberative body as in the act of naming an octogenarian for second place on the ticket.

"Freshmen" members of the national Congress are wont to lament the absence of a spirit of *cameraderie* in the House of Representatives. If this is true of the 386 members of the House elected for two years, one can readily fancy how little *esprit de corps* is to be found in an assemblage of one thousand men who exercise their group functions for less than a week and then disperse forever. Rivalry between parties is never more bitter than factional strife within parties. Nothing could have been more bitter than Mr. Rose's castigation of the Parkerites. The New York men themselves were divided. To scrutinize the faces of Murphy, Sheehan and McCarren was to read in each a different story of policies and aspirations. Outside of the southern belt there was scarcely a state that was not represented by a divided delegation. The unit rule half concealed and half revealed irreconcilable principles and preferences. Even the Massachusetts delegation, pledged to support the candidacy of a "favorite son," was, beneath the surface, divided; five of its members were bitterly opposed to Mr. Olney. The convention was indeed a jarring, disintegrate mass. For such an unorganized mass, competent leadership was a prime necessity. The biggest and most influential personality in the convention was Colonel Bryan's, but the majority of the delegates had come to St. Louis with the firm determination not to be led by Colonel Bryan. The delegates therefore turned from a personality to an abstraction in quest of leadership. They turned from Bryan to "conservatism." In the name of conservatism the Hill-Sheehan-Guffey-Gorman combination "passed around the word" for the nomination of Henry G. Davis. The delegates heard and obeyed.

The party convention is a pure evolution, and we may look to see progressive changes in the conduct of this extra-legal body. One may forecast the direction although it may be impossible to fathom the extent of these changes. The infinite folly of planting a political convention in the midst of a howling mob of ten thousand people was convincingly illustrated in the last Democratic convention. This convention could not, except by courtesy, be called a deliberative body. Men such as Senator Daniel or John Sharp Williams, who really had something to say to the convention. were not shown decent consideration, while men who had a buncombe message for the galleries were given a patient hearing. It was really the galleries that demanded the circus parades of state standards, lithographs and flags when a leading candidate was placed in nomination. One of these bogus demonstrations continued for thirty-four minutes. It was the galleries that dragged Bryan from his sick-bed to prolong the agony of the last night's session. It was the galleries that hurled insulting and indecent epithets at speakers in the Illinois contest, because they were espousing a cause which the mob did not like. With hundreds of newspaper men present and wires carrying the convention proceedings to every news center in the Union, the interests of publicity no longer demand the presence of ten thousand irresponsible people in the convention hall. In the last two Democratic state conventions of Massachusetts all spectators other than newspaper men were rigidly excluded from the hall. The step was an unpopular one, but the bear-garden features which too often have disgraced other conventions were effectively eliminated; and enlightened party opinion heartily supports the innovation.

Again, the results of the St. Louis convention can not but strengthen the growing conviction that the time is approaching for a change in the present system of representation in the convention. The anti-Parker combination had a fighting chance of success up to the moment when Colonel Guffey delivered the 68 votes of Pennsylvania to the Parkerites. A state which had never given a single electoral vote to a Democratic nominee turned the scale decisively and clinched the nomination of a man who received only 140 votes in the electoral college. It is true that the solid Democratic states of the South were behind Judge Parker's candidacy. Men such as Governor Vardaman of Mississippi were in line for the New York candidate in the hope that he might carry this and other pivotal states and so defeat Mr. Roosevelt. But reverse the situation. Suppose the Southern leaders had come into the convention solidly behind the candidacy of such a man as Senator Bailey of Texas. The Southern combination could easily have been beaten by a northern combination of Illinois, Michigan, Minnesota, Ohio, Wisconsin, Pennsylvania, Massachusetts and Maine. That is, eight northern states which ordinarily do not cast a single Democratic electoral vote could overwhelm thirteen Southern states which furnished every one of the 140 electoral votes actually received by Judge Parker. In a Republican convention the same inequality appears, though less glaringly: the southern tier, which never furnishes a Republican electoral vote, has full voting strength in determining the nominee. In the Republican convention of 1884, an effort was made to enlarge the influence of the old line Republican states and to diminish correspondingly the weight of states where the party was in a minority. The effort failed largely through the clamor and piteous appeals of the negro Republicans of the South. These men claimed, with some color of equity, that they get very little chance under state election laws, and that therefore the opportunity to take part in Republican councils on a basis of their actual numerical strength comes but once in four years. If they are shut out of the field when the harvest is indeed golden, as in the case of Mr. Hanna's campaign for the nomination of Mr. McKinley in 1896, they may justly complain that they are wounded in the house of their friends. This line of argument does not hold in the case of the Democratic convention. Democratic voters do not suffer under discriminating election laws in northern states, and the results of the last national convention suggest that a change in the basis of representation may be one of the possibilities of the future.

Finally, we may hazard the opinion that the time is approaching when national party conventions will be subjected to some species of statutory control. Parties under our governmental system are purely voluntary organizations and stand theoretically outside of the control of courts and law-making bodies. But the party has become a most important political organ, and the trend of our development is all towards the subjection of party to legal as well as to political responsibility. It may be urged that party organization implies obedience to constituted authority, and that this authority, from its very nature, must reside within and not outside of the party itself. The courts have ordinarily taken this view, and have not regarded the action of a party convention as a proper subject for judicial review. At the same time, where party machinery is used oppressively and for improper purposes, the legal organs of governmental authority have again and again successfully asserted the right of control. The commonwealth of Massachusetts, for instance, imposes a most thoroughgoing governmental control upon party action. Each party is required to elect annually a state committee, and the members of this committee are required to meet and organize at a particular time and in a particular manner. Minute directions are prescribed for the holding of party caucuses and the choice of election officials. The laws governing party machinery, as codified in 1898, fill 150 pages, containing an average of 300 words to a page. And this body of law has since been amplified by a mass of supplementary legislation. One may reasonably assert that the American party is not legally responsible, but this no longer implies that a little junta of politicians may meet at such time and place as it chooses and select nominees for public office. It can not be denied that the state is within its proper functions when it undertakes to regulate the machinery by which its governmental officers are selected. The federal government has all along conceded that the regulation of the suffrage rests primarily with the states, and has therefore not sought to exercise any direct control over the ballot, being content simply to prescribe uniform methods for the selection of federal officers in state-conducted elections. A similar species of jurisdiction might well be extended to the nomination as well as to the final selection of the chief of federal officers. In the interests of safety, decency, and due deliberation, Congress may at some future time impose regulations as to the time, place and manner of conducting national nominating conventions. A national convention hall, erected by the government at Washington, or perhaps in a more central locality, is one of the possibilities of the future. Such a hall, properly policed and provided with protection against fire and the incursion of the mob, would mark a distinct advance in the conduct of conventions. So long as all arrangements are left to a camarilla of politicians, who have friends to be rewarded and enemies to be punished; so long as the mob is present to demand the stimulating ailment of some passion-fed illusion or illusion-fed passion — so long will the proceedings of a national nominating convention fail to attain the dignity and deliberation implied in the very character of its high functions.

INDEX

847

Lightning Source UK Ltd.
Milton Keynes UK
UKHW011528040219
336710UK00013B/498/P